Nutrition and Health Series

Adrianne Bendich, PhD, FACN, FASN, Series Editor

For further volumes:
http://www.springer.com/series/7659

Victor R. Preedy • Rajaventhan Srirajaskanthan
Vinood B. Patel
Editors

Handbook of Food Fortification and Health

From Concepts to Public Health Applications
Volume 1

Humana Press

Editors
Victor R. Preedy, PhD
Department of Nutrition and Dietetics
Diabetes and Nutritional Sciences
School of Medicine
King's College London
London, UK

Vinood B. Patel, BSc (Hons), PhD
Department of Biomedical Sciences
School of Life Sciences
University of Westminster
London, UK

Rajaventhan Srirajaskanthan, MD
Department of Gastroenterology
University Hospital Lewisham
London, UK

Department of Gastroenterology
King's College Hospital
London, UK

ISBN 978-1-4939-5184-0 ISBN 978-1-4614-7076-2 (eBook)
DOI 10.1007/978-1-4614-7076-2
Springer New York Heidelberg Dordrecht London

Printed on acid-free paper

Humana Press is a brand of Springer
Springer is part of Springer Science+Business Media (www.springer.com)

Preface

In this book the Editors aim to disseminate important material pertaining to the fortification of foods from strategic initiatives to public health applications. It covers (in two volumes) policy, preclinical studies, clinical investigations, and the impact of fortification on the individual and whole communities. The importance of food fortification relates to the fact that optimal nutritional intake is an essential component of health and well-being. Unfortunately, situations arise on a local or national scale when nutrient supply or intake is deemed to be suboptimal. As a consequence, ill health occurs, for example, neural tube defects in the developing fetus, organ damage in adults, or increased rates of premature deaths. In terms of public health, malnutrition due to micronutrient deficiency can be quite profound, imposing economic and social burdens on individuals and whole communities. The complex inter-relationship between poor health outcomes and nutrient delivery can, however, be modulated by appropriate food fortification. Thereafter issues arise as to the efficacy of food fortification, what strategies should be employed and what nutrients to add. The food carrier is also important, as well as its stability. Ethical issues also arise, and the concept of potential harm also needs to be addressed in terms of cost-benefits. All of these aspects, and many others, are covered in *The Handbook of Food Fortification: From Concepts to Public Health Applications.*

This comprehensive text examines the broad spectrum of food fortification in all its manifestations.

The term *fortification* has multiple meanings and is often used synonymously in relation to the addition of any component to food to facilitate a nutritional advantage. In this book we cover fortification not only in terms of its more strict definitions, in terms of the addition of micronutrients, i.e., minerals and vitamins, but also within the context of its wider and holistic applicability. The book thus recognizes the international differences in definitions and usage of fortification. At the same time we also include chapters on novel fortificants that are contained within more complex food matrices. However, whilst some micronutrients are permitted fortificants in one country, their inclusion in some foods may be prohibited or at the "discussion" or pre-legislative stage in another country. These complexities in terminology are recognized by the Editors. In all there are two volumes with eight main parts, namely:

Volume 1

Part I: Introductory Chapters and Perspectives of Fortification
Part II: Iron Fortification
Part III: Fortified Foods and Beverages
Part IV: Biofortification: Biological Modes of Enhancing Nutrient Intake

Volume 2

Part I: Novel Food Vehicles and Agents for Fortificants
Part II: Impact on Individuals
Part III: Public Health, Concepts and Issues
Part IV: International Perspectives

Key features within each chapter include key points and, where relevant, guidance on safe levels and recommendations.

The Handbook of Food Fortification: From Concepts to Public Health Applications represents a multidisciplinary approach to food fortification and is written by many authoritative individuals, from centers and institutions around the world. It is designed for nutritionists, dietitians, medical practitioners, educationalists, health experts, epidemiologists, and other health-related professionals. It is also suitable for students, graduates, postgraduates, researchers, lecturers, teachers, and professors.

London, UK

Victor R. Preedy, PhD
Rajaventhan Srirajaskanthan, MD
Vinood B. Patel, BSc (Hons), PhD

Series Editor Page

The great success of the Nutrition and Health Series is the result of the consistent overriding mission of providing health professionals with texts that are essential because each includes (1) a synthesis of the state of the science, (2) timely, in-depth reviews by the leading researchers in their respective fields, (3) extensive, up-to-date fully annotated reference lists, (4) a detailed index, (5) relevant tables and figures, (6) identification of paradigm shifts and the consequences, (7) virtually no overlap of information between chapters, but targeted, inter-chapter referrals, (8) suggestions of areas for future research, and (9) balanced, data-driven answers to patient as well as health professionals' questions which are based upon the totality of evidence rather than the findings of any single study.

The Series volumes are not the outcome of a symposium. Rather, each editor has the potential to examine a chosen area with a broad perspective, both in subject matter as well as in the choice of chapter authors. The editor(s), whose training(s) is (are) both research and practice oriented, have the opportunity to develop a primary objective for their book, define the scope and focus, and then invite the leading authorities to be part of their initiative. The authors are encouraged to provide an overview of the field, discuss their own research, and relate the research findings to potential human health consequences. Because each book is developed de novo, the chapters are coordinated so that the resulting volume imparts greater knowledge than the sum of the information contained in the individual chapters.

The Handbook of Food Fortification: From Concepts to Public Health Applications edited by Professor Victor R. Preedy, PhD, DSc, FRIPH, FRSH, FIBiol, FRCPath, Professor Rajaventhan Srirajaskanthan, BSc (Hons), MD (Res), MRCP, and Vinood B. Patel, PhD, clearly exemplifies the goals of the Nutrition and Health Series. The major objective of this comprehensive two volume text is to review the growing evidence that food fortification has a major role in assuring adequate intake of the essential nutrients. Fortification also serves as an important vehicle for introducing newer bioactive components of food, such as carotenoids, into the diet of a population. This volume includes 63 up-to-date informative reviews of the current major fortification programs underway around the world and examines the consequences of the programs. Practicing health professionals, researchers, and academicians can rely on the chapters in this volume for objective data-driven sources about essential vitamins and minerals, proteins and fats as well as other dietary components that have been included in basic food sources. This new comprehensive review of the science behind the fortification strategies that help to assure the health of the populations at risk by providing essential nutrients is of great importance to the nutrition community as well as for health professionals who have to answer patient, client, or graduate student questions about the newest clinical research in the nutritional effects of food fortification.

The Handbook of Food Fortification: From Concepts to Public Health Applications represents the most comprehensive compilation of the recent data on the actions of specific essential nutrients and bioactive dietary components in at risk populations around the globe. It is to the credit of Drs. Preedy, Srirajaskanthan, and Patel that they have organized this volume so that it provides an in-depth overview of the critical issues involved in the determination of the best fortification strategies for infants, toddlers, school-age children, and adult populations, whether they were born in developing nations or in developed nations. The volumes' editors provide their in-depth knowledge and expertise to help the reader to understand the value of food fortification. Professor Preedy is a senior member of King's College London where he is a Professor of Nutritional Biochemistry and is also a Professor of Clinical Biochemistry at King's College Hospital. He is also Director of the Genomics Centre and a member of the School of Medicine. He is a member of The Royal College of Pathologists, a Fellow to The Institute of Biology, The Royal College of Pathologists, The Royal Society for the Promotion of Health, The Royal Institute of Public Health, The Royal Society for Public Health, and in 2012 a Fellow of The Royal Society of Chemistry. Professor Srirajaskanthan is a consultant gastroenterologist at University Hospital Lewisham and Kings College Hospital, London. He trained at the prestigious Guy's, King's and St. Thomas' Medical School where he obtained his MD (MBBS) and a B.Sc. in Neuroscience. He is a member of the Royal College of Physicians. His specialist training includes Gastroenterology, Hepatology, and Internal Medicine. Dr. Patel is a Senior Lecturer in Clinical Biochemistry at the University of Westminster and honorary fellow at King's College London. Dr. Patel obtained his degree in Pharmacology from the University of Portsmouth, his PhD in protein metabolism from King's College London, and completed postdoctoral research at Wake Forest University School of Medicine.

Each of the two volumes contains about 30 comprehensive chapters. The first volume contains four related parts. The first part provides an overview and perspective on national and international fortification strategies and policies. Five chapters examine the complexities of developing fortification initiatives and use examples of successful and not so successful fortification programs. The first chapter presents a new attempt to provide blueprint for global flour fortification with essential nutrients for countries with major population groups at risk for micronutrient deficiencies. The Flour Fortification Initiative (FFI) goal is to provide a flour fortification standard milling practice throughout the world. The focus is wheat and maize flours. The FFI model is based upon engaging partners in the public, private, and civic sectors. The chapter uses the example of how countries began fortifying flour with folic acid to prevent birth defects to illustrate the public-private-civic sector collaboration involved in flour fortification.

Micronutrient fortification of staple foods had been in place for decades before the understanding of the role of folic acid in birth defect prevention was confirmed in clinical trials. The historic perspective and current fortification programs in both developing and developed nations are examined in the next chapter. Clear definitions of terms, tables that include the countries with mandatory fortification programs, details concerning the concentration of micronutrients used in fortification, as well as a review of the positives and negatives of using food fortification to improve nutrient status are included. The following chapter examines the critical need for fortification of foods provided to the neediest populations that are consuming foods provided for humanitarian relief. Humanitarian food aid involving global food assistance utilizes organizations including the United Nations Food and Agricultural Organization (FAO), World Food Program (WFP), and the Food for Peace Act (FFP). WFP reported that over 5,000,000 metric tons of food aid was distributed to humanitarian relief efforts in 2010. The chapter includes data on diverse foods provided and the micronutrients included in the major humanitarian food programs. Food fortification programs in the Middle East are described in the next chapter that examines the vast diversity in the economic status of the 20+ countries included in the term "Middle East." The chapter examines the difficulties in reaching relatively small populations within wealthy nations that may benefit from foods fortified with micronutrients and uses national programs of flour fortification with iron as an example. Currently, ten countries in the Middle East do not have a mandatory flour fortification program in place. The last chapter in this part describes the historic development of fortification practices in Canada and begins with the establishment of mandatory uniform iodine fortification in 1949 after more than 2 decades of voluntary fortification initiatives across the country that used different concentrations of iodine. In contrast to the United States that mandated flour fortification with certain B vitamins and Iron in the early 1940s, Canada did not have mandatory flour fortification until 1976. Canada continues to examine its fortification policies especially with regard to voluntary food fortification initiatives.

The second part contains six chapters on national programs to implement iron fortification of staple foods and water. The chapter authors remind us that there may not be one mechanism that can provide iron to all populations at risk. Food fortification is a major source of iron for millions of anemic infants, children, and women worldwide. The six chapters are devoted to reviewing the multiple foods and iron compounds that have been used to enhance iron status in at risk populations. Iron has a complex chemistry as well as metabolism and reactions are dependent upon pH, potential oxidation, competition for other minerals, and presence of food components that can block or enhance its absorption. Because of these issues, and the fact that population groups consume different staple foods, many foods have been considered for iron fortification. For example, soy sauce in China, tonyu in Japan, and Nuoc-mâm (fish sauce) in Vietnam has been successfully used to reduce iron deficiency. As dairy products are widely consumed in Europe and North America, the next chapter considers the pros and cons of fortifying dairy products and milk with a number of potential iron fortificants.

Another chapter describes the use of parboiled rice to deliver both iron and zinc. Fortification of iron and zinc in the parboiling process increased iron and zinc concentrations, especially in polished rice where most of iron and zinc is usually removed during milling. Parboiled rice is produced on industrial scale and traded globally. It is commonly consumed in South Asia and Africa where iron and zinc deficiencies are widespread. Iron and zinc deficiencies have been estimated to affect 70–95 % of the population in Asia. There is also a chapter that describes the benefits of fortifying millets with iron and zinc. Millets are used chiefly as food grains in Africa, Eastern Europe, China, India, and other Asiatic countries. Finger millet, sorghum, and pearl millet are widely grown and consumed as the staple in several parts of India. The beneficial effects of fortifying millets for Indian populations are described. There is also a chapter on the clinical finding from experiments with iron fortification of drinking water that seem quite promising.

Many iron compounds are used as food fortificants. These must meet the requirements of high iron bioavailability, inertness in relation to the sensorial properties of the fortified food, absence of toxicity, resistance during storing or processing of the fortified food, and have a bioavailability similar to that found with naturally occurring iron in food. Two chapters describe specific sources of iron. One of the possible newer salts of iron that has been used to fortify food is ferric pyrophosphate and is described in the next chapter. Ferric pyrophosphate is a poorly soluble iron compound that does not change organoleptic properties of foods even when used in many difficult-to-fortify food vehicles. Reduction in the particle size of this iron salt has greatly increased its bioavailability. The second chapter describes the benefits of heme iron. Heme is a biologically important source of dietary iron because of its significantly greater bioavailability compared to non-heme iron sources. Dietary heme sources include foods containing myoglobin and hemoglobin such as meats, fish, and poultry. The positives and negatives of using heme iron as a food fortificant are described. Several studies have evaluated fortification with heme iron in different foods using biscuits, cookie fillings, weaning foods, flour, and black beans.

The third part of this volume contains 11 chapters that describe fat-soluble and water-soluble essential nutrients that are used in a number of food matrices to enhance the dietary intakes of these nutrients. Fats used as vehicles for fortification include margarine, fat spreads, cooking oils, eggs, and dairy products. Dairy products are also used as vehicles for minerals and other water-soluble nutrients. Both cow milk and soy milk products are described; commonly used fortificants include calcium, zinc, iron, iodine, and selenium. The critical issues of maintaining safe doses of minerals and at the same time assuring the palatability of the fortified milk products are discussed in each chapter. Other dairy-based foods that have been fortified with fat-soluble vitamins and certain minerals include cheeses, yogurt, fermented milk products, butter, and cream.

Additionally, corn, rice, noodles, water, and salt are reviewed as sources of added nutrients for at risk populations. Corn fortification is reviewed and indicates that it is an excellent vehicle for delivering iron, folic acid, zinc, copper, vitamins B1 and B2, and calcium. Rice, flours, and noodles have also been used to fortify their levels of folic acid and other B vitamins, and at times, vitamin C. Salt has been used as a carrier for iodine for almost 100 years and continues to be a well-accepted food source for reducing iodine deficiency disorders in at risk nations. Two detailed chapters review the biological effects of deficiencies, the choices of each fortificant and types of salts used for fortification, the complexities of maintaining the concentrations of this fortificant, assessment of bioavailability, and clinical studies of efficacy.

Margarines and fat spreads have delivered vitamins A and D in certain developed nations for more than 50 years and have also been used successfully in underdeveloped countries. Vegetable oils are also suitable vehicles for fortification with the fat-soluble vitamins A, D, and E. The fat-soluble vitamins form a true solution and are uniformly distributed in vegetable oils. The stability of vitamin A is greater in oils than in any other food, and oil facilitates the absorption of vitamin A by the body. There is a separate chapter devoted to the value of fortifying vegetable oils with vitamin A and the other fat-soluble vitamins. Newer fortificants in fats include n-3 fatty acids, plant sterols, vitamin E, vitamin C, and carotenes as well as iodine. A new potential fortificant is also described in a separate chapter. Conjugated linoleic acid (CLA) is a mixture of isomers of the essential fatty acid, linoleic acid. CLA is mainly found in food products from ruminants such as dairy products and beef. CLA is a major fat in milk fat. The reason that CLA is considered as a fortificant for nondairy sources is that recent research studies have reported anticarcinogenic, antiatherogenic, antioxidative, and immune system enhancement as well as reduction of body fat. Preliminary clinical studies are reviewed.

Enhancing the efficiency of plants to concentrate nutrients essential for human life through selective breeding is called biofortification. The uptake of certain minerals by plants is usually controlled by several genes. Choosing plants that contain higher than normal levels of the desired mineral and using the seeds of these plants for cultivation of the next generation can result in more uniform higher levels of this mineral in subsequent generations. Biofortification through genetic engineering of staple foods is a new and important avenue for fortifying staple foods. Rice, corn, and carrots have been successfully enriched with essential nutrients and carotenes. Biofortification studies of the enhancement of selenium levels in lentils are described specifically in a unique chapter. A second unique chapter describes the biofortification of eggs with tocotrienol and tocopherol, vitamin E sources, by feeding the egg laying hens with a diet high in tocotrienols and tocopherols in rice bran oil.

The fourth part, entitled Biofortification: Biological Modes of Enhancing Nutrient Intake, contains seven chapters that include discussions of genetic modifications to rice, corn, wheat, and sweet potatoes. Traditional breeding methods alone may not be a valid option for grain biofortification due to low levels of genetic variability for mineral uptake into the edible portions of the plant. Gene technology can enhance micronutrient concentrations in many grains. These chapters include detailed descriptions of the genetic vectors used to deliver new codings for mineral binding proteins, transporters, and other mechanisms to significantly enhance the concentration as well as the bioavailability of the essential nutrient. Examples reviewed include the successful biofortification of rice with vitamin A, iron, zinc, folic acid. Unlike minerals that are available in the soil, plants must synthesize vitamins, and several genes are involved in the synthesis of any vitamin. Thus, the complexity of inserting all of the genes required for the synthesis of folate, as an example, and assuring that the biochemical reactions occur in the right order and in the right place within the plant cell, is monumental. Plant scientists have, in fact, been able to biofortify rice so that its concentration of folate is significantly greater than seen with traditional breeding programs. Biofortification of corn, using genetic engineering, has resulted in significantly increased concentrations of beta carotene (provitamin A), folate, vitamin E, and ascorbic acid (vitamin C) as described in another chapter. The chapter includes a detailed description of the newest genetically engineered multivitamin corn. Another chapter describes the processes used to affect the selenium content of wheat agronomic biofortification which involves fertilizing the growing crop with the micronutrient, which the plant converts to several organic Se forms, notably selenomethionine, which are more suitable for human consumption. As exciting as the new genetic engineering research is to the scientific community, there may be many barriers to consumer and national acceptance of these new fortified products. The chapter on the potential benefits and risks of adopting folate fortified rice in Chinese communities is explored in a fully tabulated chapter. In a complementary chapter, there is an insightful discussion of the introduction of orange sweet potatoes in sub-Saharan Africa where the usual sweet potato was white and lacked any carotenoid content. The linking of agriculture to nutritional content of a staple food is reviewed. This part also contains a unique chapter that reviews the nutritional content of gluten-free foods and tabulates the essential micronutrient levels in many gluten-free products. The chapter includes a detailed discussion of the importance of biofortification in enhancing the micronutrient content of grains used in these products.

The second volume of *The Handbook of Food Fortification: From Concepts to Public Health Application* emphasizes the clinical and public health consequences of fortification programs. The four parts in this volume include chapters devoted to novel food vehicles and agents for fortification; the impact of fortification on different population groups and individuals; public health concepts and issues and finally, a critical part on international perspectives. The first part contains ten chapters that explore the potential for fortifying staple foods and commonly consumed foods including eggs, meats, yogurt, cheese, fish and fish sauces, and drink products with essential micronutrients as well as fiber and n-3 fatty acids. There is a strong rationale presented for using eggs as vehicles for fortification. Fortified eggs combine an important animal food that naturally contains high quality protein and amino acids, fats and essential fatty acids, and certain vitamins and minerals, with a unique capacity to be fortified with added essential nutrients and phytonutrients and effectively deliver these with high bioavailability. Nutrients discussed included iodine, selenium, zinc, iron, copper, manganese, chromium, fat and water-soluble vitamins and carotenoids, choline, and long chain n-3 fatty acids that are provided to the hens for transfer to the eggs. New fortificants for cheeses and new technologies to incorporate these into cheese products are included in another chapter. Microencapsulation, emulsions and gel particles, and immobilization on polymeric complexes have permitted the addition of probiotics, essential micronutrients, polyphenols, and carotenoids to be incorporated into cheeses. Other commonly consumed foods consumed daily (mainly in Asia) include fish sauce and soy sauce. In certain nations, there is mandatory fortification of these sauces with iodine. Currently, incentives are underway to also fortify with iron compounds to further enhance the nutritive value of these sauces as described in a separate chapter.

Ocean fish are an important source of long chain n-3 fatty acids; however farmed fish require sources of n-3 fatty acids in their diets to be able to incorporate these oils into their muscle tissues. New sources of n-3 fatty acids for farmed fish and enhanced production practices to assure decreased risk of oxidation are reviewed. Enhancement of long chain n-3 fatty acids in feeds has been undertaken with ruminants including beef cattle and lambs, pork, and poultry. The risks and benefits of these fortification strategies are discussed in a separate chapter. Another opportunity to deliver long chain n-3 fatty acids to the diet, especially for individuals who do not consume fish, is the development of n-3 fortified beverages. The technological issues as well as the clinical evidence of efficacy are discussed in a new meta-analysis of published data found in systematic review included in this part. Beverages that were fortified include cow and soy milks, fruit and vegetable juices, and drinks.

Four chapters describe the use of waste and/or by-products from commercial production of processed foods for the development of excellent sources of missing nutrients in relevant populations. Examples of novel source of nutrients, polyphenols, and fiber are discussed. The term "apple pomace" refers to the left-over solid biomass after extraction of juice from fresh apple fruits and this product is being used in baked goods and other applications. Bovine lung is the second example of a waste product from cattle slaughtering that is being used to successfully fortify iron levels in processed ready-to-eat foods for anemic children. Date fiber is a by-product of date syrup production and this has been incorporated into yogurt to add further value to this important staple food. Evaporated sugarcane juice, unlike refined sugar, is an important source of bioavailable iron. This by-product has been used as a natural sweetener for fruit juices and preliminary clinical studies reviewed in the chapter suggest that this fortificant is beneficial in anemic children.

The second part in this volume contains seven chapters that examine the effects of fortified food in specific populations including pregnant and lactating women, preterm infants, preschool and school-age children, postmenopausal women, and elderly living in nursing homes. A well-referenced literature review confirms that micronutrient fortified foods and beverages provided during pregnancy improved micronutrient status and reduced anemia rates in women. Also, micronutrient fortified foods, when combined with energy and essential fatty acids, resulted in improved pregnancy outcomes including increased birth weight and length. In addition, multiple micronutrient fortified foods combined with additional calories and essential fatty acids modestly improved the growth of infants and improved iron and vitamin A, but not zinc status. The effects on child development were inconsistent. One study reported an unexpected negative impact of fortification on morbidity. Malnutrition is often seen in school-age children in undeveloped communities. Two controlled studies are reviewed and confirm that intervention with a fortified lunch meal can improve iron and riboflavin blood levels in one study, and improved blood levels of many micronutrients when a multiple micronutrient powder was mixed with the food before cooking. Iodine deficiency is associated with significant declines in cognitive function in growing children. Fortification of foods with iodine and other micronutrients including iron was shown to enhance cognitive functions and school testing results in studies reviewed in another chapter in this part.

An even more at risk population for inadequate nutrient intake than young children are those that are born preterm. Moreover, human milk is an inadequate source of protein and minerals for the growing preterm infant. Neither human milk from a woman who has given birth prematurely nor human milk from a woman who has had an infant born at term is sufficient to provide all the nutritional needs of the preterm infant. Thus, human milk for the preterm infant is usually supplemented or fortified with additional protein, sodium, phosphate, calcium, magnesium, copper, zinc, and many vitamins (B2, B6, C, D, E, K, folic acid).

Another population group at risk for malnutrition is the elderly who are hospitalized or in nursing homes. Fortified foods and beverages are helpful in providing opportunities to enhance the nutritional status of these populations who are capable of consuming oral diets. One of the key nutrients that is often low in serum of immobile elderly is vitamin D. With lack of exposure to sunlight, there is a reduced ability to produce cutaneous vitamin D. This chapter reviews the other factors that can result in low vitamin D status including limited dietary intake, intestinal absorption, and kidney capacity to convert vitamin D to its active form. Fortification of bread with calcium and vitamin D enhanced blood levels of vitamin D and improved markers of bone health. Similarly, in a separate study reviewed in the next chapter, fortification of milk with calcium and vitamin D significantly enhanced bone mineral densities in elderly women.

The third part in the second volume examines the rationales used to implement food fortification strategies as public health interventions. Six chapters examine global as well as recent national initiatives to fortify foods with folic acid, vitamin B12, vitamin D, and other key nutrients. The first chapter in this part provides a broad overview of the requirements for consideration of beginning a new fortification program and also includes an in-depth analysis of potential barriers to adopting a food fortification program nationally. There is a unique chapter that examines the complexities involved with development and monitoring of a fortification program from regulatory perspective. There is a comprehensive explanation of the risk analysis process. One chapter reviews the overall use of folic acid fortification globally: 66 countries (one-third of the world's nations) have recommended mandatory folic acid fortification. Wheat or maize flour, and/or flour products such as noodles or pasta, are the food vehicles of choice used by all countries. Additional vehicles include rice and milk. Two chapters discuss the national strategies undertaken to fortify flour and/or other grains and foods with folic acid for prevention of neural tube birth defects. In Canada, the fortification program resulted in significant decreases in these birth defects as well as other benefits to infants as well as adults. It is well recognized that higher than normal folate status can block certain of the signs and symptoms of vitamin B12 deficiency. The chapter on vitamin B12 provides cogent, well-referenced arguments for consideration of food fortification with vitamin B12 in addition to folic acid fortification.

The final part of the second volume examines the current international perspectives concerning fortification and its consequences. Of great importance is the consistent lack of essential vitamins and minerals in infants, and young children under 2 years of age, women of childbearing potential and elderly populations. The following chapters provide perspectives of ways that nations cope with malnutrition and the timeframe of adoption of mandatory food fortification programs in developed as well as developing nations. Country programs from Oman, Vietnam, Pakistan, Australia, India, Brazil, and Nigeria are included. There is also a concluding chapter that summarizes the current state of food fortification programs. It is important to note, as described in the chapter, that Oman was the first country in the Middle East to make fortification of flour with folic acid a national compulsory legislation in 1996. Iron was also added to flour. Although there was an 80 % decrease in neural tube birth defects following fortification, anemia levels in preschool children remained above 10 %. However, a partial explanation may be that 9.5 % of the children suffered genetic hemoglobinopathies associated with anemia. Anemia is a serious problem for Brazilian children. In Brazil, mandatory addition of iron (30 % recommended nutritional intake (RNI) or 4.2 mg/100 g) and folic acid (70 % RNI or 150 μg) to milled wheat and corn flour was implemented in 2001. The core objective of increasing the accessibility of milled cereal grains with iron and folic acid is to reduce the prevalence of iron-deficiency and neural tube defects in Brazil. Iron-fortified water and orange juice are being explored as alternative vehicles to reduce iron deficiency in Brazil. Nigeria also has a significant issue of childhood anemia. Nigeria is one of ten countries in the world with the largest number of underweight children, with an estimated six million children under five who are underweight. Micronutrient deficiency is a direct cause of child morbidity and mortality. Micronutrients such as iron, iodine, vitamin A are missing in children's diets and 40 % of Nigerian pregnant mothers did not take any iron tablets, a recommended supplementation during pregnancy. It appears that a number of processed foods voluntarily add iron and other essential nutrients whereas mandatory programs do not appear to be in place.

A number of countries continue to have relatively high levels of childhood malnutrition. A recent survey on nutritional status of women and young children carried out in 2010 in randomly selected provinces in Vietnam confirmed that about 30 % of children under 2 years of age were stunted, 10 % were underweight, 2 % were wasted. In addition, about 15 % of children under 2 years of age had anemia. Moreover, 3 % had zinc deficiency, 12 % had vitamin A deficiency, and 50 % had marginal vitamin A status, almost 60 % had vitamin D deficiency and over 98 % had mild hypocalcaemia. Programs undertaken to provide a micronutrient fortified cereal as a complementary food for young children has resulted in a decrease in the number of malnourished children as well as increases in growth. Pakistan also has a significant number of children that suffer from iron and vitamin A deficiency. However, due to its geographical position, there is also a very high incidence of iodine deficiency and folate deficiency seen in women of childbearing potential. Salt fortification with iodine has increased over the past years and the hope is that 100 % of salt in Pakistan will contain iodine by 2013. New programs are being initiated with the primary goal of reducing the prevalence of iron-deficiency anemia among preschool children from 30 to 10 %, and in women of reproductive age from 50 to 18 %, and half the occurrence of neural tube defects among newborns from 0.4 to 0.2 % of live birth, through universal fortification of wheat flour with iron and folic acid. Indonesia also has a significant number of children with micronutrient deficiencies. Food fortification in Indonesia was initiated in 1994 with mandatory fortification of iodized salt. In 1997 trials on wheat flour fortification with iron, zinc, folate, vitamins B1 and B2 were started and as a result wheat flour fortification became mandatory in 2001. In 2011, vitamin A fortification in cooking oil was encouraged as a voluntary fortification.

Since 2001, India has implemented a school feeding program in all public primary schools. Under this program, commonly known as the "midday meal" scheme, primary schoolchildren receive free lunch meals, cooked and served at school for at least 200 days in a school year. In most States, the program has a standardized menu that consists mainly of rice and dhal (sauce prepared using pulse/lentils) or vegetables. A micronutrient intervention study in Himalayan villages in India was implemented and described in a separate chapter. The 8 month study of the intake of the micronutrient fortified food by schoolchildren was associated with significant improvements in vitamin A, folate, and vitamin B12 status as well as significant improvements in iron status but not hemoglobin levels or reductions in anemia. Although India is a sun-rich country, vitamin D deficiency has been reported in all age groups from pregnancy to late adolescence. Vitamin D deficiency is often accompanied by low calcium intakes. Reasons for this deficiency include cultural as well as genetic issues. Very few foods are fortified with vitamin D in the Indian market, and these are not commonly consumed. As there is very little vitamin D in Indian children's diet, providing vitamin D through supplementation or fortification to vulnerable groups may be the strategy of choice.

The historical account of the move from voluntary folic acid fortification of flour to mandatory fortification in 2007 in Australia is very informative, especially as Australian researchers provided seminal data showing the value of folic acid for neural tube birth defect prevention. The range of programs, initiatives, and resources available to nations and communities to help implement fortification programs is vast. The last chapter in the second volume provides readers with web addresses to hundreds of resources.

The logical sequence of the parts in each volume as well as the chapters within each part enhances the understanding of the latest information on the current standards of practice in food fortification in different countries around the world. This comprehensive two volume resource has great value for academicians involved in the education of graduate students and postdoctoral fellows, medical students, and allied health professionals and public health nutritionists who plan to interact with populations at risk for macro and/or micronutrient deficiencies.

The volume contains over 400 detailed tables and figures that assist the reader in comprehending the complexities of food technology, biological mechanisms of metabolism of essential nutrients, composition of human breast milk compared to the needs of the preterm infant, sources of infant and childhood nutrition as well as nutrition requirements through the lifespan for males and females. There are in-depth discussions of the biological significance of the microbiome and its importance in maintaining growth and health. The overriding goal of this volume is to provide the health professional with balanced documentation and awareness of the newest research and fortification approaches including an appreciation of the complexity of the interactions between genetics, maternal health, the critical role in term and preterm infants of nutrient deficiencies and new issues of bioavailability in this relatively new field of investigation. Hallmarks of the 63 chapters include key words and bulleted key points at the beginning of each chapter, complete definitions of terms with the abbreviations fully defined for the reader and consistent use of terms between chapters. There are over 2,600 up-to-date references; all chapters include a conclusion to highlight major findings. The volume also contains a highly annotated index.

This unique text provides practical, data-driven resources based upon the totality of the evidence to help the reader understand the basics of the effects of nutritional deficiencies, complexities involved in the fortification of foods with single as well as multiple micronutrients, new research using the novel sources of nutrients as well as new foods for fortification, and preventive strategies that are being implemented in the most at risk populations in developing nations across the world. Explanations are provided for the role dietary components may play in the early development of infants and the role of genetics, metabolic, or other effectors. Of equal importance, critical issues that involve, such as food preferences, nutrient interactions that affect absorption and regulatory and public health perspectives in developing and developed nations are included in well-referenced, informative chapters.

The overarching goal of the editors is to provide fully referenced information to health professionals so they may have a balanced perspective on the value of various food fortification options that are available today as well as in the foreseeable future.

In conclusion, *The Handbook of Food Fortification: From Concepts to Public Health Applications* edited by Professor Victor R. Preedy, PhD, DSc, FRIPH, FRSH, FIBiol, FRCPath, Professor Rajaventhan Srirajaskanthan, BSc (Hons), MD (Res), MRCP, and Vinood B. Patel, PhD provides health professionals in many areas of research and practice with the most up-to-date, well-referenced and comprehensive volume on the current state of the science and medical practice guidelines with regard to the value of food fortification programs. This volume will serve the reader as the most authoritative resource in the field to date and is a very welcome addition to the Nutrition and Health Series.

Morristown, NJ, USA

Adrianne Bendich, PhD, FACN, FASN
Series Editor

About Series Editor

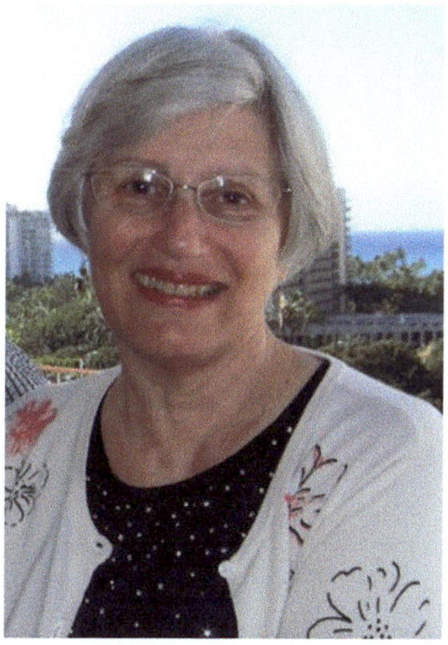

Adrianne Bendich, Ph.D., FACN, FASN. Dr. Bendich has successfully served as Series Editor for the Nutrition and Health book series for 15 years and continues to identify key areas of clinical nutrition research that can benefit from the development of targeted, objective volumes edited by the leading researchers in their fields of investigation.

Prior to retiring in September, 2010, Dr. Bendich held the position of Director of Medical Affairs at GlaxoSmithKline Consumer Healthcare where she was responsible for the Medical leadership for the Venture Group, and provided Medical support for well-known Brands including TUMS, FiberChoice, Os-Cal, Geritol, and Citrucel. Additionally, she served as a member of GSK's successful Advisory Committee team in support of FDA's Rx to OTC switch of alli®.

Dr. Bendich is internationally recognized as an expert in Women's Health, calcium and vitamin D in bone health, folic acid and pregnancy outcomes, antioxidants and carotenoid effects on immune functions. She served as the GSK corporate representative to the Women's Health Initiative (WHI) for 9 years as GSK Consumer Healthcare provided all calcium and vitamin D supplements for the WHI study.

She has held memberships and professional positions (ongoing and former): Editorial Board, *Journal of Nutrition in Gerontology and Geriatrics, Antioxidants*; an e-journal, *Journal of Women's Health and Gender-Based Medicine*; Associate Editor for *Nutrition, the International Journal*; Chair, Corporate Advisory Committee, Society for Women's Health Research; Member of the Program Advisory Committee for Helen Keller International; Advisor to the Nutrition Department, Montclair State University; member, Advisory Board, Current Topics in Nutraceutical Research; member, ASN's Industry Board and several RIS groups.

Dr. Bendich was a recipient of the Burroughs-Wellcome Fund Professorship and Roche Research Award; she is listed in Who's Who of American Women Scientists and many other Who's Who volumes; she is a recipient of the CRN Apple Award for contributions to the science of vitamin and mineral supplements. In 2012, Dr. Bendich was elected a Fellow of the American Society for Nutrition, the highest honour of the Society.

Dr. Bendich is the author of more than 100 peer-reviewed publications; Series Editor of "Nutrition and Health" for Springer/Humana Press which includes 48 volumes such as *Preventive Nutrition, Handbook of Clinical Nutrition and Aging, Diet and Human Immune Functions, Handbook of Drug-Nutrient Interactions*, and other reference volumes for health professionals as outlined at http://www.springer.com/series/7659.

About Volume Editors

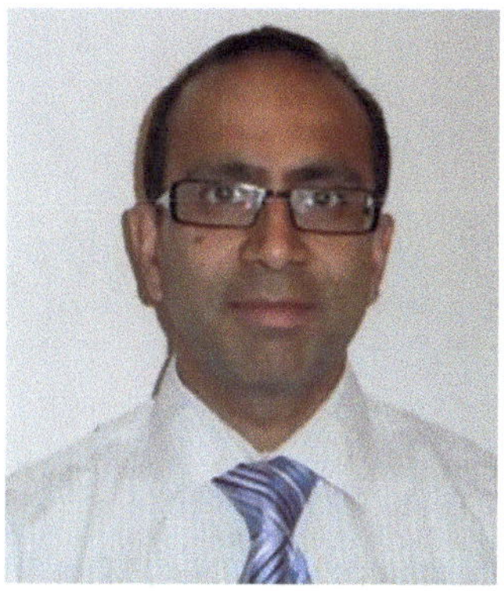

Dr. Vinood B. Patel, PhD is currently a Senior Lecturer in Clinical Biochemistry at the University of Westminster and honorary fellow at King's College London. Dr. Patel obtained his degree in Pharmacology from the University of Portsmouth, his PhD in protein metabolism from King's College London in 1997 and carried out postdoctoral research at Wake Forest University School of Medicine, USA where he developed novel biophysical techniques to characterize mitochondrial ribosomes. He presently directs studies on metabolic pathways involved in fatty liver disease, focussing on mitochondrial energy regulation and cell death. Dr. Patel has published over 150 articles, including books in the area of nutrition and health prevention.

Victor R. Preedy, BSc, PhD, DSc, FSB, FRCPath, FRSPH, FRSC is a senior member of King's College London (Professor of Nutritional Biochemistry) and King's College Hospital (Professor of Clinical Biochemistry). He is attached to both the Diabetes and Nutritional Sciences Division and the Department of Nutrition and Dietetics. He is also Director of the Genomics Centre and a member of the School of Medicine. Professor Preedy graduated in 1974 with an Honours Degree in Biology and Physiology with Pharmacology. He gained his University of London PhD in 1981. In 1992, he received his Membership of the Royal College of Pathologists and in 1993 he gained his second doctoral degree, for his outstanding contribution to protein metabolism in health and disease. Professor Preedy was elected as a Fellow to the Institute of Biology in 1995 and to the Royal College of Pathologists in 2000. Since then he has been elected as a Fellow to the Royal Society for the Promotion of Health (2004) and The Royal Institute of Public Health (2004). In 2009, Professor Preedy became a Fellow of the Royal Society for Public Health and in 2012 a Fellow of the Royal Society of Chemistry. In his career Professor Preedy has carried out research at the National Heart Hospital (part of Imperial College London) and the MRC Centre at Northwick Park Hospital. He has collaborated with research groups in Finland, Japan, Australia, USA, and Germany. He is a leading expert on the science of health. He has lectured nationally and internationally. To his credit, Professor Preedy has published over 570 articles, which includes 165 peer-reviewed manuscripts based on original research, 100 reviews and over 50 books and volumes.

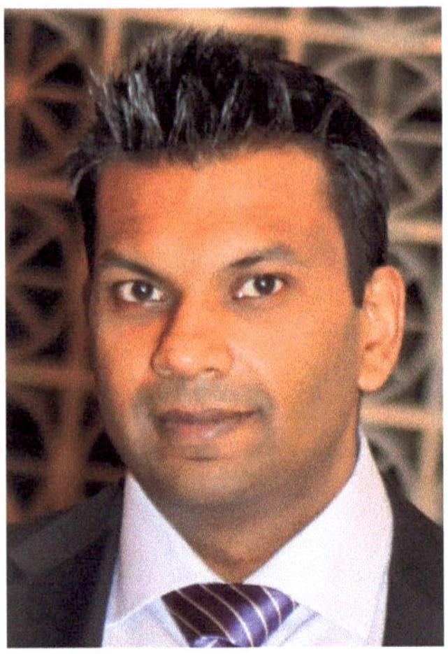

Rajaventhan Srirajaskanthan, BSc (Hons), MD (Res), MRCP is a consultant gastroenterologist at University Hospital Lewisham and Kings College Hospital, London. He trained at the prestigious Guy's, King's and St. Thomas' Medical School where he obtained his MD (MBBS) and a BSc in Neuroscience with a specialist focus in pain pathways. He has a postgraduate research degree MD (Res) was awarded by University College London. His postgraduate training was undertaken at a variety of university teaching hospitals including the John Radcliffe Hospital, Oxford, Royal Free Hospital and Kings College Hospital, London. During this time he was elected as a member to the Royal College of Physicians. His specialist training has included Gastroenterology, Hepatology, and Internal Medicine. His academic and practical fields of interests include neuroendocrine tumors, nutrition in liver disease, nonalcoholic steatohepatitis (NASH), and viral hepatitis. He has published more than 30 peer-reviewed articles, 60 abstracts, and written 6 book chapters plus coedited 3 books.

Acknowledgments

The development of this book is built upon the foundation of the excellent work provided by the staff of Humana and we are very thankful to them. In particular we wish to acknowledge the outstanding support, advice, and patience of the Series Editor, Dr. Adrianne Bendich, The Developmental Editor, Michael Griffin, and Editor, Amanda Quinn.

Contents

Contributors

Deena Alasfoor Department of Nutrition, Ministry of Health, Al Ghubra, Muscat, Oman

Olga Maria Silverio Amancio Department of Pediatrics, Paulista Medicine School, Federal University of Sao Paulo, Sao Paulo, SP, Brazil

Robert J. Baldwin Emory University, Atlanta, GA, USA

Senior Advisor, Flour Fortification Initiative, Atlanta, GA, USA

Judit Berman Department of Plant Production and Forestry Science, ETSEA, University of Lleida-Agrotecnio Center, Lleida, Spain

Navreet K. Bhullar Department of Biology, Institute of Agricultural Sciences, Swiss Federal Institute of Technology (ETH), Zurich, Switzerland

Dieter Blancquaert Department of Physiology, Ghent University, Ghent, Belgium

José Boccio Stable Isotopes Laboratory Applied to Biology and Medicine, Department of Physics, School of Pharmacy and Biochemistry, University of Buenos Aires, Buenos Aires, Argentina

Kulaporn Boonyaves Department of Biology, Institute of Agricultural Sciences, Swiss Federal Institute of Technology (ETH), Zurich, Switzerland

Josefina Aparecida Pellegrini Braga Department of Pediatrics, Paulista Medicine School, Federal University of Sao Paulo, Sao Paulo, Brazil

Lan T.T. Bui Human Protection and Performance Division, Defence Science and Technology Organisation, Scottsdale, TAS, Australia

Teresa Capell Department of Plant Production and Forestry Science, ETSEA, University of Lleida-Agrotecnio Center, Lleida, Spain

Allan Carlé Department of Endocrinology, Aalborg University Hospital, Aalborg, Denmark

Nathalie Cayot Research Unit PAM, UMR MA AGROSUP 2012.02.102, Dijon, Cedex, France

Philippe Cayot Research Unit PAM, UMR MA AGROSUP 2012.02.102, Dijon, Cedex, France

Charlotte Cerqueira Research Centre for Prevention and Health, Glostrup University Hospital, Glostrup, Denmark

Paul Christou Department of Plant Production and Forestry Science, ETSEA, University of Lleida-Agrotecnio Center, Lleida, Spain

Institució Catalana de Recerca I Estudis Avançats, Barcelona, Spain

Ross Coad Human Protection and Performance Division, Defence Science and Technology Organisation, Scottsdale, TAS, Australia

Gerald F. Combs Grand Forks Human Nutrition Research Center, ARS/USDA, Grand Forks, ND, USA

Hans De Steur Department of Agricultural Economics, Ghent University, Ghent, Belgium

Isaias Dichi Department of Internal Medicine, University of Londrina, Londrina-PR, Brazil

Levente L. Diósady Department of Chemical Engineering and Applied Chemistry, University of Toronto, Toronto, ON, Canada

Wei Dong Chinese Academy of Agricultural Sciences, Beijing, China

Michael L. Dunn Department of Nutrition Dietetics and Food Science, Brigham Young University, Provo, UT, USA

Scarlett Ewen College of Pharmacy and Nutrition, University of Saskatchewan, Saskatoon, SK, Canada

Gemma Farré Department of Plant Production and Forestry Science, ETSEA, University of Lleida-Agrotecnio Center, Lleida, Spain

Michael Fenech CSIRO Food and Nutritional Sciences, Adelaide BC, SA, Australia

Javier Fontecha Department of Bioactivity and Food Analysis, Group of Lipids, Instituto de Investigación en Ciencias de la Alimentación (CIAL; CSIC-UAM), Madrid, Spain

Xavier Gellynck Department of Agricultural Economics, Ghent University, Ghent, Belgium

Robin Graham School of Agriculture, Food and Wine, The University of Adelaide, Adelaide, SA, Australia

Alistair S. Grandison Department of Food and Nutritional Sciences, The University of Reading, Reading, UK

Tatiana Guzun-Cojocaru Research Unit EMMA, EA 581 of University of Burgundy, Dijon, Cedex, France

Izzeldin S. Hussein Research Centre (ICCIDD) MENA and Gulf Region, International Council for Control of Iodine Deficiency Disorders, Al Khuwair, Oman

Margaretha Jägerstad Department of Food Science, Swedish University of Agricultural Sciences, Uppsala BioCenter, Uppsala, Sweden

Jelena Jastrebova Department of Food Science, Swedish University of Agricultural Sciences, Uppsala BioCenter, Uppsala, Sweden

Torben Jørgensen Research Centre for Prevention and Health, Glostrup University Hospital, Glostrup, Denmark

Manuela Juarez Department of Bioactivity and Food Analysis, Group of lipids, Instituto de Investigación en Ciencias de la Alimentación (CIAL; CSIC-UAM), Madrid, Spain

Nils Knudsen Department of Endocrinology and Gastroenterology, Bispebjerg University Hospital, Copenhagen, Denmark

Willy Lambert Department of Bioanalysis, Ghent University, Ghent, Belgium

Peter Laurberg Department of Endocrinology, Aalborg University Hospital, Aalborg, Denmark

Cailin Lei Chinese Academy of Agricultural Sciences, Beijing, China

Michael J. Lewis Department of Food and Nutritional Sciences, The University of Reading, Reading, UK

Ge Liqun Rural Economy Research Institute, Liaoning Academy of Agricultural Sciences, Shenyang, Liaoning, People's Republic of China

Rubén López-Nicolás Department of Food Science and Nutrition, Faculty of Veterinary Sciences, Regional Campus of International Excellence "Campus Mare Nostrum", University of Murcia, Spain

Jan W. Low International Potato Center, Nairobi, Kenya

Graham Lyons School of Agriculture, Food and Wine, University of Adelaide, Adelaide, Australia

Lucia Helena Silva Miglioranza Department of Food Science and Technology, University of Londrina, Londrina-PR, Brazil

Teruo Miyazawa Food and Biodynamic Chemistry Laboratory, Graduate School of Agricultural Science, Tohoku University, Sendai, Japan

Kiyotaka Nakagawa Food and Biodynamic Chemistry Laboratory, Graduate School of Agricultural Science, Tohoku University, Sendai, Japan

Shaista Naqvi MRC Protein Phosphorylation Unit, College of Life Sciences, University of Dundee, Dundee, UK

Department of Plant Production and Forestry Science, ETSEA, University of Lleida-Agrotecnio Center, Lleida, Spain

Oscar Navarrete Department of Physiology, Ghent University, Ghent, Belgium

Elvan Ocak Department of Food Engineering, Yuzuncu Yil University, Van, Turkey

Lars Ovesen Department of Gastroenterology, Slagelse Hospital, Slagelse, Denmark

Pattavara Pathomrungsiyounggul Division of Food Engineering, Chiang Mai University, Chiang Mai, Thailand

Inge Bülow Pedersen Department of Endocrinology, Aalborg University Hospital, Aalborg, Denmark

Hans Perrild Department of Endocrinology and Gastroenterology, Bispebjerg University Hospital, Copenhagen, Denmark

Javier Polo APC EUROPE, S.A. R&D Department, Granollers, Spain

Kalpana Platel Department of Biochemistry and Nutrition, Central Food Technological Research Institute, Yadavagiri, Mysore, India

Chanakan Prom-u-thai Agronomy Division, Department of Plant Science and Natural Resources, Chiang Mai University, Chiang Mai, Thailand

Rajkumar Rajendram Departments of General Medicine and Intensive Care, John Radcliffe Hospital, Oxford, Oxfordshire, UK

Division of Diabetes & Nutritional Sciences, School of Medicine, King's College London, London, UK

Benjavan Rerkasem Plant Genetic Resource and Nutrition Laboratory, Chiang Mai University, Chiang Mai, Thailand

Carmen Rodríguez APC EUROPE, S.A. R&D Department, Granollers, Spain

Luis Miguel Rodríguez-Alcalá Department of Bioactivity and Food Analysis, Group of Lipids, Instituto de Investigación en Ciencias de la Alimentación (CIAL; CSIC-UAM), Madrid, Spain

Gaspar Ros Department of Food Science and Nutrition, Faculty of Veterinary Sciences, Regional Campus of International Excellence "Campus Mare Nostrum", University of Murcia, Spain

Jocelyn Sacco Department of Nutritional Sciences, University of Toronto, Toronto, ON, Canada

María Jimena Salgueiro Stable Isotopes Laboratory Applied to Biology and Medicine, Department of Physics, School of Pharmacy and Biochemistry, University of Buenos Aires, Buenos Aires, Argentina

Georgina Sanahuja Department of Plant Production and Forestry Science, ETSEA, University of Lleida-Agrotecnio Center, Lleida, Spain

Gerhard Sandmann Biosynthesis Group, Molecular Biosciences, Johann Wolfgang Goethe Universität, Frankfurt, Germany

Christof Sautter Department of Biology, Institute of Agricultural Sciences, Swiss Federal Institute of Technology (ETH), Zurich, Switzerland

Isabelle Sioen Department of Public Health, Ghent University, Ghent, Belgium

Research Foundation—Flanders, Brussels, Belgium

Darryl M. Small School of Applied Sciences, RMIT University, Melbourne, VIC, Australia

Phumon Sookwong Department of Chemistry, Chiang Mai University, Chiang Mai, Thailand

Sergei Storozhenko Department of Physiology, Ghent University, Ghent, Belgium

Christophe Stove Department of Bioanalysis, Ghent University, Ghent, Belgium

Dil Thavarajah School of Food Systems, North Dakota State University, Fargo, ND, USA

Pushparajah Thavarajah School of Food Systems, North Dakota State University, Fargo, ND, USA

Richard M. Twyman TRM Ltd., York, United Kingdom

Jeroen Van Daele Department of Bioanalysis, Ghent University, Ghent, Belgium

Dominique Van Der Straeten Department of Physiology, Ghent University, Ghent, Belgium

Hassan Vatanparast College of Pharmacy and Nutrition, University of Saskatchewan, Saskatoon, SK, Canada

M.G. Venkatesh-Mannar Micronutrient Initiative, Ottawa, ON, Canada

Jacques Viaene Department of Agricultural Economics, Ghent University, Ghent, Belgium

Antonia Villar-Tajadura Department of Bioactivity and Food Analysis, Group of Lipids, Instituto de Investigación en Ciencias de la Alimentación (CIAL; CSIC-UAM), Madrid, Spain

Meng Wang Department of Biology, Institute of Agricultural Sciences, Swiss Federal Institute of Technology (ETH), Zurich, Switzerland

Jing Wu Population Research and Outcome Studies, The University of Adelaide, Adelaide, Australia

Chunyi Zhang Chinese Academy of Agricultural Sciences, Beijing, China

Changfu Zhu Department of Plant Production and Forestry Science, ETSEA, University of Lleida-Agrotecnio Center, Lleida, Spain

Sarah Zimmerman Emory University, Atlanta, GA, USA

Flour Fortification Initiative, Atlanta, GA, USA

Uxue Zorrilla-López Department of Plant Production and Forestry Science, ETSEA, University of Lleida-Agrotecnio Center, Lleida, Spain

Part I
Introductory Chapters and Perspectives of Fortification

Chapter 1
The Link Between Organizational Bodies and Fortification Strategies and Practice: The Role of the Flour Fortification Initiative

Sarah Zimmerman and Robert J. Baldwin

Key Points

- The Flour Fortification Initiative engages partners in the public, private, and civic sectors.
- The public–private–civic sector partnership model is relevant for any group attempting to fortify a staple food.
- Representatives from the public, private, and civic sectors in each country should be involved at the beginning of fortification planning.
- Working together, these groups can achieve more than any of them could independently.
- The background of how countries began fortifying flour with folic acid to prevent major birth defects illustrates this partnership.

Keywords Partnership • Collaboration • Flour • Fortification • Nutrition • Iron • Folic acid • Neural tube defects • Birth defects • Public sector • Private sector • Civic sector

Abbreviations

EMT	Executive Management Team
FFI	Flour Fortification Initiative
MI	Micronutrient Initiative
NTD	Neural tube defect
UNICEF	United Nations Children's Fund
WHO	World Health Organization

S. Zimmerman (✉)
Emory University, 1599 Clifton Road 1599-001-1BX (SPH: Global Health), Atlanta, GA 30322, USA

Flour Fortification Initiative, Atlanta, GA 30322, USA
e-mail: Szimme2@emory.edu

R.J. Baldwin
Emory University, 1599 Clifton Road 1599-001-1BX (SPH: Global Health), Atlanta, GA 30322, USA

Senior Advisor, Flour Fortification Initiative, Atlanta, GA 30322, USA
e-mail: bobbyb@charter.net

V.R. Preedy et al. (eds.), *Handbook of Food Fortification and Health: From Concepts to Public Health Applications Volume 1*, Nutrition and Health, DOI 10.1007/978-1-4614-7076-2_1,

Introduction

At first glance, using fortified flour to address a country's vitamin and mineral deficiencies seems to be a simple proposition. Adding nutrients to flour is no more complicated than adding "improvers" that modern mills already include to enhance the flour's texture and shelf life. Flour has been fortified since the 1940s, so the technology and tools are readily available. Flour milling is usually a centralized process which simplifies quality assurance and quality control. Foods made with wheat and maize flours are commonly consumed, making flour fortification an effective tool for reaching most of the population.

In reality, however, reaching national-scale flour fortification is a complex process that requires a multi-faceted approach. The process involves identifying which nutrients are limited in people's diets, establishing standards for how much of each nutrient to add to flour, creating country-specific legislation, identifying a supply source for the nutrients to add to flour, determining distribution of the fortification costs, establishing a quality control system, and measuring the health impact among the population.

Given the variety of requirements for a successful fortification program, it is wise to involve multiple stakeholders in the process from the concept stage to implementation and evaluation. The Flour Fortification Initiative (FFI) is a network designed to facilitate that collaboration among all sectors with the goal of making flour fortification standard milling practice throughout the world. While its focus is on wheat and maize flours, the FFI model of engaging partners in the public, private, and civic sectors is relevant for any group attempting to fortify a staple food (see Fig. 1.1). Working together, these partners can achieve more than any of them could independently. The International Council for the control of Iodine Deficiency Disorders Global Network is a similar group focused on making salt iodization standard practice to prevent brain damage from iodine deficiency.

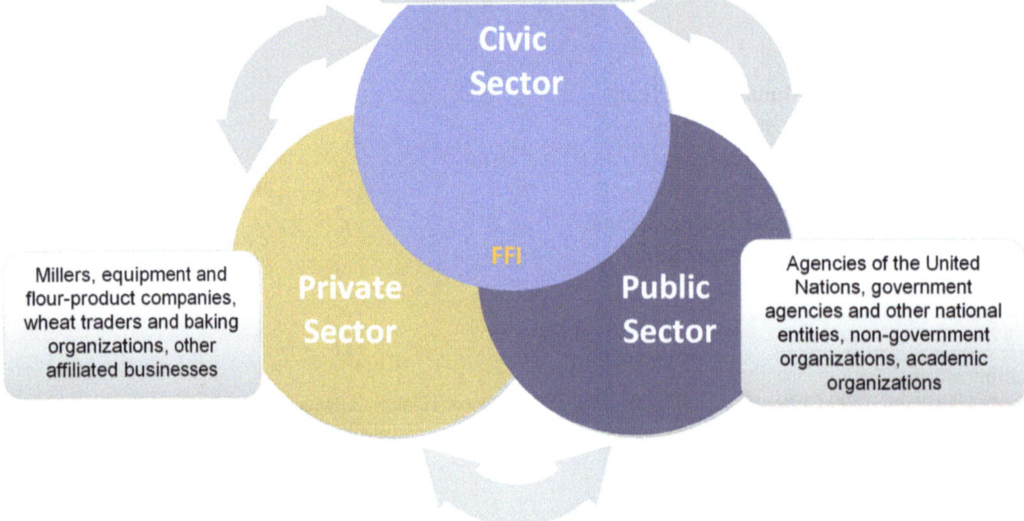

Fig. 1.1 Flour Fortification Initiative (FFI) network illustration

Flour is most commonly fortified with iron and folic acid. Iron is essential for a child's physical and mental development. As a component of hemoglobin, which carries oxygen to the body, iron is necessary for optimum physical activity and work productivity at any age. Iron is also critical for the health of a pregnant woman and her unborn child. Folic acid, a form of vitamin B9, decreases the risk of neural tube defects (NTDs) such as spina bifida and anencephaly. These birth defects are permanently disabling or fatal, but they are largely preventable if the woman has enough folic acid before she becomes pregnant and early in her pregnancy. Other vitamins and minerals that can be added to flour at each country's discretion include zinc, vitamin D, vitamin A, vitamin B12, and other B vitamins such as thiamine, riboflavin, and niacin.

This chapter will outline the role of the public, private, and civic sectors in flour fortification programs and share examples from around the world. The chapter will also describe how FFI attempts to unite its partners to achieve successful flour fortification and consequently improve nutrition status among a population. The example of how countries began fortifying flour with folic acid to prevent birth defects will illustrate the public–private–civic sector collaboration involved in flour fortification.

Public Sector

Examples of entities in the public sector include government ministries or agencies, multi-lateral agencies of the United Nations such as the United Nations Children's Fund (UNICEF), nongovernmental organizations, and academic institutions. Representatives from the public sector typically serve the following roles in flour fortification:

1. *Identify the public health problem.* Public sector groups often conduct surveys that reveal evidence of vitamin and mineral deficiencies, such as high rates of NTDs or anemia caused by iron deficiency. They can help a country identify the cause of the deficiency, including food consumption patterns, limited access to a variety of nutritious foods, and high food prices restricting purchases of foods with greater nutritional value.

   Due to cultural norms in India, for example, many people do not eat meat and consequently do not consume ample amounts of iron through their normal diets. Even among populations that do eat meat, the cost of iron-rich meat can prohibit frequent consumption. In such situations, people's diets are often high in cereal-based foods, and the phytic acid found in grains can inhibit the body's ability to absorb iron. Flour that is fortified with the appropriate iron compound and at adequate levels can overcome the phytic acid effect. The World Health Organization (WHO) offers guidelines on the form of iron to use based on the type of flour being fortified and the average consumption of that flour [1] (see Table 1.1).
2. *Recommend appropriate interventions.* Most countries use a combination of approaches to address nutrient deficiencies. Many countries in West Africa, for instance, add iodine to salt, vitamin A to vegetable oil, and iron, zinc, folic acid, and other B vitamins to flour. They might also implement nonfood strategies to improve nutrient levels, such as deworming campaigns, safe drinking water initiatives, and vitamin supplement or micronutrient powder distribution.
3. *Establish and enable the setting of standards.* When flour fortification is pursued, standards must be established for the specific levels of each chosen vitamin and mineral to be added to a kilogram of flour. In addition to the guidelines for iron, the WHO statement offers recommended levels of folic acid, vitamin B12, vitamin A, and zinc [1]. Each country sets its own standard, however, based on flour consumption patterns, the level of nutrient deficiency, and the type of flour being fortified.
4. *Ensure quality.* In most countries, the private sector conducts internal quality assurance testing. In addition, food fortification is regulated by a government entity that routinely inspects flour for

Table 1.1 Recommendations for average levels of nutrients to consider adding to fortified wheat flour based on extraction, fortificant compound, and estimated per capita flour availability

			Level of nutrient to be added in parts per million (ppm) by estimated per capita wheat flour availability (g/day)[a]			
Nutrient	Flour extraction rate	Compound	<75[b]	75–149	150–300	>300
Iron	Low	NaFeEDTA	40	40	20	15
		Ferrous sulfate	60	60	30	20
		Ferrous fumarate	60	60	30	20
		Electrolyte iron	NR[c]	NR[c]	60	40
	High	NaFeEDTA	40	40	20	15
Zinc[d]	Low	Zinc oxide	95	55	40	30
	High		100	100	80	70
Folic acid	Low or high	Folic acid	5.0	2.6	1.3	1.0
Vitamin B_{12}	Low or high	Cyancobalamin	0.04	0.02	0.01	0.008
Vitamin A	Low or high	Vitamin A palmitate	5.9	3	1.5	1

Source: World Health Organization http://www.who.int/nutrition/publications/micronutrients/wheat_maize_fortification/en/

[a]These estimated levels consider only wheat flour as main fortification vehicle in a public health program. If other mass fortification programs with other food vehicles are implemented effectively, these suggested fortification levels may need to be adjusted downwards as needed

[b]Estimated per capita consumption of <75 g/day does not allow for addition of sufficient level of fortificant to cover micronutrients needs for women of childbearing age. Fortification of additional food vehicles and other interventions should be considered

[c]*NR* Not recommended because the very high levels of electrolytic iron needed would negatively affect sensory properties of fortified flour

[d]These amounts of zinc fortification assume 5 mg zinc intake and no additional phytate intake from other dietary sources

compliance with the national standard. Public sector agencies lead the process of establishing this external inspection system.

5. *Lead program evaluation and improvement.* The public sector typically initiates efforts to determine whether the flour fortification program is having the desired impact. For example, the National Food and Nutrition Centre in Fiji conducted a nationally representative study of women of child bearing age five years after flour fortification began. The study showed statistically significant improvements in the study population's dietary intake of iron, zinc, thiamin, riboflavin, niacin and folate – all the nutrients included in Fiji's fortified flour [2].
6. *Address cost concerns.* Fortification costs for millers include one-time expenses such as purchasing and installing equipment and training staff as well as the ongoing expense of buying the premix of nutrients in accordance with established country standards. By engaging the private sector at the beginning of the fortification discussions, the public sector can determine the most acceptable way to fund these expenses. A country's healthcare savings from preventing diseases and birth defects can be significant, which leads some governments, such as Iran, to subsidize the entire fortification process. In Tanzania, the government waives import taxes on fortification equipment and nutrient premixes. Other countries require millers to bear the entire cost of fortification. In these cases, the additional cost is often passed on to consumers, but the increased price for each loaf of bread or other foods made with fortified flour is minimal.

Private Sector

The private sector encompasses businesses involved in flour fortification, including the flour mill owners and operators, equipment manufacturers, and companies that produce the vitamins and minerals added to flour. These are the groups that turn wheat berries and maize kernels into flour, carry out the fortification process, conduct internal quality control measures, and distribute and market the products. The private sector is obviously critical to implementation of flour fortification programs, and this sector is also instrumental in the fortification planning stage. The private sector roles include the following:

1. *Share in advocacy efforts.* It is often millers who recognize the potential health impact of flour fortification and lead flour fortification advocacy efforts through their individual companies or their professional associations. Millers frequently urge mandatory fortification legislation in the country so all millers incur the same expenses related to ongoing fortification. This is commonly known as "creating a level playing field" for the industry.
2. *Conduct sensory trials.* For fortified flour to be accepted by consumers, the addition of fortificants cannot change organoleptic properties (appearance, smell, or taste) of flour or foods made with flour. In Asia, private sector researchers in China, India, Indonesia, Malaysia, the Philippines, and Sri Lanka conducted a series of experiments to test whether foods commonly consumed in Asian countries would remain marketable if they were made with flour fortified in accordance with WHO recommendations [3]. They found that 15 kinds of noodles and breads could be successfully fortified with iron, folic acid, vitamin B12, vitamin A, thiamine, riboflavin, and zinc, and that the nutrients appeared to be retained throughout the food preparation process [3]. In Africa, the private industry conducted baking trials in 2010 and 2011, also with flour fortified at WHO recommended levels. The Africa trials likewise showed that typical African foods can be fortified with no adverse consequences on the food product.
3. *Provide data.* Information about the number of flour mills in a country, their production capacity, and their export practices can help a country establish appropriate fortification practices and realistic implementation timelines. Iran, for example, has more than 335 mills with a combined annual capacity of more than 23 million tons [4]. Implementing flour fortification there was very complex compared to implementation in Mauritania which has six large flour mills with a combined annual capacity of 64,000 tons [5].
4. *Guide creation of feasible standards.* While the public sector recommends optimal levels of fortification for specific nutrients in flour, the private sector can recommend a range that is feasible to accomplish. For example, a country's optimal level of folic acid in flour to prevent neural tube birth defects might be 2 mg of folic acid per kilogram of flour. The private sector may note that such a precise level is nearly impossible to achieve and instead recommend a range of 1.8–2.2 mg of folic acid per kilogram of flour. Working together, the public and private sectors can determine a range of fortification levels that will accomplish the health objective, be feasible to implement, and be simple to monitor.
5. *Conduct internal quality controls.* Mills are encouraged to keep records of the quantity of vitamins and minerals added to flour. Any variation from what is expected based on the records of premix used and flour produced will help a mill identify and correct problems in fortification procedures. Millers also regularly conduct assays known as the iron spot test to confirm that the added nutrients are in the final flour product.

Civic Sector

This group is sometimes called the voluntary or community sector in a society. When such groups adopt a cause, their influence can have significant impact. For example, Kiwanis International is devoted to helping children worldwide. When the organization looked for a global project that would give Kiwanis members in every nation a common goal and shared experience, the international group decided to partner with UNICEF to address salt iodization. In 1994, club representatives at the Kiwanis International Convention voted overwhelmingly to support the project and to raise US$80 million to meet the challenge of achieving universal salt iodization [6]. Similarly, Rotary International has adapted polio eradication as a service project. Its members worldwide are involved in fund raising and volunteer activities, including public advocacy, related to this cause [7].

With flour fortification, the main civic sector partners are those focused on preventing NTDs and supporting families with a child affected by an NTD. Examples include the March of Dimes and the International Federation for Spina Bifida and Hydrocephalus. Their role in flour fortification includes the following:

1. *Educate the public*. As community-based groups with ties to volunteers, messages from the civic sector reach an audience that may not be as easily reached by the public or private sectors. An educated public often plays a role in exerting pressure on government policy makers to enact legislation for flour fortification.
2. *Maintain urgency*. Civic sector representatives frequently have a family member with an NTD. For this reason, they are passionate about prevention and quality care for people with NTDs. Their voices add a sense of urgency to flour fortification efforts.

The Role of the Flour Fortification Initiative

Despite the critical function that the public, private, and civic sector partners each have in developing and maintaining successful flour fortification programs, they sometimes work independently and fail to harness the power of team work. The role of FFI is to encourage collaboration and facilitate dialogue among multiple stakeholders in each sector.

Globally, the FFI partnership is led by the Executive Management Team (EMT) which provides strategic direction to the network. EMT members include representatives from agencies of the United Nations, flour milling industries, academia, and government and nongovernmental organizations.

Regionally, FFI is deliberate about inviting people from each sector to meetings and workshops on varied topics such as strategic planning, technical training, quality assurance and quality control, and monitoring and evaluation. On several occasions, individuals working in one country to initiate fortification were not aware of their in-country counterparts until they attended an FFI workshop. In this respect, FFI serves as a convener to introduce partners to each other so they can work together toward the common goal of fortifying flour as a means of providing more nutrients in staple foods.

In countries seeking to begin a flour fortification program, visiting FFI staff and network partners traditionally spend a week meeting individually with stakeholders to identify each group's concerns about fortification. As a culmination activity at the end of the week, FFI moderates a meeting with all stakeholders to share their concerns with each other. During the meeting, FFI encourages the leaders to form a fortification alliance. The role of the alliance is to develop a plan to move forward with flour fortification so that all the issues are addressed. FFI continues to support the countries with advocacy and technical expertise as needed. Additionally, the national alliance may consider fortification of multiple foods as well as other strategies to benefit people who do not consume commercially produced foods.

Support for Mandatory Fortification

In bringing various sectors together, FFI occasionally finds the public sector reluctant to include the private sector for the apparent assumption that the private sector is solely motivated by profits. Instead, even though profit margins are small in the milling industry, some millers voluntarily fortify flour as a matter of corporate social responsibility. A few examples include Interflour mills in Malaysia, a Minoterie du Congo (MINOCO) mills in the Democratic Republic of Congo, and the Wheata Industrial Company Ltd., in Sudan.

The ongoing cost of buying premix to fortify a metric ton of flour with iron, folic acid, and other B vitamins is between US$2 and US$3. While the fortification cost per ton is minimal, the annual cost can be significant for mills that produce thousands of metric tons of flour a year. One reason FFI encourages mandatory flour fortification legislation is that legislation creates similar financial obligations for each miller.

Additionally, national-scale fortification distributes the health benefits equitably among the population. When fortification is voluntary, the only consumers who benefit are those who live in an area where regardless of socio-economic status or education level the fortified flour is available.

A third reason mandatory legislation is encouraged is to ensure that fortification is an ongoing initiative which will be routinely monitored for compliance and quality control. When fortification is voluntary, the levels of fortificants many change periodically or a company may choose to end fortification without notification.

Folic Acid Experience

The example of how countries began adding folic acid to flour illustrates a successful collaboration between multiple sectors. Now it is known that with 400 mg of folic acid daily at least 1 month prior to conception and in the early months of pregnancy, most of NTDs may be prevented [8]. These birth defects are permanently disabling or fatal as they affect the development of the infant's spinal cord and brain (Fig. 1.2).

Thirty years ago, the role of folic acid in preventing these birth defects was not certain. The scientific community led the way in identifying the link between folic acid (a form of vitamin B9), and preventing birth defects such as spina bifida and anencephaly. In 1991, *The Lancet* published a study showing unequivocally that folic acid can prevent NTDs [9]. The study was a randomized double blind prevention trial conducted at 33 centers in seven countries. One conclusion was that "public health measures should be taken to ensure that the diet of all women who may bear children contains an adequate amount of folic acid [9]."

With that conclusion, the civic and public sectors in North America, led by the March of Dimes and the U.S. Centers for Disease Control and Prevention, began advocacy work to change the US standard for enriched flour to include folic acid. The United States amended the existing legislation in March 1996 to require folic acid, and full implementation was required by January 1998 [10].

At the same time in the Middle East, international agencies such as the WHO, UNICEF, and the Micronutrient Initiative (MI), were leading efforts to improve nutrition in the region. Flour fortification was being considered as a possible intervention to recommend. To test the feasibility of flour fortification, the private sector became involved, and Oman Flour Mills began fortifying flour in 1996 on a trial basis. Oman Flour Mills covered 75 % of the market in Oman, and the mill was well-equipped to begin fortification without a major investment. By October 1996, when a regional workshop was held in Oman to consider multiple health interventions, the mill was fortifying flour successfully, and it continues to do so today [11].

Deciding the optimum level of folic acid to add to flour to prevent NTDs was a challenge in the early 1990s. Guatemala and El Salvador added folic acid to flour in 1992 to replace the naturally occurring vitamin that was lost in the milling process; however, the amounts added were not high enough to significantly impact the incidence of NTDs [12]. In 2002, Central American countries collectively agreed to fortify with folic acid at a rate of 1.8 parts per million (ppm) [12].

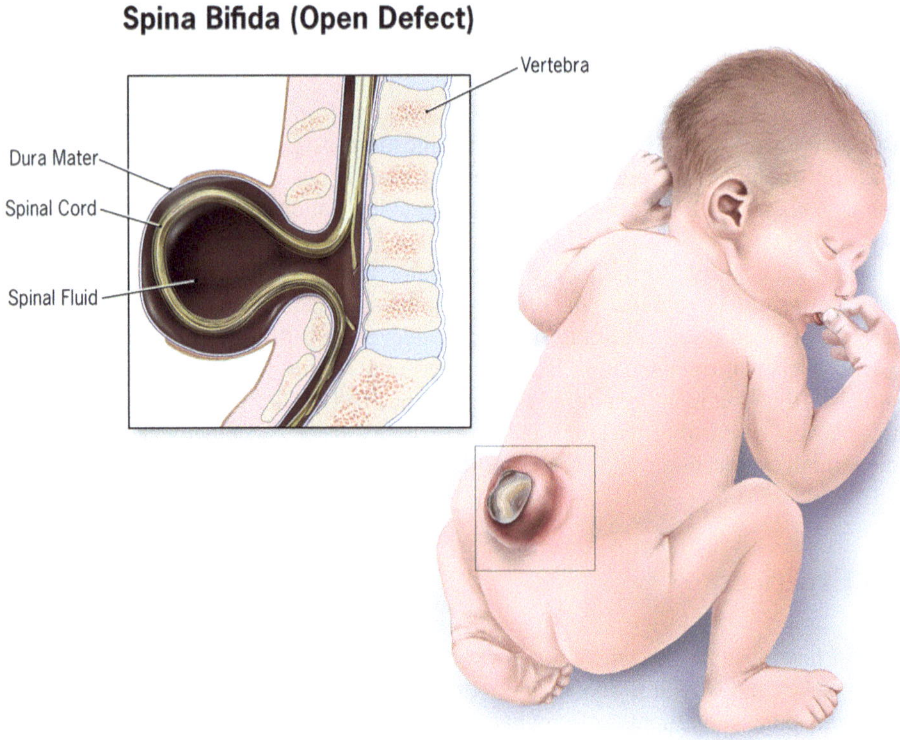

Fig. 1.2 Illustrated drawing of infant with an open defect of spina bifida. Illustration by the U.S. Centers for Disease Control and Prevention

To address the question of how much folic acid and other nutrients to add to flour, FFI convened a workshop in 2008 with more than 100 international, multi-sector experts. They developed recommendations for fortifying flour with folic acid, iron, zinc, vitamin A, and vitamin B12. The folic acid recommendations range from 1 to 5 ppm based on consumption levels of flour-based foods. The workshop results became the basis of globally recognized guidelines for adding folic acid to wheat and maize flours. These were published by the WHO in 2009 [1] and in the *Food and Nutrition Bulletin* in 2010 [13].

Once fortifying flour with folic acid became standard practice in several countries, the scientific community began to study whether this was an effective intervention. Their research shows a 30–70 % decline in NTDs when countries fortify flour with folic acid (see Table 1.2).

The March of Dimes estimates that more than 300,000 infants worldwide are affected by an NTD annually [14]. A 2008 study estimated that globally about 22,000 NTDs were prevented every year due to flour fortification [15]. That figure represented 9 % of the estimated folic acid preventable cases of spina bifida and anencephaly [15]. By 2010 more countries were fortifying flour, and an estimated 28,066 birth defects were prevented, for a total of 13.8 % of the total number of folic acid preventable spina bifida and anencephaly [16]. Eliminating the remaining birth defects that could be prevented with enough folic acid will take continued vigilance and cooperation from all sectors.

Table 1.2 Percent decrease in neural tube defects (NTDs) due to fortifying flour with folic acid

Country	NTD prevalence pre-fortification per 1,000 births	NTD prevalence post-fortification per 1,000 births	Percent decrease in NTD prevalence
Argentina [17]			
Spina bifida	1.27	0.66	48
Anencephaly	0.86	0.37	57
Brazil [17]			
Spina bifida	1.45	1.42	2[a]
Anencephaly	1.12	0.69	38
Canada [18]			
Spina bifida	0.86	0.40	53
Anencephaly	0.52	0.32	38
Chile [17]			
Spina bifida	1.02	0.46	55
Anencephaly	0.63	0.37	41
Costa Rica [19]			
Spina bifida	0.73	0.29	60
Anencephaly	0.37	0.12	68
Iran [20] (all NTDS)	3.16	2.19	31
Oman [21]	3.17	0.96	70
Spina bifida	Average 1991–1996	Average 1997–2006	
Saudi Arabia [22] King Abdul-Aziz University Hospital in Jeddah (all NTDS)	1.9	0.76	60
South Africa [23]			
Spina bifida	0.93	0.54	42
Anencephaly	0.41	0.37	10
United States [24]			
Spina bifida	0.50	0.35	30
Anencephaly	0.26	0.18	31

Some countries report spina bifida and anencephaly separately; others report all NTDs together, including encephalocele Spina bifida is malformation of the spine; anencephaly is malformation of the brain (which is always fatal); encephalocele causes sac-like protrusions of the brain and its membranes that are visible through openings in the skull. The severity of encephalocele varies, depending on its location

[a]The study in Brazil was for 3 months, and the authors concluded that a longer period of time was needed to assess fortification's effects

Conclusion

While FFI validates the role of the public, private, and civic sectors by including each group in all activities, encourages mandatory fortification, and provides technical assistance as requested, FFI does not implement flour fortification. Flour fortification is most successful when national leaders drive the process so that it conforms to local market structures and social and nutritional needs. This national leadership of the process is critical to the sustainability of the program. Multiple national stakeholders representing various sectors create win–win flour fortification strategies that are sustainable for the future.

In 2004, 33 countries had legal requirements to fortify wheat flour. By April 2013, 76 countries mandated flour fortification with at least iron or folic acid (Fig. 1.3). This progress is possible because representatives of the public, private, and civic sectors worked together to promote flour as a vehicle for delivering more nutrients to their populations.

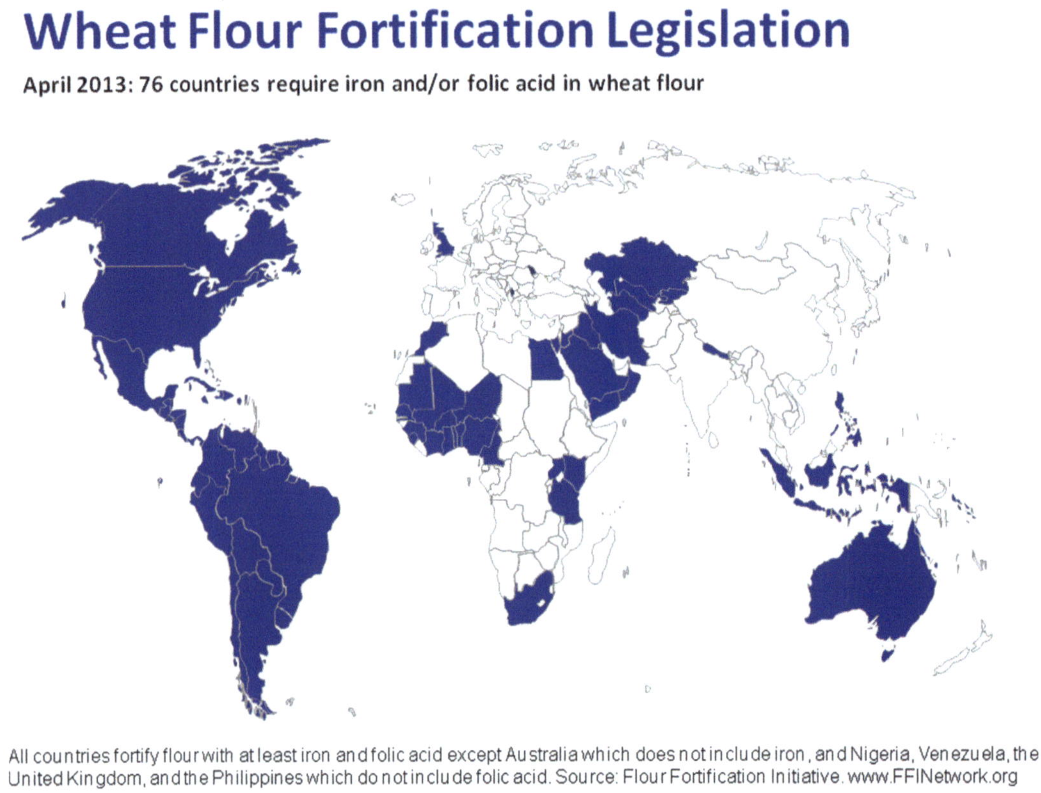

Fig. 1.3 Status of wheat flour fortification legislation (April 2013)

Guidance on Safe Levels to Be Added

Several factors influence the amount of nutrients to be added to flour for maximum health benefit. Among the considerations are average consumption of foods made with flour, type of flour, burden of diseases that can be addressed with fortified flour, and whether other foods are effectively fortified with the same nutrient.

The most recent global guidelines for flour fortification are the WHO Recommendations (see Table 1.1; [1]). The background papers that helped produce these recommendations were printed as a supplement to the *Food and Nutrition Bulletin* in 2010 [13].

Recommendations

1. *Include all sectors at the beginning of the fortification planning process.* Fortification is most successful when the public, private, and civic sectors are each involved early, and their contributions are each critical.
2. *Engage national leaders to drive the process.* International organizations can create interest in food fortification, but the program will be more appropriate for the country and more sustainable for the long-term if national stakeholders guide the process.
3. *Campaign for mandatory fortification.* Mandatory fortification creates equitable costs for the private sector, establishes beneficial standards for nutrient levels in commonly consumed foods, provides equal access to the additional nutritional benefits to all who consume the fortified food, and is easier than voluntary fortification to monitor for compliance and quality.

References

1. Recommendations on wheat and maize flour fortification meeting report: interim consensus statement. http://www.who.int/nutrition/publications/micronutrients/wheat_maize_fort.pdf. Accessed 13 June 2011.
2. National Food and Nutrition Centre. Impact of iron fortified flour in child bearing age women in Fiji, 2010 report. 2012.
3. Flour Fortification Initiative. Asian wheat flour products: impact of flour fortification on organoleptic properties, March 2011. http://www.ffinetwork.org/plan/documents/AsiaFoodImpact.pdf.
4. Dr Mahshid Lotfi. Flour Fortification in the Islamic Republic of Iran: sustainable route to improved health. http://www.ffinetwork.org/implement/documents/Iran_Case_Study.pdf.
5. FFI. Mauritania summary—April 2013. http://www.ffinetwork.org/country_profiles/country.php?record=136.
6. Kiwanis/UNICEF: History of the first worldwide service project. http://sites.kiwanis.org/Kiwanis/en/theELIMINATEproject/MNT/history/idd.aspx. Accessed 22 April 2013.
7. End polio now—the last hurdle. http://www.rotary.org/en/ServiceAndFellowship/Polio/Pages/ridefault.aspx?housead . Accessed 18 August 2011.
8. Centers for Disease Control and Prevention. Facts about folic acid. http://www.cdc.gov/ncbddd/folicacid/about.html. Accessed 3 August 2011.
9. Wald N et al. Prevention of neural tube defects: results of the Medical Research Council Vitamin Study. Lancet. 1991;338:131–7.
10. Emory University Public Health Epidemiologist Godfrey P. Oakley, Jr. is elected to Institute of Medicine. http://whsc.emory.edu/_releases/2003october/oakley.html. Accessed 19 July 2011.
11. Alasfoor D. Oman and folic acid (Zimmerman S, personal communication, 2011).
12. Dary O. When did guatemala add folic acid to flour? (Zimmerman S, personal communication, 2011).
13. Serdula M et al. Flour fortification with iron, folic acid, vitamin B12, vitamin A, and zinc: proceedings of the second technical workshop on wheat flour fortification. Food Nutr Bull. 2010;31:S3–96.
14. March of Dimes global report on birth defects: the hidden toll of dying and disabled children: executive summary. White Plains, NY: March of Dimes Birth Defects Foundation; 2006. p. 2.
15. Bell KN, Oakley GP. Update on prevention of folic acid-preventable spina bifida and anencephaly. Birth Defects Res A Clin Mol Teratol. 2009;85:102–7.
16. Youngblood ME, Bell KN, Oakley GP Jr. Global update on the prevention of folic acid-preventable spina bifida and anencephaly cases (unpublished data, 2010).
17. Lopez-Camelo JS, Castilla EE, Orioli IM. Folic acid flour fortification: impact on the frequencies of 52 congenital anomaly types in three South American countries. Am J Med Genet A. 2010;152A:2444–58.
18. Wals D et al. Reduction in neural tube defects after folic acid fortification in Canada. N Engl J Med. 2007;357:135–42.
19. Barboza Argüello MP, Umaña Solís LM. Impacto de la fortificación de alimentos con ácido fólico en los defectos del tubo neural en Costa Rica. Rev Panam Salud Publica. 2011;30(1):1–6.
20. Abdollahi Z et al. Efficacy of flour fortification with folic acid in women of childbearing age in Iran. Ann Nutr Metab. 2011;58:188–96.
21. Alasfoor D et al. Spina bifida and birth outcomes before and after fortification of flour with iron and folic acid in Oman. East Mediterr Health J. 2010;16:533–8.
22. Safdar O et al. Decline in the incidence of neural tube defects after the national fortification of flour (1997–2005). Saudi Med J. 2007;28(8):1227–9.
23. Sayed A-R et al. Decline in the prevalence of neural tube defects following folic acid fortification and its cost-benefit in South Africa. Birth Defects Res A Clin Mol Teratol. 2008;82:211–6.
24. National Birth Defects Prevention Network. Neural tube defect ascertainment project. http://www.nbdpn.org/current/2010pdf/NTD%20fact%20sheet%2001-10%20for%20website.pdf. Accessed 14 July 2011.

Chapter 2
Current Mandatory Fortificants in Developed Nations Compared to Developing Nations

Scarlett Ewen and Hassan Vatanparast

Key Points

- Micronutrient deficiencies are among the most prevalent health concerns in the world today.
- High prevalence of micronutrient malnutrition in some specific nutrients such as vitamin A, iron, iodine, and zinc are major public health issues in developed and developing countries. Thus, these four nutrients are common fortificants in a global view.
- Food fortification is considered a cost-effective, long-term population health strategy to battle the public health issues related to malnutrition and specific micronutrient(s) malnutrition.
- Fortification policies and practices have some similarities and differences across developed and developing countries and depend mainly on five key factors: (1) severity of public health need; (2) food industry sector; (3) level of awareness and knowledge; (4) political situation; and (5) consumption patterns.
- An appropriate food vehicle is one which is widely consumed and in adequate amounts by targeted populations.
- The most common food vehicles are staples including wheat flour, rice, salt, sugar, oil, and margarine.
- Monitoring systems with the cooperation of government bodies are needed to implement successful fortification programs.

Keywords Fortification • Micronutrient • Malnutrition • Public health • Mandatory fortificants

Introduction

Micronutrient malnutrition is a major global public health problem. Fortification is one of several approaches available for addressing micronutrient malnutrition. It offers a cost-effective and sustainable solution. Fortification regulations are set in place around the world in order to help improve the nutritional value of foods to ultimately improve the health of populations. The policies surrounding fortification vary from nation to nation. In this introductory chapter, evaluation of current mandatory

S. Ewen, M.Sc. • H. Vatanparast, M.D., Ph.D. (✉)
College of Pharmacy and Nutrition, University of Saskatchewan, Saskatoon, SK, Canada
e-mail: vatan.h@usask.ca

V.R. Preedy et al. (eds.), *Handbook of Food Fortification and Health: From Concepts to Public Health Applications Volume 1*, Nutrition and Health, DOI 10.1007/978-1-4614-7076-2_2,

fortification practices and policies in both developed and developing nations will be discussed. Before discussing current mandatory fortification programs in place, it is important to define some terms, and expand one's knowledge and background information on areas within the subject of fortification.

Fortification has great significance to public health as it is an approach to addressing malnutrition, which can help many populations, particularly at risk groups, achieve adequate micronutrient intakes through consumption of fortified foods. "Food fortification is a public health initiative with a long history of being used effectively to remedy nutritional deficiencies that were causing widespread national public health problems [1]." However, precautions must be taken to ensure that the intake of micronutrients through consumption of fortified foods does not exceed tolerable levels and cause adverse effects.

The factors which can lead to the unfortunate situation of a malnourished population are numerous and extensive. From a public health perspective, the determinants of health must be considered in these regards. These include and are not limited to: income, social status, social support networks, education, working conditions, both physical and social environments, and the list goes on. By addressing these factors, the ultimate goal to have healthy populations and healthy communities is possible. One aspect of being "healthy" is to be well-nourished and ensuring the body is consuming adequate intakes of micronutrients, which are essential to preventing disease. Despite the considerable progress in availability and accessibility of food in our global village, many communities are faced with malnutrition, or what has also become known as "hidden hunger [2]." "Hidden hunger" is a chronic lack of nutrients in the body, and often those who suffer from it are not aware of the deficiency until it is too late. Those most vulnerable to this hunger are from low-income groups residing in developing, less industrialized countries. Many approaches and strategies have been used to combat malnutrition or "hidden hunger." Fortification has shown promise in the past and continues to show its impact on reducing micronutrient malnutrition in at-risk populations.

The most prevalent micronutrient deficiencies in developing countries today are vitamin A, iron, iodine, and zinc; and this affects approximately one-third of the world's population [3]. A global progress report by the United Nations Children's Fund (UNICEF) evaluated 80 developing countries on prevalent micronutrient deficiencies. Ottaway [4] points to five of the major consequences of micronutrient deficiencies found from the UNICEF report:

1. Iodine deficiency is estimated to have lowered the intellectual capacity of almost all of the nations reviewed as much as 10–15 % points.
2. Iron deficiency in the 6–24-month age group is impairing the development of approximately 40–60 % of the developing world's children.
3. Severe iron deficiency anemia is responsible for the deaths in pregnancy and childbirth of more than 60,000 young women a year.
4. Vitamin A deficiency is compromising the immune system of approximately 40 % of the developing world's under-5-year-old children, leading to the death of about one million young children each year.
5. Folate deficiency is responsible for an estimated 200,000 severe birth defects each year in the 80 developing countries assessed.

With such large deficiencies in the world, it is important to employ strategies in an effort to battle these problems. There are three main approaches in helping people to meet their dietary approaches [5]. Dietary diversification, through consumer education programs helps the public to make better food choices, which will affect their overall health. The second, dietary supplementation is particularly effective towards at-risk populations; however, the concern with this approach is the risk of consuming a high amount of a micronutrient in a specific group of the population who are not really at need [6]. Lastly, food fortification is and continues to be one of the main strategies to tackle malnutrition leading to a major global issue [7, 8].

Definitions/Terminology

The Codex Alimentarius Commission (CAC) is an intergovernmental body established by the Food and Agriculture Organization (FAO) and World Health Organization (WHO) to implement the Joint FAO/WHO Food Standards Programme [9]. One of the objectives of the CAC is to provide useful guidance to governments, food industries, and others involved in implementation of food fortification programs, to ensure that fortification is carried out in a meaningful and safe manner for all [9]. It develops standards, guidelines, and other recommendations based on evidence and research [10]. The Codex General Principles for the Addition of Essential Nutrients to Foods (FAO/WHO) are intended to: (adapted by Maskeliunas and Miyagishima [10])

1. Provide guidance to those responsible for developing guidelines and legal texts pertaining to the addition of essential nutrients to foods.
2. Establish a uniform set of principles for the rational addition of essential nutrients to foods.
3. Maintain or improve the overall nutritional quality of foods.
4. Prevent the indiscriminate addition of essential nutrients to foods thereby decreasing the risk of health hazard due to essential nutrient excesses, deficits, or imbalances.
5. Facilitate acceptance in international trade of foods which contain added essential nutrients.

Codex Alimentarius [11] (1987) defines food fortification as:

> The addition of one or more essential nutrients to a food, whether or not it is normally contained in the food, for the purpose of preventing or correcting a demonstrated deficiency of one or more nutrients in the population or specific population groups.

A *fortificant* is the source of each micronutrient. For example, folic acid is a fortificant of the micronutrient, folate. Zinc oxide is the fortificant of the micronutrient, zinc. The term "enrichment" is often used interchangeably with fortification. However, enrichment refers to increasing the level of nutrients already present in a food to make it a "richer" source [4]. The term "supplementation" is used when referring to a supply of nutrients in a nonfood form such as tablets, capsules, pastilles, or a quantified amount of liquid or powder. For example, many take a calcium supplement, which is available in many forms in which the consumer may choose a preferable option that suits them. *Biofortification* is a relatively new approach that is currently being considered, and is receiving much attention. Biofortification refers to the breeding and genetic medication of plants (particularly those of staple foods) to improve their nutrient content and/or absorption [3].

Food Fortification

The aim of fortification is to increase the nutritional content of some foods by increasing the intake of one or more nutrients, which are inadequate in the food supply [3, 12]. This can be achieved by three main ways: (a) restoring the nutrient(s) lost during food processing by restoring depleted nutrients to their previous (naturally occurring) level (e.g., restoring B vitamins lost during processing); (b) increasing the level of a nutrient already present in a food (this can also be referred to as enrichment) (e.g., adding extra iron to wheat flour or extra calcium to milk); or (c) adding nutrients to a food which would make a good vehicle for delivering micronutrients to the general or targeted population (e.g., putting iodine into salt) [12].

Fortification has been a major strategy in improving the overall health of many, through improving the nutritional quality of the food supply. Several conditions are necessary for a successful food fortification program [13]. These include *surveillance procedures* to assess the prevalence of malnutrition and which micronutrients are not adequate in the food supply; an *appropriate food vehicle* which will be consumed by those most at risk for micronutrient deficiency; available and suitable *food-processing infrastructure*; availability of *fortificant*; *quality control measures* (i.e., government) to monitor addition of fortificant to food vehicle, and to protect those against excessive intake of nutrients; and *education* to inform people of the benefits of consuming fortified foods. It is ideal that all conditions be met, but realistically many developing countries often lack the resources to meet them and are thus likely to be faced with greater challenges than developed countries in implementing successful fortification programs.

Processed foods are more widely consumed in developed countries as opposed to developing countries. Thus, fortification may be more effective in developed countries since the food vehicle may reach a larger proportion of the population. There have been some major health concerns in the past, which have been resolved by fortifying particular foods [14]. For example, during the 1990s in Demark, there was a high incidence of vitamin A deficiency in young children, resulting in night blindness. After fortifying margarine with vitamin A, the deficiency in young children virtually disappeared. Similarly, after milk was fortified with vitamins A and D in Europe and North America, the prevalence of vitamin D deficiency and rickets decreased. Another example is deficiencies of the B vitamins (i.e., folate, thiamin, and riboflavin) in Newfoundland, Canada. After flour fortification with the B vitamins in 1944, the deficiencies were eliminated [14].

Micronutrients are currently being added to many staples and condiments worldwide. Some common food vehicles include different forms of milk (liquid, evaporated, powdered), margarine, vegetable oil, sugar, wheat flour, pasta, corn masa flour, maize flour, maize meal, soy/fish sauce, and salt [3].

Mandatory vs. Voluntary Fortification

Fortification can be classified as either mandatory or voluntary. Mandatory fortification occurs "when governments legally oblige food producers to fortify particular foods or categories of foods with specified micronutrients [3]." Mandatory fortification is typically used when a population (either the general population or a targeted population) is faced with, or is at risk of facing, a significant public health need which is the result of a micronutrient deficiency. With evidence and support, governments can institute mandatory fortification of particular foods. Voluntary fortification is when a "food manufacturer freely chooses to fortify particular foods in response to permission given in food law, or under special circumstances, is encouraged by government to do so [3]."

When selecting a fortification method, either mandatory or voluntary, there are five key factors that should be considered to determine which is most appropriate for the public health concern, and for the population group [3]. These five factors include:

1. *Severity of the public health need.* It is important to know the severity of the public health need or risk. This can be assessed "according to evidence of clinical or subclinical deficiency, inadequate nutrient intake, or potential health benefit [3]." If the public health need is serious, then mandatory fortification would be more appropriate than voluntary fortification.
2. *Features of the food industry sector responsible for production of the food vehicle.* Features to be considered should include the size and scale of the food industry, the presence of government support or control, and the current commercial environment. Mandatory fortification is most appropriate when there are fewer major producers in the area of concern, and is therefore easier to control and keep organized.
3. *Level of awareness and knowledge amongst the population.* Mandatory fortification may be more effective when knowledge of the population about the importance of consuming fortified foods is low, and there are few opportunities for nutrition education. On the other hand, voluntary fortification is best suited when there is high consumer interest or demand for fortified foods.

Table 2.1 Main types of food fortification programs

Type of fortification	Definition	Example(s)
Mass fortification (Also known as universal fortification)	The addition of micronutrients to foods commonly consumed by the general public	Cereals, oils, vegetable fats, milk, sugar, condiments
Targeted fortification	The addition of micronutrients to foods designed for specific population subgroups	Infant formulas; foods used for emergency situations; foods aimed for preschool and school-aged children
Market-driven fortification	The situation where the food manufacturer voluntary takes the initiative to add one or more micronutrients to processed foods, usually within regulatory limits, in order to increase sales and profitability. Usually a higher socio-economic class will purchase the products	Foods selected based on consumer demand
Other: Biofortification	The breeding and genetic medication of plants to improve their nutrient content and/or absorption Or/foods which are engineered to have greater nutrients	Plant-based staple foods

Source: Adapted from WHO report by Allen et al. [3]
The main food fortification programs are defined above. Examples of common food vehicles for each program are also shown

4. *Political environment*. Regulatory decisions are affected by two factors, the acceptable level of government intervention, and the value placed on informed consumer choice.
5. *Food consumption patterns*. The food vehicle chosen should be one that is widely available, accessible, and consumed by the population group; it should be one that will benefit the population by consuming adequate micronutrient(s) through the fortified food.

With these factors in mind, it would not be incorrect to say that fewer challenges may be faced in developed countries, while developing and implementing a food fortification program, as opposed to developing countries. Developed countries are more likely to have food processing facilities, quality control and monitoring systems, distribution infrastructure, and regulatory support [15]. Whereas the circumstances may differ greatly in developing countries whose food-processing industries are not well-established, and at-risk groups are difficult to reach and provide adequate nutrition through consumption of fortified foods.

Types of Food Fortification Programs

Fortification programs can take different forms [3] (Table 2.1). The first, *mass (or universal) fortification* is when foods that are widely consumed by the general population are fortified. Mass fortification programs are most appropriate in developing countries, where widely consumed staple foods such as cereal flour, salt, sugar, and soy sauce are found [16]. The second, *targeted fortification* is when specific foods for a specific population are fortified. Targeted groups are those who are most at-risk for micronutrient deficiencies. These types of programs are commonly seen in developing countries. For example, foods commonly consumed by children such as chocolate milk are fortified. However, we also see this type of program in developed countries. An example would be fortifying "functional foods" to prevent diseases such as osteoporosis, cancer, and heart disease [16]. The third, *market (or industry)-driven fortification* is when food manufacturers voluntarily fortify selected foods on the market.

The Advantages and Disadvantages of Food Fortification

Along with food fortification are both advantages and disadvantages. Advantages include the following (adapted from Allen et al. [3]):

- Fortified foods that are consumed on a regular and frequent basis can: (1) maintain body stores of nutrients more efficiently and effectively than intermittent supplements and (2) can lower the risk of multiple deficiencies that may result from seasonal deficits in the food supply or a poor quality diet.
- Fortified foods are likely to contain micronutrients that equate those attainable from a good, well-balanced diet.
- Fortification of widely distributed and widely consumed foods has potential to improve the nutrition status of a large proportion of the general population.
- Fortification does not require change(s) in existing food patterns nor individual compliance.
- The delivery system for fortified foods usually already exists, generally through the private sector.
- It is possible to fortify foods with multiple micronutrients simultaneously. The total cost of the food is not largely affected by the addition of more micronutrients.
- With proper regulations in place, there is a minimal risk of chronic toxicity from fortification.
- With the appropriate food system and existing technology, food fortification is more cost-effective than other strategies [8, 17].

Fortification may be a preferred approach from other strategies for the above advantages. However, there are disadvantages, or rather limitations of food fortification, which include the following (adapted from Allen et al. [3]):

- Consuming fortified foods is not a substitute for a good well-balanced quality diet—adequate energy, protein, essential fats—required for optimal health.
- Correcting micronutrient deficiencies through food fortification can be difficult because even when micronutrient-rich foods are available, they may not be consumed in sufficient quantities. All targeted groups within the general population might not consume the fortified foods.
  - Infants and young children consume smaller amounts of food and are therefore less likely to be able to obtain their recommended intakes of all micronutrients from fortified foods alone.
  - Fortified foods may not be easily accessible or available to those population groups living in remote areas.
  - Low-income groups, particularly in developing countries, often rely on a different food delivery system—locally produced or grown food—therefore are at greater risk of micronutrient deficiency, as compared to other population groups who consume processed foods.
- Poor or low-income population groups often suffer from multiple micronutrient deficiencies as a result of inadequate intake in overall diet. These groups are unlikely to obtain the recommended intake of all the micronutrients from fortified foods.
- Technological issues relating to food fortification exist, particularly the levels of added nutrients, stability of the fortificant, nutrient interaction, characteristics of physical properties, and acceptability by consumers, including cooking properties and taste.
- The nature of the food vehicle, the fortificant, or both, may limit the amount of fortificant that can be successfully added. The sensory qualities of the food such as color and flavor, and the stability of the micronutrient(s) may be affected. Also, interactions among nutrients within the food can occur (e.g., the presence of a large amount of calcium can inhibit the absorption of iron from a fortified food; the presence of vitamins has an opposing effect on iron, and thus increases absorption of iron).

- While food fortification is proven to be more cost-effective over other strategies, there are underlying costs associated with the fortification process that can limit the implementation and effectiveness of food fortification programs (e.g., start-up costs, pilot trials and testing, cost of effective monitoring, and evaluation system to ensure fortified food is effective and safe).

With food fortification populations can be protected against nutritional deficiencies, and the overall nutritional quality of the nation's food supplied can be improved. For example, fortifying milk with vitamin D can prevent deficiencies in young children. In the long term, the overall health of populations can be improved, ultimately protecting them from the risk of diet-related chronic diseases. For example, adequate calcium and vitamin D in the body can reduce the risk of osteoporosis in the future. This also puts less of a burden on the healthcare system.

When infrastructures are not ready or appropriate, and regular monitoring systems are not in place to evaluate the status of micronutrient malnutrition, the fortification programs should be implemented with some considerations. Fortification polices should be monitored based on proper periodical assessment of consumption of fortified foods and added fortificant in both the general population and at-risk populations. It is important to monitor and evaluate the progress of the food fortification program, and to be aware of possible risks of excess intakes and toxicities.

Cultural and Religious Beliefs Towards Food Fortification

Food fortification can provide reasonably fast solutions to address low micronutrient intake at a population level, while maintaining traditional dietary patterns [18]. In a comprehensive review of over 180 studies of community-based interventions for improving antenatal, perinatal, and postnatal health outcomes in developing countries [19], the researchers concluded, "there is an urgent need to adapt and evaluate culturally and regionally appropriate packages of interventions in a variety of settings." Thus, cultural barriers can be a major problem to consumption of fortified foods. A specific example is consumption rates of folic acid fortified foods by pregnant women. Rates may be low in subgroup populations due to a lack of understanding and knowledge. Also, from the program planner's side, there may be a lack of understanding of community practices and culture [19]. It is therefore important to select foods which are already present in the diet, and if not, to find a way to encourage consumption of the fortified foods while taking into account cultural and religious beliefs.

Globalization and the nutrition transition have had a great impact in shifting traditional diets consisting of local grown foods, to a diet high in industrial processed foods. This global tendency towards urbanization could lead to increasing populations consuming industrially processed foods. This provides us with a greater opportunity to reach at-risk populations through fortified foods, as we can fortify multiple food vehicles [17]. However, on the other hand, mandatory food fortification programs should continue to target staple foods and common foods consumed by targeted populations, so that these populations that continue to eat traditional foods may benefit.

Some examples of current food mandatory fortification programs around the world are presented in Table 2.2. Three common food vehicles—maize (corn) meal, rice, and wheat flour are presented. Many countries have started to fortify staples with multiple micronutrients. For example, mandatory food fortification regulations in South Africa to fortify maize (corn) meal are in place for eight multiple micronutrients (i.e., thiamin, riboflavin, folic acid, niacin, zinc, iron, vitamins B6, B12, and A).

Table 2.2 List of countries with mandatory fortification regulations, as per Fig. 2.1

Developed	Developing		
North America	Asia	Latin America	Mauritania
Canada	Indonesia	Argentina	Morocco
United States	Nepal	Belize	Oman
European Union	Philippines[a]	Bolivia	Palestine, Occupied Territory
United Kingdom	Caribbean	Brazil	Qatar
Oceania	Barbados	Chile	Saudi Arabia
Australia[b]	Cuba	Colombia	Yemen
	Dominican Republic	Costa Rica	Oceania
	Grenada	Ecuador	Fiji
	Guadeloupe	El Salvador	Sub-Saharan Africa
	Guyana	Guatemala	Benin
	Haiti	Honduras	Cameroon
	Jamaica	Mexico	Côte d'Ivoire
	Puerto Rico	Nicaragua	Ghana
	Saint Vincent	Panama	Guinea
	Trinidad & Tobago[a]	Paraguay	Mali
	Central and Eastern Europe	Peru	Nigeria[a]
	Kazakhstan	Suriname[c]	Senegal
	Kyrgyz Republic	Uruguay	South Africa
	Moldova	Venezuela[a]	Tanzania
	Turkmenistan	Middle East/North Africa	Togo
	Uzbekistan	Bahrain	Uganda
		Egypt	
		Iran	
		Iraq	
		Jordan	
		Kuwait	

Source: Flour Fortification Initiative www.FFInetwork.org
This table lists the countries with current mandatory fortification programs of wheat flour with iron and/or folic acid
Notes:
Countries fortify with at least iron and folic acid unless otherwise noted
[a]Standard includes iron but not folic acid
[b]Standard includes iron but not folic acid
[c]Unknown fortificants in country standard

Prevalence of Major Micronutrient Deficiencies in the World

In many developing countries, a diet high in cereal and legumes, and low in meat, fruits, and vegetables are common. These diets are typical for those of lower socio-economic status. These populations are particularly at risk for iron, zinc, and vitamin A deficiencies [16] (Table 2.3). Although there is no prevalence data for iron deficiency, it can be generally assumed that 50 % of anemia cases in developed countries are due to iron deficiency, and mostly all cases seen in developed countries is due to iron deficiency [20]. Anemia and vitamin A deficiencies are most prevalent in the developing areas in South-East Asia (57 % and 69 %, respectively, of total population), whereas iodine is most prevalent in the more developed region, Europe (57 %).

Iron

Iron deficiency is the most common nutritional deficiency in the world and is a public health problem in both developed and developing countries [3]. In a severe form, iron deficiency can lead to a

Table 2.3 World cereal mandatory fortification programs (as of March 2008)

Country	Micronutrient								
Food vehicle	Thiamin (ppm)	Riboflavin (ppm)	Folic acid (ppm)	Niacin (ppm)	Zinc (ppm)	Iron & type of Fe** (ppm)	Vitamin B6 (ppm)	Vitamin B12 (ppB)	Vitamin A (IU/kg)
Maize (corn) meal									
Brazil			1.5			42			
Costa Rico	4.0	2.5	1.3	45		22—FBG			
South Africa	2.19	1.69	2.0	25	15	35—E	3.1		6,943
Venezuela	2.9	2.5		48		46—FF/R			9,000
Rice									
Philippines						30—FS			
Wheat flour									
Argentina	6.3	1.3	2.2	13		30—FS			
Australia			2.0						
Bahrain			1.5			60—E			
Bolivia	4.4	2.6	1.5	35.6		60—FF			
Brazil			1.5			42			
Canada	6.4	4.0	1.5	53		44			
Chile	6.3	1.3	2.2	13		30—FS			
Columbia	6.0	4.0	1.54	55		44			
Costa Rica	6.0	4.0	1.5	55		60—FF			
Cote d'Ivoire			1.5			60—E			
Cuba	7.0	7.0	2.5	70		45—FS	6.0		
Ecuador	4.0	7.0	0.6	75		55			
El Salvador	6.2	4.2	1.8	55		55—FF			
Ghana	6.0	4.0	2.0	40	20.3	45—R		10	6,666
Guatemala	6.2	4.2	1.8	55		55—FF			
Honduras	6.2	4.2	1.8	55		55—FF			
Indonesia	2.5	4.0	2.0		30	50			
Iran			1.5			30—FS			
Jordan	3.6	3.6	1.7	35	20	34—FS	4.4	7.6	5,000
Kuwait	6.38	3.96	1.5	52.91		60—E			
Mexico			1.6			24			
Morocco	4.5	2.8	1.53	36.18		45			
Nicaragua	6.2	4.2	1.8	55		55—FF			
Nigeria	6.2	3.7		49.5		40.7—FF			30,000
Oman			1.5			30			
Palestine	2.0	2.5	1.0	25	15	25—FS	2.5	2.5	3,333
Panama	6.0	4.0	1.5	55		60			
Paraguay	4.0	2.25	2.7	31		40—FS			
Peru	4.5	2.6		35		28			
Philippines						70—R or 50—FS/FF			15,000
Qatar			1.5			60—R			
Saudi Arabia	6.38	3.96	1.5	52.9		36.3			
South Africa	1.94	1.78	1.5	23.7	15	35—R	2.63		5,947
Turkmenistan			1.5			20—FS			
Uruguay			2.4			30—FS, FF	6		
Venezuela	1.2	1.6		16		16			

Source: Adapted from Ranum and Wesley [37] (Food and Agriculture Organization of the United Nations)

This table shows examples of various micronutrient fortificant levels in cereal food vehicles (e.g., maize (corn) meal, rice, wheat flour) in selected countries

Notes:

** Iron types specified under regulations if any:

FS ferrous sulfate; *E* electrolytic iron; *FF* ferrous fumarate; *R* reduced iron (unspecified elemental iron powder); *FBG* ferrous bisglycinate; *EDTA* sodium iron EDTA

condition called anemia, which is low blood hemoglobin. According to the WHO estimates 40 % of the world's population is anemic. Children under 24 months are especially at risk of anemia, which stunts their growth and reduces their ability to resist common childhood illness [21]. Iron deficiency is also common in preschool children and pregnant women. WHO estimates that 39 % of children younger than 5 years, 48 % of children between 5 and 14 years, 42 % of all women, and 52 % of pregnant women in developing countries are anemic [3]. The WHO regions of Africa and South-East Asia have the highest risk. Iron deficiency and iron deficiency anemia are also seen and considered to be a major public health concern in many developed countries [3].

Fortification of staple foods with iron and/or folic acid has been shown to be effective and to have significant benefit for many populations in the world, but particularly in developing countries. Wheat flour is the food vehicle most often fortified with iron and/or folic acid [22]. More information regarding iron fortification can be found in various subsections of this handbook.

Iodine

The highest prevalence of insufficient iodine intake was found in Europe (57 %), and the lowest in the Americas (10 %) [3]. Salt is the most common food vehicle for delivering iodine to populations. Iodine deficiency has been reduced in most countries around the world by the implementation of Universal Salt Iodization (USI) programs [17]. More than 34 countries have reached the USI goal—to have 90 % of population consuming iodized salt—and approximately another 30 countries have 70–90 % of the population covered [17]. However, according to UNICEF [20], there are still more than 1.8 billion people in both developed and developing countries who are not covered by the USI programs and are thus still at high risk for iodine deficiency.

Vitamin A

Vitamin A deficiency affects over 130 million preschool aged children, with the most residing in the developing world [23]. Those living in South-East Asia (69 %) and rural Africa (49 %) are most at risk for vitamin A deficiency [3]. Common food vehicles used for fortification with vitamin A include oil, margarine, milk, sugar, and flour. Refer to Table 2.2 for countries with current food fortification with vitamin A.

Folic Acid

It is generally assumed that folate deficiency is prevalent in countries where the diet consists of high intake of refined cereals and low intake of leafy green vegetables and fruits [16]. This is typical of many developing countries.

Regulations for mandatory fortification of wheat flour with folic acid are currently in place in 53 countries, although in many cases these regulations have not been implemented [24]. The mandatory folic acid fortification level in select countries is illustrated in Table 2.4. In 2006, the WHO and the FAO of the United Nations published guidelines to assist countries in setting necessary levels of folic acid to be used in fortifying flour (i.e., the Target Fortification Level, the Minimum Fortification Level, the Maximum Fortification Level, the Legal Minimum Level) [3]. In the United States, mandatory fortification of enriched cereal grain products with folic acid was authorized in 1996 and fully implemented in 1998 [7]. The US program adds 140 μg of folic acid per 100 g of enriched cereal grain product and has been estimated to provide 100–200 μg of folic acid per day to women of childbearing age [25].

Table 2.4 Prevalence of the three major micronutrient deficiencies by WHO region

	Anemia		Insufficient iodine intake		Vitamin A deficiency (in preschool children)	
WHO region	No. (millions)	% of total population	No. (millions)	% of total population	No. (millions)	% of total population
Africa	244	46	260	43	53	49
Americas	141	19	75	10	16	20
South-East Asia	779	57	624	40	127	69
Europe	84	10	436	57	No data available	
Eastern Mediterranean	184	45	229	54	16	22
Western Pacific	598	38	365	24	42	27
Total	2030	36	1989	35	254	42

Source: Adapted from WHO report by Allen et al. [3]
Iron, iodine, and vitamin A are the three most prevalent deficiencies worldwide. It is important to study such deficiencies, in order to plan an efficient food fortification program, with the ultimate goal of helping to prevent micronutrient deficiencies

Highlight: Folic Acid Fortification Programs

Fortification of flour and selected grains was implemented to ensure that the majority of women of childbearing age were receiving adequate amounts of folic acid to offset the risks of neural tube defects (NTDs). Many studies have evaluated the success and issues related to folic acid fortification in Canada and the United States. Several evaluations of the folic acid fortification programs implemented in Canada and the United States have shown significant reduction in NTDs [26, 27], and thus both health and economic benefits were proven, making such programs successful. However, recent concerns have been raised that some individuals may be now exposed to higher doses of folic acid after implementation of the programs. Therefore, there is suspected possible harm for some groups from universal folic acid food fortification [28]. Concerns include a possible vitamin B12 "masking" effect, and interactions with some medications such as methotrexate and phenytoin. However, there is no strong evidence to support this yet [28]. Ray [28] stresses the need to put in place a surveillance system prior to the initiation of any fortification program. Other researchers suggest the removal of folic acid from children's supplements, to help ensure that their folic acid intakes are below the UL [29].

Success Story: The Flour Fortification Initiative

One of the most common food vehicles for food fortification is flour. The flour fortification initiative (FFI) is an example of successful initiative, which continues to show strong progress. A program status in a country for fortification may be a mandatory program, a voluntary program, a planning program, or no program activity. Around the world, there are currently 68 countries that require fortification of one or more types of flour with at least either iron or folic acid. Flour is most commonly fortified with iron, zinc, folic acid, and other B vitamins such as thiamin, riboflavin, niacin, and vitamin B12. Vitamin A and vitamin D can also be added to flour. Figure 2.1 illustrates the countries worldwide with mandatory wheat flour fortification. Table 2.5 lists the specific countries by region.

The number of countries with mandatory wheat flour fortification has increased from 33 to 68 countries since 2004. Countries are continuing to implement fortification programs. In less than 2 years, from June 2010 to May 2012, 15 countries put in place regulations for fortification of wheat

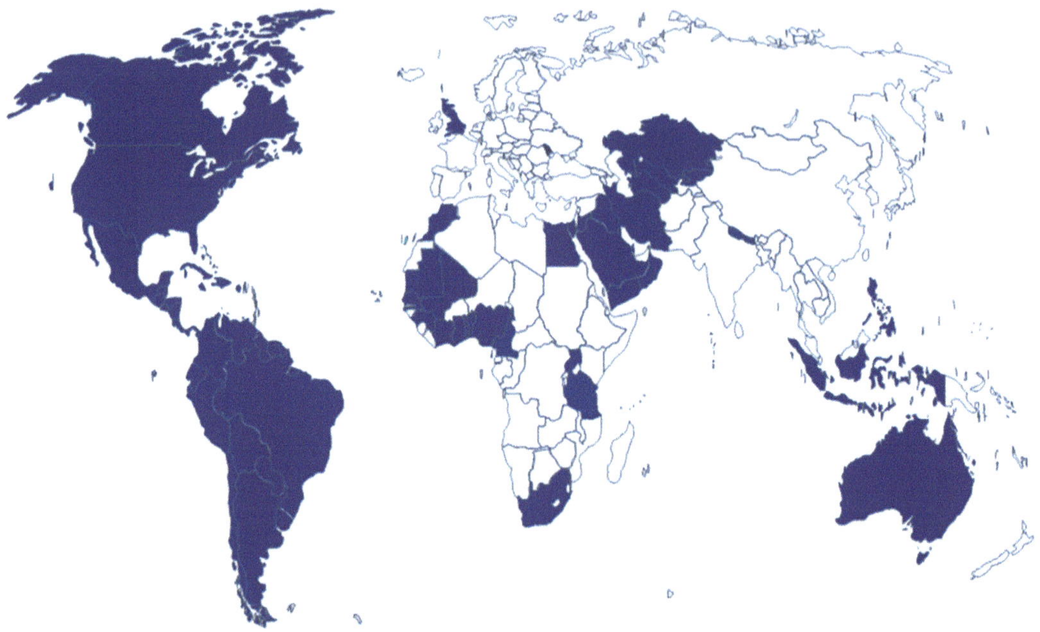

Fig. 2.1 Global progress—mandatory wheat flour fortification. This world map represents the global progress in regard to mandatory wheat flour fortification with at least iron and/or folic acid. As of May 2012, a total of 68 countries have implemented mandatory wheat flour fortification. *Source*: Flour Fortification Initiative www.FFInetwork.org

Table 2.5 Levels of folic acid fortification in five countries with mandatory fortification programs

Country	Fortification level	Date of implementation
Developed		
Canada	150 μg/100 g	1998
United States	140 μg/100 g	1998
Developing		
Chile	220 μg/100 g	2000
Costa Rica	180 μg/100 g	1998
South Africa	150 μg/100 g	2003

Source: Adapted from Crider et al. [38]

Mandatory fortification programs have been implemented around the world. This table shows two examples from developed nations and three examples from developing nations, and the mandatory fortification level, and date of implementation for folic acid

flour, for a total of 68 countries [30]. The majority of all the countries of the Americas and a large number of countries in the Middle East and Africa have successfully implemented wheat and/or maize flour fortification. For countries that aren't shaded in blue, there may be some fortification program that exists, however it is not mandatory. Currently, many countries are voluntarily fortifying, or are in the planning stages of fortification. These countries are not shown on the map for several reasons. Planning is very hard to determine and some countries that initiate plans do not follow through. Voluntary fortification is easier to determine, however with this type of program, sometimes only some flour is fortified, therefore that it can't be expected to have a public health impact [30].

Fortification Economics

Cost-effectiveness is defined as the cost of achieving a specified outcome [3]. In the case of food fortification, examples of outcomes could include the prevention of anemia in one child, or the prevention of a pregnant mother having folate deficiency and possible NTDs in her baby.

Fortification has been considered to be one of the most cost-effective approaches to addressing micronutrient deficiencies. Salt iodization, for example, is one of the most cost-effective ways to protect many populations against iodine deficiency. Adding iodine to salt costs only 2–7¢ per kilogram. This is less than 5 % of the retail price of salt in most countries [31]. According to the World Bank [8] there "... [is] probably no other technology available today [which] offers as large an opportunity to improve lives and accelerate development at such low cost and in such a short time." The start-up cost for food fortification is low for the food industry, and since the benefits from food fortification are both durable long-term solutions, it is a cost-effective approach in overcoming micronutrient malnutrition.

The economic benefits of food fortification include reduced morbidity, improved work capacity, and improved cognitive ability [23]. By increasing the consumption of specific nutrients in the body for an overall goal of preventing malnutrition will ultimately reduce health care costs. Also, the economic value of fortification is expressed in "improved work output due to increased work capacity and improved marginal productivity of labour" [23]. Lastly, fortification ultimately leads to a healthier population, and many children will have a stronger ability to learn, therefore money spent on schooling and academic performance would be increased.

Guidance on Safe Levels

Guidance on safe levels of fortificants is guided by research outcomes. Based on evidence from research, recommendations and guidelines can be drafted. The responsibilities of the health sector in many countries is to have continuous evaluation of nutrient malnutrition particularly in at-risk population and to modify the fortification policies and practices based on this. Surveillance of programs and interventions will help create healthy populations.

Surveillance of micronutrient interventions, including fortification, is crucial in effective project management, and will help to determine whether the intervention has a positive impact on the population. At a global level, WHO is highly involved with situations of micronutrients and their mandate is to assess the micronutrient status of populations, monitor and evaluate the impact of strategies for the prevention and control of micronutrient malnutrition, and to keep record of changes and trends over time. The Vitamin and Mineral Nutrition Information System (VMNIS) was established in 1991 as a way to strengthen surveillance of micronutrient deficiencies at the global level. The VMNIS is managed by the Evidence and Programme Guidance Unit of the Department of Nutrition for Health and Development which consists of WHO network of regional and country offices, and in close collaboration with national health authorities.

The specific objectives of the VMNIS [32] are to:

- Systematically retrieve and summarize data on the vitamin and mineral status of populations.
- Provide Member States with up-to-date national, regional, and global assessments of the magnitude of vitamin and mineral deficiencies.
- Track progress towards the goal of eliminating major vitamin and mineral deficiencies.
- Provide tools and resources to support efforts of Member States and their partners for assessing the vitamin and mineral nutritional status in populations.

Recommendations

The Codex Committee on General Principles (CCGP) and the Commission (CAC) make the recommendation that, for a successful fortification program, a set of five conditions should be met [10]. The first, there should be an apparent need from either clinical or subclinical evidence which indicates low levels of nutrient intake(s), or possible deficiencies. The second, the food vehicle to be selected should be one that is consumed by the population at risk. Thirdly, the lower and upper levels of food intake should be well known, and the food vehicle should be stable and uniform. The amount of nutrient(s) added to the food should be sufficient that when the population consumes the food, the nutrient deficiency should be prevented. And, lastly, the amount of the essential nutrient added should not result in excessive intakes by anyone, even if an individual has a high intake of the fortified food.

Other recommendations include the following:

- To seek innovative ways to address micronutrient deficiencies, and address the determinants of health while taking into consideration the many different environments—social, economic, and political contexts.
- To include nutrition education in food fortification programs, this is important for particular groups of people, as there is "no universally suitable vehicle for food fortification" [33].
- To possibly increase the fortification level of currently fortified foods [34] but to ensure proper monitoring and surveillance measures are in place to be aware of possible excess intakes.
- The best strategy to eliminate micronutrient malnutrition or "hidden hunger" is to use a combination of strategies including fortification, health education and promotion, dietary modification, and others.
- Food fortification programs should be implemented alongside poverty reduction programs and other interventions which promote the consumption of healthy nutritious foods among the vulnerable [17].
- To modify legislation to (1) increase the amount of micronutrients through diet by fortifying a broader range of foods, and (2) increase the amount of micronutrients added to fortified foods [34].
- In the case of mandatory flour fortification with folic acid, research has shown that it does not reach all women of reproductive age [35]. Folic acid fortification of more food products might be needed to reach all population groups effectively so they can achieve the most benefits from the added micronutrients [36].
- Reisch and Flynn [34] recommend a national public health campaign with a focus on nutrition education to health professionals as well as the general public on the importance of folic acid in the diet. Campaigns for other food fortification programs would also benefit the population at large.
- Careful monitoring of existing and proposed programs; evaluate and respond appropriately to concerns as they arise, and document the progress of these public health programs (i.e., Food fortification programs).

Conclusions

Fortification has many benefits for the health of populations around the world. It is one of the major strategies for reducing the prevalence of micronutrient deficiencies in both developed and developing countries. Enrichment and fortification play a key role in battling deficiencies and restoring health to countries around the world. The programs in place range from a mandatory program to a program which is more voluntary. Many developing countries have benefitted from mandatory programs, which have shown success in reaching the most vulnerable, whereas success has also shown from voluntary programs in developed countries.

It is noteworthy to mention that while writing this chapter and collecting the data, information on fortification policies or legislation for some countries was unavailable, or what was available is still in draft form. Therefore, an additional recommendation would be for government and monitoring surveillance systems to keep current and updated information regarding the current status of policies and legislation.

References

1. L'abbé MR, Cockell KA, Lee NS. Micronutrient supplementation: when is best and why? Proc Nutr Soc. 2003;62:413–20.
2. Kennedy E, Mannar V, Iyengar V. Alleviating hidden hunger, approaches that work. IAEA Bull. 2003;45(1):54–60.
3. Allen L, de Benoist B, Dary O, Hurrell R. Guidelines on food fortification with micronutrients. 2nd ed. Geneva, Switzerland: World Health Organization and Food and Agriculture Organization of the United Nations; 2006.
4. Ottaway B. Principles of food fortification and supplemention. In: Ottaway PB, editor. Food fortification and supplementation. Cambridge, UK: Woodhead Publishing; 2008.
5. Fletcher R, Bell I, Lambert J. Public health aspects of food fortification: a question of balance. Proc Nutr Soc. 2004;63:605–14.
6. Vatanparast H, Adolphe JL, Whiting SJ. Socio-economic status and vitamin/mineral supplement use in Canada. Health Rep. 2001;21(4):19–25.
7. Food and Drug Administration. Food standards: amendment of standards of identity for enriched grain products to require addition of folic acid. Final Rule. 21 CFR Parts 136, 137, and 139. Fed Regist. 1996;61:8781–9.
8. World Bank. Enriching lives: overcoming vitamin and mineral malnutrition in developing countries. Development in practice series. Washington, DC: World Bank; 1994.
9. Codex Alimentarius Commission. General principles for the addition of essential nutrients to foods CAC/GL 09-1987 (amended 1989, 1991). Rome: Joint FAO/WHO Food Standards Programme, Codex Alimentarius Commision; 1987. Available at http://www.codexalimentarius.net/download/standards/299/CXG_009e.pdf. Accessed 9 April 2012.
10. Maskeliunas J, Miyagishima K. Codex alimentarius standard affecting fortified foods and supplements. In: Ottaway PB, editor. Food fortification and supplementation. Cambridge, UK: Woodhead Publishing; 2008.
11. FAO/WHO: codex general principles for the addition of essential nutrients to foods (CAC/GL 09-1987).
12. Nutrition Service of the World Food Program Micronutrient fortification. WFP experiences and ways forward. Food Nutr Bull. 2006;27(1):67–75.
13. Haas J, Miller D. Overview of experimental biology 2005 symposium: food fortification in developing countries. Am J Nutr. 2006;136:1053–4.
14. Reddy V. Food fortification for reducing micronutrient deficiencies: public-private partnerships; 2003. Available at http://www.ifm.net/industry/food_fortification.htm. Accessed 13 April 2012.
15. Bishai D, Nalubola R. The history of food fortification in the United States: its relevance for current fortification efforts in developing countries. Econ Dev Cult Change. 2002;51:37–53.
16. Biebinger R, Hurrell R. Vitamin and mineral fortification of foods. In: Ottaway PB, editor. Food fortification and supplementation. Cambridge, UK: Woodhead Publishing; 2008.
17. Horton S, Mannar V, Wesley A. Best practice paper, food fortification with iron and iodine. Copenhagen Consensus Center; 2008.
18. Serra-Majem L, Ortega R, Aranceta J, Entrala A, Gil A. Fortified foods. Criteria for vitamin supplementation in Spain. Public Health Nutr. 2001;4:1331–4.
19. Bhutta ZA, Darmstadt BS, Hasan RA. Community-based interventions for improving perinatal and neonatal health outcomes in developing countries: a review of the evidence. Pediatrics. 2005;115:519–617.
20. WHO/UNICEF/UNU. Iron deficiency anemia assessment, prevention, and control. Geneva: World Health Organization; 2001.
21. Mason J et al. The micronutrient report: current progress and trends in the control of vitamin A. Ottawa, Canada: Micronutrient Initiative and International Development Research Centre; 2001.
22. Hurrell R, Ranum P, de Pee S, Biebinger R, Hulthen L, Johnson Q, et al. Revised recommendations for iron fortification of wheat flour and an evaluation of the expected impact of current national wheat flour fortification programs. Food Nutr Bull. 2010;31:S7–21.
23. Wesley A, Horton S. Economics of food fortification. In: Nutrients, dietary supplements, and nutraceuticals: cost analysis versus clinical benefits. Humana Press, 2011.
24. Centers for Disease Control and Prevention (CDC). Grand rounds: additional opportunities to prevent neural tube defects with folic acid fortification. MMWR Morb Mortal Wkly Rep. 2010;59:980–4.

25. Yang QH, Carter HK, Mulinare J, Berry RJ, Friedman JM, Erickson JD. Race-ethnicity differences in folic acid intake in women of childbearing age in the United States after folic acid fortification: findings from the National Health and Nutrition Examination Survey, 2001–2002. Am J Clin Nutr. 2007;85:1409–16.
26. De Wals P, Tairou F, Van Allen M, Uh S, Lowry R, Sibbald B, et al. Reduction in neural tube defects after folic acid fortification in Canada. N Engl J Med. 2007;357(2):135–42.
27. Mills J, Signore C. Neural tube defects rates before and after food fortification with folic acid. Birth Defects Res A Clin Mol Teratol. 2004;70(11):844–5.
28. Ray J. Efficacy of Canadian folic acid food fortification. Food Nutr Bull. 2008;29(2):S225–30.
29. Shakur Y, Garriguet D, Corey P, O'Connor D. Folic acid fortification above mandated levels results in a low prevalence of folate inadequacy among Canadians. Am J Clin Nutr. 2010;92:818–25.
30. Flour Fortification Initiative. Available at http://www.cdc.gov/immpact/projects/initiatives/flour.html. Accessed 2 April 2012.
31. Levine R, and the What Works Working Group. Millions saved: proven successes in global health, Washington, DC; 2004. Available at http://www.cgdev.org/section/initiatives/_archive/millionssaved. Accessed 2 April 2012.
32. World Health Organization. Available at http://www.who.int/vmnis/en. Accessed 11 April 2012.
33. Johnson-Down L, L'abbé M, Lee N, Gray-Donald G. Appropriate calcium fortification of the food supply presents a challenge. J Nutr. 2003;133:2232–8.
34. Reisch HS, Flynn MA. Folic acid and the prevention of neural tube defects. Challengs and recommendations for public health. Can J Public Health. 2002;93:254–8.
35. Imhoff-Kunsch B, Flores R, Dary O, Martorell R. Wheat flour fortification is unlikely to benefit the neediest in Guatemala. J Nutr. 2007;137:1017–22.
36. Dary O. Establishing safe and potentially efficacious fortification contents for folic acid and vitamin B12. Food Nutr Bull. 2008;29:S214–24.
37. Ranum P, Wesley A. World cereal fortification standards and practices, micronutrient initiative fortification handbook. Ottawa: Micronutrient Initiative; 2008. Available at http://www.sph.emory.edu/wheatflour/atlanta08/MIcountrytable2008bGAINmodifications.doc. Accessed 2 April 2012.
38. Crider K, Bailey L, Berry R. Folic acid food fortification—its history, effect, concerns, and future directions. Nutrients. 2011;3:370–84.

Chapter 3
Fortified Humanitarian Food-Aid Commodities

Michael L. Dunn

Key Points

- United Nations data indicates that over 925 million people in the world, mainly residing in seven countries, suffered from undernourishment in 2010.
- Humanitarian food aid programs are of ancient origin, but have evolved into a significant, well-organized, worldwide system coordinated by numerous collaborating state and nongovernmental organizations.
- Because cereal and legume-based products, with limited intrinsic micronutrient content, comprise the bulk of food aid donations, micronutrient fortification is critical to ensure that the needs of key vulnerable groups are met.
- Factors affecting micronutrient stability include long storage times in uncontrolled conditions during staging and transport, presence of lipid and redox active metals—such as iron—in the micronutrient premix, extended cooking times during preparation.
- Key vulnerable groups of special concern include infants and young children generally; severely, or moderately malnourished children and adolescents; the chronically ill (especially people living with HIV/AIDS or tuberculosis); pregnant and lactating women; and people of all ages suffering from micronutrient malnutrition.
- A significant challenge in micronutrient fortification of humanitarian food aid products is meeting the disparate needs of a diverse group of beneficiaries, while at the same time keeping product and manufacturing costs at a minimum.

Keywords Food aid • Fortification • Micronutrient • Vitamin • Mineral • Humanitarian

Abbreviations

CSB	Corn soy blend
DRI	Dietary reference intake
FAO	United Nations Food and Agricultural Organization

M.L. Dunn, M.S., Ph.D. (✉)
Department of Nutrition Dietetics & Food Science, Brigham Young University, S-221 ESC Provo, UT 84602, USA
e-mail: michael_dunn@byu.edu

V.R. Preedy et al. (eds.), *Handbook of Food Fortification and Health: From Concepts to Public Health Applications Volume 1*, Nutrition and Health, DOI 10.1007/978-1-4614-7076-2_3,

FBF	Fortified blended food
FFP	Food for Peace Act of the United States (Public Law 480, 7 U.S.C. 1691 et seq.)
HIV/AIDS	Human immunodeficiency virus/acquired immune deficiency syndrome
IOM	Institute of Medicine of the United States National Academies
PVO	Private voluntary organization
UL	Tolerable upper intake level
UNICEF	United Nations Children's Fund
USAID	United States Agency for International Development
WFP	World Food Program

Introduction

Many people in the world struggle to obtain sufficient sustenance for maintenance, growth, and health of the human body. Even though the global supply of food is adequate, zonal climatic events and natural disasters, wars and political turmoil, lack of resources and education, and poor environmental management repeatedly result in widespread hunger, malnutrition, and associated disease and mortality. As humanitarian D. John Shaw so succinctly stated, "The co-existence of hunger with the capacity to end it is one of the gravest paradoxes of our time" [1]. In the face of this paradox, human compassion, as well as political and economic considerations, has motivated organizations and governments to offer humanitarian assistance in cases of need.

Humanitarian food aid appears to be of ancient practice [2], but the modern system of global food assistance has its origins with the organization of the United Nations Food and Agricultural Organization (FAO) and World Food Program (WFP) [3], and specific country legislation such as the Food for Peace Act (FFP) in the United States [4]. Over time, humanitarian food aid has progressed from small-scale, largely unilateral philanthropic efforts of individual world leaders and specific relief organizations, to a massive, well-organized, multilateral system of collaborating governmental and nongovernmental agencies [1, 5]. WFP quantity reporting data indicates that over 5,000,000 metric tons of food aid were distributed to humanitarian relief efforts in 2010 [6].

The FAO estimated that 925 million people in the world were undernourished in 2010 [7]. Figure 3.1 presents FAO/WHO data [7] on distribution of the undernourished population of the world by region. Not surprisingly, people in developing countries, make up the majority of this number, with almost 16 % of the population of all developing countries considered to be undernourished [7].

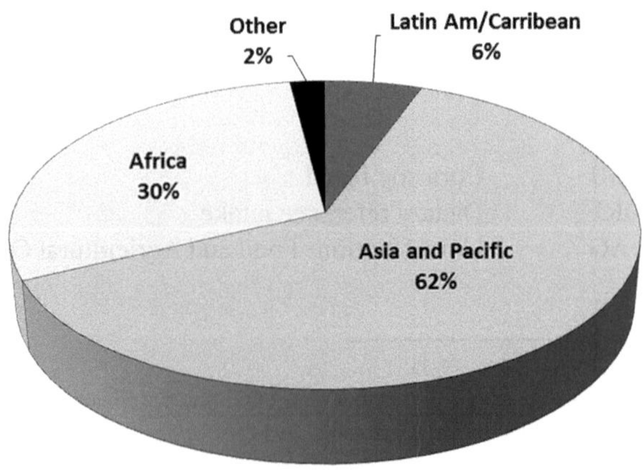

Fig. 3.1 Percent of world undernourished population by region, 2010. The chart shows that the total undernourished population of the world is distributed in only a few major geographic regions, according to FAO/WHO data [7]

Overview of Food Aid Programming and Distribution

Distribution

Although most of the undernourished people in the world live in just seven countries [7], the scope of distribution of humanitarian food aid is much more far-reaching, and varies from year to year based on actual need, as well as political and other circumstances. Statistics from the International Grains Council [8] indicate that 95 different countries received food aid in the 2009–2010 reporting year. Of humanitarian food aid distributed by member countries of the Food Aid Convention, which provides the majority of total distribution, 70 % went to countries of Africa, with the remainder going to Asia, Latin America and the Caribbean, and other regions as indicated in Fig. 3.2 [8].

Food and cash-for-food donations come from many countries across the globe, but the majority of food assistance comes from developed regions of the world, especially those areas with high cereal and leguminous crop production. Figure 3.3 shows the primary donors of food aid distributed between 1995 and 2009 [8].

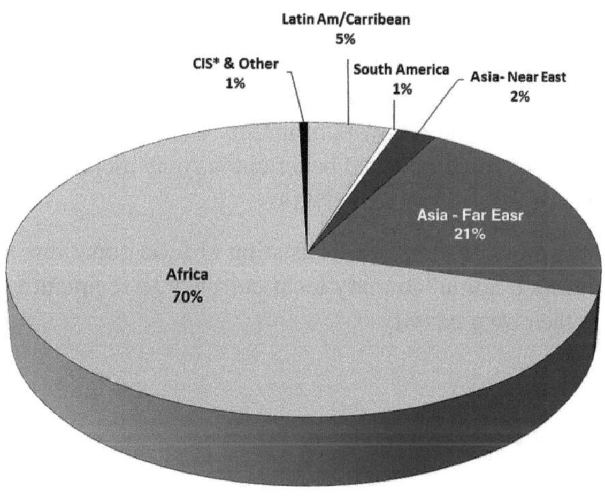

Fig. 3.2 Percent of total food aid tonnage distributed to regional beneficiaries for 2009–2010 reporting year. The chart shows that African beneficiaries received the vast majority of total food aid tonnage distributed during the 2009–2010 reporting year, while Asia received about 23 % of total distribution and the rest of the world received about 7 %. Based on data from the International Grains Council [8]. *CIS* commonwealth of independent states

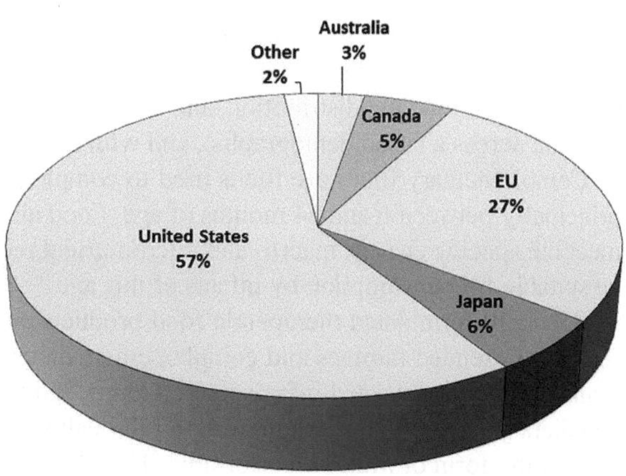

Fig. 3.3 Percent of total annual food aid donations coming from specific global food aid donors (1995–2009). Over the past 14 years, food-aid donation data provided by the International Grains Council [8] shows that the United States, the European Union, Japan, Canada, and Australia were the primary providers of food aid commodities or cash for such

While not a donor country, the United Nations World Food Programme is the primary international coordinator and distributor of multilateral food assistance. WFP relies entirely on donations from other countries for the food aid provisions themselves, as well as monetary donations for shipping, managing, and distributing them. In 2010, over 83 different donor countries and federations were listed as contributors to WFP [9]. WFP, and a large number of individual private voluntary organizations (PVOs) carry out much of the critical work of assessing needs, organizing specific programs, procuring food and associated resources, and actually distributing commodities to individuals in need.

Food Programming

Food assistance programs can be classified into three broad categories based on objective. These are defined by Barrett and Maxwell [4] essentially as follows:

Emergency/humanitarian food aid: Food assistance provided to help alleviate suffering and death associated with famine, natural disasters, wars, and other crises. Because the vulnerable populations targeted through emergency assistance invariably have the most urgent nutritional needs, and derive a significant percentage of their total caloric intake from the donated commodities, micronutrient fortified foods play a vital role in this sector.

Project-specific food aid: Food aid providing an economic or health benefit to a limited group of chronic-need beneficiaries as part of a targeted field project. Examples include maternal–child health programs, food-for-work programs, school-feeding programs, etc. Again, the specific nutrient requirements of some intended beneficiaries may dictate provision of micronutrient fortified commodities as part of the program distribution.

Programmed food aid: Consisting of food donations intended to help offset forecast shortages and to generate noninflationary local currency to recipient governments as food is sold on the open market in their own country.

Food Products

Within these broad categories, specific food products or combinations of food products, often called "food baskets," can further be defined based on usage for supplemental feeding, complementary feeding, or therapeutic feeding.

Supplemental food aid is used to supplement other foods consumed in the diet as a means of preventing or treating moderate malnutrition [10, 11]. The supplemental food assistance category makes up the bulk of food aid distribution, and is used to provide sustenance for a wide variety of adults and children across a broad demographic, and with differing nutritional needs.

Complementary foods are foods used to complement or replace breast milk in weaning children, principally between 6 and 24 months of age. Food aid products used in complementary feeding must meet the specific energy, macro- and micronutrient requirements for this vulnerable group, as well as be suitable for consumption by infants of this age

Specially formulated therapeutic food products are becoming more widely used in humanitarian feeding. Extended famines and complex emergencies inevitably lead to a sharp increase in severely malnourished and wasted infants and children. Individuals in these cases require special nutritional and dietary therapy in order to return to full health. A number of specialty [12] and therapeutic products, in the form of milk-based formulas [13], lipid-based supplements [14], biscuits [15], and other

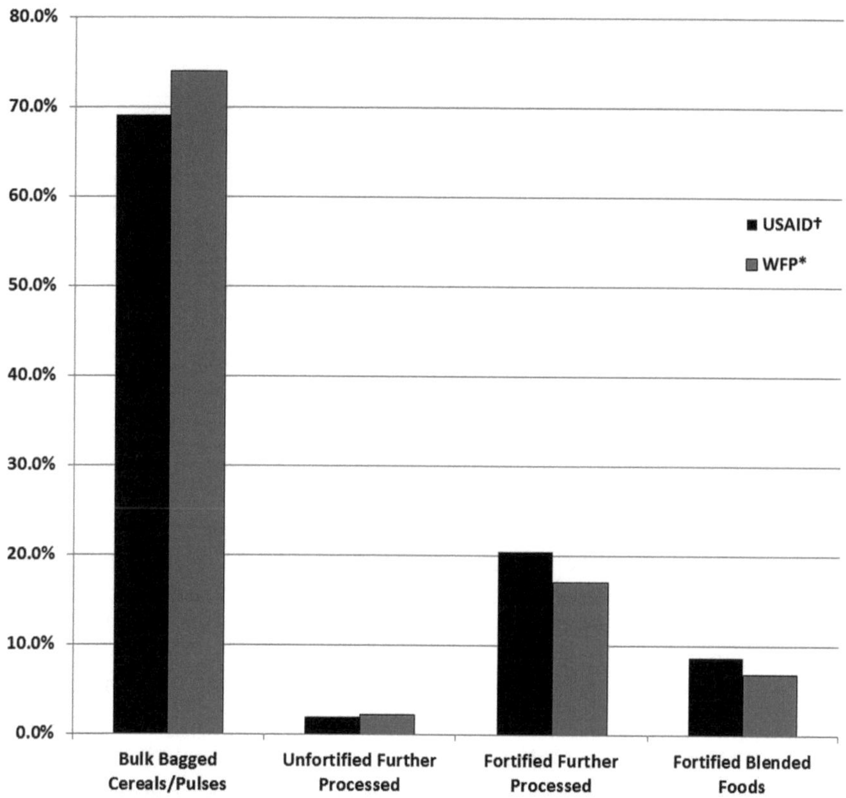

Fig. 3.4 USAID and WFP food aid distribution by commodity type [6, 16]. The graph compares the range of food aid products distributed by USAID in 2010 to the range of WFP products distributed between 2005 and 2010. Publicly available data from these, the two largest world distributors of food aid, show that micronutrient fortified products comprise between 24 and 28 % of total distribution [6, 16]. †USAID 2010 programmed food aid tonnage. *WFP 2005–2010 total distribution tonnage

products have been developed for these targeted applications. These products represented less than 0.4 % of 2005–2010 WFP total tonnage distribution [6], but are highly important in terms of the benefit they provide. Therapeutic products can also be quite costly relative to other products in the food aid offering, which is another reason for their limited application.

The overall portfolio of food aid products distributed by donor countries and WFP is rather diverse, ranging from salmon to soybeans, and includes bulk agricultural commodities, as well as value-added commodities that have been fortified with vitamins, minerals, and often soy or milk protein. Figure 3.4 indicates the percent tonnage distribution of the various products provided by WFP [6] (2005–2010 total) and USAID [16] (2010 programmed), the two largest distributors of food aid. Micronutrient fortified products comprise between 24 and 28 % of total distribution. The overall portfolio of products distributed can be categorized generally as follows: unfortified, bagged, minimally processed bulk grains and pulses; unfortified, further processed agricultural commodities; micronutrient fortified, further processed commodities; micronutrient fortified blended foods (FBFs), along with therapeutic and specialty foods.

Unfortified, bagged, minimally processed bulk grains and pulses comprise the vast majority of food aid distributed, and provide energy, protein, and other macronutrients as well as a limited range of naturally occurring vitamins and minerals—in some cases in appreciable amounts.

Table 3.1 Comparison of USAID and WFP wheat flour fortification specifications

Micronutrient	WFP target (source)	USAID minimum (source)
Thiamin	4.4 mg/kg (thiamin mononitrate)	6.4 mg/kg (not specified)
Riboflavin	2.6 mg/kg (riboflavin)	4.0 mg/kg (riboflavin)
Niacin	35.0 mg/kg (nicotinamide)	52.9 mg/kg (not specified)
Folic acid	1.0 mg/kg (folic acid)	1.5 mg/kg (folic acid)
Vitamin A	1.0 mg/kg (retinyl palmitate)	10.7 mg/kg (retinyl palmitate)
Vitamin B12	0.008 mg/kg (cyanocobalamin)	–
Zinc	30 mg/kg (zinc oxide)	–
Iron	15 mg/kg (NaFeEDTA)	44 mg/kg (not specified)
Calcium	–	1,102 mg/kg (not specified)[a]

The table shows that fortification specifications for a product as simple as enriched wheat flour can differ significantly between different distributing organizations. Data from wheat flour fortification specifications available on USAID [17] and WFP [18] websites

[a]Source must be "harmless and assimilable"

Unfortified, further processed agricultural commodities such as soya flour, dried potatoes, canned fish and meats, sugar, dates, and other products, also provide energy as well as macro- and micronutrients. These represent a minor percentage of total distribution, and consequently play more of a role in adding diversity to the beneficiary diet. Some have limited and uncertain availability, often depending on donor surpluses.

Micronutrient fortified, further processed commodities primarily include fortified cereal flours and meals, as well as vegetable oil. These products have a limited number of vitamins and minerals added—principally a standard cereal fortification blend of B-vitamins and key minerals, or vitamins A and/or D in the case of vegetable oil. Differences exist in fortification levels depending on the donor/distributor. Table 3.1 provides a comparison between fortification requirements in USAID [17] and WFP [18] specifications for wheat flour. The differences between the two specifications are representative of differences for most other standard products distributed by the two agencies.

A smaller, yet very important, food aid product category comprises the FBFs, which are grouped with therapeutic and specialty foods in Fig. 3.4. FBFs taken separately comprised about 6.5 % [6] of WFP distribution over the period 2005–2010. FBFs typically consist of cereal flour, soy, or other legume protein and/or milk powder, a more complete micronutrient premix, and sometimes include added vegetable oil and sugar. A variety of different blends are available to suit the regional food preferences of beneficiaries at the distribution site (see Table 3.2). Corn soy blend (CSB) is the most well-known and widely used of the FBFs. The original specified WFP formulation [18] for CSB comprises: 78.24 % corn (maize), 20 % whole (non-dehulled) soya beans, 0.8 % calcium phosphate, 0.76 % potassium chloride, and 0.2 % vitamin/mineral premix, which contains 12 vitamins and 6 different minerals, providing a much broader array of micronutrients than in the fortified flours alone. Table 3.3 provides a detailed description of the WFP-specified [18] micronutrient premix (FBF-V-10) for standard use in most WFP FBFs. In addition to the enhanced micronutrient profile, CSB is partially precooked to deactivate trypsin inhibitors and improve the digestibility of the starches and proteins. With addition of 12 vitamins and 6 different minerals, the FBFs are the most highly fortified of the WFP food aid products (with the exception of some of the specialty and therapeutic foods or supplements). FBFs are commonly used for complementary feeding, or to improve the diet of pregnant and lactating women, or to supplement the diet of other vulnerable groups who are at significant risk of malnutrition.

In addition to understanding the general compositional nature of food aid products, and the purposes for their use, it is also important to understand how they are distributed and prepared. The conditions of distribution and the manner of preparation can play a significant role in the nutritional benefit they deliver.

Table 3.2 Composition and specification information for common WFP [18] and USAID [17, 41] micronutrient fortified blended foods and cereals

Product/distributor	Product description	Specified formula (by weight)	Micronutrient addition	Recommended preparation
Corn soy blend/WFP [18] (USAID has similar product)	A blend of heat treated maize and soya beans, enriched with 12 vitamins and 6 minerals. It has a uniform fine texture, and is partially precooked Suitable for young children and adults	Corn 78.24 % Whole soya beans 20 % Vitamin/mineral mix 0.20 % Calcium phosphate 0.80 % Potassium chloride 0.76 % (also varieties with sugar and dairy milk added) Nutritional value/100 g dwb Energy: 380 kcal min Protein: 14 % min Fat: 6.0 % min Fiber: 5.0 % max	Thiamine Riboflavin Niacin Folic acid Pantothenic acid Vitamin B6 Vitamin B12 Vitamin A Vitamin C Vitamin D Vitamin E Vitamin K Iron Zinc Iodine Potassium Phosphorus Calcium	Add 40 g CSB to 250 g clean water Simmer for 5–10 min
Wheat soy blend/ WFP [18] (USAID has similar product)	A blend of heat treated wheat and soya beans, enriched with 12 vitamins and 6 minerals It has a uniform fine texture, and is partially precooked Suitable as a product for adults and children older than 6 months	Wheat 73.24 % Whole soya beans 25 % Vitamin/mineral mix 0.20 % Calcium phosphate 0.80 % Potassium chloride 0.76 % (also varieties with sugar, oil, and dairy milk) Nutritional Value/100 g dwb Energy: 380 kcal min Protein: 16 % min Fat: 6.0 % min Fiber: 4.0 % max	Same as CSB	Same as CSB
Rice soy blend/ RSB plus WFP [18]	A blend of heat treated wheat and soya beans, enriched with 12 vitamins and 6 minerals. Sugar and dry skim milk added. It has a uniform fine texture, and is partially precooked Preferred for young children aged 6–24 months as a complement to breast milk	Rice 52.24 % Dehulled soya beans 25 % Sugar 9 % Dry skim milk 8 % Soya oil 4 % Vitamin/mineral mix 0.20 % Calcium phosphate 0.80 % Potassium chloride 0.76 % Nutritional Value/100 g dwb Energy: 420 kcal min Protein: 16 % min Fat: 9.0 % min Fiber: 2.0 % max	Same as CSB	Same as CSB

(continued)

Table 3.2 (continued)

Product/distributor	Product description	Specified formula (by weight)	Micronutrient addition	Recommended preparation
Pea wheat blend/ PWB WFP [18]	A blend of heat treated wheat and peas, enriched with 6 vitamins and 3 minerals. Sugar and dry skim milk added. It has a uniform fine texture, and is partially precooked Intended for older infants, young children, pregnant women and nursing mothers	Wheat flour 55.5 % Peas 35 % Sugar 6 % Rapeseed oil 3.5 % Vitamin/mineral mix 0.20 % Calcium phosphate 0.80 % Potassium chloride 0.76 % Nutritional value/100 g dwb Energy: 425 kcal min Protein: 15 % min Fat: 6.0 % min Fiber: 5 % max	Thiamine Riboflavin Niacin Folic Acid Vitamin A Vitamin C Iron Zinc Calcium	Cook time same as CSB. No product/water ratio indicated
Soya fortified sorghum grits USAID [17]	A blend of bulgur wheat and soy grits, enriched with 4 vitamins and 2 minerals	Sorghum grits 85 % Soya grits 15 % Vitamin/mineral premix Nutritional value/100 g dwb Energy: 369 kcal Protein: 15 % min Fat: 2 % max Fiber: 2.1 % max	Thiamine Riboflavin Niacin Vitamin A Iron Calcium (may have folate)	Add 1 part by volume to 2 parts water. Boil 15–20 min
Soya fortified bulgur USAID [17]	A blend of bulgur wheat and soy grits, enriched with 4 vitamins and 2 minerals	Bulgur wheat 85 % Soya grits 15 % Vitamin/mineral premix Nutritional value/100 g dwb Energy: 372 kcal Protein: 17.3 % min Fat: 2.6 % max Fiber: 2.6 % max	Thiamine Riboflavin Niacin Vitamin A Iron Calcium(may have folate)	Soak 1 cup bulgur in 3 cups clean water overnight [42]. Cook in various dishes as desired
Soya fortified cornmeal USAID [17]	A blend of degermed corn meal and defatted, toasted soya flour, enriched with four vitamins and two minerals	Cornmeal 85 % Soya flour 15 % Vitamin/mineral premix Nutritional value/100 g dwb Energy: 395 kcal Protein: 13 % min Fat: 1.5 % max Fiber: 2 % max	Thiamine Riboflavin Niacin Vitamin A Iron Calcium(may have folate)	No USAID recipes provided. Similar to CSB with 10–15 min cook time

This table provides formulation and fortification information for specific food aid commodities provided by WFP [18] and USAID [17, 41] based on specifications available on each organization's website

Table 3.3 WFP-specified micronutrient premix for addition to corn-soya blend plus

Vitamin/mineral *FBF-V-10*	Target[a]	Chemical forms
Vitamins		
Vitamin A	1,664 IU	Vitamin A palmitate
Thiamine	0.128 mg	Thiamine mononitrate
Riboflavin	0.448 mg	Riboflavin
Niacin	4.8 mg	Nicotinamide
Pantothenic acid	6.7 mg	Calcium D-pantothenate
Vitamin B6	1.7 mg	Pyridoxine hydrochloride
Folate	60 μg	Folic acid
Vitamin B12	2 μg	Vitamin B12
Vitamin C	100 mg	Ascorbic acid
Vitamin D	4 μg	Vitamin D3
Vitamin E	8.3 mg	Vitamin E (form not specified, but DL-alpha tocopherol acetate is typically used)
Vitamin K	100 μg	Vitamin K1
Minerals		
Iron (a)	4 mg	Ferrous fumarate
Iron (b)	2.5 mg	Iron-sodium EDTA
Zinc	5 mg	Zinc oxide
Iodine	40 μg	Potassium iodate
Potassium	400 mg	Potassium chloride
Phosphorus	200 mg	Monocalcium phosphate
Calcium	130 mg	

The WFP website [18] provides a detailed micronutrient premix specification for use in products like corn-soya blend plus (data from WFP technical specification, CSB Plus, version 2.1, 30 Mar 2011)
[a]CSB Plus must be fortified to provide the indicated net micronutrient *supplement* per 100 g of finished product

Transportation and Storage

Based on the locations of country donors and recipients shown in Figs. 3.2 and 3.3, it is readily apparent that considerable transportation is required to get the bulk of food aid commodities to beneficiaries. While more and more emphasis is being placed on procurement of foods from the area or region of intended distribution and use, logistical considerations, and inadequate capacity make the so-called "local and regional procurement" efforts challenging [19]. Consequently, for these and other reasons, including political reasons, the status quo of shipping food aid commodities long distances from major production sites will continue into the foreseeable future.

Once food aid commodities are manufactured, packaged, and palletized, most are containerized and moved through maritime channels to major ports nearest the point of use. Once at the destination ports, the containers may sit for some time in uncontrolled conditions to await local transport, which often takes days and weeks over long distances to reach the inland point of distribution. The entire process can take 6–9 months, or even longer, from date of manufacture to arrival at the ultimate destination [20]. Because countries with high food aid usage are often located in regions of high heat and/or humidity, the environmental conditions to which these products are exposed during transportation can be extreme. Moisture migration and condensation within bags and containers can create pockets of unstable, high-moisture product which support mold growth, and lead to increased degradation reactions [21, 22].

A common practice, to help minimize the time between the advent of a food crisis and the availability of food aid at the area of need, is prepositioning. USAID, for example, has previously stockpiled food in port cities in the south Atlantic region of the United States, as well as in the Middle East and Africa to improve the timeliness of food aid delivery. Prepositioning is advantageous in many respects; however, the additional storage time opens the possibility for adverse effects on product quality. The uncontrolled nature of the storage and distribution environment and the duration of storage speaks to the need for concern regarding vitamin and lipid stability in the presence of added mineral fortificants, which can serve as catalytic pro-oxidants.

Micronutrient Stability

Several field studies [20, 23] have investigated the effects of shipping/storage and cooking on micronutrient stability in fortified food aid commodities. Even though statistically significant losses of vitamins in the dry blended food aid products were reported [20] during shipping and storage, the losses were not considered to be "serious." In addition to shipping and storage conditions, another potential cause of micronutrient degradation in food aid commodities is beneficiary preparation practices. Despite differences from region to region, water-based gruels, porridges, and pastes—ranging from very thin to very thick consistency—are the most commonly eaten food forms for FBFs and many of the fortified cereal flours and meals [23]. Most of the fortified cereal meals and FBFs cook up fairly quickly (5–15 min), but beneficiaries in one field study [23] often cooked products for much longer (around 26 min on average, and up to 53 min of boiling in one case) due to concerns with the lack of a sanitary water supply and to ensure that the products were safe to eat. Vitamin stability under these extended cook times was brought into question, and a laboratory simulation [24] showed that losses of vitamin C and E were significant (up to 53 % and 18 % loss, respectively). However, vitamin A showed relatively good retention, with no significant loss in most products, and the remaining vitamins showed no significant losses during cooking.

Formulation Issues in Micronutrition Fortification of Humanitarian Food Aid Products

Target Population for Formulation

In selecting the micronutrient profile for FBFs, the undergirding consideration is always the nutritional status and dietary need of the population of beneficiaries to be addressed; and therein lies a significant element of difficulty with respect to formulation—namely, choosing the target population.

Sadly, infants and children are usually the most seriously affected by humanitarian hunger crises [25]. Besides infants and young children generally, other vulnerable groups to which WFP FBFs are targeted include severely or moderately malnourished children and adolescents, the chronically ill (especially people living with HIV/AIDS or tuberculosis), pregnant and lactating women, and people of all ages suffering from micronutrient malnutrition [26]. Clearly, some of these groups have quite different nutritional requirements, making it improbable that a single food aid product could be formulated to meet all of their needs. One recent study [27] recommended that the FBF commodity portfolio be redesigned and divided into two product categories: one suitable for infants and children, and the other suitable for older children and adults, including pregnant and lactating women. However, a recent report [28], compiled for USAID by Webb et al. at Tufts University, rejects the idea of dual-product categories, instead proposing an improved nutrient profile for future FBF prototypes that meets most of the requirements for key vulnerable groups.

Micro- and macronutrient requirements for the key vulnerable groups expected to be users of any potentially redesigned FBF product-line have been published in the literature. These include

Table 3.4 Summary of recommended nutrient compositions for fortified blended foods targeted at specific vulnerable populations (amounts per 100 g food)

		Lutter/Dewey [29]	Golden [31]	Fleige et al. [27]	Fleige et al. [30]	Webb et al. [28]
Micronutrient	Units	BF infant[a]	MAM child[b]	NBF infant[c]	Older & PL[d]	Composite[e]
Biotin	µg	2.9	4.9	–	–	–
Choline	mg	91.8	83.8	–	–	–
Folic acid	µg	83	131.6	156	273	95
Niacin	mg	6.1	6.8	7.3	8.2	9.74
Pantothenic acid	mg	0.7	1.1	3.3	2.7	3.53
Riboflavin	mg	0.36	0.68	0.73	0.64	0.967
Thiamin	mg	0.36	0.38	0.55	0.64	0.746
Vitamin A	µg RE	500	714.4	734	377	154
Vitamin B6	mg	0.44	0.68	0.55	0.87	0.752
Vitamin B12	µg	0.52	0.98	1.27	1.29	1.5
Vitamin C	mg	140–280	37.6	55	28	40
Vitamin D3	µg	2–4	4.1	9.2	8.1	25
Vitamin E	mg	10	8.3	5.2	4.7	10.88
Vitamin K	µg	–	15.0	–	–	33
Calcium	mg	200–400	315.8	734	698	353
Copper	µg	400–800	334.6	–	–	390
Iodine	µg	180	75.2	164	113	230
Iron	mg	14	6.8	17.1	11.6	15.5
Magnesium	mg	80–120	112.8	99	111	94
Manganese	µg	1200	451.2	–	–	790
Phosphorus	mg	150–200	338.4	504	606	513
Potassium	mg	–	601.6	2,654 [30]	2,699	707
Selenium	µg	20	20.7	18.3	18.4	20
Sodium	mg	–	206.8	219 [30]	327	239
Zinc	mg	8.3	7.5	15.4	8	6.85

This table provides target vitamin and mineral levels recommended in the literature for various vulnerable groups among populations of food aid beneficiaries, including breast-fed (BF) and non-breast-fed (NBF) infants, children suffering from moderate acute malnutrition (MAM), older children and adults—including pregnant and lactating women (older & PL), and a composite group comprises infants, young children, and pregnant and lactating women

[a]Breast-fed infants, 6–23 months of age

[b]Children suffering from moderate acute malnutrition. Recommendation is for age with highest nutrient density requirement. Data presented on per 1,000 kcal basis has been converted to "per 100 g FBF" basis, using kcal density of USAID CSB

[c]Non-breast-fed infants. Recommendation is for age with highest nutrient density requirement

[d]Older children and adults, including pregnant and lactating women. Recommendation is for group with highest nutrient density requirement

[e]Composite vulnerable group, comprises infants, young children, and pregnant and lactating women

recommendations for breast-fed infants [29], for non-breast-fed infants and young children [27, 30], for moderately malnourished children [31], for older children and adults, including pregnant and lactating women [27, 30], and for a composite vulnerable group comprising infants, young children, and pregnant and lactating women [28]. Table 3.4 summarizes the recommendations of these various authors.

When trying to merge disparate groups of recommendations into a single proposal, the following guiding principles are worthy of consideration:

1. Later recommendations tend to represent more recent thinking and are typically based on the latest published research in the field.
2. Group recommendations tend to represent more consensus thinking.
3. When a range of micronutrient levels are recommended, the higher end of the range would meet the needs of more people, and would be favored, where toxicity is not an issue.

While there is a compelling case for providing two different FBF formulations, designed to meet the needs of infants and adults separately, the logistical and other problems associated with dual specifications make such a proposal unlikely to be adopted in the near term. Consequently, understanding the key differences in micronutrient recommendations presented in Table 3.4. is important for those wishing to create a single product fortification system. In keeping with the guidelines delineated above, a good starting point for formulation would be the Tufts/USAID recommendations of Webb et al., given that they represent a group consensus arrived at after a comprehensive review of the latest literature. Furthermore, their report defines a single-product FBF, designed for a composite group of infants, children, and pregnant and lactating women. Most of the Webb et al. recommendations in Table 3.4, are reasonable and well justified; however, several merit further discussion.

Guidance on Levels to Be Added

The importance of **folic acid** in the diet of pregnant women and women of childbearing age is well known. The latest recommendation [32] for pregnant women from the Institute of Medicine (IOM) is daily intake of 600 μg folate, in order to mitigate neural tube birth defects. The Tolerable Upper Intake Level (UL) established by the IOM is 1,000 μg for women and 300 μg for children. It is therefore surprising that the Webb et al. recommendation is so low (95 μg/100 g). The authors indicate that the lower value was chosen in an effort to avoid risk associated with masking of vitamin B12 deficiency. However, given that vitamin B12 is to be added simultaneously in the same premix, the risks associated with B12 deficiency would be less of a concern. A higher level, such as that proposed by Fleige et al. for pregnant women (273 μg), may be a better recommendation to minimize neural tube birth defects.

The proposal by Webb et al. of reducing **vitamin A** to 154 μg/100 g is also worth reconsidering. This reduction was recommended because of the availability of vitamin A fortified vegetable oil, which would ideally be distributed along with the FBF. However, given the possibility that the oil may or may not be added to the FBF, and given the widespread deficiency of vitamin A in beneficiary populations, a level closer to 700 μg/100 g might be a better recommendation.

Vitamin C addition is recommended by Lutter and Dewey [29] at higher than required levels (140–280 mg/100 g), on the basis that iron absorption would be enhanced. Other authors, including Webb et al. are hesitant to add higher levels of ascorbic acid because of significant cook losses reported in the literature, and the expense of ascorbic acid. Much of this concern stems from the 1997 IOM report [33] on vitamin C in food aid, wherein it was reported that vitamin C was reduced to negligible levels in some samples collected in the field and shipped on ice to analytical labs in the United States. However, a more recent laboratory simulation reported by Rowe et al. [24] indicated that only about 50 % of added vitamin C was lost when samples were analyzed immediately after cooking, rather than cooling and transporting for analysis. There is reason to believe that ascorbic acid addition at the higher levels proposed by Lutter and Dewey, would result in residual amounts of vitamin C at or above the IOM dietary reference intake (DRI). Given that vitamin C is typically sorely limiting in refugee feeding situations, the higher level of vitamin C would be recommended both to prevent scurvy and to increase iron absorption.

Vitamin D3 has received considerable attention recently, as IOM updated their DRIs in 2010 to 10 μg for infants and 15 μg for adults [34]. In addition to dietary intake, vitamin D can also be synthesized in the skin through sunlight exposure; and the IOM specifically indicated that they used minimal sun exposure by people in North America as a basis for their recommendation. Most food aid beneficiaries live in equatorial climates, with greater exposure to sunlight, albeit those with darker skin pigmentation would still benefit from added vitamin D in the diet. Consequently, fortification to a level of 10–15 μg vitamin D3/100 g product, would probably be adequate, which is more consistent with the recommendation of Fleige, et al., than the 25 μg level proposed by Webb et al.

In Table 3.4, only Golden and Webb et al. made recommendations for **vitamin K** fortification. Webb et al. suggests addition of 33 μg/100 g, in line with IOM's 30 μg DRI for children [35] but significantly lower than the 90 μg DRI for pregnant women. Per the specification data in Table 3.3, WFP requires 100 μg vitamin K per 100 g in their CSB, and this higher level would seem to be a reasonable requirement.

Webb et al. recommended a decrease in **calcium** to 353 mg/100 g to be consistent with the "new IOM recommendations." While their proposal is consistent with the recommendations of Golden and Lutter and Dewey, it is significantly lower than that of Fleige et al. and well below the IOM DRI of 1,300 mg for pregnant and lactating women. In light of this observation, a level closer to 700 mg, per Fleige et al., would not be out of line.

The IOM DRI [36] for **potassium** is quite high, ranging from 600 mg for infants to 5,100 mg for pregnant women. A common concern with potassium is the potential for bitterness imparted by potassium salts. Webb et al. indicated that they would recommend higher levels, were it not for the potential for negative impact on sensory properties. However, we have experimented with levels up to 1,500 mg/100 g in an oat-based FBF in the lab, and found sensory effects to be minimal, when using a blend of 70 % potassium chloride/30 % potassium citrate (unpublished data). The 707 mg level proposed by Webb et al. would certainly not be a problem from a palatability standpoint, and it may be possible to go even higher, depending on the product.

Given that FBFs are often given to children in various stages of malnutrition, nearly all of the authors cited in Table 3.4 agreed that **sodium** levels need to be kept relatively low to avoid problems with edema. Golden [31] discussed the phenomenon of increased retention of cellular sodium during states of malnutrition, which is significantly exacerbated by intake of dietary sodium. The modest level of between 200 and 250 mg/100 g, proposed by the authors in Table 3.4, is a reasonable approach for sodium fortification.

Other Factors to Consider

While micronutrient fortification is the primary emphasis of this handbook, additional macro-ingredient formulation issues that affect micronutrient delivery are worth consideration. One of the major concerns with food aid formulations is the presence of antinutrients and particularly phytic acid, which is abundant in grains and legumes and can bind mineral fortificants, making them unavailable for biological use. Efforts to enhance mineral bioaccessibility in these products have included use of chelated mineral fortificants. Sodium iron (III) ethylenediaminetetraacetate (NaFeEDTA), for example, has been recommended as the best iron source for fortification of whole grain or high extraction cereal products [37]. However, the higher cost of NaFeEDTA, and its potential to impart unwanted color changes in fortified products [38], have hindered its widespread use in food aid products to date. Other studies [39] have evaluated use of phytase enzyme as a pretreatment to reduce mineral binding in cereal foods. Production feasibility issues and lack of regulatory approval for phytase use in some countries have prevented this enzymatic approach from gaining a foothold in food aid production. Due to various technical/sensory and cost challenges for these and other approaches, no monumental improvements in mineral bioaccessibility have been made in plant-based FBFs to the present time.

Yet another macro-ingredient problem that affects micronutrient delivery is the thick consistency of most of the FBFs, when prepared at concentrations meeting target energy requirements. USAID CSB, for example, contains up to 70 % corn, and is consequently very high in starch. A 20 % (w/w) initial concentration of CSB in water is required in order for the cooked porridge to deliver the recommended [29] energy density of 0.8 kcal/g suggested for infants. At this concentration the cooked CSB is thick and paste-like in consistency [40]. Many mothers consequently dilute the CSB to a thin gruel consistency to facilitate feeding to weaning infants [40]. The end result is a product that not only fails to meet the child's energy requirements but also has severely diminished micronutrient density. Proposals to remedy this potential issue include increased extrusion pressure/time during manufacture [30], as well as addition of amylase-rich barley malt [30] to dextrinize the starch, resulting in a thinner consistency. Webb et al. [28], address this issue by recommending an addition of 15 g vegetable oil to 50 g dry FBF during beneficiary preparation. A previous study [40] has shown that addition of 12.2 g oil to 50 g dry CSB was sufficient to achieve acceptable viscosity, but care needs to be taken with the formulation to avoid micronutrient dilution from the added oil.

Recommendations

1. Approaches to redesigning the FBF portfolio to include two product fortification categories—one suitable for infants and children, and the other suitable for older children and adults, including pregnant and lactating women—should be further explored. Viscosity of products targeted at infants should be low enough that further dilution with water will not be required.
2. In the meantime, most of the micronutrient recommendations of Webb et al. in Table 3.4 are excellent proposals for fortification of a composite FBF targeting the range from infants to pregnant and lactating women. Alternative recommendations for a number of micronutrients are listed herein, and are suggested as means of better meeting the nutritional needs of this broader range of beneficiaries.
3. The serious problem of limited mineral bioaccessibility in cereal–legume-based FBFs should be a major focus of attention; and funding of research into cost-effective, feasible solutions should be a priority. Mineral chelates, alone or blended with ferrous sulfate, provide the highest level of bioavailability in FBFs at present.

Conclusion

In conclusion, it is evident that development of micronutrient fortified food aid products is a complex undertaking. The challenges are significant, and largely stem from the diversity of beneficiary populations being served, from a cultural, as well as a physiological/demographic standpoint. These challenges are made more difficult by the critical need to maintain product and distribution costs as low as possible, which limits opportunities to create the "ideal" product for each beneficiary group. Finally, there is little opportunity for control over a food aid product once it has been placed into the hands of the beneficiary. The product may be traded, improperly prepared, shared with others in the household, or fed to animals—all of which can minimize the potential nutritional benefits to the recipients. Given these challenges, the past success of fortified food aid has been limited to some degree, but the beneficial effects are nonetheless significant and far reaching. Much research is presently being undertaken in the field, and new and improved products are now being developed and tested as a matter of regular course. Many are the individuals whose lives have been improved and even saved through the timely delivery of humanitarian food aid; and it is hoped that those who find themselves in need in the future will benefit to an even greater extent as nutritionists and food scientists continue to expand the body of knowledge and experience in this critical area.

Acknowledgements The author would like to thank Dr. James Hansen, M.D., Ph.D., for his careful review of the manuscript and his invaluable insights and additions.

References

1. Shaw DJ. The UN World Food Programme and the development of food aid. New York: Palgrave; 2001.
2. Garnsey P. Famine and food supply in the Graeco-Roman world: responses to risk and crisis. Cambridge: University Press; 1988.
3. Shaw DJ. Global food and agricultural institutions. New York: Routledge; 2009.
4. Barrett CB, Maxwell DG. Food aid after fifty years, recasting its role. New York: Routledge; 2005.
5. Shaw J, Clay E, editors. World food aid. Rome: World Food Programme; 1993.
6. World Food Programme. Quantity reporting. Available at: http://www.wfp.org/fais/reports. Accessed 24 September 2011.
7. Food and Agriculture Organization of the United Nations. The state of food insecurity in the world 2010. 2010. http://www.fao.org/docrep/013/i1683e/i1683e.pdf. Accessed 12 September 2011.
8. International Grains Council. Food aid operations. Available at: http://www.igc.int/en/publications/foodaidshipments.aspx. Accessed 24 September 2011.
9. World Food Programme. Contributions to WFP 2010. Available at: http://www.wfp.org/about/donors/year/2010. Accessed 26 September 2011.
10. World Food Programme. WFP's food basket. Available at: http://www.wfp.org/nutrition/WFP-foodbasket. Accessed 17 September 2011.
11. de Pee S, Manary M, Ashorn P. The devil is in the details [letter]. Nutr Rev. 2011;69(2):116–7.
12. de Pee S, Bloem MW. Current and potential role of specially formulated foods and food supplements for preventing malnutrition among 6- to 23-month-old children and for treating moderate malnutrition among 6- to 59-month-old children. Food Nutr Bull. 2009;30(3 Suppl):S434–63.
13. Desjeux JF, Briend A, Prudhon C, Greletty Y, Golden MH. Definition and assessment of a therapeutic food for severely malnourished children in situation of humanitarian crisis. Bull Acad Natl Med. 1998;182(8):1679–95.
14. Chaparro CM, Dewey KG. Use of lipid-based nutrient supplements (LNS) to improve the nutrient adequacy of general food distribution rations for vulnerable sub-groups in emergency settings. Matern Child Nutr. 2010;6:1–69.
15. Therapeutic food for malnutrition treatment. Compact for life. Available at: http://www.compactforlife.com/malnutrition-treatment/. Accessed 2 November 2011.
16. USDA Foreign Agricultural Service. Food aid reports. Available at: http://www.fas.usda.gov/excredits/FoodAid/Reports/reports.html. Accessed 27 September 2011.
17. USDA Farm Service Agency. Commodity requirements. Available at: http://www.fsa.usda.gov/FSA/webapp?area=home&subject=coop&topic=pas-ex-cr. Accessed 27 September 2011.
18. World Food Programme. Food specifications. Available at: http://foodquality.wfp.org/FoodSpecifications/tabid/56/Default.aspx. Accessed 25 September 2011.
19. U.S. Government Accountability Office. International food assistance: local and regional procurement report. Available at: http://www.gao.gov/products/GAO-09-570. Accessed 28 September 2011.
20. Ranum P. Final report of the micronutrient assessment project. Washington, DC: SUSTAIN; 1999. Available at: www.sustaintech.org.
21. Milton RF, Pawsey RK. Spoilage relating to the storage and transport of cereals and oil seeds. Int J Food Microbiol. 1988;7(3):211–7.
22. Wareing PW, Boxall RA, Gough MC, Phillips SI. Changes in the mycoflora of UK wheat shipped to tropical regions. Int Biodeterior Biodegradation. 1993;32(1):175–85.
23. Rowe JP, Brodegard WC, Pike OA, Steele FM, Dunn ML. Storage, preparation, and usage of fortified food aid in the diet of Guatemalan, Ugandan, and Malawian beneficiaries: a field study report. Food Nutr Bull. 2008;29(3):213–20.
24. Rowe JP, Ogden LV, Pike OA, Steele FM, Dunn ML. Effect of end-user preparation methods on vitamin content of fortified humanitarian food-aid commodities. J Food Compost Anal. 2009;22(1):33–7.
25. United Nations Children's Fund. The state of the world's children 2008. 2008. Available at: http://www.unicef.org/sowc08/docs/sowc08.pdf. Accessed 17 September 2011.
26. World Food Programme. Improving the nutritional quality of WFP's food basket—an overview of nutrition issues, commodity options and programming choices. Available at: http://documents.wfp.org/stellent/groups/public/documents/newsroom/wfp197188.pdf. Accessed 17 September 2011.
27. Fleige LE, Sahyoun NR, Murphy SP. A new simulation model estimates micronutrient levels to include in fortified blended foods used in food aid programs. J Nutr. 2010;140(2):355–65.
28. Webb P, Rogers BL, Rosenberg I, et al. Improving the nutritional quality of U.S. food aid: recommendations for changes to products and programs. Boston, MA: Tufts University; 2011.
29. Lutter CK, Dewey KG. Proposed nutrient composition for fortified complementary foods. J Nutr. 2003;133(9 Suppl):S3011–20.

30. Fleige LE, Moore WR, Garlick PJ, et al. Recommendations for optimization of fortified and blended food aid products from the United States. Nutr Rev. 2010;68(5):290–315.
31. Golden MH. Proposed recommended nutrient densities for moderately malnourished children. Food Nutr Bull. 2009;30(3 Suppl):S267–342.
32. Institute of Medicine. Recommended dietary allowance and adequate intake values, vitamins and elements. 11 September 2011. Available at: http://www.iom.edu/Activities/Nutrition/SummaryDRIs/DRI-Tables.aspx. Accessed 31 October 2011.
33. Institute of Medicine. Vitamin C fortification of food aid commodities. Washington, DC: National Academy Press; 1997.
34. Institute of Medicine. Dietary reference intakes for calcium and vitamin D. 30 November 2010. Available at: http://www.iom.edu/Reports/2010/Dietary-Reference-Intakes-for-Calcium-and-Vitamin-D/DRI-Values.aspx. Accessed 31 October 2011.
35. Institute of Medicine. Dietary reference intakes for vitamin A, vitamin K, arsenic, boron, chromium, copper, iodine, iron, manganese, molybdenum, nickel, silicon, vanadium, and zinc. Washington, DC: National Academy Press; 2001.
36. Institute of Medicine. Dietary reference intakes: water, potassium, sodium, chloride, and sulfate. Washington, DC: National Academy Press; 2004.
37. Hurrell R, Ranum P, de Pee S, et al. Revised recommendations for iron fortification of wheat flour and an evaluation of the expected impact of current national wheat flour fortification programs. Food Nutr Bull. 2010;31 (1 Suppl):S7–21.
38. Richins AT, Burton KE, Pahulu HF, Jefferies LK, Dunn ML. Effect of iron source on color and appearance of micronutrient-fortified corn flour tortillas. Cereal Chem. 2008;85(4):561–5.
39. Rimbach G, Pallauf J, Moehring J, Kraemer K, Minihane AM. Effect of dietary phytate and microbial phytase on mineral and trace element bioavailability—a literature review. Curr Top Nutraceutical Res. 2008;6(3):131–44.
40. Black CT, Pahulu HF, Dunn ML. Effect of preparation method on viscosity and energy density of fortified humanitarian food-aid commodities. Int J Food Sci Nutr. 2009;60(S7):219–28.
41. USAID. Commodities reference guide. Available at: http://www.usaid.gov/our_work/humanitarian_assistance/ffp/crg/sec2.htm. Accessed 26 September 2011.
42. USAID. PL 480 Title II recipes. 8 July 2004. Available at: http://www.usaid.gov/our_work/humanitarian_assistance/ffp/50th/recipes.html. Accessed 29 September 2011.

Chapter 4
Middle East Perspectives of Food Fortification: Implementation Dynamics and Policy Factors

Deena Alasfoor

Key Points

- The Middle East Region is composed of countries that are variable in population size, demographics, wealth, health, and nutritional status.
- Health and nutritional status are dependent on the economic and infrastructure development of countries.
- Fortification is a cost-effective strategy for the management and control of anemia in developed countries.
- Important factors in successful implementation of fortification are identification of the problem, advocacy, alliance, consultation, responsive industry, and resources.
- Pockets of population subgroups continue to have high rates of anemia in-spite of over-all improvement in a country.
- Anemia continues to be a public health problem in developing countries.
- Implementation of fortification contributes to reduction of iron deficiency, but anemia should be managed through multiple interventions.
- Almost half of the countries in the Middle East do not require flour fortification.
- Anemia helped improve anemia status in countries where trend data are available.
- Development of reliable and sustainable program indicators should be integrated into fortification initiatives.

Keywords Middle East • Fortification • Flour fortification • Anemia • Iron deficiency anemia • Oman • Kuwait • Morocco • Qatar • KSA • Algeria • Bahrain • UAE • Somalia • Egypt • Sudan • Afghanistan • Tunisia • Libya • Jordan • Occupied territories of Palestine • Lebanon • Syria • Djibouti • Iran • Iraq • Yemen

D. Alasfoor, M.Sc. (✉)
Department of Nutrition, Ministry of Health, 18th November Street,
Al Ghubra, Muscat, Oman 100
e-mail: deena1@omantel.net.om

V.R. Preedy et al. (eds.), *Handbook of Food Fortification and Health: From Concepts to Public Health Applications Volume 1*, Nutrition and Health, DOI 10.1007/978-1-4614-7076-2_4,

Abbreviations

CDC	Centers for Disease Control
DALY	Disability-adjusted life years
FFI	Flour Fortification Initiative
GNI	Gross national income
HDI	Human Development Index
KSA	Kingdom of Saudi Arabia
MI	Micronutrients initiative
MT	Metric tonnes
PPP$	Purchasing power parity
UAE	United Arab Emirates
UNDP	United Nations Development Program
UNICEF	United Nations Children Fund
WHO	World Health Organization

Introduction

The Middle East countries have the same geography and history but are very different in many other aspects. The term started in 1850 when the British India Office named the Arab gulf countries (Middle East) during the British occupation. After the second world war, it became synonymous with the region that included all countries west of India to the Mediterranean sea [1].

Middle East countries are variable in land size and population characteristics. Some of these such as Somalia, Iraq, and the Occupied Territories of Palestine are home to political unrest, and/or natural disasters while others enjoy political stability and high national income. For example, the Gulf Cooperation Council countries (Qatar, Saudi Arabia, UAE, Kuwait, Bahrain, and Oman) are considered among the world wealthiest nations, compared to Yemen and Sudan that have the world lowest Human Development (HDI) and income indices as defined by the UNDP [2, 3].

The World Health Organization (WHO) developed flour fortification guidelines in 2006, for which a revision was published in 2010. The 2006 guidelines included human requirements, iron bioavailability, and anemia rates factors. Additionally, the 2010 revision factored in population groups targeted, anemia rates, as well as amount, bioavailability, and type of fortificant [4, 5].

Flour fortification program spread gradually since the middle of the twentieth century when the United States was the first country to start it. In May 2012, the Four Fortification Initiative reported that flour fortification is mandatory in 68 countries worldwide [6, 7]. Anemia, however, persists to be a public health problem in many countries of the world, mostly affecting the needy and vulnerable. The impact of fortification on iron status of population is most probably defined by a combination of population (human), agent (food vehicle), and fortificant characteristics. Documented literature is available on the food and fortificant vehicle factors, but very little information is available on population characteristics. Moreover, the magnitude by which fortification is expected to reduce anemia, or other iron status indicators is not known, and possible confounding factors are recognized but not fully understood. Unsurprisingly, rate of improvement of iron status and anemia is inconsistent [8].

Impact of fortification cannot be considered in isolation of health, development, or economic status. In this chapter the development status of countries of the Middle East will be explored; how and when fortification was initiated with emphasis on iron in flour. Anemia trend in Middle East countries will be explored in relation to fortification. Given the lack of comparable data, it is difficult to arrive at a conclusive evidence for the effectiveness of fortification in the Middle East.

Status of Development of Middle Eastern Countries

The HDI of the UNDP is defined according to three dimensions: Long and healthy life (life expectancy index), Knowledge (Education index), and a decent standard of living (GNI). Countries of the region are distributed over the developmental spectrum with Qatar, UAE, and Bahrain among the highest ranked, and Yemen, Sudan, and Afghanistan are among the lowest. Qatar tops the world income at 107,721 PPP$ in 2011 [9].

Life expectancy ranges between 74 years in Qatar and 48 in Afghanistan; whereas the mean number of schooling is highest at 9.4 in Bahrain and lowest at 2.3 and 3.3 years in Yemen and Somalia, respectively. All other countries are spread in the middle ranges of education, income, life expectancy, and the composite HDI indicator.

Anemia is associated with income; low-income population groups were found to have lower iron status [10, 11]. A descriptive study of 46 African countries showed that the decline in the national financial situation led to an increase in food and medicine prices and cut in health expenditure. In East Asia, using mathematical modeling and information from 1997 financial crisis, it was estimated that the economic situation setback that started in 2009 would result in 10–20 % increase in maternal anemia [12, 13].

Development indicators factors can interfere with fortification outcome. Hypothetically speaking, if the same fortification program was implemented, anemia in a population with low income, access to food, and high illiteracy rates is unlikely to improve at the same rate as a more developed population.

Flour Fortification in the Middle East

Fortification was initiated through the collaborative efforts of the Eastern Mediterranean Region office of the WHO with CDC, UNICEF, MI, and FFI in response to requests from member countries in 1996 [14, 15]. Prior to that, Kingdom of Saudi Arabia (KSA) started fortifying flour with iron and vitamins in 1994 and Afghanistan started on a small scale in the same year. Oman followed in 1996, and in 2001 the program was initiated in Kuwait in 2002 in Bahrain, Jordan, and Qatar. Flour was fortified in Yemen in 2005 and in Iran, Iraq, Morocco, and Palestine in 2006 [16].

At the time of writing this chapter, ten countries in the region did not establish flour fortification and these are: Libya, Somalia, Sudan, Syria, UAE, Tunisia, Algeria, and Lebanon. A number of factors were identified for successful implementation [17], (Fig. 4.1) and these are:

- Identification of the anemia as a public health problem: In 1996 estimates of anemia from national surveys were published for 15 countries in the region. Those indicated moderate to severe public health problem among women and children. Since then most countries have implemented periodic national surveys and collected monitoring data for various population groups. Currently, national data on anemia are published for most countries except Algeria and Syria. Some have subnational or dated national data such as KSA, Somalia, Sudan, Qatar, and Libya [18, 19]. This illustrates that anemia is well established as a public health problem in the region. It was identified in 1995, and consistently it is being investigated as evidence accumulated from the large number of studies carried out in the region.
- Advocacy and communication: Since the regional workshop in 1996, scientists and authorities raised anemia as a public health problem, as well as fortification as a solution. In some cases they were faced with fierce arguments against the program. Fortification advocates were requested to demonstrate the need for intervention. Medical specialists had unfounded concerns regarding iron overdose among thalassemia patients in Lebanon. An initial regional meeting to promote flour

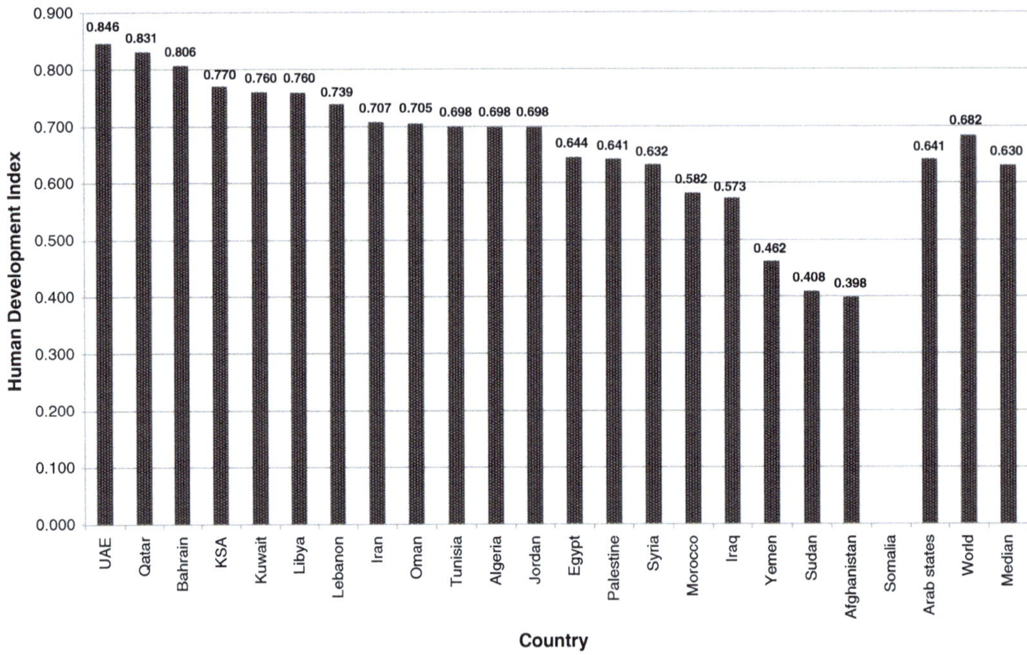

Fig. 4.1 Human Development Index 2011 of the Middle East countries

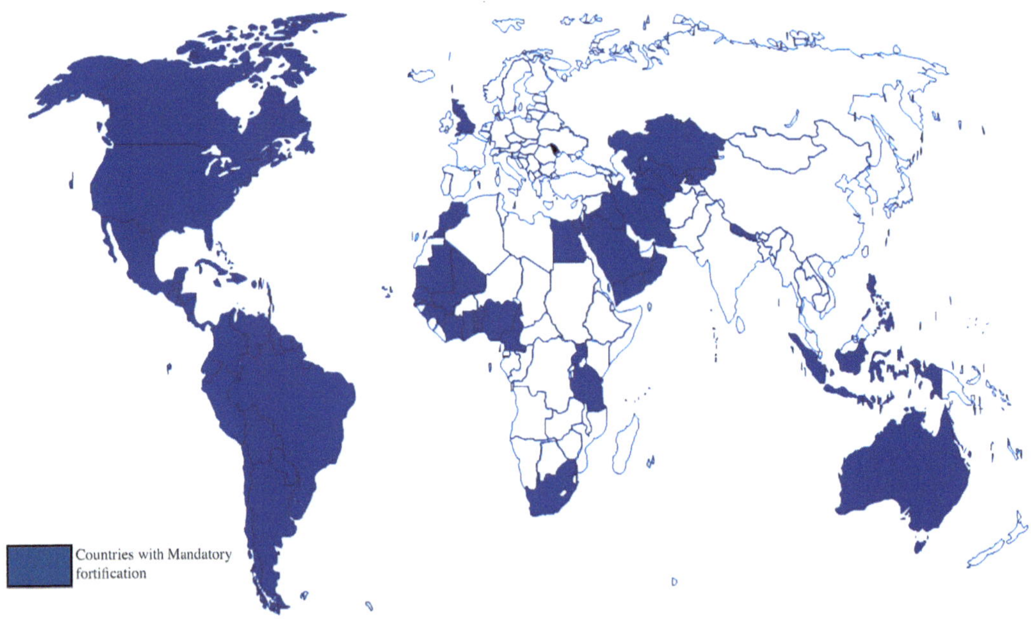

Fig. 4.2 Map of global progress in flour fortification with iron or iron and folic acid [44]

fortification in Iran October 1995 was attended by seven countries and was followed by a technical multi-agency consultation in Muscat in which 15 milling and food technology experts from 15 countries participated and contributed evidence to the feasibility of fortification in EMRO. After several technical and logistical questions by counties of the region, WHO-EMRO organized a follow-up meeting in Beirut [14, 15, 20] (Fig. 4.2).

Table 4.1 List of Middle East classified countries according to various UN and International Organization [33, 41–43]

World Health Organization (Eastern Mediterranean)	UNDP (Arab states)	UNICEF (Middle East and North Africa)	Food and Agriculture Organization (Near East)
Afghanistan			
Bahrain	√	√	√
Djibouti	√	√	√
Egypt	√	√	√
Iran		√	√
Iraq	√	√	√
Jordan	√	√	√
Kuwait	√	√	√
Lebanon	√	√	√
Libya	√	√	√
Morocco	√	√	
Oman		√	√
Pakistan			
Qatar		√	√
Saudi Arabia (KSA)	√	√	√
Somalia	√		√
Sudan (and South Sudan since 2011)	√	√	√
Syria	√	√	√
Tunisia	√	√	
United Arab Emirates	√	√	√
Yemen	√	√	√
Others	Algeria	Algeria, occupied Palestine territories	Algeria, Kyregystand, and Turkimestan

The presence of International organizations such as the WHO, UNICEF, MI, FFI, CDC, and more recently Global Alliance for Improved Nutrition had a detrimental contribution to the program. These organizations played an important role in capacity building for surveys (Oman, Jordan); surveillance systems (Kuwait); advocacy and provision of fortificant and mixers (Egypt), as well as contributions to developing standards and guidelines [21] (Table 4.1).

- Alliance and consultation: It is unclear whether there were formal alliances in most of the countries that adopted fortification in the region. However, regional and national cooperation between public health authority, industry, and the legal authority is clearly a prerequisite for establishing fortification standards and guidelines. In most countries legal authorities, i.e., Ministries of commerce issue fortification standards, whereas technological and financial issues and their solutions were put forth by the milling industry.
- Responsive industry: This may be the most important driving force for flour fortification in the region. Informed and motivated management in the Milling industry helped ease the way to successful implementation. There are 1–2 mills in each of the GCC countries; Palestine, Somalia, and Syria, whereas flour from all other countries is produced by a number of mills that range between 5 in Yemen and over 300 in Iran (Table 4.2).

  Bahrain started fortifying flour on a pilot basis before the health authorities took it into consideration. In Oman and KSA, millers obtained guidelines and expertise from their contacts in the milling industry and started fortification with minimal, if any contribution from the government.

  The international association for operative millers is an organized and structured network that brings together multimillion industries. Open lines of communications between the regional and international millers made it easier to acquire the know-how. In addition, the comparatively low cost and high credibility of the intervention made it an attractive option. In 2003 a regional meeting for the International Association of Operative Millers in Dubai adopted a resolution to support the

Table 4.2 Number of mills and fortification status of the Middle Eastern Countries

Country	Number of Mills	Fortification Status	Year fortification started
Algeria	250	None	–
Afghanistan	17	Voluntary, partial	1994
Bahrain	1	Mandatory	2002
Egypt	>145	Partial	2007
Jordan	13	Mandatory	2002
Iran	330	Mandatory for larger mills	2006
Iraq	NA	All imported	2006
Kuwait	1		2001
Lebanon	12	None	–
Libya	>9		
Morocco	121	80 mills fortifying	2006
Oman	2	Mandatory	1996
Occupied territories of Palestine	2	Mandatory	2006
Qatar	1	Mandatory	2002
KSA	4	Mandatory	1981
Yemen	>5	Mandatory	2005
Somalia	1	None	–
Sudan	7	None	–
Syria	1	None	–
UAE	1	None	–
Tunisia	36	None	–

Flour Fortification Initiative. The Flour Fortification Initiative is a partnership between more than 23 private companies and 26 public/educational institutions worldwide to advance flour fortification [17, 21, 22].

- Resources: Financial and technical resources are needed for several components of the program. Among those: iron assessment for populations, communication, and advocacy, establishing the program and finally monitoring the program. Countries that established the program had access to those resources either through support of international organizations or local funds; the program advances much faster in countries where a small number of mills have most of the market share such as KSA, Kuwait, Bahrain, and Oman. Where there are large mills, advanced technology and large production volume helps to reduce cost, which is estimated to be 0.25$ per capita [23].

Anemia Before and After Fortification

Fortification as a preventive and control measure for anemia and iron deficiency is well known [24]; and the biological factors that enhance or decrease iron absorption are established. However, reliable trend data on anemia in the Middle East are not available, and therefore it is not possible to monitor fortification outcomes. Logistical issues such as access to equipment and fortificant, ability to introduce the technology into the milling process, and large number of mills are factors that contribute to lack of adequate establishment of fortification. In addition some populations may have non-optimum dietary habits that include reliance on non-fortified imported products, or low bioavailable diet [8, 25, 26].

Other factors could render iron fortification less effective and these are the health status, presence of infection, and presence of other interventions. It is difficult to account for these factors in the region

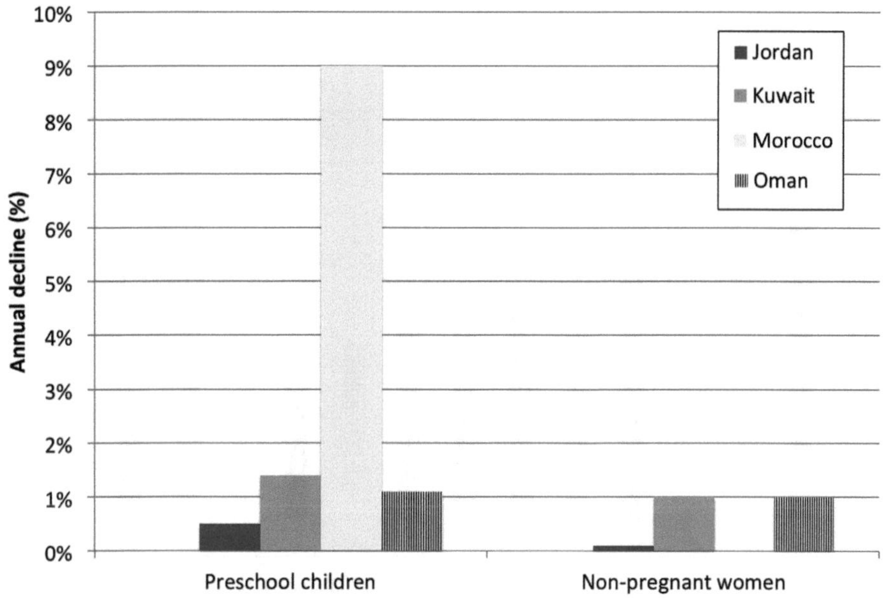

Fig. 4.3 Annual rate of anemia decline in some countries of the Middle East

because of the lack of country comparable data. Trend data from Oman and Kuwait show consistent decline in anemia rates among pregnant women in Oman, non-pregnant women in Kuwait (personal communication, Quentin Johnson) (Fig. 4.3).

In Egypt there was an increase in anemia rates from 2000 to 2005, where preschool children went up by an annual rate of 8 % and nonpregnant women anemia rate went up by 6.4 % annually; however, there are no available data on the rates after fortification. In Algeria, rates of anemia among pregnant women were reported to be 46.9 % in 2011. Post-fortification rates in Afghanistan were 37.9 %, 24.7 % for preschool children and pregnant women, respectively, with no baseline to compare with. Bahraini nonpregnant women showed an increased anemia rates from 37.3 % in 1999 to 51.4 % in 2002; however, post-fortification data was collected after 6 months of fortification only [27–30].

Countries that had data to permit pre- and post-fortification anemia status were Kuwait, Jordan, Oman, and Morocco. Data from Morocco and Jordan are based on cross-sectional studies before and after flour fortification, whereas data form Oman is based on institution based surveillance of pregnant women at first visit from 1992 to 2011 (refer to chapter 64: Oman perspective this book). Data from Kuwait is based on institution-based surveillance of Hemoglobin levels for nonpregnant women from 2001 to 2010.

Morocco showed the largest improvement in anemia status at 9 %, annually which was possibly magnified because the study was conducted under controlled conditions, and children were monitored, which may create a bias.

Jordan showed a negligible annual decline in anemia; which is explained by low flour fortification coverage; as 44.1 % of the households only had fortified bread. In addition, the flour was fortified at 30 ppm as opposed to the recommended 60 ppm.

Both Oman and Kuwait had a rate of 1 % for pregnant women, and comparable rates for preschool children at 1.4 % for Kuwait and 1.1 % for Oman (refer to chapter 64) [31–33]. In Kuwait the fortificant used was changed in 2007 from elemental to the more bioavailable electrolytic iron. When comparing the rates of decline before and after this change, it is observed that anemia among women of childbearing age in Kuwait declined from 30 % in 2001 to 20 % in 2007, and 18 % in 2010, whereas anemia among adolescents was found to be 32.5, 28, and 24 % in the years 2001, 2007, and 2010 in the

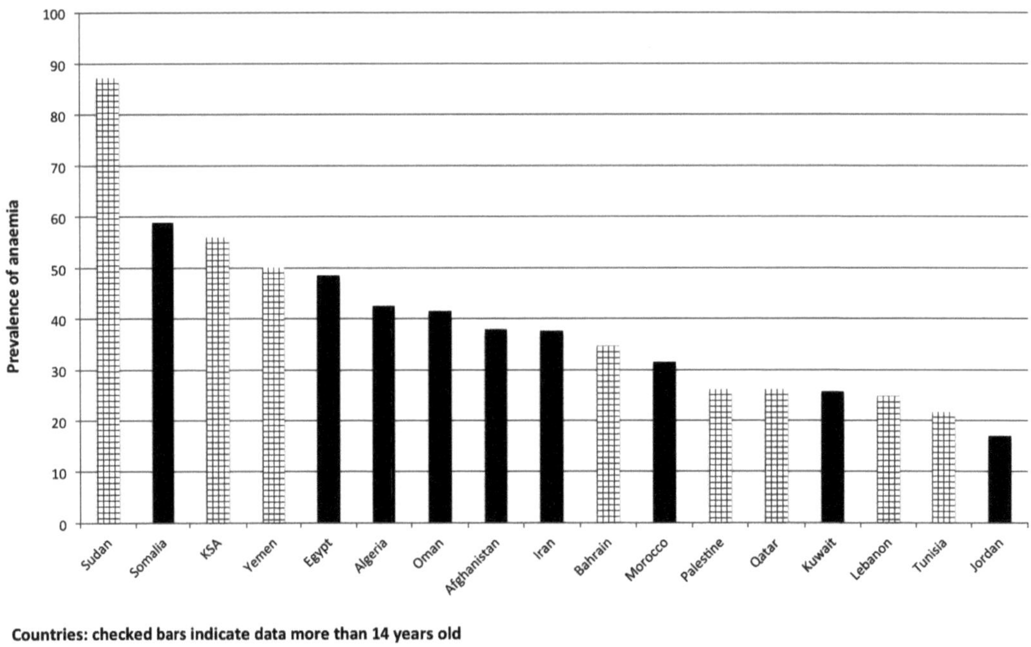

Fig. 4.4 Prevalence estimates of anemia among preschool children in the Middle East

same order. This indicates annual decline rates of 1.7 % and 0.7 % before and after 2007, respectively, for women of childbearing age, compared to 0.75 and 1.3 % before and after 2007 for adolescents (Dr. Ali Jaffer, GCC Executive Health Board, personal communication). A conclusion regarding efficacy of electrolytic versus elemental iron at the population level at this stage is not possible based on these findings.

Anemia among preschool children in the region ranges between 59 % in Somalia and to 17 % in Jordan. There is not enough data to generate powerful statistical analysis, however as shown in Fig. 4.4 countries that implemented fortification continue to have anemia rates above 20 % [34].

Conclusions

Fortification is being widely advocated as a cost-effective strategy for the prevention and control of anemia. Despite low anemia rates observed in developed countries, presumably as a result of fortification, the risk of anemia remains high in developing countries and among population subgroups in developed countries. In addition, low iron status in low-income populations and immigrants cannot be explained by diet alone; therefore, a holistic public health approach should be taken when managing anemia in populations. Factors other than iron consumption and bioavailability should be considered; including those that are contextual such as health conditions, development indicators, and the environment [24].

Anemia could be nutritional and this is caused by reduced iron intake, or due to low folic acid, vitamin B12, vitamin A status, or secondary to protein energy malnutrition. Genetic hemoglobin disorders could reduce the impact of fortification on anemia; and an array of infectious diseases can increase blood loss. It is important to have realistic evidence-based expectations when designing a fortification program. It is highly unlikely that fortification would significantly reduce anemia in countries with high rates of malaria or schistosomiasis without a complementary prophylaxis program; nor it is expected to reach a national prevalence estimate lower or close to the rate of genetic hemoglobin disorders [11].

Monitoring systems with close observation of vulnerable groups is essential. Hemoglobin assessment is useful to detect trend of anemia but an additional indicator of iron status is needed to measure the change in iron reserves and anticipate possible outcome. In Iran and Jordan fortification was found to improve Ferritin but not hemoglobin levels.

The impact study conducted in Bahrain found increased anemia rates based on hemoglobin after 6 months of fortification. These unexpected findings could be due to a combination of factors that include short time from fortification to assessment and that does not permit the reserves to reflect in circulating hemoglobin in addition to inadequate assessment and quality assurance procedures for measurement of biological indicators [30, 35, 36].

Fortification has a benefit/cost ratio of 8:1; and the cost/person/year is about $0.12. This makes it an important opportunity especially in light of the accommodating industry situations in the Middle East. Fortification is estimated to reduce perinatal and maternal mortality by one-third for cost per disability-adjusted life years (DALY) calculations, significantly lesser than supplementation that reduces mortality by two thirds. Fortification remains, however, a cost-effective sustainable approach by virtue or its consistent delivery systems and low implementation cost that is mostly taken up by the industry [37–39].

Recommendations

Public health authorities and international organizations should consider anemia a major public health problem and take a public health muti-intervention approach for its management and control.

Fortification is a cost-effective strategy; however, the magnitude by which it is expected to control anemia is limited. Countries are advised to develop and maintain indicators of anemia as well as iron status of various population groups especially women and children, the poor and displaced.

It is important to understand the risk factors of anemia in the region and build coalition, gain political support, and engage the industry in public health plans. Consideration should be given to classifying countries according to the magnitude of risk factors and develop a clear framework for management that considers modifiable and non-modifiable risk factors, equity considerations, and the social determinants that may be responsible for anemia, dietary composition, and flour consumption [40].

References

1. Anderson EW, Fisher WB. The Middle East: geography and geopolitics. London: Routledge; 2000. p. 342.
2. UNDP. Indices and data: Human Development Index. United Nations Development Program; 2011 [cited 2012 February 5]. Available from: https://docs.google.com/viewer?url=http%3A%2F%2Fhdr.undp.org%2Fen%2Fmedia%2FHDR_2011_EN_TechNotes.pdf.
3. GCC. The Cooperation Council of the Arab States of the Gulf: charter; 2012 [cited 2012]. Available from: http://www.gcc-sg.org/eng/indexfc7a.html?action=Sec-Show&ID=1.
4. Hurrell R, Ranum P, de Pee S, Biebinger R, Hulthen L, Johnson Q, et al. Revised recommendations for iron fortification of wheat flour and an evaluation of the expected impact of current national wheat flour fortification programs. Food Nutr Bull. 2010;31(1 Suppl):S7–21.
5. Allen LH, De Benoist B, Dary O, Hurrell R; World Health Organization. Department of Nutrition for Health and Development. Guidelines on food fortification with micronutrients. Geneva: World Health Organization; 2006. p. 341.
6. FFI. Map of global progress. Flour Fortification Initiative; 2012 [cited 16 May 2012]. Available from: http://www.sph.emory.edu/wheatflour/globalmap.php.

7. Cordain L. Cereal grains: humanity's double-edged sword. World Rev Nutr Diet. 1999;84:19–73.
8. Lynch SR. Why nutritional iron deficiency persists as a worldwide problem. J Nutr. 2011;141(4):763S–8.
9. UNDP. Human development report 2011. Sustainability and equity: a better future for all. New York: United Nations Development Program; 2011. p. 176.
10. Oliveira JS, de Lira PI, Osorio MM, Sequeira LA, Costa EC, Goncalves FC, et al. [Anemia, hypovitaminosis A and food insecurity in children of municipalities with Low Human Development Index in the Brazilian Northeast]. Anemia, hipovitaminose A e inseguranca alimentar em criancas de municipios de Baixo Indice de Desenvolvimento Humano do Nordeste do Brasil. Braz J Epidemiol. 2010;13(4):651–64.
11. Balarajan Y, Ramakrishnan U, Ozaltin E, Shankar AH, Subramanian SV. Anaemia in low-income and middle-income countries. Lancet. 2011;378(9809):2123–35.
12. Kirigia JM, Nganda BM, Mwikisa CN, Cardoso B. Effects of global financial crisis on funding for health development in nineteen countries of the WHO African region. BMC Int Health Hum Rights. 2011;11(1):4.
13. Bhutta ZA, Bawany FA, Feroze A, Rizvi A, Thapa SJ, Patel M. Effects of the crises on child nutrition and health in East Asia and the Pacific. Glob Soc Policy. 2009;9(1):119–43.
14. Verster A; World Health Organization. Regional Office for the Eastern Mediterranean. Guidelines for the control of iron deficiency in countries of the Eastern Mediterranean, Middle East and North Africa. Alexandria: WHO Regional Office for the Eastern Mediterranean; 1996. p. 65.
15. Verster A; World Health Organization. Regional Office for the Eastern Mediterranean. Fortification of flour with iron in countries of the Eastern Mediterranean, Middle East and North Africa. Alexandria: WHO Regional Office for the Eastern Mediterranean; 1998. p. 64.
16. FFI. Algeria summary January 2011–2012. 23 April 2012. p. 3. Available from: http://www.sph.emory.edu/wheatflour//Africa.php—countryprofiles.
17. Tyler VQ. Reducing iron deficiency through wheat flour fortification in the middle east, lessons from efforts in Bahrain, Jordan and Iran [qualitative research]. Atlanta: Emory University; 2005.
18. Verster A, van der Pols JC. Anaemia in the Eastern Mediterranean region. East Mediterr Health J. 1995;1(1):9.
19. WHO. Vitamin and mineral nutrition information system (VMNIS). Geneva: World Health Organization; 2012 [cited 2012 April 25; Anemia data by country]. Available from: http://www.who.int/vmnis/database/anaemia/countries/en/index.html.
20. WHO/EMRO, UNICEF, MI, ILSI. Fortification of flour to control micronutrient deficiencies in the Eastern Mediterranean, Middle East and North Africa: report of a joint WHO/UNICEF/MI/ILSO workshop, Beirut, Lebanon, 13–16 June 1998. Alexandria: WHO Regional Office for the Eastern Mediterranean; 1999.
21. Amad R. Assessment and update of iron deficiency anemia in the MENA region. (Assignment Report), unpublished, UNECEF - MENA 2002.
22. FFI. Who we are. Online Flour Fortification Initiative; 2012 [cited 2012 April 23]. Available from: http://www.sph.emory.edu/wheatflour/partnerlinks.php.
23. Jere R. Behrman HA, Hoddinot J. Hunger and malnutrition. Copenhagen Consensus; February 2004. Copenhagen: Copenhagen Consensus Center; 2004. p. 58.
24. Ramakrishnan U, Yip R. Experiences and challenges in industrialized countries: control of iron deficiency in industrialized countries. J Nutr. 2002;132(4 Suppl):820S–4.
25. Lynch SR. The impact of iron fortification on nutritional anaemia. Best Pract Res Clin Haematol. 2005;18(2):333–46.
26. Berger J, Dillon JC. [Control of iron deficiency in developing countries]. Strategies de controle de la carence en fer dans les pays en developpement. Sante. 2002;12(1):22–30.
27. FFI. Egypt, summary January 2011–2012 [cited 23 April 2012]. p. 2. Available from: http://www.sph.emory.edu/wheatflour//Africa.php-countryprofiles.
28. WHO. Vitamin and mineral nutrition information system (VMNIS); Egypt. WHO; 2012 [cited 23 April 2012]. Available from: http://who.int/vmnis/anaemia/data/database/countries/egy_ida.pdf.
29. Demmouche A, Lazrag A, Moulessehoul S. Prevalence of anaemia in pregnant women during the last trimester: consequence for birth weight. Eur Rev Med Pharmacol Sci. 2011;15(4):436–45.
30. Al Dallal ZS, Hussain KM. Impact of the national flour fortification program on the prevalence of iron deficiency and anemia among women at the reproductive age in the Kingdom of Bahrain. Manama-Bahrain: Ministry of Health, Kingdom of Bahrain; 2003.
31. El Hamdouchi A, El Kari K, Rjimati L, El Haloui N, El Mzibri M, Aguenaou H, et al. [Impact of flour fortification with elemental iron on the prevalence of anaemia among preschool children in Morocco]. Impact de l'enrichissement de la farine en fer elementaire sur la prevalence de l'anemie chez les enfants en age prescolaire au Maroc. East Mediterr Health J. 2010;16(11):1148–52.
32. National micronutrient survey. Amman, Jordan: Ministry of Health, Jordan; Global Alliance for Improved Nutrition (GAIN); Centers for Disease Control (CDC); and United Nations Children Fund (UNICEF)-Jordan; 2010.

33. Johnson Q. Information on fortification in the middle east. In: Alasfoor D, editor. electronic mail ed. 2012; 1. Personal communication through e mail with Quentin Johnson, Miller Expert.
34. WHO. Worldwide prevalence of anaemia 1993–2005: WHO global database on anaemia. Geneva: World Health Organization; 2008. p. 40.
35. Sadighi J, Mohammad K, Sheikholeslam R, Amirkhani MA, Torabi P, Salehi F, et al. Anaemia control: lessons from the flour fortification programme. Public Health. 2009;123(12):794–9.
36. Zimmermann MB, Hurrell RF. Nutritional iron deficiency. Lancet. 2007;370(9586):511–20.
37. Horton S. The economics of food fortification. J Nutr. 2006;136(4):1068–71.
38. Sue Horton VMAW. Micronutrient fortification; food fortification with iron and iodine. Copenhagen consensus 2008. Copenhagen: Copenhagen Consensus Center; 2008
39. Baltussen R, Knai C, Sharan M. Iron fortification and iron supplementation are cost-effective interventions to reduce iron deficiency in four subregions of the world. J Nutr. 2004;134(10):2678–84.
40. Cotta RM, Oliveira Fde C, Magalhaes KA, Ribeiro AQ, Sant'Ana LF, Priore SE, et al. Social and biological determinants of iron deficiency anemia. Cad Saude Publica. 2011;27 Suppl 2:S309–20.
41. Bowley A. Mandatory floof enrichment. Nutriview [Internet]. 2003;Special Issue:19.
42. Zimmerman S. Information of fortification in the middle east. In: Alasfoor D, editor. 2011. e-mail personal communication with Sara Zimmerman.
43. Sharif IEA. Information on fortification in the middle east. In: Alasfoor D, editor. Description of the fortification program in Sudan; 2011. p. 3. e-mail personal communication with Izzeldin Sharif.
44. FFI. Cartographer map of global progress, fortification status 2012. Atlanta: FFI; 2012.

Chapter 5
Food Fortification Policy in Canada

Jocelyn Sacco

Key Points

- Food fortification has a long history of use in Canada to address public health needs.
- The earliest evidence of food fortification in Canada was the iodization of salt; other major fortification policies include the mandatory addition of B vitamins and iron to flour, the fortification of milk and margarine with vitamin D, and the folic acid fortification of enriched cereal grains.
- The desire to harmonize with the fortification policies of major trading partners was often an important consideration in the decision to fortify.
- The addition of vitamins and minerals to foods without evidence of public health need is increasing in Canada.
- The implications of expanded voluntary food fortification for population health are unclear.

Keywords Fortification • Voluntary • Mandatory • Discretionary • Enrichment • Dietary patterns • Adequacy • Excess • Natural health products

Abbreviations

CCHS	Canadian Community Health Survey
DRI	Dietary reference intakes
FDR	Food and drug regulations
IMA	Interim Marketing Authorization
NHPs	Natural health products
TMAL	Temporary Marketing Authorization Letters
UL	Tolerable upper intake level

J. Sacco, B.Sc. (✉)
Department of Nutritional Sciences, University of Toronto,
Fitzgerald Building, 150 College Street, Toronto, ON, Canada M5S 3E2
e-mail: jocelyn.sacco@mail.utoronto.ca

V.R. Preedy et al. (eds.), *Handbook of Food Fortification and Health: From Concepts to Public Health Applications Volume 1*, Nutrition and Health, DOI 10.1007/978-1-4614-7076-2_5,

Introduction

This chapter presents a brief history of food fortification policy in Canada, with emphasis on some of the major developments in this practice. The guiding principles and regulatory framework for food fortification in Canada are then outlined and current directions in food fortification policy are discussed. Readers are encouraged to refer to other authors for additional reviews of this history [1–3].

A summary of the major developments in food fortification policy in Canada can be found in Table 5.1.

A number of themes arise when considering Canada's experience with food fortification. These include questions about the most appropriate foods to use as vehicles for nutrient additions and the need to balance reductions in nutrient inadequacy with the potential for excessive nutrient intake. There has also been ongoing tension over whether the addition of nutrients to foods is the best approach to correct nutrient inadequacies, compared with shifts in dietary patterns.

History of Food Fortification in Canada

Salt and Iodine

One of the first instances of food fortification in Canada was the iodization of salt. Iodine deficiency resulting in goitre was known to exist in parts of Canada in the 1920s, resulting from soils naturally poor in iodine [4]. Following the work of Marine and Kimball, who demonstrated a dramatic impact of salt iodization on goitre prevention among schoolgirls in Ohio [5, 6], salt iodization began to be practiced in Canada [7]. Iodization was initially indiscriminate, resulting in large variation in the iodine content of salt, often at levels thought to be in excess of nutritional needs [7]. Following a review directed by the National Research Council, optimal levels of iodine addition, including a minimum and maximum level, were defined for addition to salt [7]. The iodization of salt was made mandatory in 1949 [3].

Table 5.1 Summary of major developments in food fortification policy in Canada[a]

Year	Mandatory fortification	Year	Indiscriminate fortification
1944	Enrichment of flour mandated in Newfoundland (prior to entry into Canada) to address nutrient deficiencies	1964	Liberal addition of vitamins and minerals to unstandardized foods prohibited; Canada restricts food fortification to certain standardized foods, at defined levels of nutrient addition
1949	Iodization of salt is mandated to prevent goitre	2004	Introduction of NHP directorate; permits discretionary addition of nutrients to foods following approval of NHP status
1975	Mandatory fortification of milk and margarine with vitamin D to prevent rickets	2005	Discretionary food fortification proposed, no action taken
1976	Enrichment of bread and flour with thiamine, niacin, riboflavin, and iron were made mandatory to address suboptimal nutrient intakes	2011	Interim marketing authorization permits addition of vitamin D to bread and yeast-leavened bakery products
1998	Folic acid fortification of enriched cereal grain implemented to prevent neural tube defects		

[a]Unpublished

Some indication of the success of this policy was observed following a large national nutrition survey (*Nutrition Canada*) conducted in 1970–1972, which suggested that on the basis of iodine excretion alone, iodine intake was adequate, with only small prevalences of goitre still observed in some areas [8]. However these were not attributed to inadequate iodine intake [8, 9]. Generally, the iodization of salt is thought to be responsible for eliminating goitre in Canada [3].

Nutrition in Newfoundland

Some of the early development of food fortification practices began in Newfoundland, a large island off the eastern coast of Canada, prior to its entry into Canada. This is further described in Box 5.1.

Box 5.1 Nutrition in Newfoundland

In Newfoundland, a reliance on fishing and land ill-suited for agriculture led to poor dietary practices [84]. Prior to its entry into Canada in 1949, widespread symptoms of nutrient deficiency had been reported, leading to the organization of a large nutrition study of the area, including clinical evaluations, to better evaluate the extent of the problem [84]. The study revealed high prevalences of vitamin A, C, and riboflavin deficiency, and some indication of thiamine and niacin deficiency.

In 1943, prior to the release of the study findings, the Government of Newfoundland mandated the enrichment of white flour with thiamine, niacin, riboflavin, and iron; this had taken effect by 1944, just after the study had been completed [17]. In 1947, calcium was added to enriched flour in Newfoundland [17]. This enrichment policy was made possible by the recent synthesis of thiamine in 1935, followed by the synthesis of riboflavin and niacin shortly thereafter [16, 85, 86]. It was recognized that milling of white flour resulted in large losses of thiamine and other B vitamins in the flour and that the addition of vitamins to flour may correct these inadequacies [15]. Although changes in dietary patterns also had the potential to correct these deficiencies, it was generally perceived that Canadians were resistant to increasing their intakes of whole wheat flour and bread [15].

Because much of the land in Newfoundland was not suitable for agriculture [84], milk production was very limited. This fostered the growth of the margarine industry [87]. In 1945 margarine was fortified with vitamin A in Newfoundland to make it a better substitute for butter [17].

A follow-up survey in Newfoundland in 1948 noted marked improvements in the symptoms of thiamine, vitamin A, niacin, and riboflavin deficiencies, and this was attributed to the fortification of flour and margarine [17]. Although margarine had been historically banned for sale in Canada, when Newfoundland joined Canada in 1949, margarine became permitted for sale in the rest of the country [87].

Enrichment of Bread and Flour in Canada

In 1939, dietary surveys conducted in Halifax, Quebec, Toronto, and Edmonton suggested that poor intake of thiamine, among other nutrients, was a problem in Canada [10–14]. An assessment of other B vitamins was not conducted, but intakes were presumed to be poor because thiamine, niacin, and riboflavin were thought to be found together in most foods. Although beriberi, or acute thiamine deficiency, was not widespread, milder clinical presentations were of concern and action was felt to be warranted [15].

The enrichment of bread and flour was taking place in the United States by 1941 [16], and in Newfoundland, by 1944 [17]. However in Canada there was some argument against the addition of only a few nutrients to flour, when it was apparent that other nutrients were being lost in the milling of white flour, not all of which could be synthesized and added back [18]. At this time the addition of synthetic nutrients was perceived to be a form of adulteration [19], and Canada instead opted to encourage retention of these nutrients in flour through different milling processes [15, 20]. This process, developed by F.F. Tisdall in 1941 produced flour that was soon standardized in Canada as "Canada Approved Vitamin B White Flour" [19]. This flour was not widely taken up for use by industry because of perceived challenges in production and difficulty marketing, and by 1944 it was estimated that only 7 % of flour consumed in Canada was "Canada Approved" [19].

In the mid- to late-1940s, nutrition surveys were conducted across Canada by the Department of National Health and Welfare that measured dietary intake and conducted physical examinations (including blood analyses) [21–23]. These surveys documented signs of micronutrient deficiencies for a number of nutrients, particularly for vitamin D and riboflavin, and to a lesser extent vitamin C, iron, and vitamin A. These deficiencies rarely led to advanced nutrient deficiency diseases but often resulted in milder clinical symptoms [21–23]. While some were critical of the need for enrichment in Canada, given that thiamine and niacin deficiency (mild or severe) were not widely reported [21, 24], voluntary enrichment of white flour with thiamine, riboflavin, niacin, and iron was permitted in Canada by 1953, in part due to a push from the baking and milling industries to harmonize with the United States [25, 26]. Allowing flour enrichment also harmonized practices with Newfoundland, which was now a part of Canada and employing mandatory enrichment of flour [27].

Following the Nutrition Canada survey, nutrient intakes were perceived to be suboptimal and a number of mandatory enrichment options were proposed, including the addition of thiamine, riboflavin, niacin, and iron to flour [8, 28, 29]. By 1976 the addition of thiamine, riboflavin, niacin, and iron at specified levels became mandatory [30].

Vitamin D Fortification in Canada

Canada has historically had a high incidence of rickets [23]. This can be attributed to poor vitamin D intake because of the limited food sources of this nutrient, coupled with the low synthesis in the skin due to insufficient sunlight exposure for much of the year [31].

In 1929 the number of deaths reported due to rickets was 203, and this declined to 34 by 1944 [23]. This followed the introduction of irradiated yeast which was fed to cows, increasing the vitamin D content of milk [8]. By 1946, vitamin D insufficiency remained a problem, as evidence of "definite" or "past" rickets was noted among a large proportion of children 5 years and younger in surveys in British Columbia and Saskatchewan [23].

By 1964, vitamin D addition to foods was widespread, and was being added to such foods as fluid milk (although the practice varied widely by province), evaporated milk, milk powder, chocolate drink powders, fruit drinks, breakfast cereals, baby biscuits, and margarine [2, 32]. The widespread voluntary addition of vitamin D to such foods was thought to contribute to a large number of children 1–5 years with excessive vitamin D intakes, while at the same time, rickets persisted [2]. In 1964, the Food and Drug Directorate amended the food and drug regulations (FDR) to ban the addition of vitamin D to all foods except for evaporated milk, margarine, and infant foods [33–35], although fluid milk was added to the list of foods permitted for vitamin D addition in 1965 [2]. The move to restrict vitamin D fortification followed reports of hypercalcemia among infants in the UK and Switzerland, which were attributed to excessive vitamin D intake from fortified foods and dietary supplements [33]. Similar concerns of excessive vitamin D intakes among infants in Canada had also been expressed [36]. However, because the addition of vitamin D to these foods was voluntary, exposure was variable and rickets remained a problem among children [37, 38]. Acknowledging the increase in rickets in the country, the Canadian Council on Nutrition *recommended* that it should be mandatory that all forms of milk be fortified with vitamin D (within minimum and maximum levels) [38]. It was perceived that this would not pose risk of excess within the permitted range of nutrient addition, given current milk consumption patterns and common use of vitamin D supplements [35, 38]. It appears that some provinces began adopting this practice right away by making the addition of vitamin D at the dairy level permissible [39], but poor vitamin D intakes among infants, children, and adolescents were still reported in the Nutrition Canada survey [40]. The addition of vitamin D to milk and margarine was made mandatory in Canada in 1975 [27], and this policy is credited with eliminating rickets in Canada [27]. The addition of vitamin D to milk and margarine was made mandatory in Canada in 1975 [27], and is believed to have dramatically reduced the prevalence of rickets [27]. However, this problem appears to persist in Canada. In 2004–2006, 104 cases of vitamin D deficiency rickets were reported in young children across Canada [41], suggesting that alternative strategies may be needed to address this problem.

Indiscriminate Addition of Vitamins and Minerals to Foods in Canada

By 1939 there were a variety of nutrition-related claims appearing on foods in Canada that were perceived to be misleading or exaggerated [42]. This resulted in revisions to the FDR in 1941 that restricted the types of claims that may be made and set a minimum amount of nutrient that must be present for any claim to be made (these corresponded with amounts thought to reflect "good" or "excellent" sources of the nutrient per reasonable daily intake of the food), and set minimum amounts for nutrient addition [3, 42, 43]. In 1949, maximum permitted levels of nutrient addition were established [3].

The addition of vitamins and minerals to foods as a marketing tool was common in the early 1960s [2, 25, 32, 34]. After 1964, the indiscriminate addition of vitamins and minerals to foods was prohibited in order to prevent consumer deception [2, 34]. These regulations continued to permit the addition of certain vitamins and minerals to certain foods (e.g., breakfast cereals), at predefined amounts. Nutrient addition to unstandardized foods was prohibited [34].

Following evidence of suboptimal nutrient intakes from the Nutrition Canada Survey, voluntary breakfast cereal fortification was expanded to permit the restoration of nutrients lost during processing [44, 45]. In response to industry requests, zinc was added to this list in 1989 [46].

Folic Acid Fortification

In the 1980s a growing body of evidence suggested a potential link between increasing intake of folic acid and a reduction of neural tube defects. This was supported by many observational studies and by the early 1990s, a number of large randomized controlled trials [47–49].

Folic acid is required for the proper formation of the neural tube during prenatal development, which occurs early in the first trimester; often before a woman knows she is pregnant [47]. Although encouraging supplementation of folic acid among women of childbearing age had been identified as an option to prevent neural tube defects, there are many challenges to this approach, including the potential for poor compliance [50], therefore food fortification was pursued as a way to reduce the prevalence of neural tube defects.

The voluntary fortification of enriched bread, flour, pasta, cornmeal, rice, and other grain products with folic acid was implemented in the United States in March 1996 and fortification was made mandatory

Jan 1, 1998 [51, 52]. In order to reduce barriers to trade, and to prevent neural tube defects, Canada moved to permit voluntary folic acid fortification shortly after the United States (December 1996) [53–55]. Voluntary fortification of enriched cereal grains was made mandatory in December 1998.

A large reduction in the incidence of neural tube defects in Canada has been observed since the implementation of the policy. There is evidence that neural tube defects have declined by as much as 46 % in Canada [56], and this decline was even greater in provinces with higher baseline prevalences, for example reductions in Newfoundland and Labrador reached 78 % by 2003 [54, 56].

Although this policy has been successful, concerns about adverse effects of mandatory folic acid fortification have been expressed. One concern, recognized prior to the implementation of the policy, was the potential for masking the hematologic signs of vitamin B12 deficiency, which could allow the neurological symptoms to progress unnoticed [47]. More recently, there is emerging evidence of a relationship between high folic acid intake and an increased risk of colorectal cancer [53, 57, 58], although at this stage the research is equivocal [59].

Recent estimates of red blood cell folate levels from a nationally representative sample of Canadians suggest that the prevalence of folate inadequacy in the population falls below 5 % and the proportion of women of childbearing age with red blood cell folate levels below the cut-off considered optimal to prevent neural tube defects is 22 % [60]. However, a large proportion of the population has a red blood cell folate status considered to be "high," which is far in excess of need [60]. Whether or not these levels translate into adverse effects for health is unclear, but it highlights the challenges associated with implementing population-wide fortification in order to address nutrient intakes in a subset of the population, and reinforces the need to continue monitoring the impact of this policy on health.

Current Framework for Food Fortification Policy in Canada

Guiding Principles

Canada uses food fortification in a manner consistent with the guidance in the Codex Alimentarius [27, 61], a set of internationally recognized food standards developed by the Codex Alimentarius Commission, which was established by the Food and Agriculture Organization and World Health Organization. These guiding principles are described in Box 5.2.

Box 5.2 Codex Basic Principles for the Addition of Essential Nutrients to Foods

The Codex Alimentarius guidelines for the addition of nutrients to foods describe the use of fortification:

- To address documented nutritional needs
- To maintain the nutritional equivalence of substitute foods (e.g., nondairy milk beverages)
- To restore nutrients lost during processing, handling, or storage
- For special purpose foods (e.g., meal replacements)

Furthermore, the Codex guidelines specify that the nutrient added should be available in nutritionally significant amounts that do not lead to excessive intakes, is stable in the food and biologically available. The guidelines also discourage the addition of vitamins and minerals to foods that may mislead or deceive consumers [61].

Current Regulatory Framework

The addition of vitamins and minerals to foods in Canada is currently regulated under the Food and Drugs Act. Part D division 3 of the Food and Drugs Regulations (FDR) outlines a list of nutrients that can be added to foods, and to which foods they can be added [62]. Standards of identity for these foods in the FDR prescribe the maximum and minimum amounts at which the specific nutrients can be added. A regulatory amendment to the FDR is required for additional foods to be fortified or nutrients to be added. However, in some cases (e.g., calcium fortified orange juice), a Temporary Marketing Authorization Letters (TMAL) or Interim Marketing Authorizations (IMAs) has been issued, which permits a product to be sold temporarily, before the regulatory change is finalized. Requests for IMAs for the addition of nutrients to foods must be consistent with Codex Alimentarius principles (FDR, B.01.056).

Expansion of Voluntary Food Fortification in Canada

Proposal for Discretionary Fortification

In 2005, Health Canada proposed a food fortification policy that, if adopted, would amend the Food and Drugs Regulations to permit manufacturers to add vitamins and minerals to a wide variety of foods at their discretion, a practice referred to at the time as "discretionary fortification" [63]. The policy was designed to facilitate trade harmonization, recognizing more liberal fortification policies in the United States and Europe, and to provide Canadians with a greater variety of food sources of nutrients. Outlined in the policy proposal was a list of nutrients to be permitted to be added to foods, and the maximum and minimum levels at which they could be added. These amounts correspond with those needed for nutrient content claims (e.g., "good" or "excellent" source claims) on food labels. Consistent with similar policies in other jurisdictions [64, 65], Health Canada's proposed discretionary fortification policy excluded standardized and staple foods and beverages from being fortified. Because they are so widely consumed, permitting their indiscriminate fortification was thought to pose unacceptable risk of excessive nutrient intake. Additional regulations were proposed to permit the expansion of breakfast cereal fortification to encompass a greater variety of nutrients, often at higher levels of addition.

Since its release, Health Canada's proposed policy has been shrouded in controversy largely because of concerns that discretionary fortification will function to reinforce poor dietary patterns and contribute to obesogenic diets [66–68]. Although consultations continue [69], it appears that Health Canada's discretionary fortification policy, as proposed in 2005, is no longer planned for adoption in its current form, although the changes to breakfast cereal fortification are thought to be moving forward [68].

Importantly, this policy direction reflected a shift away from the guiding principles, outlined by the Codex Alimentarius, that Canada has traditionally followed, towards food fortification without a public health rationale. Health Canada has since proposed the incorporation of discretionary fortification principles into Codex guidelines [61, 70].

Three evaluations of the health implications of the proposed discretionary fortification policy have been conducted. Although this policy has not been implemented, food fortification at the discretion of the manufacturer is expanding in Canada via alternative regulatory avenues (described in the subsequent section) and insights gained from examinations of the original policy proposal can inform current developments.

In order to explore the implications of the policy for dietary patterns in Canada, Sacco and Tarasuk conducted an analysis of the consumption of foods eligible to be fortified under the proposed discretionary fortification policy using nationally representative dietary intake data from the Canadian

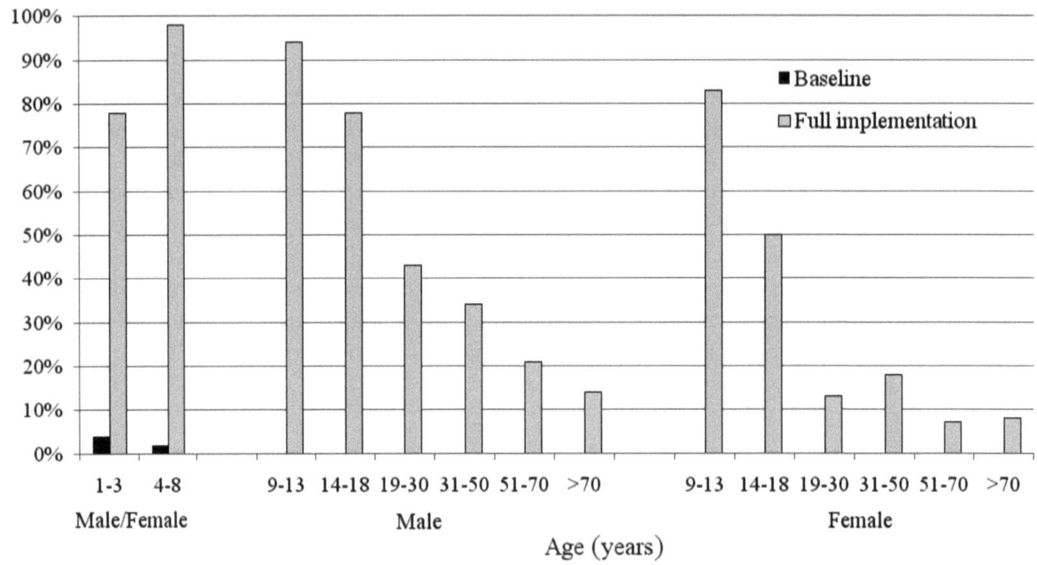

Fig. 5.1 Impact of discretionary fortification, as modeled in the CCHS (2004), on the proportion of the population that exceeds the tolerable upper intake level for niacin (adapted from Sacco and Tarasuk J Nutr. 2009;139(10):1980–6)

Community Health Survey (CCHS), Cycle 2.2 (2004) [71]. They found that the consumption of these foods is negatively associated with intake of fruits and vegetable, milk products, fiber, and other indices of healthy eating [71]. Furthermore, many of these eligible foods are highlighted in Canada's Food Guide as "foods to limit" [72].

Further concerns arise regarding the slate of nutrients proposed to be eligible for addition, and the amounts at which they could be added. Health Canada conducted modeling of the proposed policy in order to prevent risks of excessive intake [63]. However, they used data from provincial nutrition surveys that were not nationally representative of the population, assessed a limited number of nutrients, and did not assess the potential for benefit as well as risk [63].

Using the CCHS (2004), and applying the criteria outlined in the proposed policy, Sacco and Tarasuk modeled the potential impact of the discretionary fortification policy and the proposed expansion to breakfast cereal fortification on the nutrient intakes of Canadians [73]. These results highlighted the mismatch between the proposed nutrient additions and Canadians' actual needs. While the addition of some nutrients permitted under the proposed policy could potentially reduce the prevalence of inadequate intakes in the population, some other nutrients slated for addition (e.g., niacin, thiamine, riboflavin) are already being consumed in adequate amounts by most of the population, so there would be no discernible benefit from their addition. In some instances, depending on uptake of the policy by both manufacturers and consumers, the permitted nutrient additions could increase risk of excessive nutrient intakes, particularly among children and adolescents [73]. Figure 5.1 shows the potential impact of full implementation of discretionary fortification, as modeled in the CCHS (2004), on the proportion of the population that exceeds the tolerable upper intake level (UL) for niacin.

Natural Health Products as Voluntarily Fortified Foods

The Natural Health Products Regulations is another more recent regulatory avenue through which foods can be fortified [74]. Under these regulations, foods can apply for Natural Health Product

(NHP) status. An example of an NHP currently fortified with vitamins or minerals and sold in Canada is Red Bull Energy Drink.

Although the proposed discretionary fortification policy has not been formally adopted, the voluntary addition of vitamins and minerals to foods without a public health rationale has begun to occur through NHP regulations [74]. These regulations, introduced in 2004, were designed to create standards for safety and efficacy for products such as herbal remedies, vitamins, minerals, homeopathic, and traditional Chinese medicines. The regulations do not expressly exclude NHPs from assuming a "food-format"; hence foods adding nutrients or making certain claims prohibited for foods under the FDR may be eligible for NHP status, and legally sold in Canada. Acknowledging that ambiguities exist with respect to whether certain foods can be considered NHPs, Health Canada has published a guidance document on this issue [75]. Whether such products are regulated as foods or NHPs depends on how they are represented, public perception and traditional use of the food, as well as its composition and format [75].

A major concern surrounding this new direction in Canadian food fortification policy is that there are no apparent restrictions on the maximum permitted levels of nutrient addition or on the types of foods permitted for fortification. This is particularly concerning because one fortified beverage was recently available in Canada containing retinol at the level at which the UL is set. (The critical adverse effect for which the UL was established is hepatotoxicity among the general population and teratogenicity among women of childbearing age [76].) Very recently, following concerns expressed by nutrition experts [77], the beverage manufacturer has indicated that the retinol will be reduced to one-third of the original amount.

Interim Marketing Authorization for the Addition of Vitamin D to Bread

In recent years there has been increasing interest in the relationship between vitamin D and health, with a growing body of literature linking this nutrient to chronic disease risk. Revised Dietary Reference Intakes (DRI) for vitamin D (and calcium) were established in 2010 which outline updated requirement estimates that take into consideration this new literature base [31]. Recent evaluations of vitamin D intake and status among Canadians found that intake of this nutrient is inadequate for optimal bone health for 26 % of the population [78, 79]. This suggests that there is potential benefit to be gained by the addition of this nutrient to foods, particularly because there are so few foods in which vitamin D is found naturally. This has resulted in some discussion of expanding the existing vitamin D fortification practices in Canada [79, 80].

In February 2011, in response to a submission by a member of the baking industry [81], an IMA was issued for the voluntary addition of vitamin D to bread and "unstandardized yeast-leavened bakery products." This would allow a maximum of 90 IU (2.25 μg) of vitamin D to be added per 100 g of product, permitting a product to display a "source of vitamin D" claim. The rationale for this IMA is that it will allow for a broader range of vitamin D fortified products, which would be of benefit to both consumers and the food industry [82].

Although an increase in vitamin D intake for many Canadians would likely be of some benefit, adopting voluntary fortification as an approach to addressing this public health problem raises some concerns. Specifically, benefit can only be realized by those purchasing these products, and it is unclear if those consuming them are likely to be those in need. Although bread is widely consumed and has been a successful vehicle in delivering other nutrients to Canadians under mandatory fortification policies, the voluntary nature of this policy suggests that not all manufacturers will take up this opportunity. Additionally, the fact that other bakery products would be eligible for fortification (e.g., doughnuts), raises some concerns over the implications of adding nutrients to foods otherwise considered unhealthy [72, 82].

Conclusion

In Canada, food fortification practices have evolved in response to public health needs. In many cases these practices began as short-term voluntary fortification policies that later became mandatory. These mandatory food fortification policies have been responsible for correcting a variety of nutrient deficiencies over the last century. Although there was a period prior to 1964 when fortification of unstandardized foods was voluntary and largely unrestricted, Canada has since tightly regulated the addition of vitamins and minerals to foods. However, in recent years regulatory changes have allowed for an increase in fortification practices at the discretion of the manufacturer.

As food fortification evolved in Canada, the goal was often one of achieving balance between addressing nutrient needs and preventing excessive nutrient intakes. It has also been shaped by the desire to harmonize with other regulatory jurisdictions, which resulted in the need to weigh industry and trade considerations against public health concern. The literature on food fortification in Canada also raises questions about the necessity of some nutrient additions and the impact of food fortification on dietary patterns.

Recommendations

Dietary assessment methodology has advanced dramatically over the past few decades, improving our ability to assess the impact of food fortification policies on nutrient intakes and delineate population health implications. For example, the establishment of ULs provided, for the first time, benchmarks against which the potential for excessive nutrient intake can be evaluated [83]. In order to facilitate evaluation and monitoring of fortification policies and practices, nutrient composition databases for use in future nutrition surveys should be better designed to capture food fortification, particularly voluntary food fortification.

It is important that we continue to monitor the implications of food fortification policies in Canada, both mandatory and voluntary, on population health, particularly in the context of changing dietary patterns and our evolving understanding of the role of nutrients in health and disease.

References

1. Nathoo T, Holmes C, Ostry A. An analysis of the development of Canadian food fortification policies: the case of vitamin B. Health Promot Int. 2005;20(4):375–82.
2. Cheney MC. Canadian experience with food fortification. Public Health Rev. 2000;28(1–4):171–7.
3. Institute of Medicine (IOM). Dietary reference intakes: guiding principles for nutrition labeling and fortification. Washington, DC: National Academies Press; 2003.
4. Graham D. The use and abuse of iodine in the treatment of goitre. Can Med Assoc J. 1924;14(9):821.
5. Kimball OP, Rogoff JM, Marine D. The prevention of simple goiter in man: third paper. J Am Med Assoc. 1919;73(25):1873–4.
6. Marine D, Kimball OP. Prevention of goiter in man. J Lab Clin Med. 1917;3:40–3.
7. Lathe FE. The use of iodized salt in Canada. Can Med Assoc J. 1936;34(6):711.
8. Bureau of Nutritional Sciences. Nutrition Canada—Ontario survey. Ottawa: Health and Welfare Canada; 1975.
9. Murray TK. Prevalence of goiter in Canada. Am J Clin Nutr. 1977;30:1573–5.
10. Patterson JM, McHenry EW. A dietary investigation in Toronto families having annual incomes between $1,500–$2,400. Can J Public Health. 1941;32(2):251.
11. Young EG. A dietary survey in Halifax. Can J Public Health. 1941;32(2):236.
12. Hunter G, Pett LB. A dietary survey in Edmonton. Can J Public Health. 1941;32(2):259.
13. Sylvestre JE, Nadeau H. Enquete sur l'alimentation habituelle des familles de petits-salaries dans la ville de Quebec. Can J Public Health. 1941;32(5):241.

14. Pett LB. Canadian nutrition around 1950. Can J Public Health. 1972;63(2):161.
15. Tisdall FF, Jackson SH, Drake TGH, et al. The retention of the wheat vitamins in flour and bread, a problem of national importance. Can Med Assoc J. 1941;45(2):101–5.
16. Sebrell WH. Recollections of a career in nutrition. J Nutr. 1985;115(1):23–38.
17. Aykroyd WR, Jolliffe N, Lowry OH, et al. Medical resurvey of nutrition in Newfoundland 1948. Can Med Assoc J. 1949;60(4):329.
18. McHenry EW. Observations on the nutritive value of bread. Can J Public Health. 1940;31:428.
19. Wilder RM, Williams RR. Enrichment of flour and bread: a history of the movement. Bulletin of the National Research Council. Washington, DC: National Academy of Sciences; 1944.
20. Tisdall FF. High extraction wheaten flour. Can Med Assoc J. 1944;50:564.
21. Pett LB. Are there nutritional problems in Canada? Can Med Assoc J. 1948;59:326.
22. Pett LB, Hanley FW. A nutrition survey on a Nova Scotian island. Can Med Assoc J. 1948;59(3):230–6.
23. Pett LB, Hanley FW. A nutrition survey among school children in British Colombia and Saskatchewan. Can Med Assoc J. 1947;56:187.
24. Pett LB. Ottawa newsletter: flour and bread. Can Med Assoc J. 1956;75(9):777.
25. Curran RE. Regulatory control in Canada under the Food and Drugs Act. Food Drug Cosmet Law J. 1962;17:312.
26. Wilder RM. A brief history of the enrichment of flour and bread. JAMA. 1956;162(17):1539–41.
27. Bureau of Nutritional Sciences, Food Directorate, Health Protection Branch. The addition of vitamins and minerals to foods: proposed policy recommendations. Ottawa: Health Canada; 1999.
28. Chapman DG. Current topics in Canadian food regulatory affairs. Food Drug Cosmet Law J. 1975;30:654.
29. Bureau of Nutritional Sciences, Health Protection Branch, Department of National Health and Welfare. Nutrition Canada—food consumption patterns report. Ottawa: DNHW; 1975.
30. Robbins L, Barewal S. The apparent nutritive value of food available for consumption in Canada, 1960–75. Canada: Information Services Agriculture; 1981.
31. Institute of Medicine (IOM). Dietary reference intakes for calcium and vitamin D. Washington, DC: National Academies Press; 2011.
32. Beaton GH, McHenry EW, editors. Nutrition: a comprehensive treatise. Nutritional status: assessment and application. New York: Academic; 1966. p. 3.
33. Broadfoot BVR, Trenholme MA, McClinton EP, Cowan EJ. Vitamin D intakes of Ontario children. Can Med Assoc J. 1966;94:332.
34. Chapman RA, Morrison AB. Regulatory agencies and food safety. Can Med Assoc J. 1966;94(12):609–13.
35. Campbell ME. Vitamin D—too much or too little. N S Med Bull. 1966;45(8):201.
36. Mott GA, Ross RH, Smith DJ. A study of vitamin C and D intake of infants in the metropolitan Vancouver area. Can J Public Health. 1964;55:341–5.
37. Barsky P. Rickets: Canada: 1968. Can J Public Health. 1969;60:29.
38. Evidence in support of the desirability of the addition of vitamin D to milk. Can J Public Health. 1968;59(8):328.
39. Barsky P. Vitamin D, and rickets. Manit Med Rev. 1967;47(6):291.
40. Sabry ZI, Campbell E, Campbell JA, Forbes AL. Nutrition Canada—a national nutrition survey. Nutr Rev. 1974;32(4):105–11.
41. Ward LM, Gaboury I, Ladhani M, Zlotkin S. Vitamin D-deficiency rickets among children in Canada. Can Med Assoc J. 2007;177(2):161–6.
42. Davidson AL. The genesis and growth of food and drug administration in Canada. Ottawa: Ministry of National Health and Welfare; 1949.
43. Government of Canada. Orders in council. Canada Gaz. 1941;74(51):4491–3.
44. Regulations amending the food and drug regulations: breakfast cereals (SOR/83-858). Canada Gazette Part II. 1983;117(22):95. Available at: http://www.collectionscanada.gc.ca/databases/canada-gazette/093/001060-119.01-e.php?document_id_nbr=10795&image_id_nbr=525909&f=p&PHPSESSID=1enp9kdu2sk05bqsgfhlhub045
45. Regulatory agendas: addition of vitamins and mineral nutrients to breakfast cereals. Canada Gazette Part I. 1983;117(47), Supplement 2, p. 296. Available at: http://www.collectionscanada.gc.ca/databases/canada-gazette/093/001060-119.01-e.php?image_id_nbr=698019&document_id_nbr=11446&f=p&PHPSESSID=1enp9kdu2sk05bqsgfhlhub045
46. Food and Drug Regulations. Amendment (SOR/89-145). Canada Gaz II. 1989;123(7):1849.
47. Institute of Medicine (IOM). Dietary reference intakes for thiamin, riboflavin, niacin, vitamin B6, folate, vitamin B12, pantothenic acid, biotin and choline. Washington, DC: National Academies Press; 1998.
48. Czeizel AE, Dudas I. Prevention of the first occurrence of neural-tube defects by periconceptional vitamin supplementation. N Engl J Med. 1992;327:1832–5.
49. MRC Vitamin Study Research Group. Prevention of neural tube defects: results of the medical research council vitamin study. Lancet. 1991;338(8760):131–7.
50. Nestle M. Folate fortification and neural tube defects: policy implications. J Nutr Educ. 1994;26(6):287–92.

51. White Junod S. Folic acid fortification: fact and folley. 2009. Available at: http://www.fda.gov/AboutFDA/WhatWeDo/History/ProductRegulation/SelectionsFromFDLIUpdateSeriesonFDAHistory/ucm091883.htm. Accessed 31 Aug 2011.
52. Food and Drug Administration. Food standards: amendment of standards of identity for enriched grain products to require addition of folic acid. Fed Regist. 1996;61:8781–97.
53. Kim YI. Will mandatory folic acid fortification prevent or promote cancer? Am J Clin Nutr. 2004;80(5):1123.
54. Public Health Agency of Canada. Evaluation of food fortification with folic acid for the primary prevention of neural tube defects (1997–2003): executive summary. 2004. Available at: http://www.phac-aspc.gc.ca/publicat/faaf/index-eng.php. Accessed 7 Oct 2011.
55. Regulations amending the food and drug regulations (SOR/96-527). Canada Gazette Part II. 1996;130(26):40–43. Available at: http://www.collectionscanada.gc.ca/databases/canada-gazette/093/001060-119.01-e.php?image_id_nbr=952245&document_id_nbr=14922&f=p&PHPSESSID=1enp9kdu2sk05bqsgfhlhub045
56. De Wals P, Tairou F, Van Allen MI, et al. Reduction in neural-tube defects after folic acid fortification in Canada. N Engl J Med. 2007;357(2):135–42.
57. Mason JB, Cole BF, Baron JA, Kim YI, Smith AD. Folic acid fortification and cancer risk. Lancet. 2008;371(9621):1335; author reply 1335–6.
58. Mason JB, Dickstein A, Jacques PF, et al. A temporal association between folic acid fortification and an increase in colorectal cancer rates may be illuminating important biological principles: a hypothesis. Cancer Epidemiol Biomarkers Prev. 2007;16(7):1325–9.
59. Kennedy DA, Stern SJ, Moretti M, et al. Folate intake and the risk of colorectal cancer: a systematic review and meta-analysis. Cancer Epidemiol. 2011;35(1):2–10.
60. Colapinto CK, O'Connor DL, Tremblay MS. Folate status of the population in the Canadian Health Measures Survey. Can Med Assoc J. 2011;183(2):E100–6.
61. Codex Alimentarius Commission. General principles for the addition of essential nutrients to foods. CAC/GL 09-1987. Rome: WHO and the FAO of the United Nations; 1991.
62. Food and Drugs Regulations (FDR). Part D. Vitamins and minerals. Division 3. Addition of vitamins, mineral nutrients or amino acids to foods. Available at: http://laws-lois.justice.gc.ca/eng/regulations/C.R.C.%2C_c._870/. Accessed 7 Oct 2011.
63. Health Canada. Addition of vitamins and minerals to foods: health Canada's proposed policy and implementation plans. 2005. Available at: http://www.hc-sc.gc.ca/fnan/nutrition/vitamin/fortification_final_doc_1-eng.php. Accessed 30 Aug 2011.
64. European Parliament. Regulation (EC) no 1925/2006 of the European Parliament and of the Council of 20 December 2006 on the addition of vitamins and minerals and of certain other substances to foods. Off J Eur Union. 2006;49:26–38.
65. Food and Drug Administration. 21 Code of federal regulations, Subpart B. Section 104.20. Fortification policy. Washington, DC: FDA; 1993. Available at: http://www.accessdata.fda.gov/scripts/cdrh/cfdocs/cfcfr/CFRSearch.cfm?fr=104.20. Accessed 7 Oct 2011.
66. Dieticians of Canada. Position on discretionary fortification of foods with vitamins and minerals. 2009. Available at: http://www.dietitians.ca/Downloadable-Content/Public/foodfortification-position-paper.aspx. Accessed 7 Oct 2011.
67. Beauchesne E, Kondro K. Health Canada contemplates providing food industry with 'discretionary' authority to fortify junk foods. Can Med Assoc J. 2009;180(12):1196.
68. Freedhoff Y. Fortified food loophole or natural health product? Can Med Assoc J. 2010;182(8):E333–4.
69. Yan W. Invitation letter to stakeholders: think-tank on expanded voluntary addition of vitamins and minerals to foods; 2010.
70. Codex Alimentarius Commission. Discussion paper on the proposal for new work to amend the codex general principles for the addition of essential nutrients to foods. CAC/GL 09–1987. Rome: WHO and the FAO of the United Nations; 2007.
71. Sacco JE, Tarasuk V. Discretionary addition of vitamins and minerals to foods: implications for healthy eating. Eur J Clin Nutr. 2010;65(3):313–20.
72. Health Canada. Canada's food guide. 2007. Available from: http://www.hc-sc.gc.ca/fn-an/food-guide-aliment/index-eng.php. Accessed 7 Oct 2011.
73. Sacco JE, Tarasuk V. Health Canada's proposed discretionary fortification policy is misaligned with the nutritional needs of Canadians. J Nutr. 2009;139(10):1980–6.
74. Health Canada. Natural health products directorate. Available at: http://www.hc-sc.gc.ca/dhp-mps/prodnatur/index-eng.php. Accessed 7 Oct 2011.
75. Natural Health Products Directorate and Food Directorate. Classification of products at the natural health product interface: products in food formats, version 1.0. Ottawa: Health Canada; 2009.
76. Institute of Medicine (IOM). Dietary reference intakes for vitamin A, vitamin K, arsenic, boron, chromium, copper, iron, manganese, molybdenum, nickel, silicon, vanadium, zinc. Washington, DC: National Academy Press; 2002.

77. Schmidt S. Coca-Cola alters drink in response to experts concerns. 2011. http://www.canada.com/health/Coca+Cola+alters+drink+response+experts+concerns/5444192/story.html. Accessed 7 Oct 2011.
78. Whiting SJ, Langlois KA, Vatanparast H, Greene-Finestone LS. The vitamin D status of Canadians relative to the 2011 dietary reference intakes: an examination in children and adults with and without supplement use. Am J Clin Nutr. 2011;94(1):128–35.
79. Vatanparast H, Calvo MS, Green TJ, Whiting SJ. Despite mandatory fortification of staple foods, vitamin D intakes of Canadian children and adults are inadequate. J Steroid Biochem Mol Biol. 2010;121(1–2):301–3.
80. Calvo MS, Whiting SJ. Overview of the proceedings from experimental biology 2004 symposium: vitamin D insufficiency: a significant risk factor in chronic diseases and potential disease-specific biomarkers of vitamin D sufficiency. J Nutr. 2005;135(2):301–3.
81. Baking Association of Canada. Health Canada approves voluntary fortification of bakery products with vitamin D. 2011. http://www.bakingassoccanada.com/pdf/Newsletter%20-%202011.04.pdf. Accessed 7 Oct 2011.
82. Food and drug regulations—amendments. Interim marketing authorization HYPERLINK "http://www.gazette.gc.ca/rp-pr/p1/2011/2011-02-19/html/notice-avis-eng.html" \l "d103" \o "To permit the optional addition of vitamin D2-yeast to yeast-leavened bakery products (Project 1694) (external link)"to permit the optional addition of vitamin D2-yeast to yeast-leavened bakery products. Canada Gazette Part 1. 2011;145(8). Available at: http://www.hc-sc.gc.ca/fn-an/legislation/ima-amp/index-eng.php.
83. Institute of Medicine (IOM). Dietary reference intakes: applications in dietary assessment. Washington, DC: National Academy Press; 2000.
84. Adamson JD, Jolliffe N, Kruse HD, et al. Medical survey of nutrition in Newfoundland. Can Med Assoc J. 1945;52(3):227–50.
85. Baldwin RS, Robert R. Williams (1886–1965):—a biographical sketch. J Nutr. 1975;105(1):1–14.
86. Hogan AG. Riboflavin: physiology and pathology. JAMA. 1938;110(15):1188.
87. Heick WH. Margarine in Newfoundland history. Newfoundland Labr stud. 1986;2(1):29–37.

Part II
Iron Fortification

Chapter 6
Iron Fortification of Milk and Dairy Products

Philippe Cayot, Tatiana Guzun-Cojocaru, and Nathalie Cayot

Key Points

- Anaemia is a worldwide health problem, mainly due to the low availability of iron in food products.
- The bioavailability of heme iron is far greater than the one of non-heme iron.
- Dairy products consumed together with iron-rich food decrease the availability of iron but the competition between calcium and iron ions is not clear.
- Iron is naturally present in milk under the form of lactoferrin, but lactoferrin may undergo thermal denaturation during process.
- Iron salts, cheaper than lactoferrin, are preferably used to fortify dairy products. The bioavailability of iron depends on the solubility and the dissociation constant of the salts.
- To administer iron as a medicine or through iron-enriched foodstuffs is potentially dangerous because it can induce peroxidation, which increases oxidation stress.
- Encapsulation and/or stable iron complex could be a good solution to protect iron against oxidation.

Keywords Anaemia • Dairy products • Iron fortification • Iron salts • Lactoferrin • Iron-bis-glycinate • Lipid oxidation • Peroxidation

Introduction: Iron Status in Human Nutrition

World Prevalence of Iron

Blood haemoglobin level is used to define anaemia. Thresholds are given by category of age, of sex, and also of physiological status such as pregnancy. For example, the threshold is 120 g L^{-1} of haemoglobin in blood for a nonpregnant adult woman, 110 for a pregnant woman, 130 for a man older than

P. Cayot (✉) • N. Cayot
Research unit PAM, UMR MA AGROSUP 2012.02.102, Bâtiment Nord, AgroSup Dijon,
26 Boulevard du Docteur Petitjean BP 87999, 21079 Dijon, Cedex, France
e-mail: p.cayot@agrosupdijon.fr

T. Guzun-Cojocaru
Research unit EMMA, EA 581 of University of Burgundy, Bâtiment Nord, AgroSup Dijon,
26 Boulevard du Docteur Petitjean BP 87999, 21079 Dijon, Cedex, France

V.R. Preedy et al. (eds.), *Handbook of Food Fortification and Health: From Concepts to Public Health Applications Volume 1*, Nutrition and Health, DOI 10.1007/978-1-4614-7076-2_6,

15 years, 110 for a child under 5 years... Iron deficiency constitutes the most important worldwide problem of human nutrition. In 2005, 1.62 billions of people were concerned by iron deficiency. Iron deficiency is encountered mostly in poor countries and particularly in Western Pacific, except Australia and New Zealand, in India and Pakistan, in the great majority of countries in Africa, in South America, more precisely in Brazil, Peru, and Bolivia. Iron deficiency is also spread in developed countries where 26–28 % of preschool children and nonpregnant women are deficient in iron [1]. The prevalence of iron deficiency is higher for women than for men and higher for children than for adults [2]. Iron deficiency comes from diverse origins but mainly related to the low availability of iron in food products. All types of supplementation and especially pharmaceutical forms—neutraceutical—give lower results than iron fortification of foodstuffs [3]. Iron fortification of foodstuffs remains the cheapest way to avoid iron deficiency and insure the daily intake over a long period. It is also better than tablet supplements that are known for causing digestive intolerance. Pregnant women consuming iron tablets have experienced morning sickness, nausea, and vomiting [4, 5]. These side effects explain partly the low observance of pharmaceutical correction against anaemia.

Physiologic Role of Iron

Iron is present in very low quantities in human body (2.3 g for 60 kg woman, 3.8 g for a 70 kg man that is nearly 0.005 % w/w) but iron plays a capital physiologic role. Iron allows the exchange with oxygen (haemoglobin, myoglobin) and activates numerous enzymes [6].

Enzymes containing iron or enzymes using iron as a cofactor enable:

- The production of citrate (in its isocitrate form) in Krebs cycle (catalysis by aconitase)
- The synthesis of catecholamines that are useful for the development of brain (catalysis by monooxygenases such as phenylalanine hydroxylase, tyrosine hydroxylase, tryptophanehydroxylase)
- The synthesis of desoxyribonucleoside diphosphate, which constitutes DNA from ribonucleoside diphosphate (catalysis by the ribonucleotide reductase)
- The peroxidation in cells, owing to lipoxygenase

Iron is stored in the body and carried in blood plasma mainly by transferrin, ferritin, and lactoferrin.

The metabolism of iron is unusual because nearly in closed circuit. The absorption of iron takes place within the duodenal mucosal cells, but the regulation of its absorption and the existence of specific biochemical pathways are not fully elucidated. Two pathways of iron uptake have been identified. The major pathway for iron absorption uses a carrier-mediated process involving a transmembrane protein transporter for non-heme iron. Heme iron, principally haemoglobin and myoglobin from animal food products, represents only a small fraction of the iron found in diet but it is well absorbed because of a specific pathway and it can remain intact when entering the mucosal cells [7].

Guidance on Safe Levels and on Levels of Fortification in Iron

Daily Requirements of Iron Intake

Human being needs to compensate the daily loss in iron. Daily loss is quite low for a man: 14×10^{-3} mg kg^{-1} of body weight, which corresponds to 1 mg day^{-1} or so. Nonmenopausal women have to face more important losses, 1.5 mg day^{-1} on average, and even more for pregnant women. The recommended daily intake is 25 mg day^{-1} for women, 12 for men, and 6–10 for children and infants to ensure the iron requirement (1–2 mg day^{-1}) because only about 10–15 % of the consumed iron is absorbed.

Consequences of a Too Low Intake

The diseases occurring when intake is too low are numerous: decrease in immune defense [8]; retard in cognitive development of children [9]; anomalous development of children brain [10, 11]. As a consequence, low school performances of children and teenagers [12] may be observed. Anaemic adults have reduced physical and intellectual performance compared to healthy people [13], and anaemic pregnant women have a higher risk of premature infant [14]. Surprisingly, anaemia of nursing mothers and iron supplementation of nursing mothers do not change the iron concentration or the lactoferrin concentration in mother's milk [15].

Otherwise, iron deficiency increases the risk factor for increased lead absorption. Due to absorption mechanisms for lead and iron [16], lead level in children's blood may be decreased by iron supplementation.

Danger of a Too Great Intake

The acute toxicity of iron is generally set at 250 mg day^{-1} but the Medical Institute of Canada sets the limit at 100 mg day^{-1} [17]; 400 mg day^{-1} could be lethal. Chronic iron overload would increase the risk of cirrhosis, hepatitis and liver cancer, induces intestinal irritation, vomiting and diarrhoea, articular pain, hormonal disturbance, heart disorder, and osteoporosis [18–20].

Bioavailability of Iron

Different Sources of Iron; Efficient Forms

Two forms of iron exist in the human body or in foodstuffs: heme iron and non-heme iron. Heme iron is constituted by all the hemoproteins (haemoglobin, myoglobin), non-heme iron by all the transport-proteins (transferritin, ferritin, lactoferrin), some enzymes (aconitase, hydrolases, lipoxygenase), and the iron salts. Non-heme iron, Fe(II) or Fe(III)-salts, are in a non-negligible quantity (3–8 mg/100 g) in grain legumes such as chickpea, cowpea, or lentil compared to other vegetable products [21, 22]. The iron contained in grain legumes is hardly assimilated by the human body: less than 1–5 % at a maximum of the iron consumed. Anti-nutritional factors such as phytates (inositol-hexaphosphate), polyphenols, and also calcium ions are heavily decreasing the bioavailability of iron. Due to their diet, vegetarians have not only a lower intake of iron but also a very low quantity of assimilated iron [23]. Nonvegetarians may have a good iron intake and the total absorption of iron may vary between 5 and 15 %. Meat, liver, or black pudding contain not only greater quantities of iron than grain legumes but the bioavailability of the hemic-iron (myoglobin, haemoglobin) present in these animal foodstuffs is high. Compared to iron(II)sulphate, which is selected as a reference and whose bioavailability is set at 100 by definition, the bioavailability of lactoferrin scales from 100 to 800, the one of haemoglobin from 100 to 700, the ones of iron gluconate and iron phosphate are 89 and 25, respectively [24].

The Assimilation of Iron Is Decreased by the Consumption of Dairy Products

Dairy products consumed together with iron-rich food decrease the availability of iron [24]. A positive dose–response effect was observed between milk consumption and prevalence of anaemia: the more important the cow milk consumption by 6–12-month-old children, the more frequent the anaemia [25]. Two explanations can be put forward: high concentration in calcium ion could compete with iron ion for a receptor; phosphate groups of casein can complex iron ions. This second explanation is enforced by the fact that the hydrolysis of proteins lessens the inhibiting effect of casein for iron absorption [26]. Additionally, the uptake of Fe–β-CN (1–25) has been demonstrated to be greater than the uptake of Fe gluconate, which makes Fe–β-CN (1–25) a good candidate for food fortification [27].

Even if nutritionists recommend avoiding the consumption of milk products in the same meal together with iron-rich dishes (e.g., kidney pie, roast beef with potatoes but not Yorshire pudding—because of milk in its composition!), competition between calcium and iron ions is not clear. Numerous papers are discussing about calcium/iron absorption. A 2-week food intake of iron-fortified infant cereals and addition of calcium hydrogenophosphate at two levels have had no significant effect on haemoglobin levels [28]. Another work has nevertheless shown that phosphate supplements (orthophosphate or hexametaphosphate) caused significant decreases in iron absorption and retention at the lower level of calcium intake. Simultaneously supplementing the diet with calcium and orthophosphate caused a similar reduction in iron absorption [29]. Phosphate and especially hexametaphosphate could be suspected to complex iron ion. It was demonstrated that calcium carbonate and calcium salt of citric and malic acid had a more pronounced effect on iron bioavailability than Ca in dairy products (milk, cheese), and that Fe–Ca interactions were influenced by the physiological state of the animal [30]. Yoghurt, used as substituting material in diet (in order to add 1 % of Ca), did not change iron absorption. Generally, in most of published works, it seems that calcium ions do not change iron absorption. Casein seems to be responsible of the low bioavailability of iron.

Iron Naturally Present in Milk

Depending of the period of lactation, the iron content in human milk is between 0.52±0.14 (corresponding to 9.3 μmol L^{-1}) and 0.38±0.12 mg L^{-1} (corresponding to 6.8 μmol L^{-1}), respectively for colostrum and 90-day mature milk [31].

Most of the iron is complexed with lactoferrin, protected in the core of this protein. The affinity of lactoferrin for iron is very high [32]: *K*a = 1E30. Human milk generally contains 1–3 g L^{-1} of lactoferrin (corresponding to 12.5–37.5 μmol L^{-1}), which is more than cow milk (0.1–0.4 g L^{-1}) [33]. As a comparison, iron content in pork liver, beef meat, and egg yolk is respectively 220, 110, and 70 mg kg^{-1} and Camembert contains only 0.6 mg kg^{-1} of iron. Dairy products are poor in iron and fortified dairy products are elaborated despite the fact that a dairy matrix decreases iron availability [26].

Fortification in Iron for Dairy Baby Food

The efficiency of iron fortification of milk formulas is subjected to controversy. No clear evidence of clinical benefit of iron fortification has been demonstrated for 6 month infants [34]. Other authors reported an increase of the blood haemoglobin level of infants and children after 6 and 12 months treatments [35, 36]. These results are not necessarily incompatible and depend greatly on the formula: factors such as type of iron carrier, oxidation degree of iron (Fe II more bioavailable than Fe III) [37], promoting (vitamin C) or inhibiting molecules (phytate, phenols) for the assimilation of iron, calcium level, and protein type are all able to influence the results.

Dairy Products Fortified with Lactoferrin

Despite the low content of iron and lactoferrin in cow milk, lactoferrin is isolated from milk and commercialized by companies. Due to its cationic nature ('basic protein'; $pI = 8.7$), lactoferrin can be purified by cation-exchange chromatography [38, 39]. This purification method is the most popular procedure in factories producing isolated milk proteins.

The fortification in iron with lactoferrin is more expensive than the fortification with iron salt; nevertheless the isolated lactoferrin is commonly used for supplementation of infant formula [33]. In the future, transgenic cows could offer the opportunity to obtain a great quantity of human lactoferrin [40] and the possibility of a general fortification of infant formula with human lactoferrin.

It is generally admitted that lactoferrin uses a specific adsorption receptor in human body, which allows good iron assimilation. This hypothesis has not yet been verified [41]. Human milk (rich in lactoferrin compared to bovine milk) seems to be well adapted to infant up to 4 months: healthy full-term breastfed infants have been susceptible to iron anaemia due to late introduction of complementary food (after 4 months).

During the second half of infancy (after 4 months), the diet should be enriched in iron [42, 43] but not necessarily with lactoferrin. Because of Maillard reactions or protein denaturation during the process, lactoferrin addition is not the best strategy for a good iron intake [44]. Lactoferrin denaturation by heating could occur in pasteurization process but more probably during sterilization. The temperature of maximum heat absorption in DSC analysis is 72.4 °C for human lactoferrin, 70.2 for sheep lactoferrin, and 69.3 for goat lactoferrin [45]. The denaturation temperature of bovine lactoferrin was found 60.4 °C (first endothermic peak) with an onset temperature near 50 °C [46]. These values from calorimetric measurements indicate the high sensitivity of bovine lactoferrin to thermal denaturation. It is thus wise to wonder if the denatured lactoferrin allows a good iron bioavailability for infants nourished with baby food enriched with lactoferrin.

On the contrary, the addition of vitamin C in a formula can really increase iron absorption. In fact, vitamin C betters the iron assimilation for infants, children, or adults [6] without increasing the solubilisation of iron [26].

Dairy Products Fortified with Iron Salts; Products Nowadays Available in Developed Countries

It is easier to find iron-enriched breakfast cereals or diet bars than iron-fortified dairy products on the current market. Dairy products are preferably enriched in ω3 oils, in calcium or in probiotics. The only examples of iron-fortified dairy products are milk and petit Suisse cheese for infant or very young children. Milk formulas for infants and young children generally contain iron sulphate (0.7–1.3 g/100 g) whereas petit Suisse cheese formulas integrate ferrous phosphate, pyrophosphate, diphosphate, or lactate (1.1–1.2 g/100 g). Other dairy products, such as different types of cheese and yoghurts, have been considered by researchers for iron fortification [47].

Numerous salts are available to enrich food in iron (see Table 6.1). The choice of the iron salt to be used is generally based on a good solubility, no precipitation, no change of pH. Some salts, such as citrate or phosphate, are also good buffers. Generally the more soluble the iron form is, the more available it is. Nevertheless, this is not an absolute rule since ferrous chloride, for instance, is very soluble but not totally bioavailable. Ferrous chloride is very quickly oxidized just after solubilisation, what is easily observed by the rapid appearance of orange colouring. It explains why ferrous chloride is not as available as foreseen considering its solubility.

Table 6.1 Solubility and bioavailability of different iron salts

Iron salts	Solubility in water	Bioavailability	Sensitivity to peroxidation
Ferrous sulphate	High	100[a]	Very high
Ferrous lactate		89–106	
Ferrous chloride		50	
Ferrous fumarate	Low	100	High
Ferrous succinate		92	
Ferrous citrate		74	
Ferrous tartrate		62	
Ferrous phosphate	Insoluble	27	Relatively low
Ferrous pyrophosphate		30	

[a]Ferrous sulphate has been chosen as reference and its bioavailability is 100 by definition

Some Chemistry Bases to Keep in Mind Before Formulating an Iron-Fortified Dairy Product

Some black spots are sometimes observed in milk powder enriched in iron salts. These black spots have different origins such as change in valence of iron ion (Fe^{2+}/Fe^{3+}) or the fact that iron salts are becoming insoluble. For example, if sulphate is added in a matrix where $pH \geq 7$, iron hydroxide will be produced and a decrease of the iron solubility will be observed [48].

Products of Solubility, pKa Values of Counter-Ion and Precipitation of Iron

The addition of an iron salt has to be done according to the p*K* values (see Table 6.2). For sulphate or chloride, the value of the dissociation constant is very low. As a consequence, iron sulphate or iron chloride can be used in foodstuffs in a large range of pH. For other iron salts, the values of dissociation constant have to be studied before addition to a foodstuff. The salts have buffer capacity around their p*K*.

In presence of a high protein concentration (as in dairy products) and because of the great buffer capacity of proteins, the addition of a limited quantity of iron salt has not effect on pH. In yoghurt (pH 4.4) or in more acidic foodstuffs, pH is near or under the p*K*a value and the counter-ion of iron ion is partially protonated. There is then a change of salts that could sometimes induce precipitation of iron salts (see after, low soluble iron salt).

The solubility of ferrous salts varies a lot (see Table 6.3). Ferrous chloride is highly soluble, ferrous sulphate is very soluble, but the solubility of ferrous fumarate is very low. As a comparison, calcium and sodium salts are far more soluble (see Table 6.3).

Calcium and ferrous salts have not always the same level of solubility: calcium hydroxide, calcium carbonate, and calcium phosphate are more soluble than their corresponding iron salts, but iron tartrate is more soluble than calcium tartrate (see Table 6.3).

Iron precipitation may also occur by exchange of calcium and iron with citrate at $4 < pH < 6.4$ which is a common value encountered in dairy products. Calcium citrate is far more soluble than ferrous citrate (see Table 6.3). By addition of iron salts, there is a production of iron citrate and, if the concentration is above 0.5 g L^{-1}, precipitation occurs whereas there is no calcium citrate precipitate. Addition of a soluble iron salt in dairy product could also produce precipitate of iron phosphate.

It is risky to simply relate the iron solubility of salts to the corresponding iron bioavailability in foodstuffs. Ferrous fumarate solubility is very low in water but increases in acidic solution and in physiologic acid buffer. This explains the good bioavailability of iron in the fumarate form. As another example, despite their low solubility and low availability, as indicated in Table 6.1, iron phosphate

Table 6.2 Dissociation constant of different salts

Salts	Acid–base couples	Dissociation constants p*K*
Chloride	HCl/Cl^-	−9.3
Sulphate	$H_2SO_4/HSO_4^-/SO_4^{2-}$	−3; 1.9
Phosphate	$H_3PO_4/H_2PO_4^-/HPO_4^{2-}/PO_4^{3-}$	2.1; 7.2; 12.3
Lactic acid/lactate	$H_3C–CH(OH)–COOH/H_3C–CH(OH)–COO–$	3.9
Fumaric acid/fumarate	HOOC–(CH=CH)–COOH/…/-OOC–(CH=CH)–COO–	3; 4.4
Citric acid/citrate	$HOOC–CH_2–C(OH)(COOH)–CH_2–COOH/…/^-OOC–CH_2–C(OH)(COO^-)–CH_2–COO$	3.1–4.8–6.4

Table 6.3 Water solubility of sodium, calcium, and ferrous salts

	Solubility in water	
Salts	K_{sp}	Threshold of solubility mol L^{-1} (g L^{-1})
Sodium chloride	39	6.1 (359)
Calcium chloride	1,210	6.7 (745)
Ferrous chloride	630	5.4 (685)
Ferrous sulphate	3 (heptahydrate salt)	1.7 (486)
Ferrous fumarate	6.9×10^{-5}	8.3×10^{-3} (1.4)
Ferrous citrate	4×10^{-6}	2×10^{-3} (0.5)
Calcium citrate	4.4×10^{-9}	14.9×10^{-3} (8.5)
Ferrous tartrate	5.9×10^{-9}	15.8×10^{-3} (8.77)
Calcium tartrate	1.96×10^{-10}	1.4×10^{-5} (0.032)
Ferrous (iron(II)) carbonate	3.2×10^{-11}	
Calcium carbonate	3.8×10^{-9}	
Ferrous (iron(II)) hydroxide	8×10^{-16}	
Calcium hydroxide	5.5×10^{-6}	
Ferric (iron(III)) phosphate	1.3×10^{-22}	
Ferrous (iron(II)) phosphate	1.07×10^{-29}	
Calcium phosphate	2×10^{-29}	

salts had iron bioavailability estimated respectively at 61 % and 69 % (ferrous sulphate alone as reference) in fortified low-fat fluid milk and petit suisse cheese fortified with micronized ferric orthophosphate (Fe (III)) [49].

Components exist in foodstuffs that influence clearly the bioavailability; for example, anti-nutritional factors such as phytic acid have a negative effect on bioavailability whereas ascorbic acid has a positive effect. Ascorbic acid addition was shown to enhance the iron absorption of adult women fed with cereals fortified with iron sulphate or fumarate [50]. In another study, 15 healthy adult men received a treatment with ferrous ascorbate or pasteurized milk fortified with 15 mg L^{-1} of ferrous sulphate microencapsulated using phospholipids: 14 men showed higher iron absorption with ascorbic acid (mean iron absorption of 8.65 % towards 1.99 % with the fortified milk) [51]. An over-fortification in ascorbic acid should be recommended to compensate the loss during storage of infant milk powder [52] but a limit of such over-fortification has to be defined because of the pro-oxidant activity of ascorbic acid in high concentration. Another pitfall of the use of ascorbic acid to enhance the iron bioavailability is the decrease of the nutritional value of proteins by loss of lysine and tryptophan which are two very essential amino acids for infant. The reduction of the nutritional value is due to the alkylation of lysyl residues (ascorbylation by iron catalyzed Maillard reaction) and to the oxidation of tryptophanyl residues [53].

Prebiotic and probiotics addition in formula could be an alternative strategy to improve the iron bioavailability as colon can function as a significant site of iron absorption. Prebiotic and probiotics may have different actions such as possible reduction of Fe(III) to Fe(II) by probiotics, stimulation of proliferation of the epithelial cells and expansion of the absorptive surface area, stimulation of the expression of mineral-transport proteins in epithelial cells [54].

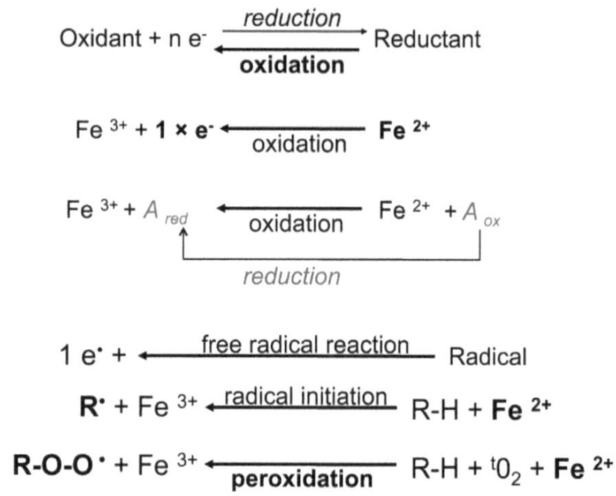

Fig. 6.1 Relation between redox chemistry of ionic iron (ferrous, Fe^{2+} and ferric, Fe^{3+} ions) and peroxidation of molecules in presence of oxygen. $^{t}O_2$ (or $^{3}O_2$ or <O=O>) is the ground state of the oxygen molecule. R–O–O• is the peroxide produced in presence of ferrous ion and oxygen

Peroxidation of Lipids with Iron Ions

To administer iron as a medicine or through iron-enriched foodstuffs is potentially to use retarding bomb. The iron form which allows the absorption of this micronutrient is the ferrous ion (Fe^{2+}). The ferrous ion is very unstable and is oxidized in ferric ion (Fe^{3+}) that gives an electron. A radical gives a radical electron as a reducer gives a ground state electron. A radical with ground state oxygen (none excited oxygen molecule) induces the peroxidation as a reductive molecule induces oxidation (see Fig. 6.1).

It is not necessary to produce singlet oxygen molecule ($^{s}O_2$ or $^{1}O_2$ or •O-O• that is an excited oxygen molecule) such as in photoxidation (light, sensitizer and triplet—normal—oxygen) to produce peroxide. Copper ion (Cu^{2+}) initiates peroxidation of lipid, in the same way as ferrous ion does and even more strongly than iron does. Ferrous ion but also ferrous–ferric complex, and heme iron have the power to induce peroxidation [55, 56]. Lactoferrin is an iron-binding protein (transferrin family) and can chelate metal in the extent of two moles of iron bound per mole of protein, which makes a distinction with iron transport structure. For this reason, lactoferrin is considered as an antioxidant like EDTA, a very powerful complexing agent [57]. This antioxidant activity depends on the following factors: the lipid system, the concentration in protein, the type of buffer, the presence of metal ions and heterocyclic antioxidants. Additionally, γ-tocopherol, ferulic acid, coumaric acid, tyrosol, and natural phenolic extracts from olive oil can modulate the antioxidative activity of the lactoferrin [58].

It is thus very important to verify if the treatment against anaemia using nutraceutical or iron-fortified foodstuffs may avoid peroxidation of lipids of the tract cells, such as intestinal brush cells. Models of ω3-fat peroxidation have shown that fat globules stabilized by proteins at the oil/water interface were not peroxidised at the same level using Fe–Na–EDTA, ferrous bis-glycinate, or ferrous sulphate [59]. Iron-EDTA did not induce peroxidation and its addition even decreased the slow peroxidation of lipids in the emulsion stabilized by milk protein (sodium caseinate or isolated β-lactoglobulin). This was probably due to a complexation of metallic traces by EDTA. The addition of the traditional ferrous sulphate or of iron-bis-glycinate [14, 60, 61] (the new promising iron complex), gave no difference on the peroxide value (PV) when the emulsion was stabilized by sodium caseinate. In this case, peroxide value was around 2.6 mmol of peroxide produced per kilogramme of oil, what is quite high after 7 days of storage (see Fig. 6.2). After the same duration of storage,

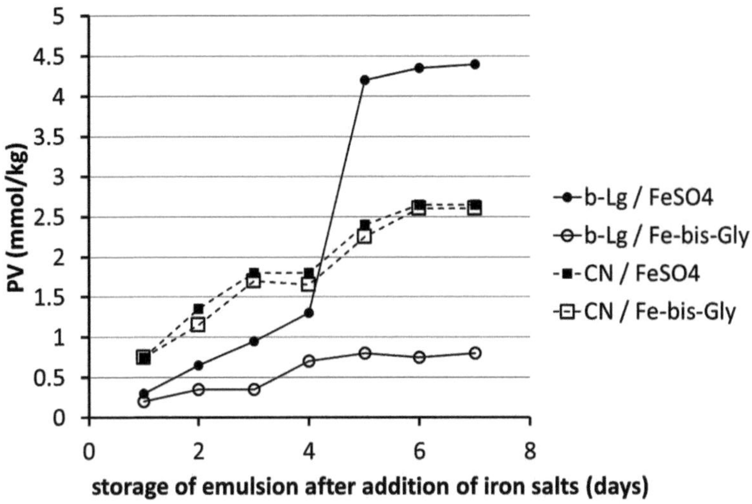

Fig. 6.2 Peroxide value of canola oil emulsions stabilized with β-lactoglobulin (b-Lg) or sodium caseinate (CN) in aqueous buffers containing ferrous sulphate ($FeSO_4$) or ferrous bis-glycinate (Fe-bis-Gly) during a storage following the mixing of the emulsion and the iron buffer (pH 6.5). Adapted from ref [60]

when the emulsion was stabilized by β-lactoglobulin, peroxide value was 4.4 mmol $kg^{-1}$when using iron sulphate and 0.8 mmol kg^{-1} when using iron-bis-glycinate. Iron-bis-glycinate induced a slow increase of PV during the storage of the W-O emulsion stabilized using a whey protein whereas PV increased more sharply with caseinate that possessed phosphate groups (phosphoseryl residues). Phosphate groups of caseinate have destabilized the iron-bis-glycinate chelate because of their high affinity for iron ions (see previously the maximum solubility of iron phosphate; the lower the solubility, the higher the affinity). Ferrous was released from the complex salts and the free ferrous ions induced peroxidation of lipids at the O-W interface. On the opposite, carboxylate groups did not destabilize the iron-bis-glycinate chelate and the release of free iron ions at the interface was avoided. β-lactoglobulin (no phosphate group) in mixture with iron-bis-glycinate induced a limited quantity of peroxide. Ferrous sulphate induces more peroxide because this salt is very soluble, is not a complex and gives free ferrous ions.

Except in the case of Fe–Na–EDTA, it is well founded to imagine that ingestion of iron salt with fortified food or nutraceutical could induce peroxidation of lipids of the membranes in stomach and intestinal cells. Iron-EDTA has to be avoided because of the risk of heavy metal accumulation in liver [62, 63].

Free radical damages include lipid peroxidation, but also DNA hydroxylation, protein hydroxylation, isoprostanes production, and their effects on body should not be neglected. Radicals such as peroxide lead to cell injury and cell death that create diseases [64]. The peroxidation of lipids in intestinal cells could lead to intestinal irritation or inflammation. Lactoferrin was shown to induce no side effects on rat gastric mucosa, whereas ferrous sulphate and ferrous citrate caused some serious injuries [65]. Iron supplementation using ferrous fumarate did not increase oxidative stress, checked at postnatal age of 5–6 weeks, in healthy preterm infants with very low birth weight (inferior to 1,500 g) and born at a gestational age under 32 weeks [66]. The type of fortification chosen for dairy products has to evaluate the risk linked with free radicals. Commercial infant milk powders are often fortified with ferrous sulphate and, moreover, formulas are mixing very reactive iron salts together with ω3-rich oils that are highly sensitive to peroxidation!

Perspective of New Iron-Enriched Formulas

Iron Salts and Complexes

Iron sulphate leads to precipitated iron hydroxide when pH is above 6. For pH around 7, it would be better to use ferric peptides derivate from the hydrolysis of casein [48]. Proteins such as lactoferrin or protein fractions (peptides) are good candidates to carry iron in dairy products but protein can also be used as encapsulating material. β-lactoglobulin used to encapsulate iron in filamentous gel would be able to limit iron release in gastric phase (pH 1.2 and pepsin) and would be able to release iron thanks to pancreatin during the intestinal phase at pH 7.5 [67].

Iron complexes avoiding free iron in solution but giving highly bioavailable iron are scarce. EDTA avoids perfectly the oxidation of ω-3 oil [59] but this solution is not authorized in every country because of the risk of heavy metal accumulation in the body. Phytic acid salt gives unavailable iron, oxalic acid salts is rapidly toxic (kidney stones), and iron-bis-glycinate is not compatible with $pH<5$ nor with phosphoprotein in the medium [59, 68].

Iron casein micelles have been prepared by partial exchange of calcium within the casein micelles by pH-cycles. The milk composed with iron casein micelles remains able to produce curd by rennet [69]. The colour of this type of iron(II) fortified milk is darker than the one of regular milk, indicating may be a change of the oxidation degree of Fe. This solution could be used in hard cheese production where the milk is not much acidified before clotting. Moreover, in such products, fat milk is most of the time saturated and that reduces considerably the risk of fat peroxidation.

For processed cheese, phosphate and polyphosphates used as technological agents have a high capacity of complexing iron, which would reduce the risk of iron oxidation. Hexametaphosphate was used with copper ion that is a strong oxidative agent and gave promising results against peroxidation in presence of copper or iron ions [70]. Processes using long duration of heating have to be studied regarding the stability of iron phosphate salts.

Control of Iron Transfer to Interface in Presence of ω-3 Oil

For a dairy baby formula enriched in ω-3 oil and iron, it is a strict requirement to avoid contact between oil and iron ion in aqueous phase. The pH of the aqueous phase controls the stability of the iron complex and the type of protein used on the interface (with or without chemical function having a high affinity towards bivalent ions, that is to say serylphosphate residues) controls the transfer of iron to the interface [59, 68]. Yoghurts (pH around 5) fortified with iron-bis-glycinate could avoid the destabilization of the iron-bis-glycinate chelate in stomach thanks to a strong buffer effect and thus avoid an acidic transit before intestine. A multilayer around an emulsion could also protect against peroxidation and avoid contact with iron at the O/W interface. Such a system is presented in Fig. 6.3. A first layer near the surface of fat globule is shown with surface active acid proteins (negatively charged) then a second layer is added using positively charged macromolecules such as chitosan or basic protein such as lysozyme or lactoferrin [71, 72]. Chitosan or lysozyme could be more efficient than lactoferrin in this system because they allow avoiding proximity of iron with the oil surface.

Encapsulation of Iron

The value of iron absorption in milk obtained with encapsulated ferrous sulphate in phospholipid micelles is 2.3 times higher than in milk fortified with 'classical' ferrous sulphate—simply dissolved

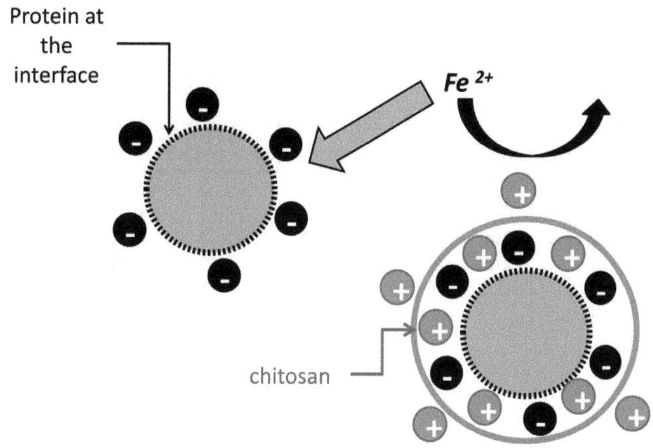

Fig. 6.3 Multilayer interface of an emulsion made with negatively and positively charged macromolecules to avoid iron contact with oil. The oil–water multilayer interface is positively charged (same charge of iron ion whereas simple interface prepared with usual milk proteins would have been negatively charged)

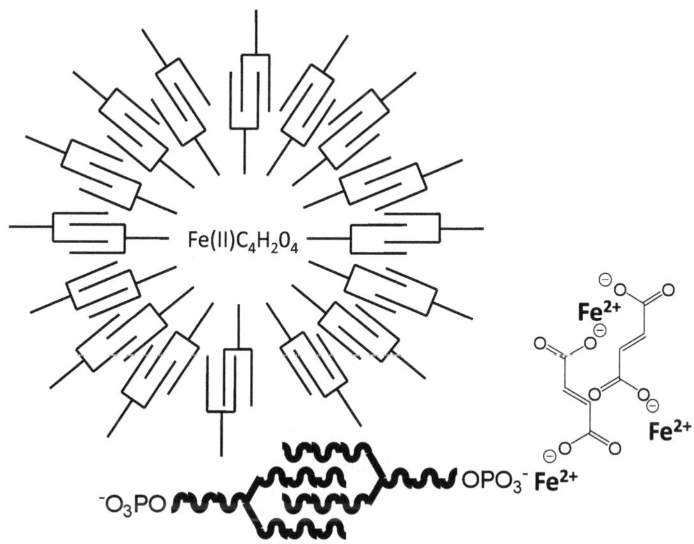

Fig. 6.4 Phospholipid micelle entrapping fumarate salts of low soluble iron(II)

in milk [51] (see Fig. 6.4). Ferrous ascorbate in water is nevertheless 4 times more efficient than ferrous sulphate encapsulated in micelles in milk. In milk, casein and calcium probably decrease the iron bioavailability. A more sophisticated encapsulation system has been imagined: a water-in-oil-in-water emulsion was used to encapsulate at the same time iodine, retinol, and iron (see Fig. 6.5). The W-O-W emulsion allowed separating two incompatible components (ferrous ion produces retinol radical) and has given good results to correct deficiency in a poor children population [73, 74]. These capsules of iron could be added to milk just before coagulation of rennetted milk to produce iron-fortified cheese.

The iron fortification of dairy desserts is more complicated than the fortification of yoghurts or cheeses. Colouring compounds act as sensitizer and induce peroxidation via photoxidation. Photoxidation can change the valence of iron and produce dark colouring or black points. Iron could also oxidise aroma precursors or aroma molecules and change the aromatic profile of the foodstuff. Strong and persistent metallic flavours, bitter taste, or astringency may be encountered when using ferrous salts [75]. Ferrous salts stimulate complex oral and retronasal sensations but

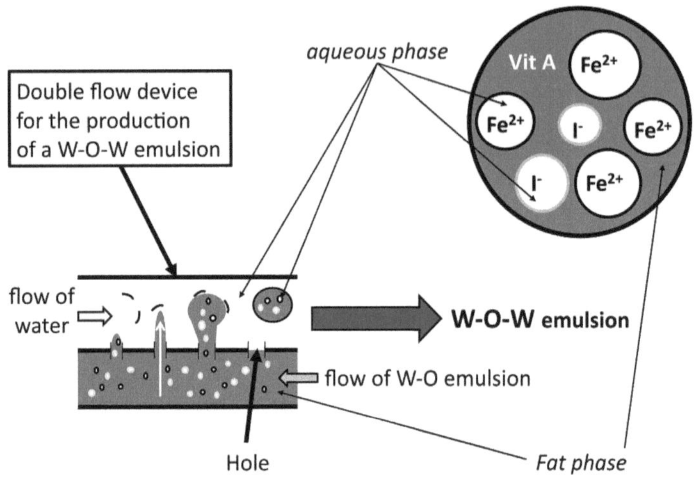

Fig. 6.5 Encapsulation of iron ions in the water-in-oil-in water emulsion (W-O-W). Fat has a high melting point because W-O-W emulsion is dried to obtain a powder. Chitosane is obtained by deacetylation of crustaceans' chitin

also tactile cues. They particularly evoke metallic sensations. Sensory perception of ferrous salts may be roughly described as a combination of the four basic tastes as well as metallic and astringent perception [76]. Desserts are pleasure foodstuffs and pleasure is not consistent with flavour defect. This problem must be handled by the marketing staff when designing a fortified food taken as a functional food.

Conclusion

Are dairy products well adapted to iron fortification despite calcium/iron competition? A good vehicle for iron must be a very commonly consumed foodstuff. Soy sauce in China [77], tonyu in Japan, and Nuoc-mâm (fish sauce) in Vietnam [78] were successfully used for correction of iron deficiency. As dairy products are widely consumed in Europe and North America, they can be a good vehicle for iron, though the possible competition between calcium and iron absorption. Milk fat is saturated and is not sensitive to peroxidation. In case of addition of ω3-oil (for example for baby food), encapsulation and/or stable iron complex could be a good solution to protect iron against oxidation.

References

1. De Benoist B, McLean E, Egli I, Cogswell M. Worldwide prevalence of anemia 1993–2005: WHO global database on anaemia. World Health Organization. Geneva, Switzerland: WHO Press; 2008. http://whqlibdoc.who.int/publications/2008/9789241596657_eng.pdf
2. Thomas D, Frankenberg E. Health, nutrition and property: a microeconomic perspective. Bull World Health Organ. 2002;8:106–13.
3. Zhengxing C, Wilna O-T. Food fortification to prevent and control iron deficiency. Afr J Food Sci. 2002;2:751–60.
4. Nguyen P, Einarson A. Managing nausea and vomiting of pregnancy with pharmacological and non pharmacological treatments. Womens Health. 2006;2:753–60.
5. Nguyen P, Nava-Ocampo A, Levy A, O'Connor DL, Einarson TR, Taddio A, et al. Effect of iron content on the tolerability of prenatal multivitamins in pregnancy. BMC Pregnancy Childbirth. 2008;8:17–25.
6. Hercberg S. La carence en fer et nutrition humaine. (Iron deficiency and human nutrition). France Paris: Lavoisier; 1988.

7. Benito P, Miller D. Iron absorption and bioavailability: an updated review. Nutr Res. 1998;18:581–603.
8. Berger J, Dyck JL, Galan P, Apologan A, Schneider D, Traissac P, et al. Effect of daily iron-supplementation on iron status, cell-mediated immunity, and incidence of infections in 6-36-month-old Togolese children. Eur J Clin Nutr. 2000;54:29–35.
9. Lozoff B, Brittenham GM, Wolf AW, Urrutia JJ. Developmental deficits in iron deficient infants: effects of age and severity of iron lack. J Pediatr. 1982;101:948–51.
10. Guesry P. The role of nutrition in brain development. Prev Med. 1998;27:189–94.
11. Shafir T, Angulo-Barroso R, Jing Y, Angelilli ML, Jacobson SW, Lozoff B. Iron deficiency and infant motor development. Early Hum Dev. 2008;84:479–85.
12. Halterman JS, Kaczorowski JM, Aligne CA, Auinger P, Szilagyi PG. Iron deficiency and cognitive achievement among school-aged children and adolescents in USA. Pediatrics. 2001 Jun;107(6):1381–6.
13. Walter T, Olivares M, Pizarro F, Munoz C. Iron, anemia, and infection. Nutr Rev. 1997;55:111–24.
14. Allen LH. Advantages and limitations of iron amino acid chelates as iron fortificants. Nutr Rev. 2002;60:18–21.
15. Zavaleta N, Nombrera J, Rojas R, Hambraeus L, Gislason J, Lönnerdal B. Iron and lactoferrin in milk of anemic mothers given iron supplements. Nutr Res. 1995;15:681–90.
16. Wolf AW, Jimenez E, Lozoff B. Effects of iron therapy on infant blood lead levels. J Pediatr. 2003;143:789–95.
17. Trumbo P, Yates AA, Schlicker S, Poos M. Dietary reference intakes: vitamin A, vitamin K, arsenic, boron, chromium, copper, iodine, iron, manganese, molybdenum, nickel, silicon, vanadium, and zinc. J Am Diet Assoc. 2001;101:294–301.
18. Edwards CQ, Griffen LM, Goldgar D, Drummond C, Skolnick MH, Kushner JP. Prevalence of hemochromatosis among presumably healthy blood donors. N Engl J Med. 1988;318:1355–62.
19. Sempos CT, Looker AC. Iron status and the risk of coronary heart disease. Nutr Metab Cardiovasc Dis. 1999;9:294–303.
20. Schumann K. Safety aspects of iron in food. Ann Nutr Metab. 2001;45:91–101.
21. Quinteros A, Farré R, Lagarda MJ. Optimization of iron speciation (soluble, ferrous and ferric) in beans, chickpeas and lentils. Food Chem. 2001;75:365–70.
22. Iqbal A, Khalil IA, Ateeq N, Khan MS. Nutritional quality of important food legumes. Food Chem. 2006;97:331–5.
23. Hunt JR. Bioavailability of iron, zinc, and other trace minerals from vegetarian diets. Am J Clin Nutr. 2003;78(3 Suppl):633S–9.
24. Hurrell RF. Bioavailability of iron. Eur J Clin Nutr. 1997;51:4–8.
25. Hadler M-C, Colugnati F, Sigulem DM. Risks of anemia in infants according to dietary iron density and weight gain rate. Prev Med. 2004;39:713–21.
26. De Souza NC, Colli C, Silverio Amancio OM. Infant formula iron dialysability related to other nutrients. Food Chem. 2005;90:779–83.
27. Ani-Kibangou B, Bouhallab S, Mollé D, Henry G, Bureau F, Neuville D, et al. Improved absorption of caseinophosphopeptide-bound iron: role of alkaline phosphatise. J Nutr Biochem. 2005;16:398–401.
28. Shah BG, Belonje B. The lack of effect of added dibasic calcium phosphate on the bioavailability of electrolytic iron in infant cereals. Nutr Res. 1985;5:181–8.
29. Steinhardt Bour NJ, Soullier BA, Zemel MB. Effect of level and form of phosphorus and level of calcium intake on zinc, iron and copper bioavailability in man. Nutr Res. 1984;4:371–9.
30. Minotti PL, Buchowski MS, Miller DD. Effects of calcium supplementation, calcium source and lactose on iron absorption in the rat. Nutr Res. 1993;13:1173–81.
31. Silvestre MD, Lagarda MJ, Farré R, Martínez-Costa C, Brines J. Copper, iron and zinc determinations in human milk using FAAS with microwave digestion. Food Chem. 2000;68:95–9.
32. Lönnerdal B. Chap 3. Whey protein in human milk. In: Atkinson SA, Lönnerdal B, editors. Protein and non-protein nitrogen in human milk. Boca Raton, FL: CRC Press; 1989. p. 29–42.
33. Wakabayashi H, Yamauchi K, Takase M. Lactoferrin research, technology and applications. Int Dairy J. 2006;16:1241–51.
34. Hemminki E, Nemet K, Horvàth M, Malin M, Schuler D, Hollan S. Impact of iron fortification of milk formulas on infant's growth and health. Nutr Res. 1995;15:491–503.
35. Wang YY, Chen CM, Wang FZ, Jia M, Wang KA. Effects of nutrient fortified complementary food supplements on anemia of infants and young children in poor rural of Gansu. Biomed Environ Sci. 2009;22:194–200.
36. Walter T, Pino P, Pizarro F, Lozoff B. Prevention of iron-deficiency anemia: comparison of high- and low-iron formulas in term healthy infants after six months of life. J Pediatr. 1998;132:635–40.
37. Wapnir RA. Effect of food sources and processing on protein and mineral absorption. In: Protein nutrition and mineral absorption. New York: CRC Press; 1990. p. 61–76.
38. Law BA, Reiter B. The isolation and bacteriostatic properties of lactoferrin from bovine milk whey. J Dairy Res. 1977;44:595–9.

39. Yoshida S, Wei Z, Shinmura Y, Fukunaga N. Separation of lactoferrin-a and -b from bovine colostrums. J Dairy Sci. 2000;83:2211–5.
40. Simojoki H, Hyvönen P, Orro T, Pyörälä S. High concentration of human lactoferrin in milk of rhLf-transgenic. cows relieves signs of bovine experimental Staphylococcus chromogenes intramammary infection. Vet Immunol Immunopathol. 2010;136:265–71.
41. Jovaní M, Reyes B, Farré R. Effect of lactoferrin addition on the dialysability of iron from infant formulas. J Trace Elem Med Biol. 2003;17:139–42.
42. Dube K, Schwartz J, Mueller MJ, Kalhoff H, Kersting M. Iron intake and iron status in breastfed infants during the first year of life. Clin Nutr. 2010;29:773–8.
43. Verrall T, Gray-Donald K. Impact of a food-based approach to improve iron nutrition of at-risk infants in northern Canada. Prev Med. 2005;40:896–903.
44. Viadel B, Perales S, Barberá R, Lagarda MJ, Farré R. Ferritin synthesis by Caco-2 cells as an indicator of iron bioavailability: application to milk-based infant formulas. Food Chem. 2007;102:925–31.
45. Conesa C, Sánchez L, Rota C, Pérez M-D, Calvo M, Farnaud S, et al. Isolation of lactoferrin from milk of different species: calorimetric and antimicrobial studies. Comp Biochem Physiol B Biochem Mol Biol. 2008;150:131–9.
46. Bengoechea C, Peinado I, McClements DJ. Formation of protein nanoparticles by controlled heat treatment of lactoferrin: factors affecting particle characteristics. Food Hydrocoll. 2011;25:1354–60.
47. Martínez-Navarrete N, Camachoa MM, Martínez-Lahuerta J, Martínez-Monzó J, Fito P. Iron deficiency and iron fortified foods—a review. Food Res Int. 2002;35:225–31.
48. Chaud MV, Izumi C, Nahaal Z, Shuhama T, Pires Bianchi Mde L, de Freitas O. Derivatives from casein hydrolysates as a potential source in the treatment of iron deficiency. J Agric Food Chem. 2002;50:871–7.
49. Salgueiro J, Leonardi N, Segal M, Shafran N, Carasso Y, Zubillaga M, et al. Iron bioavailability from fortified fluid milk and petit suisse cheese determined by the prophylactic-prevention method. Biol Trace Elem Res. 2006;109:91–6.
50. Fidler MC, Davidson L, Zeder C, Walczuk T, Hurrel RF. Iron absorption from ferrous fumarate in adult women is influenced by ascorbic acid but not by Na_2EDTA. Br J Nutr. 2003;90:1081–5.
51. Uicich R, Piio F, Ahneida C, Diaz M, Boccio J, Zubillaga M, et al. Bioavailability of microencapsulated ferrous sulfate in fluid cows milk. Studies in human beings. Nutr Res. 1999;19:893–7.
52. Chávez-Servín JL, Castellote AI, Rivero M, López-Sabater MC. Analysis of vitamins A, E and C, iron and selenium contents in infant milk-based powdered formula during full shelf-life. Food Chem. 2008;107:1187–97.
53. Leclère J, Birlouez-Aragona I, Melib M. Fortification of milk with iron-ascorbate promotes lysine glycation and tryptophan oxidation. Food Chem. 2002;76:491–9.
54. Yeung CK, Glahn RP, Welch RM, Miller DD. Prebiotics and iron bioavailability—is there a connection? J Food Sci. 2005;70:R88–92.
55. Cheng Z, Li Y. What is responsible for the initiating chemistry of iron-mediated lipid peroxidation: an update. Chem Rev. 2007;107:748–66.
56. Baron CP, Andersen HJ. Myoglobin-induced lipid oxidation. A review. J Agric Food Chem. 2002;50:3887–97.
57. Nielsen NS, Petersen A, Meyer AS, Timm-Heinrich M, Jacobsen C. Effects of lactoferrin, phytic acid, and EDTA on oxidation in two food emulsions enriched with long-chain polyunsaturated fatty acids. J Agric Food Chem. 2004;52:7690–9.
58. Medina I, Tombo I, Satueä-Gracia MT, German JB, Frankel EN. Effects of natural phenolic compounds on the antioxidant activity of lactoferrin in liposomes and oil-in-water emulsions. J Agric Food Chem. 2002;50:2392–9.
59. Guzun-Cojocaru T, Koev C, Yordanov M, Karbowiak T, Cases E, Cayot P. Oxidative stability of oil-in-water emulsions containing iron chelates: transfer of iron from chelates to milk proteins at interface. Food Chem. 2011;125:326–33.
60. Olivares M, Pizarro F, Pineda O, Name JJ, Hertrampf E, Walter T. Milk inhibits and ascorbic acid favors ferrous bis-glycine chelate bioavailability in humans. J Nutr. 1997;127:1407–11.
61. Jeppsen RB, Borzelleca JF. Safety evaluation of ferrous bisglycinate chelate. Food Chem Toxicol. 1999;37:723–31.
62. Hurrell RF, Lynch S, Bothwell T, Cori H, Glahn R, Hertrampf E, et al. Enhancing the absorption of fortification iron a sustain task force report. Int J Vitam Nutr Res. 2004;74:387–401.
63. Zhu L, Miller DD. Tissue iron distribution and urinary mineral excretion vary depending on the form of iron ($FeSO_4$ or NaFeEDTA) and the route of administration (oral or subcutaneous) in rats given high doses of iron. J Agric Food Chem. 2007;55:8793–9.
64. De Zwart LL, Meerman JHN, Commandeur JNM, Vermeulen NPE. Biomarkers of free radical damage applications in experimental animals and in humans. Free Radic Biol Med. 1999;26:202–26.
65. Uchida T, Taishi Oda, Kaoru Sato, Hiroshi Kawakami. Availability of lactoferrin as a natural solubilizer of iron for food products. Int Dairy J. 2005;16:95–101.
66. Braekke K, Bechensteen AG, Halvorsen BL, Blomhoff R, Haaland K, Staff AC. Oxidative stress markers and antioxidant status after oral iron supplementation to very low birth weight infants. J Pediatr. 2007;151:23–8.

67. Remondetto GE, Beyssac E, Subirade M. Iron availability from whey protein hydrogels: an in vitro study. J Agric Food Chem. 2004;52:8137–43.
68. Guzun-Cojocaru T, Cayot P, Loupiac C, Cases E. Effect of iron chelates on oil–water interface, stabilized by milk proteins: the role of phosphate groups and pH. Prediction of iron transfer from aqueous phase toward fat globule surface by changes of interfacial properties. Food Hydrocoll. 2010;24:364–73.
69. Raouche S, Dobenesque M, Bot A, Lagaude A, Marchesseau S. Casein micelles as vehicle for iron fortification of foods. Eur Food Res Technol. 2009;229:929–35.
70. Alexa RI. In development of fortified reduced-fat spreads using microgel delivery systems, PhD thesis, University College of Dublin, Ireland. (Alexa RI, O'Kennedy BT, Mounsey SJ, Jacquier JC. Oxidative stability of hydrocolloid-stabilised water/oil emulsions as influenced by free Cu^{2+} or Cu-hexametaphosphate complexes in neutral and acidic conditions. Submitted to Food Chemistry. 2011).
71. Gudipati V, Sandra S, McClements DJ, Decker EA. Oxidative stability and in vitro digestibility of fish oil-in-water emulsions containing multilayered membranes. J Agric Food Chem. 2010;58:8093–9.
72. Lesmes U, Sandra S, Decker EA, McClements DJ. Impact of surface deposition of lactoferrin on physical and chemical stability of omega-3 rich lipid droplets stabilised by caseinate. Food Chem. 2010;123:99–106.
73. Zimmermann MB, Weqmueller R, Zeder C, Chaouki N, Beibinger R, Hurrell RF, et al. Triple fortification of salt with microcapsules of iodine, iron and vitamin A. Am J Clin Nutr. 2004;80:1283–90.
74. Wegmüller R, Zimmermann MB, Bühr VG, Windhab EJ, Hurrell RF. Development, stability, and sensory testing of microcapsules containing iron, iodine, and vitamin a for use in food fortification. J Food Sci. 2006;71:S181–7.
75. Yang HH-L, Lawless HT. Time–intensity characteristics of iron compounds. Food Qual Prefer. 2006;17:337–43.
76. Lim J, Lawless HT. Detection thresholds and taste qualities of iron salts. Food Qual Prefer. 2006;17:513–21.
77. Mannar V, Galleyo EB. Iron fortification: country level experiences and lessons. J Nutr. 2002;132:8565–85.
78. Thuy P, Berger I, Davidsson L, Khan NC, Lam NL, Cook JD, et al. Regular consumption of NaFeEDTA-fortified fish sauce improves iron status and reduces the prevalence of anemia in anemic Vietnamese women. Am J Clin Nutr. 2003;78:284–90.

Chapter 7
Ferric Pyrophosphate as an Alternative Iron Source for Food Fortification

María Jimena Salgueiro and José Boccio

Key Points

- Food fortification has been shown to be an efficient strategy to prevent iron deficiency.
- Many efforts are still made to provide an adequate iron source for food fortification.
- Ferric pyrophosphate, which is a white-coloured poorly soluble iron compound, does not change organoleptic properties of foods even when used in many difficult-to-fortify food vehicles.
- Some strategies were implemented in order to increase ferric pyrophosphate bioavailability, such as protect it, solubilize o stabilize it and/or reduce its particle size.
- Contrary to earlier concerns, evidence does not indicate significant differences in its bioavailability compared to that of water soluble compounds.

Keywords Fortification • Iron • Anaemia • Bioavailability • Ferric pyrophosphate • Ferrous sulphate

Abbreviations

FDA	Food and Drug Administration
GRAS	Generally recognized as safe
mo	Months
RBV	Relative bioavailability values
WHO	World Health Organization
y	Years
mm	Micrometers

M.J. Salgueiro, Ph.D. (✉) • J. Boccio, Ph.D.
Stable Isotopes Laboratory Applied to Biology and Medicine, Department of Physics,
School of Pharmacy and Biochemistry, University of Buenos Aires,
Junín 956, Piso Bajo, 1113 Buenos Aires, Argentina
e-mail: jsalgueiro@ffyb.uba.ar

V.R. Preedy et al. (eds.), *Handbook of Food Fortification and Health: From Concepts to Public Health Applications Volume 1*, Nutrition and Health, DOI 10.1007/978-1-4614-7076-2_7,

Introduction

Food fortification has been shown to be an efficient strategy to prevent iron deficiency [1]. Many iron compounds are at our disposal to be used as potential sources for food fortification. However, only a few of them completely meet the requirements of high iron bioavailability, inertness in relation to the sensorial properties of the fortified food, absence of toxicity, resistance during storing or elaboration processes of the fortified food, and absorption mechanism following the same pattern as dietary iron. For these reasons, many efforts are still made to provide an adequate iron source for food fortification.

Iron is found in foods in two different groups: one of haemic iron and the other one of non-haemic iron [2]. The haem-type iron is a part of haemoglobin, myoglobin, cytochromes and many other haem proteins, which are present principally in animal foods. The haem group, which is present in all these proteins, is formed by a complex organic ring, called protoporphyrin, to which a divalent iron atom is bound, which is able to form six coordinated bounds—four of them with the protoporphyrin, one with a nitrogen atom of the protein fraction, and the last remaining free as a binding site for an oxygen molecule [2]. The non-haemic iron type corresponds to iron that is not bound to a haem group; it includes basically inorganic salts of this metal and they are found principally in vegetal foods as well as in the principal pharmaceutical preparations utilized for the therapy against iron deficiency or available as fortification sources [2].

Iron Compounds

Relative bioavailability values (RBV) from animal and human studies have proven valuable in the choice of iron compounds to fortify foods [for revision of methods, see [3–5]]. In fact, the RBV is classically used to divide iron compounds into three groups (see Table 7.1) [6]. The first group is that of water-soluble compounds with an RBV close to that of ferrous sulphate which is considered the reference standard iron source. Iron compounds in this group are highly reactive thus, although they have high bioavailability they modify sensorial characteristics of food vehicles and this limits their use for food fortification [6]. The second group includes iron compounds poorly soluble in water but

Table 7.1 Iron compounds classified as their RBV

Group characteristics		Iron compounds
Group I	Soluble in water	Ferrous sulphate[a,b]
	Highly reactive	Ferrous gluconate[a]
	High RBV	Ferrous lactate[a]
		Ferrous ammonic citrate[a]
Group II	Poorly soluble in water	Ferrous fumarate[a,b]
	Soluble in diluted acid solutions	Ferrous succinate
	Less reactive than group I	Ferrous saccarate
	Medium RBV	
Group III	Insoluble in water	Ferric orthophosphate
	Poorly soluble in diluted acid solutios	Ferric ammonic orthophosphate
	Practically non-reactive	Ferric pyrophosphate[a,b]
	Variable RBV depending on type of compound, particle size, food matrix	Elemental iron[a] powder (electrolytic[b], carbonilic, reduced)

RBV relative biological value
[a]Listed as generally recognized as safe (GRAS) by the FDA [6]
[b]Recommended for food fortification by the WHO [7]

that dissolve more or less completely in the gastric juice, thus RBV of compounds in this group are lower than that of ferrous sulphate. Even though their poor solubility makes them less reactive, they can still provoke rancidity, mostly because of their humidity. Therefore, their use for food fortification is also limited. On the other hand, their solubility is affected by secretion of hydrochloric acid; therefore, they might not be suitable for food fortification in those regions with high prevalence rates of *Helicobacter pylori* infection [6]. The third group includes iron compounds insoluble in water and poorly soluble in diluted acid solutions. Thus, these iron sources although less bioavailable, are mostly stable in food vehicles. This is why they are extensively used for food fortification even in vehicles such as infant formulas and cereals [6]. Bioavailability reports of members of this group have shown a variety of results with regard to rates of absorption (5–95 %) depending on the food matrix and the iron source as assayed in humans or animals [8, 9]. Therefore, at least for poorly water-soluble iron compounds, the use of a single RBV value to set a fortification level and predict potential efficacy in all food vehicles may be of limited value [10]. Because of their low reactivity, they are commonly used to fortify cereals, infant formulas and flours.

Ferric Pyrophosphate

One of the best examples of the above discussion about iron compounds of group III is ferric pyrophosphate. Ferric pyrophosphate, which is a white-coloured poorly soluble iron compound, does not change organoleptic properties of foods even when used in many difficult-to-fortify food vehicles [11]. First reports about its bioavailability showed that it was only about 30–50 % of ferrous sulphate [12] which reduced its nutritional value. Nevertheless, some strategies were implemented in order to overcome this problem, such as protect it, solubilize o stabilize it and/or reduce its particle size.

Strategies for Improving Bioavailability

Particle size is an important determinant of iron absorption from poorly soluble iron compounds in foods. Decreasing the particle size of elemental iron powders increases their absorption as it was demonstrated in many reports [13–16]. Therefore this strategy was employed in the development of ferric pyrophosphate micronized sources where this parameter was modified from regular (21 μm) to 2.5 or 0.5 μm or even nanoparticles [17, 18]. In this way, some micronized dispersible ferric pyrophosphate sources were developed, potentially useful in food vehicles that readily undergo adverse sensory changes when fortified with soluble iron, such as rice, infant cereals and salt [8]. The effect of reducing the particle size on the bioavailability of this insoluble iron compound was tested in different studies (which are summarized in Table 7.2).

Conclusions derived from these results clearly show that the possibility of obtaining dispersable ferric pyrophosphate when reducing its particle size improves its bioavailability. Fidler et al. [19] reported an RBV in humans of 82 % from a wheat-milk infant cereal using a ferric pyrophosphate of ~0.3 μm whereas Moretti et al. [10] published 62 % because of the greater particle size (0.77 μm) of their iron source. Another interesting conclusion is that, for the same particle size of ferric pyrophosphate the food matrix is an important factor which affects bioavailability. For example, the same batch of micronized ferric pyrophosphate (same particle size) was assayed in wheat-milk infant formula with an RBV of 62 % while RBV for rice resulted only of 15–24 % [10]. On the other hand, reduction of particle size not only accounted for improving ferric pyrophosphate bioavailability in food vehicles as powders but also developments were made in order to consider it as an alternative fortificant for

Table 7.2 Bioavailability assays for ferric pyrophosphate

References	Strategy	Population—vehicle	Results
Hurrell et al. [9]	Ferric pyrophosphate (compared to ferrous sulphate)	Women 20–40 y; chocolate drink	
	Added in test meal immediately before consumption		RBV 75 %
	Processed during the manufacture of the chocolate drink powder		RBV 21 %
Moretti et al. [10]	Reduced particle size 0.77 μm micronized dispersible ferric pyrophosphate	Young women fed with: wheat-milk infant cereal given with and without ascorbic acid; processed and unprocessed rice meal	RBV 62 % vs. 39 % RBV 15 % vs. 24 %
Wegmüller et al. [17]	Reduced particle size regular 21 μm vs. 2.5 μm Protection 2.5 μm encapsulated in hydrogenated palm oil vs. 0.5 μm mixed with emulsifiers	Vehicle AIN93G diet for laboratory animals	RBV 59 % vs. RBV 69 % RBV 43 % vs. RBV 95 %
Fidler et al. [19]	Reduced particles size + protection 0.3 μm mixed with emulsifiers (compared to ferrous sulphate)	Adult women fed with: Wheat-based infant cereal yoghurt drink	RBV 87 % RBV 97 %
Tsuchita et al. [20]	Protection (powder vs. suspension)	Diets for laboratory animals	
	Mixed with skim milk and dehydrated		RBV 100 %
	Directly dehydrated		RBV 66 %
	Directly dehydrated mixed with skim milk and dehydrated		RBV 82 %
Salgueiro et al. [21]	Protection ferric pyrophosphate stabilized and solubilized with glycine (compared to ferrous sulphate)	Animals fed with a modified AIN93G; iron supplied in:	
		Water	RBV 106 %
		Yoghurt	RBV 114 %
Hurrell et al. [22]	Solubilization	Experimental diets fed to laboratory animals female 20–46 y fed with an infant cereal	
	Ferric pyrophosphate		RBV 58 %
	Ferric pyrophosphate solubilized with sodium citrate		RBV 103 %
	Ferric pyrophosphate solubilized with ammonium citrate		RBV 83 %
	Ferric pyrophosphate		RBV 39 %
Moretti et al. [23]	Reduced particle size 2.5 μm micronized ground ferric pyrophosphate (vs. placebo)	6–13-y-old children fed with fortified rice (7 mo)	Prevalence of iron deficiency and iron deficiency anaemia Baseline: 78 % and 29 %, respectively End of treatment: 25 % vs. 49 % and 15 % vs. 28 %, respectively

(continued)

Table 7.2 (continued)

References	Strategy	Population—vehicle	Results
Radhika et al. [24]	Reduced particle size 3.14 μm (vs. placebo)	5–11-y-old children fed with fortified extruded rice kernels (8 mo)	Prevalence of iron deficiency decreased significantly (33–14 %) and increased marginally in the placebo group (31–37 %)
Zhu et al. [25]	Soluble ferric pyrophosphate effects of ascorbic acid, tannic acid, Ca, Zn, Mg, citrate, cysteine, incorporation to rice and to non-fat milk	Caco-2 cell culture model with or without the combination of in vitro digestion	Bioavailability affected in similar directions but in smaller scale than ferrous sulphate and ferric chloride
Davidsson et al. [26]	Infant cereal fortified with: ferrous fumarate, ferric pyrophosphate, ferrous sulphate	Infant cereal fortified fed to children aged 7–24 mo (9 mo)	No differences were observed for haemoglobin, plasma ferritin or plasma C-reactive protein among groups
Hurrell et al. [27]	Ferric pyrophosphate	Males and females 18–40 y fed with a fortified wheat cereal	RBV 15 %

Guidance on levels to be added
For most food vehicles ferric pyrophosphate, as an iron fortificants, is added at twice the amount (for details, see Guidelines on food fortification with micronutrients/edited by Lindsay Allen, Bruno de Benoist, Omar Dary and Richard Hurrell. ©World Health Organization and Food and Agriculture Organization of the United Nations 2006. ISBN 92 4 159401 2. Available: http://www.who.int/nutrition/publications/guide_food_fortification_micronutrients.pdf)
RBV relative biological value; *y* years; *mo* months

liquid foods. In this case, processing of fortified foods is crucial for determining iron bioavailability from ferric pyrophosphate as demonstrated by Hurrel et al. [9]. In this study the RBV of ferric pyrophosphate fell from 75 to 21 % when it was processed into a vacuum-dried chocolate drink. Tsuchita et al. [20] showed similar results depending on the processing of dehydratation and rehydratation of fortified milk.

Protection and encapsulation of iron compounds are other general strategies to overcome major challenges in food fortification with iron [28]. Thus, protected forms of ferrous sulphate were extensively investigated for reducing its interaction and reactivity with the food matrix. Microencapsulation with liposomes and stabilization or chelation with aminoacids are some of the examples in literature [29–35]. In the case of insoluble iron compounds, like ferric pyrophosphate, protection strategies are referred mostly to the process of avoiding agglomeration of reduced particle size by adding some kind of emulsifiers. The objective is to assure the dispersion of micronized ferric pyrophosphate for improving its bioavailability. Studies performed in animals showed that the quality of the emulsifier affects iron absorption since RBV using hydrogenated palm oil was 43 % vs. 95 % when using a mix of dextrin, glycerol esters of fatty acids, sodium chloride and enzymatically hydrolyzed lecithin [17]. In the same way, solubilization of ferric pyrophosphate was an alternative to increase its bioavailability as reflected in some studies where addition of aminoacids such as glycine during manufacture of the iron compound [21], as well as solubilization with sodium citrate and ammonium citrate were performed [22]. A remark that appeared from these results is that protection is not only useful to improve ferric pyrophosphate bioavailability in dry vehicles but also makes it an attractive source to fortify liquid foods or drinks such as milk. First ferric pyrophosphates used for food fortification were insoluble in liquid vehicles but new micronized and emulsified compounds are dispersible.

Conclusions

Food fortification with iron can be an effective strategy to control iron deficiency anaemia, but adding iron to food still remains a challenge. Non-water-soluble iron compounds have been reported to be less well absorbed than ferrous sulphate. Thus, concerns about their usefulness as food fortificants has been raised in the past, especially when young children are the target of them. Ferric pyrophosphate is one of these iron compounds that has been extensively assayed in many vehicles difficult to fortify because of many reasons, such as salt, cereals, infant formulas, rice and even dairy products. Contrary to earlier concerns, the results do not indicate significant differences in its bioavailability compared to that of water soluble compounds. Furthermore, ferric pyrophosphate does not interact with the nutritional matrix and does not change sensory characteristics of foods. Reducing the particle size, sometimes employing some emulsifier to prevent agglomeration, has demonstrated excellent results for improving ferric pyrophosphate bioavailability up to RBV similar to ferrous sulphate. Food-fortification practices vary nationally and the need to adjust the dietary iron bioavailability factor for fortification iron will depend on the proportion of fortification iron in the total iron intake and the iron compounds used [36]. Nonetheless, these data about ferric pyrophosphate will be important in the development of food-fortification strategies to combat anaemia and iron deficiency in highly vulnerable population [26].

References

1. Bothwell T, McPhail P. Prevention of iron deficiency by food fortification. In: Fomon SJ, Zlotkin S, editors. Nutritional anemias. Nestlé nutrition workshop series 30. New York: Raven; 1992. p. 183–92.
2. Boccio J, Salgueiro J, Lysionek A, Zubillaga M, Weill R, Goldman C, et al. Current knowledge of iron metabolism. Biol Trace Elem Res. 2003;92:189–212.
3. Wienk KJ, Marx JJ, Beynen AC. The concept of iron bioavailability and its assessment. Eur J Nutr. 1999;38:51–75.
4. Dutra-de-Oliveira JE, Freitas MLS, Ferreira JF, Gonçalves AL, Marchini JS. Iron from complex salts and its bioavailability to rats. Int J Vitam Nutr Res. 1995;65:272–5.
5. Fritz JC, Pla GW, Harrison BN, Clark GA, Smith EA. Measurement of the bioavailability of iron, using the rat hemoglobin repletion test. J Assoc Off Anal Chem. 1978;61:709–14.
6. Salgueiro MJ, Zubillaga MB, Lysionek A, Caro R, Weill R, Boccio J. Fortification strategies to combat zinc and iron deficiency. Nutr Rev. 2002;60:52–8.
7. World Health Organization. Guidelines on food fortification with micronutrients. Geneva, Switzerland: World Health Organization; 2006.
8. Moretti D, Lee TC, Zimmermann MB, Nuessli J, Hurrell RF. Development and evaluation of iron-fortified extruded rice grains. J Food Sci. 2005;70:S330–6.
9. Hurrell RF, Reddy MB, Dassenko SA, Cook JD. Ferrous fumarate fortification of a chocolate drink powder. Br J Nutr. 1991;65:271–83.
10. Moretti D, Zimmermann MB, Wegmüller R, Walczyk T, Zeder C, Hurrell R. Iron status and food matrix strongly affect the relative bioavailability of ferric pyrophosphate in humans. Am J Clin Nutr. 2006;83:632–8.
11. Wegmüller R, Zimmermann MB, Hurrell RF. Dual fortification of salt with iodine and encapsulated iron compounds: stability and acceptability testing in Morocco and Côte d'Ivoire. J Food Sci. 2003;68:2129–35.
12. Hurrell RF. How to ensure adequate iron absorption from iron-fortified food. Nutr Rev. 2002;60:S7–15.
13. Motzok I, Pennell MD, Davies MI, Ross HU. Effect of particle size on the bioavailability of reduced iron. J Assoc Off Anal Chem. 1975;58:99–103.
14. Verma RS, Motzok I, Chen SS, Rasper J, Ross HU. Effect of storage in flour and of particle size on the bioavailability of elemental iron powders for rats and humans. J Assoc Off Anal Chem. 1977;60:759–65.
15. Cook JD, Minnich V, Moore CV, Rasmussen A, Bradley WB, Finch CA. Absorption of fortification iron in bread. Am J Clin Nutr. 1973;26:861–72.
16. Swain JH, Newman SM, Hunt JR. Bioavailability of elemental iron powders to rats is less than bakery-grade ferrous sulfate and predicted by iron solubility and particle surface area. J Nutr. 2003;133:3546–52.

17. Wegmüller R, Zimmermann MB, Moretti D, Arnold M, Langhans W, Hurrel RF. Particle size reduction and encapsulation affect the bioavailability of ferric pyrophosphate in rats. J Nutr. 2004;134:3301–4.
18. Rhoner F, Ernst FO, Arnold M, Hilbe M, Biebinger R, Ehrensperger F, et al. Synthesis, characterization and bioavailability in rats of ferric phosphate nanoparticles. J Nutr. 2007;137:614–9.
19. Fidler MC, Walczyk T, Davidsson L, Zeder C, Sakaguchi N, Juneja LR, et al. A micronised, dispersible ferric pyrophosphate with high relative bioavailability in man. Br J Nutr. 2004;91:107–12.
20. Tsuchita H, Kobayashi A, Kojima T, Kuwata T, Noguchi T, Koto K, et al. Bioavailability of iron from ferric pyrophosphate. J Agric Food Chem. 1991;39:316–21.
21. Salgueiro MJ, Arnoldi S, Kaliski MA, Torti H, Messeri E, Weill R, et al. Stabilized-solubilized ferric pyrophosphate as a new iron source for food fortification. Bioavailability studies by means of the prophylactic-preventive method in rats. Biol Trace Elem Res. 2009;127:143–7.
22. Hurrell RF, Furniss DE, Burri J, Whittaker P, Lynch SR, Cook JD. Iron fortification of infant cereals: a proposal for the use of ferrous fumarate or ferrous succinate. Am J Clin Nutr. 1989;49:1274–82.
23. Moretti D, Zimmermann MB, Muthayya S, Thankachan P, Lee TC, Kurpad AV, et al. Extruded rice fortified with micronized ground ferric pyrophosphate reduces iron deficiency in Indian schoolchildren: a double-blind randomized controlled trial. Am J Clin Nutr. 2006;84:822–9.
24. Radhika MS, Nair KM, Kumar RH, Rao MV, Ravinder P, Reddy CG, et al. Micronized ferric pyrophosphate supplied through extruded rice kernels improves body iron stores in children: a double-blind, randomized, placebo-controlled midday meal feeding trial in Indian schoolchildren. Am J Clin Nutr. 2011;94:1202–10.
25. Zhu L, Glahn RP, Nelson D, Miller DD. Comparing soluble ferric pyrophosphate to common iron salts and chelates as sources of bioavailable iron in a Caco-2 cell culture model. J Agric Food Chem. 2009;57:5014–9.
26. Davidsson L, Sarker SA, Jamil KA, Sultana S, Hurrell R. Regular consumption of a complementary food fortified with ascorbic acid and ferrous fumarate or ferric pyrophosphate is as useful as ferrous sulfate in maintaining hemoglobin concentrations >105 g/L in young Bangladeshi children. Am J Clin Nutr. 2009;89:1815–20.
27. Hurrell RF, Reddy MB, Burri J, Cook JD. An evaluation of EDTA compounds for iron fortification of cereal-based foods. Br J Nutr. 2000;84:903–10.
28. Hurrell RF. Fortification: overcoming technical and practical barriers. J Nutr. 2002;132:806S–12.
29. Boccio J, Zubillaga M, Caro R, Lysionek A, Salgueiro J, Calmanovici G, et al. Microencapsulated ferrous sulfate to fortify cow milk absorption and distribution in mice. J Nutr Sci Vitaminol. 1998;44:381–9.
30. Lysionek A, Zubillaga M, Salgueiro J, Sarabia M, Caro R, Weill R, et al. Study of industrial microencapsulated ferrous sulfate by means of the prophylactic-preventive method to determine its bioavailability. J Nutr Sci Vitaminol. 2000;46:125–9.
31. Lysionek A, Zubillaga M, Salgueiro J, Caro R, Weill R, Boccio J. Bioavailability study of dried microencapsulated ferrous sulfate SFE-171 by means of the prophylactive-preventive method. J Trace Elem Med Biol. 2001;115:255–9.
32. Lysionek A, Zubillaga M, Salgueiro J, Piñeiro A, Caro R, Weill R, et al. Bioavailability of microencapsulated ferrous sulfate in powdered milk produced from fortified fluid milk: a prophylactic study in rats. Nutrition. 2002;18:279–81.
33. Zimmermann MB. The potential of encapsulated iron compounds in food fortification: a review. Int J Vitam Nutr Res. 2004;74:453–61.
34. Zimmermann MB, Zeder C, Chaouki N, Saad A, Torresani T, Hurrell RF. Dual fortification of salt with iodine and microencapsulated iron: a randomized, double-blind, controlled trial in Moroccan schoolchildren. Am J Clin Nutr. 2003;77:425–32.
35. Zimmermann MB, Zeder C, Chaouki N, Torresani T, Saad A, Hurrell RF. Addition of microencapsulated iron to iodized salt improves the efficacy of iodine in goitrous, iron-deficient children: a randomized, double-blind, controlled trial. Eur J Endocrinol. 2002;147:747–53.
36. Hurrell R, Egli I. Iron bioavailability and dietary reference values. Am J Clin Nutr. 2010;91(Suppl):1461S–7.

Chapter 8
Iron- and Zinc-Fortified Parboiled Rice

Chanakan Prom-u-thai and Benjavan Rerkasem

Key Points

- Fortification of iron and zinc in parboiling process effectively increased iron and zinc concentrations compared with those in non-fortified parboiled rice, especially in the polished rice where most of iron and zinc is usually removed during milling process.
- Parboiled rice is already produced on industrial scale and traded globally as well as within each country.
- It is commonly consumed in South Asia and Africa where iron and zinc deficiencies in human population are widespread.
- Iron and zinc-fortified parboiled rice can easily and rapidly reach rice consumers in these countries without the need to alter consumption habits of local populations and establishing new market network and access.
- It offers highly cost-effective tool to reduce the incidences of iron deficiency in developing countries within an immediate future if it is adopted by the current parboiled rice industry.

Keywords Rice • *Oryza sativa* • Parboiled rice Fortification • Parboiling process • Polishing process • Iron • Zinc

Abbreviations

DAE Dilute acid extractable
DTZ Diphenyl thiocarbazone
Fe Iron

C. Prom-u-thai, Ph.D. (✉)
Agronomy Division, Department of Plant Science and Natural Resources,
Chiang Mai University, Chiang Mai 50200, Thailand
e-mail: chanakan.p@cmu.ac.th

B. Rerkasem, Ph.D.
Plant Genetic Resource and Nutrition Laboratory, Chiang Mai University,
Chiang Mai 50200, Thailand
e-mail: benrerkasem@gmail.com

V.R. Preedy et al. (eds.), *Handbook of Food Fortification and Health: From Concepts to Public Health Applications Volume 1*, Nutrition and Health, DOI 10.1007/978-1-4614-7076-2_8,

Fe-EDTA	Iron-ethylene diamine tetraacetic acid
PPB	Pearl Prussian blue
Zn	Zinc

Introduction

Iron (Fe) and zinc (Zn) deficiency have been estimated to affect 70–95 % of the population in Asia [1, 2], where rice is the staple food for most people. Iron deficiency induces anemia, impairs growth, development and immunity, especially in infants and young children [3, 4], while Zn deficiency adversely affects the immune system, increases susceptibility to infections, restricts growth in young children and impairs the senses for taste and smell, memory and spermatogenesis in adults [5, 6]. Increasing Fe and Zn concentration in rice grain (in polished rice) is expected to promote Fe and Zn intake by rice consumers and decrease incidences of Fe and Zn deficiency among the poor, especially in developing countries where access to Fe- and Zn-rich foods such as animal products is limited [7, 8].

To alleviate Fe and Zn deficiency in human populations, several strategies have been suggested, including supplementation, dietary modification and food fortification [9], as well as genetic and agronomic biofortification during production of staple food crops [10–12]. Supplementation schedules, however, are not cost-effective in the long term and the efficacy also depends on reeducating consumers who have limited knowledge on nutrition and health. Dietary modification may promote increased consumption of Fe and Zn from food sources, which are produced through cropping high Fe and Zn cultivars and improved Fe and Zn fertilizer management [10, 13]. This strategy is promising, but requires expertise in fertilizer management and its effectiveness in boosting Fe and Zn density in grains can vary a great deal, with changing seasonal conditions and other agronomic practices. The wide range of Fe and Zn in the grain of different varieties of rice [14, 15] offers an opportunity to increase Fe and Zn content by rice breeding, but it is time consuming and expensive [16] and may not be feasible for economically disadvantaged in developing countries. Iron concentration of the genetically modified "golden rice" has been successfully boosted several folds [12, 17]. However, vigorous opposition to genetically modified or GM food has led to the golden rice to face stiff resistance from consumers and governments in many countries. In the mean time, alternative cost-effective means to deliver improved Fe and Zn nutrition through the staple food system are urgently needed to address this Fe and Zn deficiency problem. Cost-effective fortification methods that can be readily deployed need to be easily integrated into existing rice processing, marketing, and distribution network.

Fortification of Fe and Zn in the flour of wheat, corn, and rice has been successfully established [1, 6]. Iron and Zn fortification in rice flour has also been promoted in Sri Lanka and the Philippines [1]. However, the practice is far from common in most developing countries. Unlike wheat which is mostly polished into flour before further processing into bread, pasta, or noodle, the volume of rice used as flour constitutes a miniscule fraction of all rice consumed. Therefore, as a means to boost Fe and Zn intake in rice eaters, rice needs to be fortified with Fe and Zn in the form of whole grains that people commonly eat. The Fe- and Zn-fortified rice must also meet the sensory standard of the target consumers, and the nutrient density is sufficiently robust against normal procedure for rice cooking. Thus fortification in rice by mixing Fe surface coated grain with ordinary rice has not been well received as the off-color of Fe coated grains are readily detected and tend to be removed along with other impurities [7]. Moreover, Fe in the surface coating tends to be lost when rice is washed, another common precooking procedure.

This review looks at parboiled rice, a form of processed rice, which accounts for a sizable share of the global rice harvest and is the major form of rice consumed in South Asia and Africa, as a possible vehicle for delivering Fe and Zn nutrition, especially among low income rice eaters in developing countries.

Rice Processing and Potential for Fortification

The ripe rice seed consists of the caryopsis enclosed in a tough siliceous hull (husk). The first step of rice milling is to remove the husk, which subtracts about 20 % from the paddy weight, and produces unpolished rice [18]. The next step is mechanical polishing to produce polished rice, the form of rice most commonly consumed, and bran which consists of the outer layers of the caryopsis including pericarp, testa, nucellus, part of the aleurone layer and some endosperm along with the germ or embryo. The bran fraction constitutes about 10 % of unpolished rice weight [18], and up to 85 % of the Fe and Zn content of unpolished rice [14, 19]. Because of its content of many nutrients unpolished rice is becoming increasingly popular among health conscious rice eaters. In much major rice growing regions the paddy is also processed by parboiling, by steaming of wet paddy, before milling.

Parboiling rice is a traditional practice that has been established for more than 20 centuries. Parboiled rice is produced in many parts of the world including India, Bangladesh, Pakistan, Myanmar, Malaysia, Sri Lanka, Guinea, South Africa, Italy, Spain, Thailand, Switzerland, USA, and France [20]. The production of parboiled rice is currently about >100 million tons annually which accounts for about half of the world rice crop [21]. People in many countries such as India (60 %) and Bangladesh (90 %) consume parboiled rice as the staple food [22]. Thailand, where practically no parboiled rice is consumed, exports 2–3 million tons of polished parboiled rice each year to the countries in Middle East and Africa [23]. Production and marketing system of parboiled rice, including processing facilities and trading network, is established in producing and consuming countries.

The process of rice parboiling involves soaking the unhusked paddy rice in warm water at 40–60 °C to reach the moisture content about 30 %. Harvesting at such high grain moisture content is the norm in off-season rice which reaches maturity at the start of the monsoons. It also helps to shorten the turn-around time between crops in modern rice farming with two to three rice crops are grown on the same land in each year. Parboiling allows farmers to sell their paddy rice at high moisture contents of 20–30 % without drastic price deduction of substandard grade rice, as it would have been polished into very low grade raw rice or otherwise required costly drying. Without drying facility, thc wct rice seed could also begin to germinate and produce undesirable odor. Soaking in warm water helps to prevent paddy rice from fermentation which can cause strong offensive odor. The soaked paddy rice is steamed under low pressure for a period of time which result in gelatinization of the endosperm starch, making the grain more resistant against milling breakage. The milling yield of whole grain as percentage of paddy weight, head rice yield, ranges from 80 to 100 % in parboiled rice, compared with 20–60 % in raw rice [24, 25]. Slight pressure at 0.8–1.0 kg cm^{-2} during steaming helps to shorten steaming time which can be expensive in a longer process. The steamed paddy rice is then dried in the sun or power driers depending on available facility of each mill. De-husking and polishing are applied to the dried parboiled rice in the same way as the processing of ordinary, non-parboiled, or raw rice to produce white (polished) parboiled rice, a preferred form among parboiled rice consumers, and occasionally unpolished parboiled rice. Polished parboiled rice is usually slightly yellowish although the color largely fades after cooking and the texture is a bit harder than raw rice because of gelatinization of the starch grains. Parboiled rice is generally reported to be more nutritious than raw rice as most of nutrients located in the outer layers of the caryopsis have moved inwards in to the endosperm during parboiling [26].

The parboiling therefore prevents losses in and adding to the value of rice harvested at high moisture contents in three ways. Firstly, steaming kills the seed and prevents it from germinating. Secondly, gelatinization of the starch grain reduces grain breakage after milling. Thirdly, it saves the production cost of rice by saving the cost of drying. Fourthly, if saves time and allow more rice crops to be grown on the same land with earlier harvest and shorter turn-around time between crops. We now examine how fortification with Fe and Zn may be incorporated in to the parboiling process, by first reviewing the commercial parboiling process in Thailand, the world's largest exporter of parboiled rice and then exploring laboratory procedures for effective fortification of Fe and Zn through parboiling.

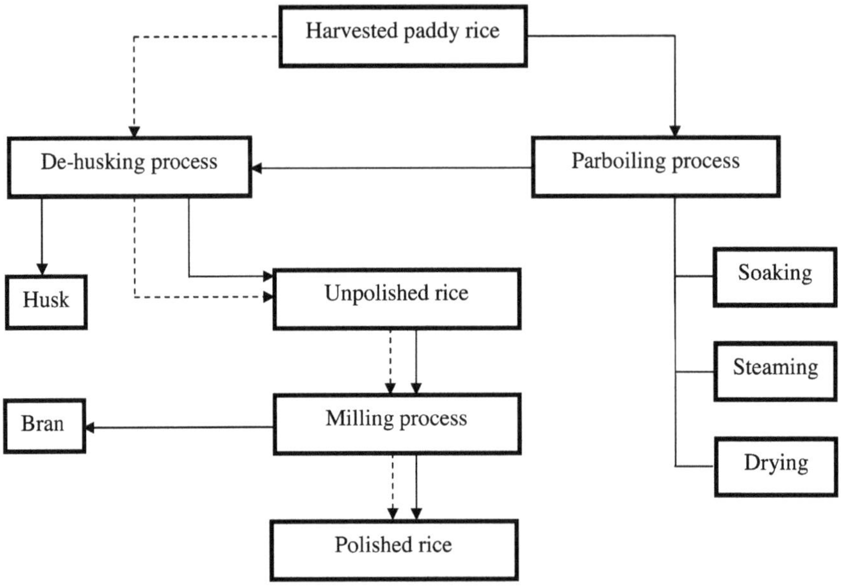

Fig. 8.1 The process of raw (*broken line*) and parboiled rice (*full line*) from farmer's harvest to product for export

Interviews with parboiled rice mill operators in the Central and Lower Northern Regions of Thailand provided information on the parboiling process in an industry that produces 2–3 million tons of polished rice for export each year (Fig. 8.1). The rice varieties considered most suitable for parboiling were CNT1, SPR1, and PSL2, with amylose content of 26–29 %. Low amylose content rice varieties are not usually recommend to use in parboiling process due to the problem of too soft and sticky texture during parboiling process. Paddy arriving from the farm with high moisture (25–30 %) may go straight to the parboiling processes, shipment is usually does with lower moisture but >14 % is dried in the sun or in power drier. The parboiling process begins with cleaning rice seed as it may be dirty during harvesting processes in the field. Then the process is continuing with soaking of the paddy at 60 °C for 4–6 h. This warm soaking stops fungal growth which can develop undesirable odor as well as the seed from germinating. Soaked paddy rice is then steaming at low pressure, depending on technique available at each mill. Slight pressure at 0.8–1.0 kg cm^{-2} during steaming helps to shorten steaming time, while normal steaming without pressure is requiring longer period. The duration of soaking and steaming is also well known as the technique to control the final color and texture of the parboiled rice product as it can be controlled depending on the order from customers. Therefore, it is most likely as secrete among each parboiled rice mills. The steamed paddy rice is then dried in the sun or power driers depending on available facility of each mill.

Incorporating Iron and Zinc Fortification into Rice Grain in the Parboiling Process

In laboratory scale, parboiling was processed by using paddy rice grains of the selected cultivars. Approximately 200 g of paddy rice were rinsed thoroughly in three changes of filtered water and then three changes of distilled water before applying treatments to prevent it from contamination from Fe and Zn.

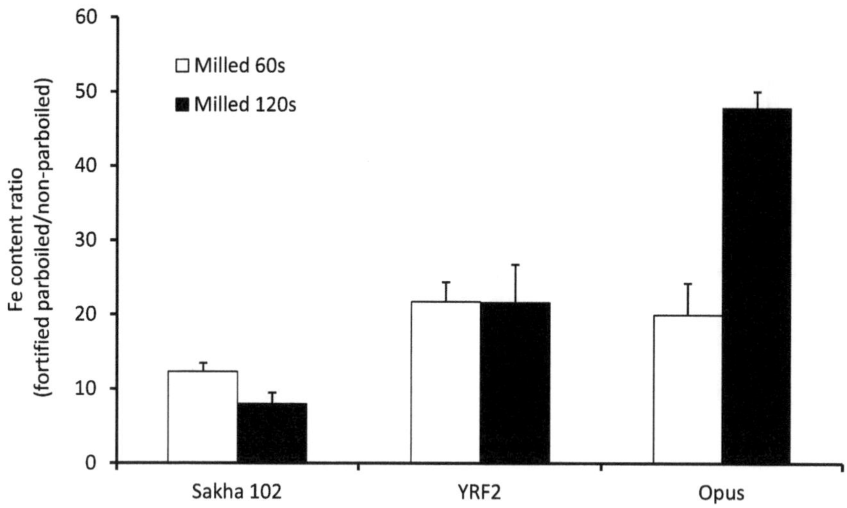

Fig. 8.2 The ratio of Fe content in fortified rice grain to that of unfortified rice grain. The parboiled and raw grains were polished for 60 and 120 s. The *bars* represent standard errors of corresponding means from three replicates. Flow chart shows the process of raw (*broken line*) and parboiled rice (*full line*) from farmer's harvest to product for export

For fortification process, rinsed paddy rice was soaked in 200 mL of Fe solution containing 150, 250, 350, and 450 mg Fe kg^{-1} of paddy rice, at acidic (3.0–3.5) pH values for Fe fortification and 50, 100, 150, 200, 250, 300, 350, and 400 mg Zn kg^{-1}, as $ZnSO_4$ or ZnO for zinc fortification. Zinc sulfate and oxide are commonly used in food fortification due to their chemical stability and cost effectiveness [5, 6]. For the control treatment, unfortified parboiled rice, rinsed paddy rice, was soaked with 200 mL of distilled water. The above soaked paddy rice grains were steamed under the low pressure (0.8 kg cm^{-2}) at 119 °C for 10 min in a pressure steamer (Megafeta, model-supernova, Spain). The steamed paddy rice was cooled and sun-dried to the moisture level of 10–12 %. The dried paddy rice with Fe and Zn fortification was de-husked to yield unpolished rice and then polishing to produce polished rice as for a common practice in the industry.

Adding Fe and Zn to the paddy rice in the parboiling process significantly increases total Fe and Zn concentration in the polished rice grain, which is potentially, highly bioavailable based on an in vitro evaluation [24, 27]. Under laboratory simulated parboiling conditions, Fe and Zn fortification increased Fe and Zn concentrations in polished rice for up to 50- and 5-folds, respectively, compared to the background level of 4–7 mg Fe kg^{-1} and 10–12 mg Zn kg^{-1} dry weight, but the increase was also influenced by variety, milling time, and fortification rate (Figs. 8.2 and 8.3). This means that differences of variety, milling time, and fortification rate will be need to be considered for the potential of Fe fortification in parboiling process. For Zn fortification, $ZnSO_4$ and ZnO gave similar results in the Zn enrichment of polished rice, while grain Zn concentration increased with increasing rate of Zn fortification. This means that the ratio of Zn fortification in parboiling process is much more significant than Zn form.

On the other hand, the concentration of Fe in polished rice exponentially increased with increasing rate of Fe fortification with variation among varieties, indicating the different potential of Fe penetration into the inner layer of rice grain among rice varieties (Fig. 8.4). This means that rate of fortification many need to be adjusted accordingly for different rice varieties for the potential of Fe fortification in parboiling process.

Current findings also indicate that the optimum condition for Fe and Zn fortification in parboiling process is soaking paddy rice grains (unhusked) in acidic (pH 3.0–3.5) iron-ethylene diamine tetraacetic acid (Fe-EDTA) for Fe and $ZnSO_4$ or ZnO for Zn solution containing 250 mg Fe and Zn kg^{-1} paddy rice at 60 °C for 6 h. Under this set of conditions, Fe and Zn concentration in parboiled rice

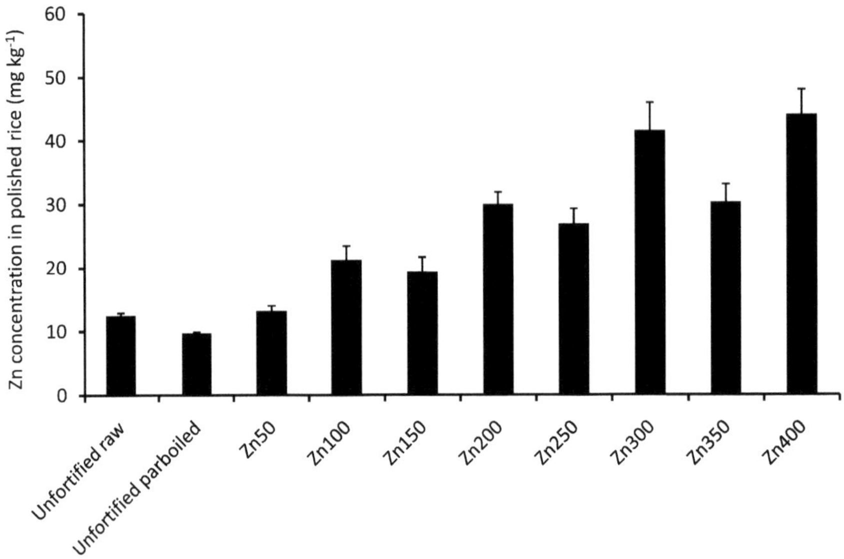

Fig. 8.3 Zinc concentration in polished rice treated with different rates of Zn fortification. The Zn values were pooled together from two forms of Zn treatments. The histogram shows the mean + SEM of Zn concentration in polished rice treated with different rates of Zn fortification from the *Journal of Food Chemistry* with permission from Elsevier. *Source*: Prom-u-thai et al. [25], License no. 2775940066915, Issue date: 25 October 2011

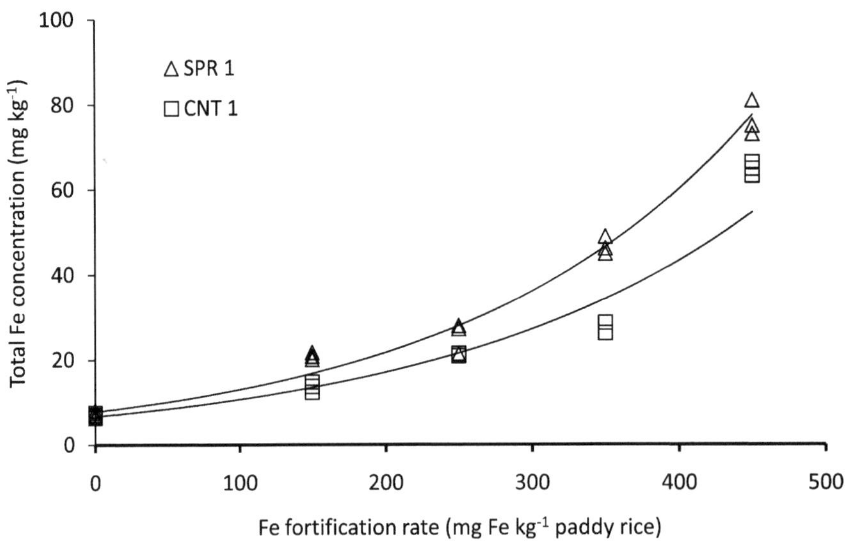

Fig. 8.4 Relationship between Fe fortification rates and total Fe concentrations in polished rice of Fe-fortified parboiled rice and unfortified and raw/parboiled rice in two rice varieties pooled ($n = 18$). The relationship between Fe fortification rates and total Fe concentrations in polished rice of Fe-fortified parboiled rice and unfortified and raw/parboiled rice from the *Journal of Food Chemistry* with permission from Elsevier. *Source*: Prom-u-thai et al. [25], License no. 2775930865488, Issue date: 25 October 2011

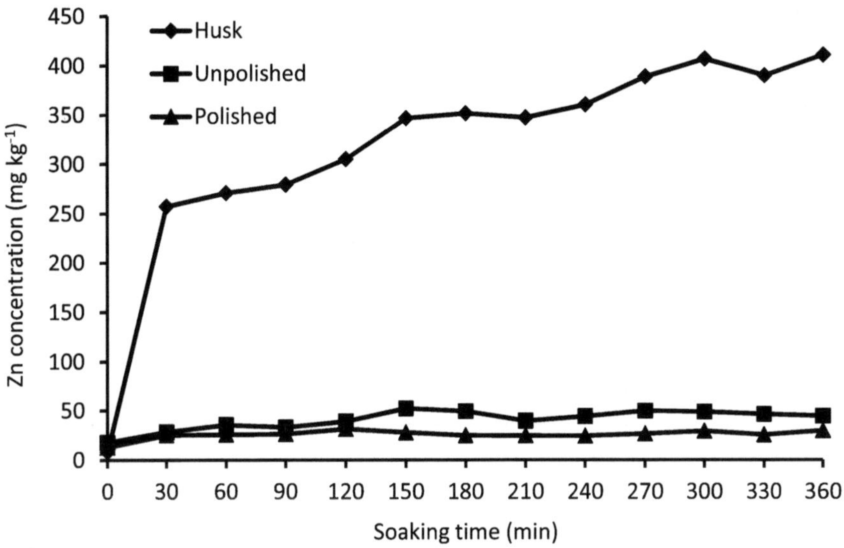

Fig. 8.5 Zinc concentrations in husk, unpolished and polished rice treated with 200 mg Zn kg^{-1} paddy rice over different soaking time during fortification process. The line graph shows Zn concentrations in husk, unpolished and polished rice treated with 200 mg Zn kg^{-1} paddy rice over different soaking time during fortification process from the *Journal of Food Chemistry* with permission from Elsevier. *Source*: Prom-u-thai et al. [25], License no. 2775940066915, Issue date: 25 October 2011

increased to 27 mg Fe kg^{-1} and 30 mg Zn kg^{-1}, the levels considered desirable to correct deficiency in rice eaters (Ross Welch, personal communication), from the base of 5 mg Fe kg^{-1} and 10–12 mg Zn kg^{-1} in unfortified parboiled and raw polished rice, without adverse impact on rice cooking qualities such as color, flavor, and textures [28].

The fortified Fe and Zn effectively penetrated into the interior of the endosperm, which was clearly demonstrated localization staining with Perls' Prussian blue (PPB) for Fe and Diphenyl thiocarbazone (DTZ) for Zn. In the grains polished for 60 s, unfortified raw rice grains only had a very low intensity of staining in the surface layer of the endosperm, while in Fe-fortified and parboiled grain, a high intensity of staining was found in the outer layers (20–30 % of the cross-section distance) of the endosperm of the fortified grains [24]. Zinc penetration in rice grain increased with increasing Zn fortification rate. By examining Zn concentrations in husk, unpolished and polished rice grains after fortification process, it was shown that the added Zn penetrated across the rice grain within 30 min after soaking (Fig. 8.5). There was a high rate of Zn retention in the husk which contained up to 257 mg Zn kg^{-1} dry matter. In comparison, Zn concentrations in unpolished rice increased from 17 to 28 and in polished rice from 13 to 25 mg kg^{-1}, after 30 min of soaking. The results indicated that the distribution of the staining tended to diffuse through the dorsal region of the grain and gradually towards the opposite pole of the grain. From visual observation, the parboiling process achieved a significant penetration through the inner layers of the endosperm of the parboiled rice grains. The Fe and Zn penetration into the inner layer of the endosperm after fortification process ensure the retention of adequate Fe and Zn after polishing for optimum cooking qualities of rice grain. In addition, the penetration of fortified Fe and Zn into the inner layer of rice grain after parboiling process is confirmed by the positive linear relationship between unpolished and polished rice, in which Fe and Zn concentration in polished rice of the fortified, parboiled rice increased linearly with those of the unpolished rice (Figs. 8.6 and 8.7).

When dealing with the low income sector of the population, for whom efforts to overcome Fe and Zn deficiency problem are directed, cost of rice is a matter of concern. The quality of polished rice,

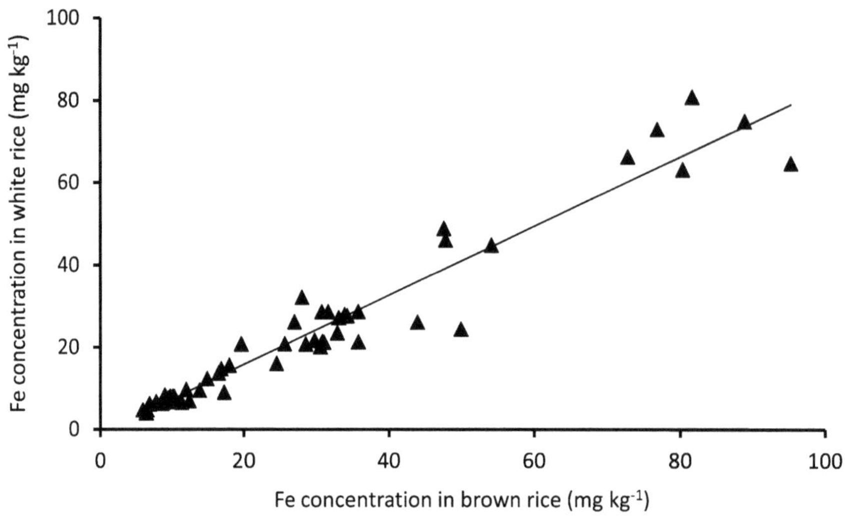

Fig. 8.6 Relationship between Fe concentration in unpolished and polished rice in unfortified raw/parboiled rice and Fe-fortified parboiled rice with different rates of Fe loading among three rice varieties. The relationship between Fe concentration in unpolished and polished rice in unfortified raw/parboiled rice and Fe-fortified parboiled rice from the *Journal of Food Chemistry* with permission from Elsevier. *Source*: Prom-u-thai et al. [25], License no. 2775930865488, Issue date: 25 October 2011

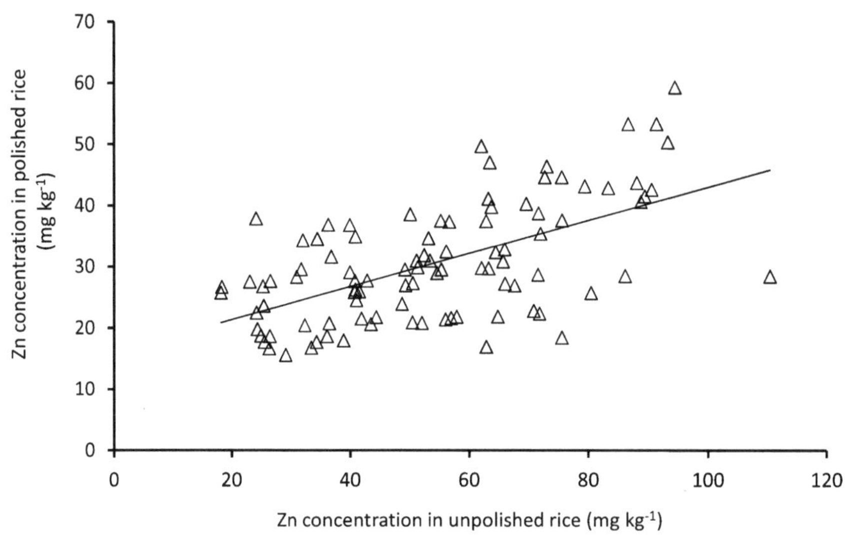

Fig. 8.7 Relationship between Zn concentration in unpolished and polished rice of parboiled rice fortified with different rates of Zn of two Zn forms in two rice cultivars. The relationship between Zn concentration in unpolished and polished rice of parboiled rice fortified with different rates of Zn from the *Journal of Food Chemistry* with permission from Elsevier. *Source*: Prom-u-thai et al. [25], License no. 2775940066915, Issue date: 25 October 2011

and so the price, are generally determined by the percentage of whole grain. Broken rice generally sells at one quarter to half of the price of premium grade full grain rice, with the market for broken parboiled from Thailand is among low income earners in various countries. The fact that broken rice is preferred among lower income consumers, for economic reason also brings an unexpected nutritional advantage. The Fe concentration in unfortified parboiled rice in the broken grain was more than

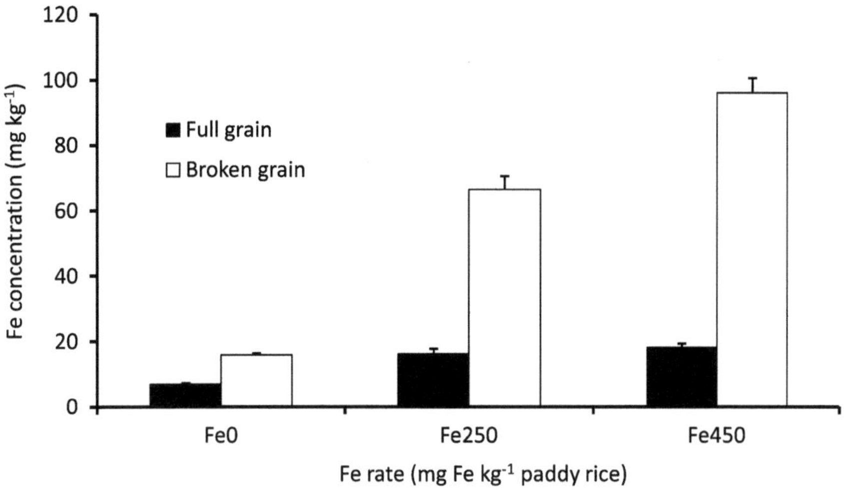

Fig. 8.8 Fe concentrations in full and broken grains in cultivar CNT1 of unfortified (Fe0) and fortified parboiled rice at 250 (Fe250) and 450 (Fe450) mg Fe kg^{-1} paddy rice. The histogram shows the mean + SEM of Fe concentrations in full and broken grains in cultivar CNT1 of unfortified (Fe0) and fortified parboiled rice from the *Journal of Food and Nutrition Science* with permission from Scientific Research Publishing. *Source*: Prom-u-thai et al. [32]

twice as much as in the full grain; the difference became magnified to 4–5 times in fortify parboiled rice (Fig. 8.8). The reason for this appears to be higher concentration of Fe in the grain tips that break off to constitute to broken grain. This concentration of Fe at the grain tips that becomes even more intensified in Fe-fortified parboiled rice fortified with Fe can be seen by the more intense staining of Fe by Perls' Prussian blue.

Even though, the concentration of Zn in broken fortified parboiled rice has not been evaluated as for Fe, but the results so far indicated that it is a real advantage that the cheaper broken rice already contains much more Fe means that low income rice consumes are already benefiting. Work on rice grain Fe should focus more on the cheaper broken grain and less on the more expensive whole grain. Fortification of Fe during parboiling therefore appears very promising as a means of improving Fe nutrition among parboiled rice consumers, including those with low income who buys broken rice, and so reducing the risk of Fe deficiency anemia among rice eaters.

Cooking and Acceptability to Consumers of Iron- and Zinc-Fortified Parboiled Rice

Washing rice in several rinses of water before cooking is a common practice among rice consumers. The fact that fortified Fe and Zn penetrate into the inner layers of rice grain ensures retention of the Fe and Zn during this precooking treatment. However, the degree of Fe and Zn loss from rinsing in the Fe and Zn-fortified parboiled rice grains may vary with cultivars, milling time and fortification rate (Figs. 8.9 and 8.10).

One of the most significant findings for Fe and Zn fortification through parboiling process is that the fortified Fe and Zn in the parboiled rice remained highly bioavailable, as measured by an in vitro digestion of cooked rice samples and Fe uptake at the intestinal surface by ferritin formation in cultured Caco-2 cells [29] as well as the dilute acid extraction of Fe and Zn as indirect method to measure Fe and Zn bioavailability [27]. This means that the enriched nutrients can be expected to have real

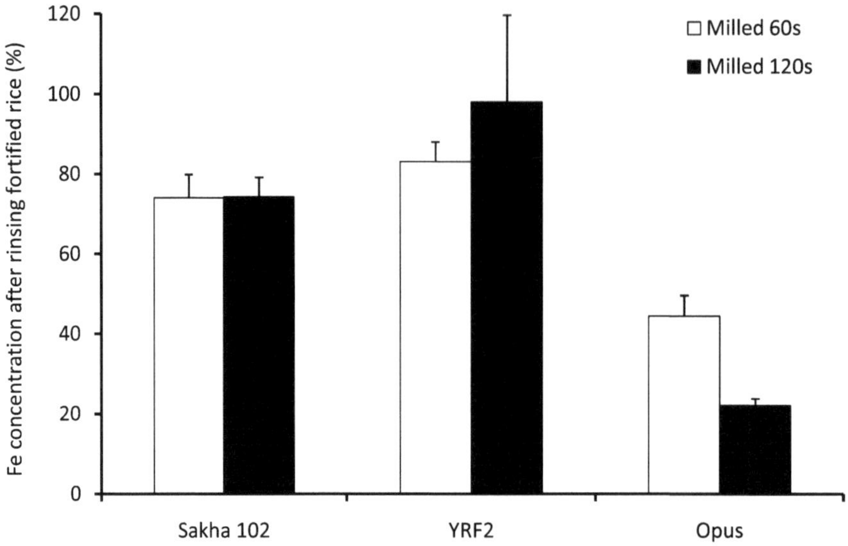

Fig. 8.9 Iron retention rate (as % of the un-rinsed) after rinsing (simulating rice washing) in the Fe-fortified parboiled rice grains polished for 60 and 120 s, respectively, in the three rice cultivars tested. The histogram shows mean + SEM of Fe retention rate (as % of the un-rinsed) after rinsing in the Fe-fortified parboiled rice grains milled for 60 and 120 s from the *Journal of Food Chemistry* with permission from Elsevier. *Source*: Prom-u-thai et al. [27, 28], License no. 2775940328307, Issue date: 25 October 2011

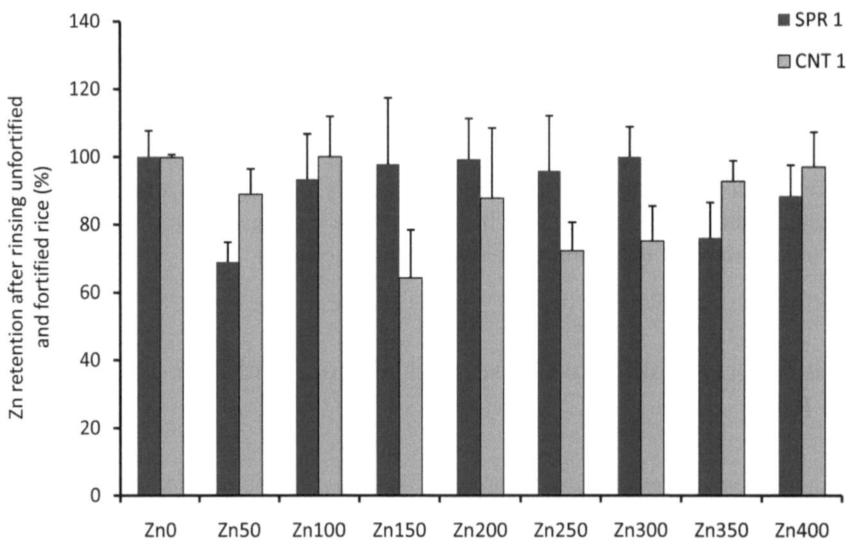

Fig. 8.10 Zinc retention rate (the amount of Zn remained after rising treatments/the total amount of Zn before rinsing) in parboiled rice after rinsing with three changes of water, which was fortified with different rates of $ZnSO_4$. The histogram shows the mean + SEM of Zn retention rate in parboiled rice after rinsing with three changes of water from the *Journal of Food Chemistry* with permission from Elsevier. *Source*: Prom-u-thai et al. [25], License no. 2775940066915, Issue date: 25 October 2011

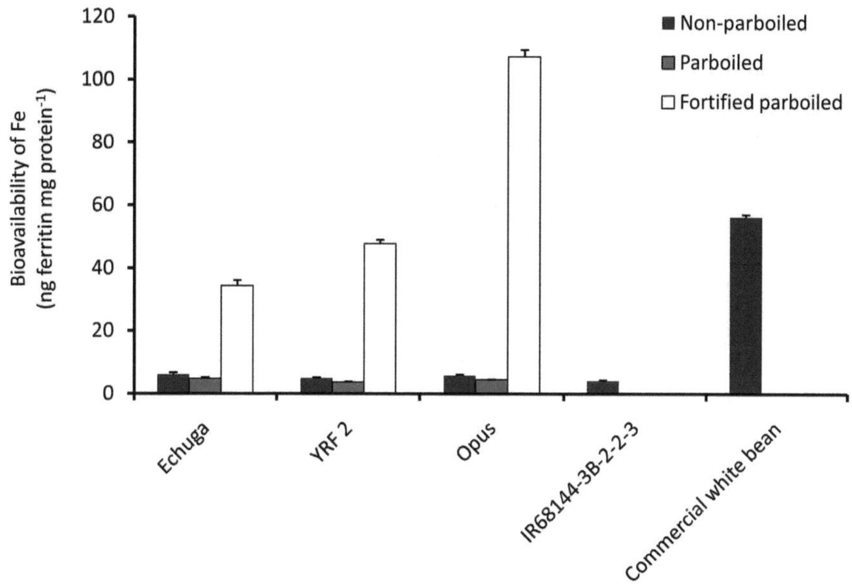

Fig. 8.11 Bioavailability of Fe from digests of rice samples in three cultivars after milling for 120 s and commercial Thai parboiled rice, IR68144-2B-3-2-2, KDML 105 and a commercial US white bean were included. Values are mean ± SEM ($n=3$). $FeCl_3$ with ascorbic acid (50 μm L^{-1} Fe with 1 mmol L^{-1} ascorbic acid) served as a positive control to verify responsiveness of the Caco-2 cells to bioavailable Fe. The histogram shows the mean + SEM of bioavailability of Fe from digests of rice samples in three cultivars after milling for 120 s and commercial Thai parboiled rice from the *Journal of Food Chemistry* with permission from Elsevier. *Source*: Prom-u-thai et al. [27, 28], License no. 2775940328307, Issue date: 25 October 2011

benefits to the consumers. Even though this method can rise up the level of Fe and Zn concentration in parboiled rice, but it would not be successful if fortified parboiled rice with Fe and Zn is not in bioavailable form for human diets.

The uptake of Fe by Caco-2 cells in the polished grains increased significantly with increasing levels of Fe loaded in the parboiled rice (Fig. 8.11). The fortified parboiled rice of cultivar Opus (107.3 ng ferritin mg $protein^{-1}$) had higher Fe uptake than in YRF 2 (47.7 ng ferritin mg $protein^{-1}$) and Echuga (34.2 ng ferritin mg $protein^{-1}$), respectively, which related with the order of the fortified Fe density in their parboiled rice grains. In comparison, the unfortified raw or parboiled rice of these cultivars had very low levels of Fe uptake, 4–7 ng ferritin mg $protein^{-1}$ as well as the cultivar IR68144-2B-3-2-2 (a selected high Fe line from conventional breeding). Commercial US white bean as a comparing sample, which is well known to be rich in bioavailable Fe, had about 57 ng ferritin mg $protein^{-1}$. This means that the method Fe and Zn fortification during parboiling process is not only significantly increasing Fe and Zn concentration in rice grain, but it is also enhancing bioavailability of Fe and Zn in human diets.

The advantage of parboiled rice fortified with Fe and Zn is that almost to all of the fortified Fe and Zn is in bioavailable form as it was observed from a close positive correlation between Fe uptake and total Fe concentrations in the rice samples tested: the unfortified raw and parboiled rice and Fe-fortified parboiled rice of the three cultivars tested ($r=0.96^{**}$) (Fig. 8.12). However, milling time and rinsing fortified parboiled rice also affected on Fe uptake. Increasing milling time decreased the level of Fe loaded in the Fe-fortified parboiled rice and their Fe uptake, but the Fe uptake remained relatively high at 35–120 ng ferritin mg $protein^{-1}$ after milling for 120 s, which was well above that of the unfortified raw and parboiled rice grains, the high Fe rice, and remained comparable to that of the legume sample. Rinsing the Fe-fortified, parboiled grains of YRF 2 decreased total Fe concentrations

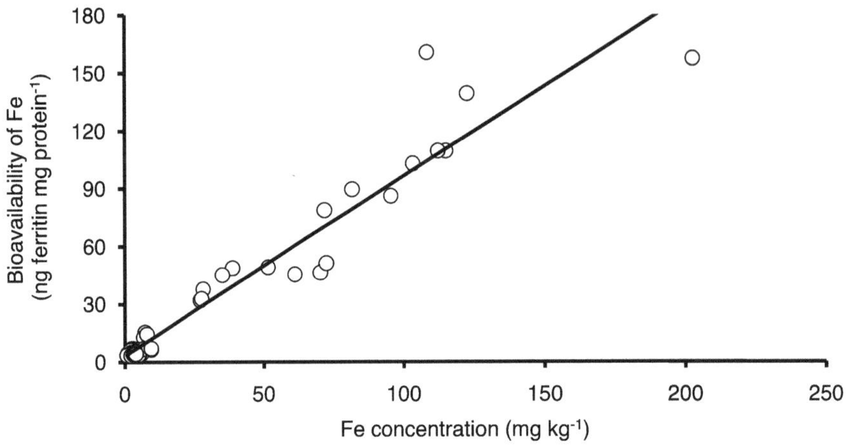

Fig. 8.12 Relationship between bioavailability of Fe and total Fe concentration in unfortified raw and parboiled rice and Fe-fortified parboiled rice of the three cultivars. The dataset was from test results with grains polished for 60 and 120 s ($n=54$). The relationship between bioavailability of Fe and total Fe concentration in unfortified raw and parboiled rice and Fe-fortified parboiled rice from the *Journal of Food Chemistry* with permission from Elsevier. *Source*: Prom-u-thai et al. [27, 28], License no. 2775940328307, Issue date: 25 October 2011

in the grains and thus the amount of bioavailable Fe in the grain, based on the Fe uptake test by Caco-2 cells. However, this effect was not strong enough to decrease the enhanced levels of bioavailable Fe in the Fe-fortified parboiled grain, resulting in 85 ng ferritin mg protein^{-1} Fe uptakes in rinsed grains, compared to about 100 ng ferritin mg protein^{-1} of non-rinsed grains in cultivar YRF 2. This level of Fe uptake in rinsed grains remained well above unfortified raw and parboiled rice. The rinsing effects were also observed in unfortified raw and parboiled rice grains in cultivar Opus. Therefore, fortification of Fe and Zn in parboiled rice is a promising approach to increase both Fe and Zn concentration in rice grain as well as its Fe and Zn uptake.

There is also a significant finding in this study, it was found that there was a close positive linear correlation between the uptake of Fe and dilute acid-extractable (DAE) Fe in polished grain of Fe-fortified parboiled rice grains of the three rice cultivars ($r=0.90^{**}$) (Fig. 8.13). This means that the method of DAE which is an easy and rapid method to determine the uptake of Fe can be used as an indirect method to evaluate the uptake of fortified Zn in parboiled rice. The uptake of fortified Zn was depending on rice cultivar and fortification rate (Fig. 8.14). There was also a linear correlation between the dilute acid-extractable (as an indirect index of bioavailable Zn pool) Zn and total Zn concentrations in the parboiled rice (Fig. 8.15). Even though, there is a convenient method to determine the level of bioavailability of Fe and Zn in fortified parboiled rice, an in vivo study is requiring in the future study.

The changes of precooking quality, cooking quality and consumers' acceptance are critical reasons that have contributed to the lack of success of Fe and Zn fortification of raw rice [30, 31]. The study of consumer acceptability has been investigated for Fe and it was found that these fundamental problems have not been found with Fe-fortified parboiled rice at optimal Fe density. Two sensory panels, one in parboiled rice eating Bangladesh and one in Thailand where parboiled rice is hardly ever consumed, found the cooked parboiled rice fortified with appropriate rate of Fe to be indistinguishable from commercially available and locally produced parboiled rice. The sensory test among 19 panelists in Bangladesh gave an overall acceptability of 100 % to the parboiled rice fortified with 250 mg Fe kg^{-1} paddy rice, while 95 % was given in unfortified parboiled rice. On the other hand, fortification with 450 mg Fe kg^{-1} paddy rice was given lower acceptability (63 %), probably due to the

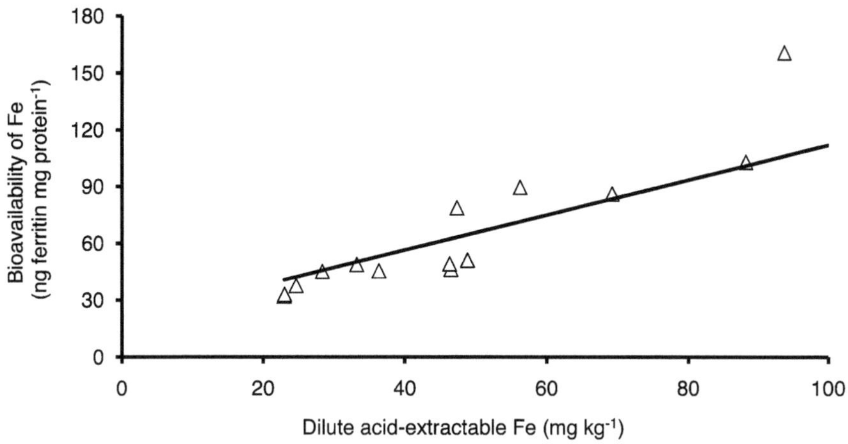

Fig. 8.13 Relationship between the dilute acid-extractable Fe and Fe bioavailability (in vitro test) in three cultivars of Fe-fortified parboiled rice. The dataset was pooled from test results with grains polished for 60 and 120 s ($n = 18$). The relationship between the dilute acid-extractable Fe and Fe bioavailability (in vitro test) of Fe-fortified parboiled rice from the *Journal of Food Chemistry* with permission from Elsevier. *Source*: Prom-u-thai et al. [27, 28], License no. 2775940328307, Issue date: 25 October 2011

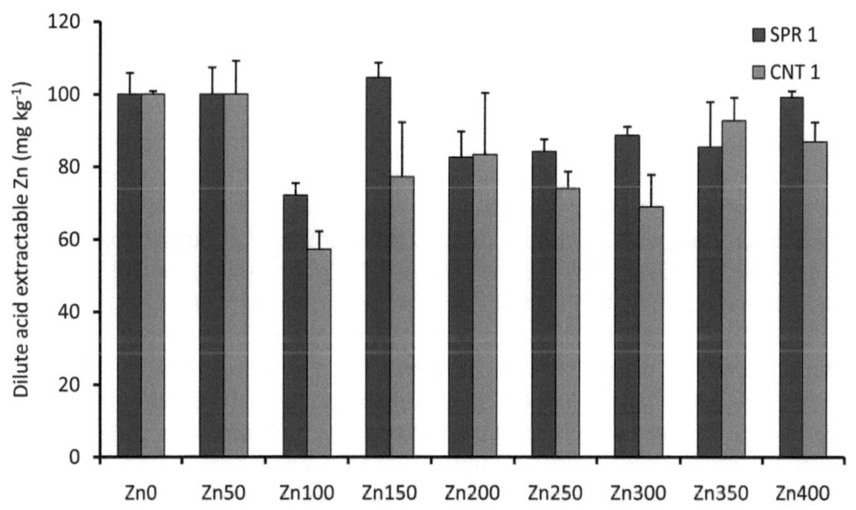

Fig. 8.14 The concentration of dilute acid-extractable (DAE) Zn (the potential bioavailable pool of Zn in polished rice of parboiled rice fortified with different rates of $ZnSO_4$). The histogram shows the mean + SEM of concentration of dilute acid-extractable Zn from the *Journal of Food Chemistry* with permission from Elsevier. *Source*: Prom-u-thai et al. [25], License no. 2775940066915, Issue date: 25 October 2011

changing of cooking quality such as color and/or flavor when fortified with very high rates of Fe [28]. The consumer acceptability has not been investigated for Zn-fortified parboiled rice. However, with the initial results from consumer's acceptability of parboiled rice fortified with Fe provide a great confidence of marketability and consumer acceptance of the Fe-fortified parboiled rice. However, the initial findings with Fe-fortified parboiled rice establish the information that the optimal rate of Fe and Zn fortification should be care as it is a great impact in consumer acceptability.

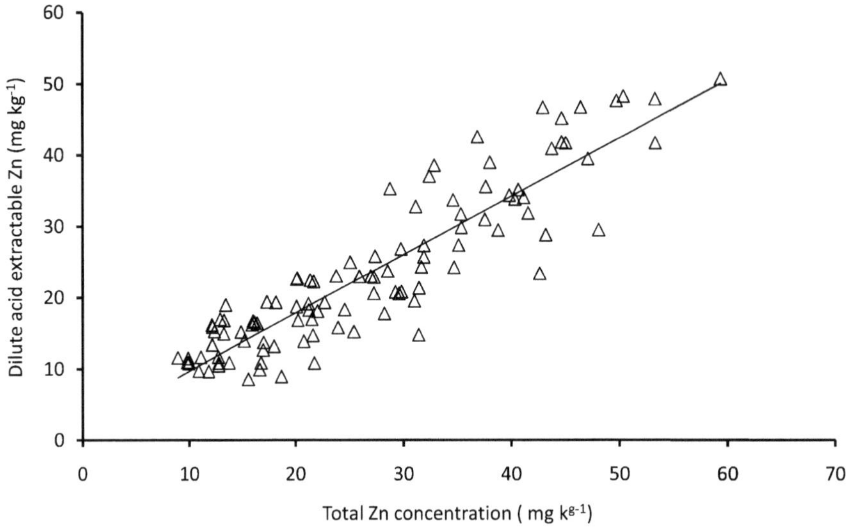

Fig. 8.15 The relationship between total Zn and DAE Zn concentration in parboiled rice treated with increasing rates of Zn. The data were pooled from the two cultivar tests. The relationship between total Zn and DAE Zn concentration in parboiled rice treated with increasing rates of Zn from the *Journal of Food Chemistry* with permission from Elsevier. *Source*: Prom-u-thai et al. [25], License no. 2775940066915, Issue date: 25 October 2011

Guidance on Levels to Be Added

Fortification of Fe and Zn through parboiling process is different from other direct food fortification processes as not all of Fe and Zn applied during fortification is retained inside fortified parboiled rice. This is because the fortifying nutrients are applied to the paddy rice with husk which is then removed before cooking and consumption in the husking process. Following fortification, parboiled-paddy rice is de-husked to yield unpolished rice and then the polishing process is applied to produce polished rice. Even though, much of fortified Fe and Zn is located in the husk of paddy rice, but significant level of fortified Fe and Zn is moved inwards into the inner grain layers during parboiling process. Therefore, the appropriate level of Fe and Zn concentration in polished parboiled rice will depend on amounts of the nutrients that penetrate into the endosperm interior during parboiling. However, since the penetration rate of Fe and Zn in fortified parboiled rice varied somewhat with rice cultivar, form of Fe and Zn, fortification rate and polishing time, adjustments may need to be made accordingly. So far, the suggested level of Fe and Zn fortification in parboiling process is 250 mg Fe and Zn kg^{-1} paddy rice to get the desired amount of Fe and Zn which should result in 25–30 mg Fe and Zn kg^{-1} considered desirable concentration in white parboiled rice. Evaluation of penetration of the fortified Fe and Zn into the interior of the rice embryo for specific parboiling condition and rice variety may lead to considerable savings in the cost of chemicals used for parboiling.

Recommendations

Fortification of parboiled rice with Fe and Zn, by introducing the nutrients into industrial process already in existence offers an ideal opportunity for increasing Fe and Zn intake and alleviating Fe and Zn deficiency among rice consumers. A fortification pilot in collaboration with small scale parboiling mills in areas with acute Fe and Zn deficiency should be conducted, in order that efficacy of the methodology on increasing concentration of the nutrients in the rice that people consume, and impact on their health can be evaluated. Special attention should also be paid to Fe and Zn fractions of the rice grain that are expected to be greatly elevated by fortification, such as the rice husk, broken rice normally consumed by the poor and bran which is extracted for oil and used as animal feed. Furthermore, there are two concerns related to health of consumers and the environment. Firstly, there is an urgent need for safety limits of Fe and Zn concentration in foods consumed in large amounts such as rice, especially for those sectors of the population with special health problems such as thalassemia which can be exacerbated by excessive Fe. Secondly, the waste solution from the soaking process in parboiling rice which contains huge amounts of Fe and Zn requires proper management as it could be toxic to animals and/or plants. Further research is needed to determine how the remaining Fe and Zn can be reused.

The husk from de-husking process of fortified parboiled rice has 80–100 times higher Fe and Zn concentration than fortified unpolished and polished rice. It is usually valueless for rice mills as it is not consumable. In fact, it could be use as a mixture for plant growing media and/or the supplement for animal feeding. Beside this, there is also the bran fraction from the polishing process of unpolished to polished rice which consists of the outer layers of the caryopsis including pericarp, testa, nucellus, part of the aleurone layer and some endosperm along with the germ or embryo and it is usually sell it for animal feeding purpose or extracted for rice bran oil. It would be useful to evaluate how the quality of these by-products, including the many nutritional compounds such as antioxidants and vitamins, are affected by the elevated levels of Fe and Zn achieved by fortification during parboiling. These are areas of research that could be fruitfully explored.

Conclusion

Parboiled rice is already produced on industrial scale and traded globally as well as within each country. It is commonly consumed in South Asia and Africa where Fe and Zn deficiencies in human population are widespread. The parboiling process offers an ideal opportunity for Fe and Zn fortification during the soaking of paddy before steaming. The effectiveness of Fe and Zn fortification in parboiling process in the laboratory that satisfies (a) the levels of Fe and Zn in polished rice that people eat, (b) retention of the fortified Fe and Zn in normal process of rice cooking, (c) tests for bioavailability and thus potential for the fortification to benefit the target population and (d) found accepted by regular consumers of parboiled rice. These conditions together suggest that fortifying parboiled rice with Fe and Zn may be a rapid and cost-effective mean to improve the amount of Fe and Zn intake in the sector of population who are most at risk from Fe and Zn deficiency. With an established industry infrastructure and half of the world's rice production already parboiled, Fe- and Zn-fortified parboiled rice offers a ready tool for significantly improving Fe and Zn nutrition in economically disadvantaged populations in South Asia and Africa. Iron- and Zn-fortified parboiled rice can easily and rapidly reach rice consumers in these countries without the need to alter consumption habits of local populations and establishing new market network and access. It offers highly cost-effective tool to reduce the incidences of Fe deficiency in developing countries within an immediate future if it is adopted by the current parboiled rice industry. Moreover, the infrastructures for production and market distribution have been well established in each location and no major additional investment is required for Fe and Zn fortification through parboiling.

Acknowledgement We acknowledge University of Queensland for postdoctoral research fund, McKnight Foundation, Thailand Research Fund, International Foundation for Science and Office of the Higher Education Commission under National Research University project for financial supported.

References

1. Hettiarachchi M, Hilmers DC, Liyanage C, Abrams SA. Na(2)EDTA enhances the absorption of iron and zinc from fortified rice flour in Sri Lankan children. J Nutr. 2004;134(11):3031–6.
2. Pinstrup-Andersen P, Pandya-Lorch R, Rosegrant MW. World food prospects: Critical issues for the early twenty-first century. Food Policy Report. International Food Policy Research Institute, Washington, D.C. 1999. pp. 1–30.
3. WHO. The world food summit: micronutrient malnutrition: half of the world affected. Geneva: World Health Organization; 1996.
4. WHO. The world health report 2002. Geneva, Switzerland: World Health Organization; 2002.
5. Hotz C, Brown K. Assessment of the risk of zinc deficiency in populations and options for its control. Food Nutr Bull. 2004;25:S94–203.
6. Rosado J. Zinc and copper: proposed fortification levels and recommended zinc compounds. J Nutr. 2003;133: 2985S–9.
7. Hurrell RF, Cook JD. Strategies for iron fortification of foods. Trends Food Sci Technol. 1990;9:56–61.
8. Juliano BO. Rice in human nutrition "Prepared in collaboration with FAO". Rome: Food and Agriculture Organization of the United Nations; 1993
9. Brown K, Peerson J, Rivera J, Allen L. Effect of supplemental zinc on the growth and serum zinc concentrations of prepubertal children: a meta-analysis of randomized controlled trials. Am J Clin Nutr. 2002;75:1062–71.
10. Cakmak I. Enrichment of cereal grains with zinc: agronomic or genetic biofortification? Plant Soil. 2008;302:1–17.
11. Pfeiffer W, McClafferty B. HarvestPlus: breeding crops for better nutrition. Crop Sci. 2007;47:S-88–105.
12. Vasconcelos M, Datta K, Oliva N, Khalekuzzaman M, Torrizo L, Krishnan S, et al. Enhanced iron and zinc accumulation in transgenic rice with the *ferritin* gene. Plant Sci. 2003;164:371–8.
13. Gregorio GB, Senadhira D, Mendoza RD, Manigbas NL, Roxas JP, Guerta CQ. Progress in breeding for salinity tolerance and associated abiotic stresses in rice. Field Crop Res. 2002;76(2–3):91–101.
14. Prom-u-thai C, Fukai S, Godwin DI, Huang L. Genotypic variation of iron partitioning in rice grain. J Sci Food Agric. 2007;87:2049–54.
15. Senadhira D, Gregorio G, Graham RD. Breeding iron and zinc dense rice. In: Paper presented at the international workshop on micronutrient of rice for developing countries. Philippines: International Rice Research Institute; 1998.
16. Bouis HE. Enrichment of food staples through plant breeding: a new strategy for fighting micronutrient malnutrition. Nutr Rev. 1996;54(5):131–7.
17. Goto F, Yoshihara T, Shigemoto N, Toki S, Takaiwa F. Iron fortification of rice seed by the soybean ferritin gene. Nat Biotechnol. 1999;17(3):282–6.
18. Juliano BO, Bechtel BD. Rice: chemistry and technology. St. Paul, MN: American Association of Cereal Chemists; 1985.
19. Prom-u-thai C, Sanchai C, Rerkasem B, Jamjod S, Fukai S, Godwin DI, et al. The effect of grain morphology on degree of milling and iron loss in rice. Cereal Chem. 2007;84:384–8.
20. Pillaiyar P. Household parboiling of parboiled rice. Kishan World. 1981;8:20–1.
21. Bhattacharya KR. Parboiling of rice. 3rd ed. St. Paul, MN: American Association of Cereal Chemists; 2004.
22. Choudhury NH. Parboiling and consumer demand of parboiled rice in South Asia. Manila: International Rice Research Institute; 1991.
23. Rerkasem B. Having your rice and eating it too: a view of Thailand's green revolution. ScienceAsia. 2007;33 Suppl 1:75–80.
24. Prom-u-thai C, Fukai S, Godwin DI, Rerkasem B, Huang L. Iron-fortified parboiled rice—a novel solution to high iron density in rice-based diets. Food Chem. 2008;110:390–8.
25. Prom-u-thai C, Rerkasem B, Fukai S, Huang L. Key factors affecting Fe density in Fe-fortified parboiled rice: parboiling conditions, storage duration, external Fe loading rate and genotypic differences. Food Chem. 2010;123:628–34.
26. Doesthale YG, Devara S, Rao S, Belavady B. Effect of milling on mineral and trace-element composition of raw and parboiled rice. J Sci Food Agric. 1979;30(1):40–6.
27. Prom-u-thai C, Glahn PR, Cheng Z, Fukai S, Rerkasem B, Huang L. The bioavailability of iron fortified in whole grain parboiled rice. Food Chem. 2009;112:982–6.
28. Prom-u-thai C, Rerkasem B, Fukai S, Huang L. Iron-fortification and parboiled rice quality: appearance, cooking quality and sensory attributes. J Sci Food Agric. 2009;89(15):2565–71.
29. Glahn RR, Lee OA, Yeung A, Goldman MI, Miller DD. Caco-2 cell ferritin formation predicts nonradiolabeled food iron availability in an in vitro digestion/Caco-2 cell culture model. J Nutr. 1998;128:1555–61.
30. Cook JD, Reddy MB, Burri J, Juillerat MA, Hurrell RF. The influence of different cereal grains on iron absorption from infant cereal foods. Am J Clin Nutr. 1997;65(4):964–9.
31. Li Y, Diosady LL, Jankowski S. Stability of vitamin B1 in Ultra Rice in the presence of encapsulated ferrous fumarate. Int J Food Sci Nutr. 2008;59(1):24–33.
32. Prom-u-thai C, Huang L, Rerkasem B. Iron fortification in parboiled rice – a rapid and effective tool for delivering Fe nutrition to rice consumers. Food Nutr Sci. 2011;2:323–8.

Chapter 9
Millet Flours as a Vehicle for Fortification with Iron and Zinc

Kalpana Platel

Key Points

- Fortification of staples with micronutrients is a feasible strategy to combat micronutrient deficiencies.
- Cereals have been commonly used as vehicles for fortification with minerals and vitamins since more than 8 decades.
- Millets are widely grown and consumed by the lower economic segments of the population especially in the developing countries.
- In spite of their extensive consumption, millets are less explored as vehicles for fortification with minerals.
- Finger millet, sorghum, and pearl millet, which are widely grown and consumed as the staple in several parts of India were examined for their feasibility as vehicles for fortification with iron and zinc.
- These millet flours were found suitable for fortification with iron and zinc, providing significant amounts of bioaccessible minerals.
- EDTA, a known metal chelator, when included as a co-fortificant significantly improved the bioaccessibility of both iron and zinc from the fortified flours.
- Fortification of millet flours with ferrous fumarate and zinc stearate along with EDTA did not have any adverse effect on the shelf-life of the fortified flours, or on the sensory quality of the products prepared from them.
- It would be worthwhile to examine other millets consumed as a staple in several parts of the world for feasibility as vehicles for fortification with micronutrients.
- Fortification of millet flours with minerals therefore seems to be a feasible strategy to combat micronutrient deficiency.

Keywords Fortification • Millets • Iron • Zinc • EDTA

K. Platel, Ph.D. (✉)
Department of Biochemistry and Nutrition, Central Food Technological Research Institute, Yadavagiri, Mysore 570020, India
e-mail: kalpanaplatel@gmail.com

V.R. Preedy et al. (eds.), *Handbook of Food Fortification and Health: From Concepts to Public Health Applications Volume 1*, Nutrition and Health, DOI 10.1007/978-1-4614-7076-2_9,

Introduction

Deficiency of micronutrients, especially iron, iodine, vitamin A, and zinc, are widely prevalent not only in developing countries, but also in the developed countries. Micronutrient deficiencies are often known as "hidden hunger," since they are less visible than protein energy undernutrition. For the last 2 decades, micronutrient deficiencies especially nutritional anemia, iodine deficiency disorders, and vitamin A deficiency have been a subject of concern in developing countries. Deficiency of iron is a public health problem, particularly in developing countries such as India, where 79 % of children between 6 and 35 months and women between 15 and 49 years of age are anemic [1]. In recent years, the deficiency of zinc is also being recognized as a global health problem [2]. Both iron and zinc deficiency have several functional consequences such as impairment of cognitive function, linear growth impairment, behavioral problems, mood changes, memory impairment, problems with spatial learning, and neuronal atrophy. In addition, iron deficiency anemia is found to be associated with reduced work capacity in adults, an increased risk of maternal and neonatal mortality and premature birth, and altered immune function [3, 4].

Fortification is a cost-effective method that can be used at the national level to prevent deficiency of both iron and zinc without any change in existing dietary patterns or any personal contact with the recipients [2]. Fortification of foods is often regarded as the most cost-effective long-term approach to reducing the prevalence of mineral deficiency [5]. The concept of food fortification with micronutrients was documented as early as 1923, when Switzerland introduced the iodization of salt to prevent goiter and cretinism. Rickets caused by deficiency of vitamin D in children living in the Northern Hemisphere was prevented by addition of vitamin D to infant formula and dairy products [6]. In 1941, United States was the first country to enrich wheat flour with iron and vitamins and subsequently, virtually all white wheat flour and wheat bread, most corn meal, grits, and macaroni products were fortified with iron, as were a large proportion of other cereal products. Mandatory enrichment of white wheat flour with iron was introduced in the United Kingdom and Canada in 1953 and many other countries have since introduced either mandatory or voluntary enrichment (UK) [3]. Fortification with iron has been successfully adopted for wheat flour, rice, sugar, salt, milk, fish sauce, and curry powder. Other foods like wheat biscuits, wheat flour noodles, and maize meal have also been tried [7–15].

In India, food fortification was used in the early years as a strategy to improve the intake of macronutrients, in order to combat protein energy malnutrition [6]. In this direction, wholesome foods were blended to improve the protein content. The Indian multipurpose food is one such blend of edible peanut flour and chickpea flour that provides high protein with added minerals and vitamins. Blending of wheat flour with peanut flour to raise the protein content was another strategy tried in India [6].

While fortification of wheat flour, sugar, and salt with iron is a common strategy in industrialized countries [6], fortification of millet flours with minerals has gained little attention. Millets are used chiefly as food grains in Africa, Eastern Europe, China, India, and other Asiatic countries [16]. In developing countries such as India where a majority of the population consume plant-based foods, cereals, millets, and pulses are major dietary sources of iron and zinc.

In the Indian scenario, this country is the largest producer and consumer of millets, sharing nearly 60 % of the area and output of the millets grown in the world [17]. According to recent statistics, the production of pearl millet in India is about 8.89 million tons, that of sorghum is 7.25 million tons, and of coarse cereals including finger millet is 40.04 million tons [18].

Finger millet is predominantly cultivated in Karnataka, Andhra Pradesh, and Tamil Nadu, where this millet is the staple to a large section of the rural population. Finger millet is also grown in the Himalayas, but its cultivation there is scattered [19].

Pearl millet is consumed predominantly in western and central states of India, and is the staple mainly in Gujarat and Rajasthan. Across income classes, pearl millet is consumed mainly by the low and middle income groups; about 46 % of pearl millet in urban India is consumed by the low income groups.

Sorghum is primarily produced in Maharashtra and southern states of Karnataka and Andhra Pradesh, these three states together accounting for nearly 80 % of the all-India production. Madhya

Pradesh, Gujarat, and Rajasthan are the other states producing sorghum. India is the third largest producer of sorghum in the world. The low income consumers account for 35 and 49 % of sorghum consumption in rural and urban areas of India respectively [20].

In view of the extensive production and consumption of millets especially among the lower economic groups of the population, their fortification with minerals such as iron and zinc is certainly a rational strategy to enhance the intake of these minerals thereby reducing their deficiency.

Millet Flours as Carriers of Iron

While cereal flours are common vehicles for fortification with micronutrients, millets are less explored in this context. Fortification of millet flours with iron would be a feasible public health strategy to combat iron deficiency, since millets form the staple for large segments of the population, especially the poorer sections, in developing countries. Finger millet (*Eleucine coracana*) is widely consumed in the southern parts of India and is a good source of minerals. Sorghum (*Sorghum bicolor*) is an important food crop providing energy, protein, vitamins, and other nutrients to millions people living in semi arid tropical regions of the world [21]. Although millets such as pearl millet (*Pennisetum glaucum*), finger millet, and sorghum are generally good sources of trace minerals [22], the bioavailability of these minerals may be limited because of the presence of high levels of phytates and fiber which are major inhibitors of bioavailability of iron and zinc [23]. Inclusion of promoters of iron absorption in addition to the mineral would thus be beneficial in providing higher amounts of bioavailable iron.

Finger millet, sorghum, and pearl millet were recently examined for feasibility of fortification with iron [24, 25]. Initially, ferrous fumarate and ferric pyrophosphate added at levels to provide 6 mg iron per 100 g flour, were examined for fortification of finger millet flour [24]. Both the salts were found to be equally effective with respect to iron bioaccessibility; however, the bioaccessible iron content declined in the ferric pyrophosphate fortified flour after 30 days of storage. Therefore ferrous fumarate was subsequently used as the fortificant, and was added to the millet flours a level that provided 60 mg iron per kg flour. EDTA, a known metal chelator, was added along with ferrous fumarate at levels equimolar to the added iron. The bioaccessible iron content of the fortified flours was determined by the in vitro simulated gastrointestinal digestion method, involving equilibrium dialysis [24]. Bioaccessibility of iron was determined periodically from the fortified flours stored at ambient temperature for a period of 60 days [24, 25].

Bioaccessibility of iron from the fortified millet flours: Fortification of the millet flours with ferrous fumarate to provide 6 mg of iron per 100 g of the flour brought about an increase in the bioaccessible iron content of the fortified flours. Finger millet flour had a bioaccessible iron content of 0.23 mg/100 g, which increased to 0.29 mg/100 g upon fortification (27 % increase). Similarly, fortification of sorghum and pearl millet flours brought about 41–44 % increase in the bioaccessible iron content (Table 9.1). There was no significant decline

Table 9.1 Bioaccessible iron content of iron-fortified millet flours

	Bioaccessible iron (mg/100 g)		
	Days of storage		
Flour	0	30	60
Finger millet	0.23	0.21	0.20
Finger millet + iron	0.29[a]	0.26[a]	0.24[a]
Sorghum	0.39	0.37	0.35
Sorghum + iron	0.56[a]	0.53[a]	0.42[a,b]
Pearl millet	0.39	0.35	0.32[b]
Pearl millet + iron	0.55[a]	0.53[a]	0.44[a,b]

Adapted from [20, 21]
Values are average of five replicates
[a]Significantly higher than control (unfortified grain)
[b]Significantly lower than initial (day 0) value

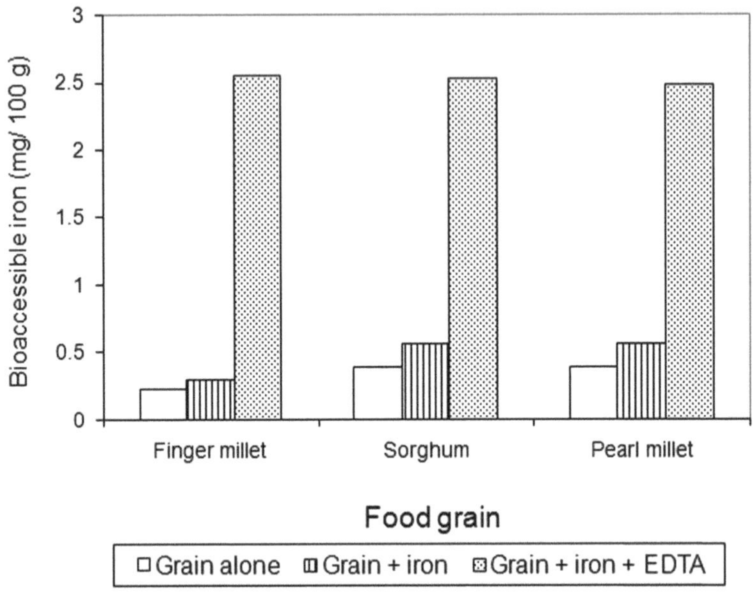

Fig. 9.1 Effect of EDTA on the bioaccessibility of iron from iron-fortified millet flours

in the iron bioaccessibility from the finger millet and sorghum flour upon storage, but the bioaccessible iron content in the pearl millet flour reduced significantly over the period of storage both in the unfortified as well as the fortified flour (Table 9.1). Thus, addition of iron increased the bioaccessible iron content to different extents in the three millet flours. Despite similar total iron content, the bioaccessibility of the native iron from sorghum flour was higher than that from finger millet flour. Fortification of these flours with iron at the same level significantly enhanced the bioaccessible iron content of sorghum flour, but that of finger millet flour was only marginally increased. Both sorghum and pearl millet flour had similar bioaccessible iron content, in spite of a higher amount of total iron in the latter. This could probably be attributable to the higher amounts of inhibitory factors such as phytate and tannin present in pearl millet flour [26].

Influence of EDTA on iron bioaccessibility from the fortified millet flours: Addition of EDTA at levels equimolar to the added iron significantly increased the bioaccessibility of the iron from the fortified millet flours. EDTA brought about a six to eightfold increase in the bioaccessible iron content of the fortified flours (Fig. 9.1). However, this increase tended to decline over the period of storage. Incidentally, EDTA also significantly increased the bioaccessibility of iron from the unfortified flours. Thus, EDTA successfully countered the negative effects of the inhibitory factors inherently present in the millet flours. In spite of the decline in bioaccessible iron content during storage, it continued to be much higher than that of the unfortified flours as well as with the flours fortified with iron alone, even at the end of 60 days of storage [24, 25].

Effect of fortification of millet flours with iron on the bioaccessibility of the native zinc: Iron–zinc interaction is a matter of concern in the case of iron fortification; since the molar ratio of iron to the inherent zinc will be altered several fold as a result of addition of exogenous iron. However, the addition of exogenous iron to millet flours did not negatively influence the bioaccessibility of the native zinc, despite a significant decrease in the Zn:Fe molar ratio as a result of iron fortification. On the other hand, the addition of EDTA as a co-fortificant significantly enhanced the bioaccessibility of the native zinc from all the millet flours examined [24, 25].

Shelf-life of the iron-fortified millet flours: Fortification of finger millet, sorghum, and pearl millet flours did not seem to affect the keeping quality of the flour under ambient conditions up to a period of 60 days, as indicated by their moisture and free fatty acid content that were monitored during the period of storage [24, 25].

As mentioned earlier, millet flours are less explored as vehicles for fortification with micronutrients, and the two reports mentioned above have suggested that millet flours can indeed be employed as carriers of iron. Such qualitatively rich flours can be a part of the nutrition intervention programs to overcome the deficiency of iron.

Millet Flours as Carriers of Zinc

The importance of zinc in human health has been widely recognized in recent years, and zinc deficiency is included as a major risk factor to the global burden of diseases along with iron, vitamin A, and iodine deficiencies since 2002 [26]. Although the major source of zinc in our diet is animal foods, a majority of the population in developing countries derive this micronutrient from plant foods, especially grains. Staple foods in developing countries include cereals and legumes, which are the main sources of zinc for most of the population but even if net zinc intake appears adequate, compromised zinc status is common [27]. Recent evidence from National Food Balance Sheets suggests that the food supply of nearly 50 % of the global population is low in absorbable zinc because of limited availability of animal products and a higher intake of cereals and legumes [28]. Thus, fortification of staple food grains with zinc may be a suitable approach to prevent zinc deficiency in developing countries.

Bioaccessibility of zinc from the fortified millet flours: In a recent study, finger millet, sorghum, and pearl millet that are commonly consumed as the staple in several parts of India, were fortified with zinc. Two zinc salts, namely zinc stearate and zinc oxide were initially used for fortifying finger millet flour with zinc at levels that provided 5 mg zinc/100 g flour. Zinc stearate was found to provide significantly higher amounts of bioaccessible zinc as compared to zinc oxide [29]. Fortification of the flours of finger millet, sorghum, and pearl millet with zinc stearate to provide 5 mg zinc per 100 g flour brought about a significant increase in the bioaccessible zinc content [29, 30]. The native zinc content in finger millet, sorghum, and pearl millet flours was 1.72, 1.68, and 4.04 mg/100 g, respectively, and the bioaccessible zinc content was 0.18, 0.37, and 0.69 mg/100 g, respectively. Addition of zinc stearate at the level mentioned above increased the bioaccessible zinc content to 0.49, 0.61, and 0.79 mg/100 g in finger millet, sorghum, and pearl millet flours, respectively. These levels remained stable during a 60-day period of storage in finger millet and sorghum flours, but tended to decline slightly after 30 days of storage in the pearl millet flour (Table 9.2). Among the three millet flours, pearl millet flour had the highest native as well as bioaccessible zinc content, but despite fortification with zinc stearate which more than doubled the native zinc content, the increase in bioaccessible zinc content was only marginal (0.70–0.79 mg/100 g). Similarly, despite comparable zinc content in fortified finger millet and sorghum flour, the latter provided higher amount of bioaccessible zinc (0.61 mg/100 g). Thus, it is evident that fortification with zinc has

Table 9.2 Bioaccessible zinc content of zinc-fortified millet flours

	Bioaccessible zinc (mg/100 g)		
	Days of storage		
Flour	0	30	60
Finger millet	0.18	0.17	0.15
Finger millet + zinc	0.49[a]	0.45[a]	0.44[a]
Sorghum	0.37	0.33	0.32
Sorghum + zinc	0.61[a]	0.59[a]	0.58[a]
Pearl millet	0.70	0.68	0.63
Pearl millet + zinc	0.79	0.77	0.72

Adapted from [25, 26]
Values are average of five replicates
[a]Significantly higher than control (unfortified grain)

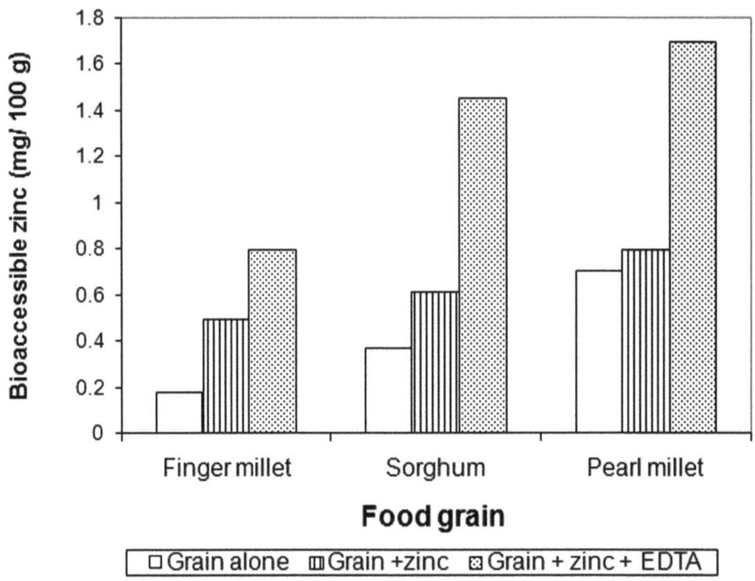

Fig. 9.2 Effect of EDTA on the bioaccessibility of zinc from zinc-fortified millet flours. Values are average of five replicates

a more pronounced effect on sorghum as compared to either finger millet or pearl millet flour with respect to the increase in bioaccessible zinc content. Further, the bioaccessible zinc content in the fortified sorghum flour was more stable as compared to that in pearl millet flour, which tended to decline after a period of 30 days [29, 30].

Influence of EDTA on zinc bioaccessibility from the fortified millet flours: As in the case of iron-fortified millet flours, addition of EDTA at levels equimolar to the added zinc significantly enhanced the bioaccessible zinc content of all the three millet flours examined (Fig. 9.2). The bioaccessible zinc content was increased to an extent of 1.6-fold in finger millet, while in sorghum and pearl millet flours there was more than twofold increase in the same. In addition to enhancing the bioaccessibility of zinc, EDTA also countered the slight reduction in the same during storage that was seen in finger millet and sorghum flours where EDTA was not included; however, the decrease in bioaccessible zinc content of fortified pearl millet flour on storage beyond 30 days was not countered by the addition of EDTA. As in the case of iron fortification, EDTA also increased the bioaccessibility of the native zinc from all the three millet flours. A significant decrease in the iron:zinc ratio as a result of fortification of the millet flours with zinc did not adversely affect the bioaccessibility of the native iron in these flours.

Effect of fortification of millet flours with zinc on the bioaccessibility of the native iron: The iron:zinc ratio of the zinc-fortified millet flours was significantly reduced as a result of addition of exogenous zinc. However, this reduction did not result in any compromise in the bioaccessibility of the native iron from the zinc-fortified millet flours. On the other hand, inclusion of EDTA as a co-fortificant was beneficial in increasing the bioaccessibility of the native iron [29, 30]. Thus, addition of exogenous zinc to the millet flours does not have any negative influence on the bioaccessibility of the inherent iron.

Shelf-life of the zinc-fortified millet flours: Moisture and free fatty acid contents of the stored fortified flours indicated that the fortified finger millet and sorghum flours can be stored up to 60 days under ambient conditions. Pearl millet flour seems to have limited shelf-life as indicated by the FFA content, which increased marginally at the end of 60 days of storage [29, 30]. Thus, millet flours seem to be suitable for fortification with zinc, and inclusion of EDTA as a co-fortificant further improved the bioaccessibility of zinc from these flours.

Double Fortification of Millet Flours with Iron and Zinc

In the view of widespread multiple mineral deficiencies, it would be appropriate to fortify staple foods with two or more minerals simultaneously. In this context, finger millet and sorghum were double fortified with iron and zinc [31]. Ferrous fumarate and zinc stearate were added at levels that provided 6 mg iron and 5 mg zinc per 100 g of flour, respectively. EDTA was used as a co-fortificant, and was added at a level equimolar with the added iron.

The bioaccessible iron content of the finger millet and sorghum flour was 0.33 and 0.37 mg Fe/100 g, respectively (Table 9.3). When the flour was double fortified including iron at the level of 6 mg Fe/100 g flour along with EDTA the bioaccessible iron increased to 2.39 and 2.63 mg Fe/100 g flour in finger millet and sorghum flour respectively. Thus fortification of the millet flours with ferrous fumarate and EDTA led to a significant (sevenfold) increase in bioaccessible iron content of both the millet flours. There was a marginal (13.8 %) decline in the bioaccessible iron content in of the fortified sorghum flour stored for 60 days, while that in the fortified finger millet flour was negligible [31].

Double fortification of the millet flours also resulted in an increase in the bioaccessibility of zinc, the same being enhanced from 0.22 to 0.83 mg/100 g in finger millet flour and from 0.39 to 1.63 mg/100 g in sorghum flour, which amounts to about 3.5- to 4-fold increase (Table 9.4). However, there was a significant decline in the bioaccessible zinc content from the fortified millet flours on the 60th day of storage, the extent of this decline being 14 and 33 % in the finger millet and sorghum flours, respectively. Despite this decline, the bioaccessible zinc content of the fortified millet flours remains fourfold higher than the unfortified flours in either case [31].

Fortification with both iron and zinc would alter the molar ratios of these minerals. Significant alteration of the molar ratios of iron and zinc in the millet flours as a result of double fortification did

Table 9.3 Bioaccessible iron content (mg/100 g) of the double-fortified millet flours

	Bioaccessible iron (mg/100 g)		
	Days of storage		
Flour	0	30	60
Finger millet	0.33	0.31	0.29
Fortified finger millet	2.39[a]	2.27[a]	2.06[a,b]
Sorghum	0.37	0.36	0.35
Fortified sorghum	2.63[a]	2.61[a]	2.57[a]

Adapted from [27]
Values are average of five replicates
[a]Significantly higher than control (unfortified grain)
[b]Significantly lower than initial (day 0) value

Table 9.4 Bioaccessible zinc content (mg/100 g) of the double-fortified millet flours

	Bioaccessible iron (mg/100 g)		
	Days of storage		
Flour	0	30	60
Finger millet	0.22	0.21	0.16
Fortified finger millet	0.83[a]	0.77[a]	0.71[a]
Sorghum	0.39	0.37	0.35
Fortified sorghum	1.63[a]	1.35[a,b]	1.09[a,b]

Adapted from [27]
Values are average of five replicates
[a]Significantly higher than control (unfortified grain)
[b]Significantly lower than initial (day 0) value

not compromise the bioaccessibility of these two minerals, since the bioaccessible iron and zinc values were similar to those in the flours fortified with either of the minerals alone [24–26, 30]. This indicates that the addition of these two minerals together does not interfere with the bioaccessibility of either of them. The shelf-life of the double-fortified flours was also satisfactory up to a period of 60 days, as indicated by their moisture and free fatty acid contents [31].

Millet flours are normally consumed after heat processing; in India, these millet flours are most commonly consumed in the form of dumpling and *roti* (unleavened bread). Sensory analysis of these two products prepared from fortified millet flours indicated that these products were sensorily acceptable [32, 33]. Bioaccessibility of iron and zinc from the cooked products was comparable to that from the raw flour [20, 21, 25–27]. This indicates that fortification with iron and zinc both individually and in combination does not alter the sensory characteristics of heat processed products prepared from fortified millet flours, and that the bioaccessibility of the minerals is not compromised by subjecting the fortified flours to heat processing.

Conclusion

Millet flours seem to be suitable candidates for fortification with iron and zinc, both individually and in combination. Addition of EDTA has a significant beneficial influence on the bioaccessibility of these minerals. Given the fact that diets in India and probably other developing countries are predominantly plant-based with poor mineral bioavailability, any improvement in the bioaccessibility of essential minerals from the same would be significant in the context of improving their intake. Fortification of millet flours with iron and zinc therefore is a feasible strategy to increase the intake of these important micronutrients. Since millets are consumed as the staple, fortification of the same would not call for any drastic change in food habits, and the fortified millet flours would be easily accepted by the target population. Such qualitatively rich flours could also be used in supplementary feeding programs, and promoted through the public distribution systems for a wide outreach.

The studies mentioned above examined the feasibility of fortifying three millet flours that are commonly consumed in India, with iron and zinc. These millets were found suitable for mineral fortification, providing significant levels of bioaccessible iron and zinc, and were also cost-effective. These studies merit extension to other millets that form the staple in several developing countries world over.

Millet flours thus seem to be promising candidates for fortification with minerals, and if successfully employed for this purpose, would have a wide outreach in combating iron and zinc deficiency.

References

1. Krishnaswamy K. The problem and consequences of the double burden—a brief overview. In: Programme and abstracts, symposium on nutritional security for India—issues and way forward. New Delhi: Indian National Science Academy; 2009. p. 5–6.
2. Hotz C, Brown KH. Assessment of the risk of zinc deficiency in populations and options for its control. Food Nutr Bull. 2004;25:94–204.
3. Hurrell R, Bothwell T, Cook JD, et al. The usefulness of elemental iron for cereal flour fortification: a SUSTAIN Task Force report. Nutr Rev. 2002;60:391–406.
4. Tran CD. Micronutrients in health research. In: Yoshida T, editor. Advances of zinc in health research. New York: Nova; 2008. p. 23–70.
5. Drago SR, Valencia ME. Effect of fermentation on iron, zinc and calcium availability from iron fortified dairy products. J Food Sci. 2002;67:3130–3.
6. Subbulakshmi G, Naik M. Food fortification in developing countries—current status and strategies. J Food Sci Tech. 1999;36:371–95.

7. Cook JD, Reusser M. Iron fortification: an update. Am J Clin Nutr. 1983;38:648–59.
8. Arroyave G. Food nutrition with emphasis on the addition of micronutrients to wheat flour. Washington, DC: VITAL/ISTI; 1992.
9. Florentina RF, Pedro MR. Rice fortification in the Philippines. In: Combating iron deficiency anemia through food fortification. Washington, DC: INACG; 1990.
10. Zoller JM, Wolinsky I, Paden CA, et al. Fortification of non food items with iron. Food Technol. 1980;32:38–47.
11. Molina MR. Foods considered for nutrient additions: sugar. In: Bauerfieind JD, Lachance PA, editors. Nutrient additions to foods. Trumbull, CT: Food and Nutrition Press; 1991.
12. Anon. Use of iron fortified salt to combat anemia in Indian experience. Nutr Rev. 1980;41:302–3.
13. Mannar V. Fortification of salt with iron—a status report. In: Combating iron deficiency anemia through food fortification technology. Washington, DC: INACG; 1990.
14. Bauerfeind JC. Foods considered for nutrient additions in condiments. In: Bauerfieind JD, Lachance PA, editors. Nutrient additions to foods. Trumbull, CT: Food and Nutrition; 1991.
15. Walter T. Combating iron deficiency: Chile: a case study. In: Combating iron deficiency anemia through food fortification technology. Washington, DC: INACG, 1990.
16. Bookwalter GN, Lyle SA, Warner K. Millet processing for improved stability and nutritional quality without functionality changes. J Food Sci. 1987;52:399–402.
17. Nagaraj N, Basavaraj G, Parasarthy RP. Policy brief on future outlook and options for target crops: the sorghum and pearl millet economy of India. ICRISAT; 2011. http://www.icrisat.org
18. Agricultural statistics at a glance, 2010. Directorate of Economics and Statistics, Department of Agriculture and Cooperation.
19. Krishna KR. Agroecosystems in South India: nutrient dynamics, ecology and productivity. Florida: Brown Walker; 2010. p. 281.
20. Basavaraj G, Parthasarathy RP, Bhagavatula S, et al. SAT eJournal. 2010;8. http://ejournal.icrisat.org
21. Zhang G, Hamaker BR. Sorghum (*Sorghum bicolor* L. Moench) flour pasting properties influenced by free fatty acids and protein. Cereal Chem. 2005;82:534–40.
22. Gopalan G, Ramasastri BV, Balasubramanian SC. Nutritive value of Indian foods. Hyderabad: National Institute of Nutrition, Indian Council of Medical Research; 1999.
23. Murty DS, Kumar KA. Traditional uses of sorghum and millets. In: Dendy DAV, editor. Sorghum and millets: chemistry and technology. St. Paul, MN: AACC International; 1995. p. 185–221.
24. Tripathi B, Platel K. Iron fortification of finger millet (*Eleucine coracana*) flour with EDTA and folic acid as co-fortificants. Food Chem. 2011;126:534–47.
25. Tripathi B, Platel K. Feasibility of fortification of sorghum (*Sorghum bicolor L. Moench*) and pearl millet (*Pennisetum glaucum*) flour with iron. LWT Food Sci Technol. 2012 (in press).
26. Ezzati M, Loez AD, Rodgers A, et al. Selected major risk factors and global and regional burden of disease. Lancet. 2002;360:1347–60.
27. Gibson RS, Yeudall F, Drost N, et al. Dietary interventions to prevent zinc deficiency. Am J Clin Nutr. 1998;68(Suppl):481s–7s.
28. Brown KH, Wuelher SE, Peerson JM. The importance of zinc in human nutrition and estimation of global prevalence of zinc deficiency. Food Nutr Bull. 2001;22:113–25.
29. Tripathi B, Platel K. Fortification of finger millet (*Eleucine coracana*) flour with zinc. J Trace Elem Med Biol. 2010;24:46–51.
30. Tripathi B, Chetana, Platel K. Fortification of sorghum (Sorghum vulgare) and pearl millet (Pennisetum glaucum) flour with zinc. J Trace Elem Med Biol. 2010;24:257–62.
31. Tripathi B, Platel K, Srinivasan K. Double fortification of sorghum (*Sorghum bicolour L. moench*) and finger millet (*Eleucine coracana L. Gartn*) flour with iron and zinc. J Cereal Sci. 2011;55:195–201.
32. Tripathi B, Ravi R, Prakash M, et al. Sensory characteristics of zinc fortified millet products. Int J Food Properties. 2011 (in press).
33. Tripathi B, Ravi R, Prakash M, et al. Sensory acceptability of iron-fortified millet products. Int J Food Sci Nutr. 2011;62:651–9.

Chapter 10
Iron-Fortified Drinking Water

Olga Maria Silverio Amancio and Josefina Aparecida Pellegrini Braga

Key Points

- Prevalence, at-risk groups, consequences, and predisposing factors of iron deficiency anemia as a problem of public health.
- Strategies to combat iron deficiency.
- Importance of food fortification in the battle against micronutrient deficiency.
- Technological difficulties of fortification with iron.
- Experience of fortifying drinking water with iron, dealing with guidance on the levels to be added.
- Recommendations for fortifying drinking water with iron.

Keywords Iron • Anemia • Iron deficiency • Potable water • Iron salts

Abbreviations

FDA	Food and Drug Administration, USA
FeNaEDTA	Iron sodium ethylenediaminotetraacetate
GDP	Gross domestic product
WHO	World Health Organization

Introduction

Iron Deficiency Anemia

Iron deficiency anemia is the most frequent nutritional deficiency in the world and it constitutes one of the greatest problems for public health especially in developing countries, where it coexists with predisposing factors as much biological, as social and economic. It is estimated that two billion people

O.M.S. Amancio, Ph.D. (✉) • J.A.P. Braga, Ph.D.
Department of Pediatrics, Paulista Medicine School, Federal University of Sao Paulo, Sao Paulo, SP, Brazil
e-mail: amancio.olga@gmail.com; pgpediatria@gmail.com

V.R. Preedy et al. (eds.), *Handbook of Food Fortification and Health: From Concepts to Public Health Applications Volume 1*, Nutrition and Health, DOI 10.1007/978-1-4614-7076-2_10,

are anemic and that iron deficiency affects 3.5 billion people. In industrialized countries incidence of anemia has been diminishing in recent decades, coinciding with recognition of the nutritional problem and the generation of health actions [1–3].

It is important to point out that although anemia and iron deficiency are often used as interchangeable terms, anemia represents the most serious form of iron deficiency and is only one of the many adverse consequences of this deficiency. This leads us to believe that the problem of iron deficiency is even greater, estimating that the number of individuals with this deficiency may be at least double that estimated for anemia [1, 4].

Children, pregnant women, and women of childbearing age are considered to be at greater risk for iron deficiency. The consequences of anemia for the body are well established, such as anorexia, apathy, adynamia, even negative repercussions are described in mental and motor development in infants and decreased scholastic development. In adults, it results in reduced capacity for work, with a decrease in productivity [1, 4]. In this context, as well as being a public health problem, anemia is an economic problem, because it results in lower work capacity, lower monetary gain and greater costs with health and education, resulting in high cost for countries. Studies from the World Bank show that there are losses in GDP up to 5 % in countries whose population suffers from micronutrient deficiency [5, 6].

Factors that favor the onset of iron deficiency anemia are complex and may be related to a combination such as low iron reserves at birth, periods of accelerated growth, consumption of food sources with low iron bioavailability, little control on health conditions of the population, other associated nutritional deficiencies, repeated infections, and low socioeconomic status. In adults, repeated pregnancies and more frequent bleeding in women of childbearing age are associated with these factors [1, 4].

Strategies to Combat Iron Deficiency

The World Health Organization—WHO has pledged to try to find a solution to this problem and in this manner, has proclaimed strategies to combat iron deficiency, amongst them, nutritional education associated with measures to increase consumption of this mineral, parasitic infection control, supplementation with iron-based compounds and food fortification with iron [1, 4].

Nutritional education is the ideal way to prevent iron deficiency, through the consumption of a balanced diet, with high iron bioavailability, the presence of foodstuffs enhancing iron absorption and reduction in the ingestion of iron absorption inhibitors. In practice this solution does not happen in the short term, since the feeding of a population is an expression of their cultural habits and is related to the environment, socioeconomic status and food production in the region, in other words, no matter what the preventive measure to be adopted may be, it is of fundamental importance that it respects the characteristics of the population to be affected [1].

Medicinal supplementation involves the supply of medicinal iron, in prophylactic doses to age groups at greater risk. Although its efficiency in the control of anemia has been demonstrated, it presents adherence difficulties for the population due to forgetfulness or the low importance that is attributed to it. As well as this, the need for prolonged use, access difficulty to the medicament, inadequate distribution by the health network, a metallic taste and a possibility of side effects such as the darkening of teeth and feces, and gastrointestinal changes restrict the effectiveness of this prevention method [7–9].

Prophylactic iron supplementation is a useful method that should be indicated when the at-risk population does not have access to foodstuffs fortified with this nutrient or when the needs might be very high; in this case, it should be used for a short period of time. There should also be adequate motivation and education, as a necessary measure to increase the effectiveness of this strategy [8–10].

Weekly supplementation has also been used as an alternative, although its efficiency has not been duly proven in some studies [11, 12].

Food Fortification with Micronutrients

Food fortification has been an alternative used by industrialized countries for more than 50 years. Within the context of solutions for the problem of micronutrient deficiencies, it is indicated as the most sustainable measure as having the best cost-benefit ratio. Although the primary role of fortification is deficiency prevention, in the medium term, it may lead to the reduction and control of the deficiency in question, guaranteeing, in this manner, an adequate ingestion of micronutrients for the population [2, 13, 14].

The importance of this procedure is obvious and unquestionable for the whole population, especially for the pediatric age group, whose nutritional needs are relatively greater due to growth needs. On top of this importance the Food and Drug Administration—FDA [15] highlights that, "the scope and maintenance of a desirable level of nutritional quality in the nation's food supply are important public health objectives. The addition of nutrients to specific foods can be an effective way of maintaining and improving the overall nutritional quality of the food supply." In turn, the World Bank [5] referring to food fortification as a strategy to combat micronutrient deficiency in the world affirms that, "probably no other technology offers the opportunity to improve lives at such low cost and in such a short space of time."

The main advantages of fortification rest on the fact that the population receives the micronutrient without modifying their routine eating habits, does not require individual cooperation, can reach all social sectors, besides presenting a relatively low cost.

The level of consumption necessary for fortification should be efficient but should not exceed the individual's needs. It is important to point out that universal fortification is not exempt from risks if the exposition period continues to last for years.

Technological Difficulties of Iron Fortification

Iron is the micronutrient used in fortification that presents great technical complexity and which produces sensory changes more easily in the product.

The greatest difficulty is found in the selection of the iron salt, since cost, bioavailability, and acceptability should be taken into account with color, taste, odor, and texture still being duly observed [8, 16, 17].

A wide variety of iron salts can be used, the most common is ferrous sulfate; other iron salts such as fumarate, lactate, and gluconate may be used but are more expensive than sulfate. Aminochelated iron and FeNaEDTA have been used with success in the fortification of foodstuffs [1, 18, 19].

The iron salts (sulfate, fumarate, gluconate), more soluble forms, have rapid absorption and a low cost. However, they lead to alterations in color and taste of the foodstuff. These salts have their absorption impaired by the foodstuff, being better absorbed when administered an hour before meals. They cause gastrointestinal side effects, such as diarrhea, epigastralgia, nausea, and constipation [18, 19].

On the other hand, compounds with lower solubility in water, ferric salts, though classically they do not cause organoleptic alterations in the fortified product, are little absorbed as they do not dissolve in the gastrointestinal tract during digestion. They do not suffer the influence of foodstuffs on their absorption, enabling them to be administered as much in fasting as with the diet. Their greatest inconvenience is cost [19].

FeNaEDTA does not display turbidity, color alteration, and does not present a metallic taste, having cost as a disadvantage. Both, FeNaEDTA as much as aminochelated iron produce results in hemoglobin concentration similar to those of ferrous sulfate, whereas ferric orthophosphate has a lower biological value [20].

Color and turbidity increase with the presence of chloride in iron-fortified water, nevertheless the addition of ascorbic acid or citric acid diminishes turbidity [20].

Other than the fortification with iron of solid foods, liquid foodstuffs, milk, juice, and water, has been used successfully by some authors in reducing the prevalence of iron deficiency anemia [21–23].

The Experience of Water Fortification with Iron

The fortification of water with iron, applied in at-risk populations, during a determined period, has been proven to be of easy applicability, effective and low cost, being one alternative for developing countries, linked to other measures to prevent iron deficiency anemia. Its success, as with all fortification, depends on producing few symptoms, and not being recognized on account of alterations in taste or the color of the vehicle by the population in question.

Experimental studies held in laboratories, tested different iron salts diluted in water, in different concentrations, evaluating color, taste, and turbidity, by means of chemical and physical tests. The solution that contains the salt FeNaEDTA remains clear and transparent, without modification in color or taste. Also, a study with aminochelated iron was carried out yielding good results [24]. A comparison with rats on the effect of different iron salts on weight gain, hemoglobin, hematocrit, and transferrin saturation showed that FeNaEDTA and aminochelated iron produced effects similar to of those ferrous sulfate [25].

Guidance on Levels to Be Added

Several controlled studies on water fortification with iron used various concentrations of elemental iron as ferrous sulfate, adding ascorbic acid or not and they report an increase in hemoglobin concentrations, whether in children or in adults of low economic status.

Thus, 10 mg elemental Fe/L water plus 100 mg ascorbic acid was used on children aged 1–6 years and adults from low-income families; [26] on children aged 1–6 years enrolled in day-care centers [27], on children enrolled in day-care centers aged from 6 months to 6 years [28]. Ten milligrams of elemental Fe/L water plus 90 mg ascorbic acid was used in children at day-care centers aged 1–6 years (Table 10.1).

Arcanjo et al. [31] in Sobral, municipality of Ceara—Brazil, carried out a randomized, controlled, double-blind study, proving the effectiveness of iron-fortified drinking water. This study involved children aged 2–5 years, from four public schools, each school composing one group. For fortification, ferrous sulfate was used, in concentrations of 5 mg of elemental iron per liter of water (group A), 7.5 mg (group B), and 10 mg (group C), during a period of 4 months. These concentrations were determined after a pilot study. In group D, control, a placebo (*Bixa orellana*) was added. Hemoglobin and hematocrit values were checked before and after intervention. The study concluded that the consumption of drinking water fortified with 7.5 mg of elemental iron/L water, resulted in greater adhesion on behalf of the children and a significant increase in hemoglobin values, with a reduction in the anemia prevalence (Table 10.2).

Intervention times, which vary from 4 to 8 months, do not show influence on the results.

Recommendations for Iron Fortification of Water

It is important to highlight that fortification must be used in a safe manner, in a place where it is possible to control water fortification, as reported in published studies. Enrichment of water with iron should be made daily, using containers with filtered water, which should be adequately washed each day to avoid

Table 10.1 Studies on water fortification with iron

Local	*N*	Age (years)	Iron salt	Intervention time (months)	Experimental group (EG)		Control group (CG)		References
					Initial Hb g/dL	Final Hb g/dL	Initial Hb g/dL	Final Hb g/dL	
Day-care center	31	2–6	$FeSO_4$ 20mgFe/L	8	10.6	13.7	–	–	Dutra de Oliveira et al. [30]
Low-income families	EG: 44	1–6 Adults	$FeSO_4$ 10mgFe/L + ascorbic acid 100 mg/L Ascorbic acid 100 mg/L	4	Children: 10.9 Adults: 12.9	Children: 11.7 Adults: 13.7	Children: 1.,3 Adults: 13.3	Children: 10.9 Adults: 12.5	Dutra de Oliveira et al. [26]
Day-care center	321	0.5–6	$FeSO_4$ 10mgFe/L+ Ascorbic acid 100 mg/L	5	11.8	12.9	–	–	Lamounier et al. [29]
Day-care center	EG: 74 CG: 76	1–6	$FeSO_4$ 10mgFe/L+ Ascorbic acid 100 mg/L Ascorbic acid 100 mg/L	6	10.98	11.54	11.13	11.95	Almeida et al. [27]
Day-care center	160	1–6	$FeSO_4$ 10mgFe/L + Ascorbic acid 90 mg/L	8	11.8	12.4	–	–	Beinner et al. [28]

Table 10.2 Hemoglobin and hematocrit mean values of schoolchildren in schools A, B, C and D before and after water fortification with iron

	Hemoglobin (g/dL)			Hematocrit (%)		
	Fortification		p[1]	Fortification		p[1]
Schools	Before	After	Value	Before	After	Value
A 5mg Fe *n*=64	10.8 (0.9)	11.2[a] (0.9)	0.001	33.8 (2.3)	35.8[a] (3.0)	<0. 0001
B 7.5 mg Fe *n*=89	10.5 (0.8)	11.5[b] (0.9)	<0. 0001	31.9 (2.9)	34.7[a] (2.8)	<0. 0001
C 10 mg Fe *n*=77	10.7 (1.2)	11.4[b] (1.0)	<0. 0001	33.5 (4.1)	36.1[b] (3.1)	<0. 0001
D placebo *n*=77	10.8 (1.1)	11.5[b] (0.7)	0.112	32.9 (4.7)	37.2[c] (2.6)	<0. 0001
p Value	0.09	0.002[2]		0.008	<0.001[3]	

Fe: elemental iron/L of water.
Different superscript letters in each column represent statistically significant results: $p < 0.05$
p[1] Descriptive level of paired student t-test
[2] Descriptive level of 1-way analysis of variance complemented by the Dunn multiple comparisons test
[3] Descriptive level of 1-way analysis of variance criterion complemented by the Tukey multiple comparisons test

impregnation with the element, impeding in this way any possible intoxication with the element (either acute through an increase in daily concentration, or chronic possibly leading to iron overload, especially in at-risk populations such as those with thalassemia and sufferers of hemochromatosis). A reason for which the fortification of piped water with iron, with currently available technology, is not used and is not advisable.

In relation to the concentration of elemental iron in water, it is believed that a pilot study will determine the best accepted and efficient concentration for a determined population group.

With regard to the length of intervention, in accordance with a review of literature, 4 months would be sufficient.

Conclusion

In conclusion, iron-fortified drinking water is an effective measure, having the best cost-benefit ratio in preventing deficiency of this mineral. It has the advantage of easy procedures and applicability, and daily consumption of the target population.

References

1. De Maeyer EM, Dallman P, Gurney JM, et al. Preventing and controlling iron deficiency anaemia through primary health care. A guide for health administrators and program managers. Geneva: WHO; 1989.
2. Hurrell RF. Preventing iron deficiency through food fortification. Nutr Rev. 1997;55:210–22.
3. World Health Organization. Worldwide prevalence of anaemia 1993–2005: WHO Global database on anaemia. Geneva: WHO; 2008.
4. World Health Organization/United Nations Children's Fund/United Nations University. Iron deficiency anaemia. Assessment, prevention and control. A guide for programme managers. Geneva: WHO/UNICEF/UNU; 2001.

5. The World Bank. Enriching lives. Overcoming vitamin and mineral malnutrition in developing countries. Washington, DC: World Bank; 1994.
6. Horton S, Ross J. Corrigendum to: "The economics of iron deficiency". [Food Policy. 2003;28:51–75]. Food Policy. 2007;32:141–3.
7. Le HT, Brower ID, Burema J, et al. Efficacy of iron fortification compared to iron supplementation among Vietnamese schoolchildren. Nutr J. http://www.nutritionj.com/content/5/1/32. Accessed 15 Sept 2011.
8. Braga JAP, Barbosa TNN, Ferreira AMA. Anemia ferropriva. In: Palma D, Escrivão MAMS, Oliveira FLC, editors. Nutrição Clínica na Infância e na Adolescência—Guias de Medicina Ambulatorial e Hospitalar da UNIFESP–EPM. São Paulo, SP: Manole; 2009. p. 219–42.
9. Braga JAP, Vitalle MS. Deficiência de ferro na criança. Rev Bras Hematol Hemoter. 2010;32:38–44.
10. Olivares MG. Suplementación con hierro. Rev Chil Nutr. 2004;31:272–5.
11. Arcanjo FPN, Arcanjo C, Amancio OMS, et al. Weekly iron supplementation for the treatment of anemia in preschool children: randomized, double-blind, placebo-controlled trial. J Trop Pediatr. 2011;57(6):433–8.
12. Beaton G, McCabe G. Efficacy of intermittent iron supplementation in the control of iron deficiency anaemia in developing countries. An analysis of experience final report to micronutrient initiative. http://idl-bnc.idrc.ca/dspace/bitstream/10625/29662/3/117067.pdf. Accessed 15 Sept 2011.
13. Germani R. Enriquecimento e Restauração da Farinha de Trigo. In: Nutti MR, editor. Enriquecimento e Restauração de Alimentos com Micronutrientes: Uma Proposta para o Brasil. São Paulo, SP: ILSI Brasil; 2000. p. 89–96.
14. Dary O, Hainsworth M. The food fortification formulator: technical determination of fortification levels and standards for mass fortification. http://www.a2zproject.org/pdf/Food-Fortification-Formulator.pdf. Accessed 15 Sept 2011.
15. Food and Drugs Administration (USA). Code of Federal Regulations, 21 CFR 100.1. Fortification Policy. Washington, DC: US Government Printing Office; 1994. p. 179–82.
16. Hurrell RF. Prospects for improving iron fortification of foods. In: Fomon S, Zlotkin S, editors. Nutritional anemias. New York, NY: Raven; 1992. p. 193–201.
17. Gaitán DC, Olivares MG, Arredondo MO, et al. Biodisponibilidade de hierro en humanos. Rev Chil Nutr. 2006;33:142–8.
18. Fisberg M, Bueno M, Lacerda JMS, et al. Fortificação de Ferro em Alimentos. In: Braga JAP, Amancio OMS, Vitalle MSS, editors. O Ferro e a Saúde das Populações. São Paulo, SP: Roca; 2006. p. 213–23.
19. Velloso EP, Fisberg M. The impact of food fortification on the prevention of iron deficiency. Rev Bras Hematol Hemoter. 2010;32:134–9.
20. Dutra-de-Oliveira JE, Marchini JS, Lamounier J, et al. Iron-fortified drinking water studies for the prevention children's anemia in developing countries. Anemia; 2011:1–5; doi: 10.1155/2011/815194.
21. Giorgini E, Fisberg M, De Paula RAC, et al. The use of sweet rolls fortified with iron bis-glycinate chelate in the prevention of iron deficiency anemia in preschool children. Arch Latinoam Nutr. 2001;51:48–53.
22. Hertrampf E, Olivares M, Walter T, et al. Anemia ferropriva en el lactante: erradicación com leche fortificada com hierro. Rev Med Chile. 1990;118:1330–7.
23. Almeida CAN, Crott GC, Ricco RG, et al. Control of iron-deficiency anaemia in Brazilian preschool children using iron-fortified orange juice. Nutr Res. 2003;23:27–33.
24. Olivares MG, Pizarro FA. Bioavailability of iron bis-glycinate chelate in water. Arch Latin Am Nutr. 2001;51:22–5.
25. Dutra-de-Oliveira JE, Freitas ML, Ferreira JF, et al. Iron from complex salts and its bioavailability to rats. Intern J Vitam Nutr Res. 1995;65:272–5.
26. Dutra-de-Oliveira JE, Scheid MM, Desai ID, et al. Iron fortification of domestic drinking water to prevent anemia among low socioeconomic families in Brazil. Int J Food Sci Nutr. 1996;47:213–9.
27. Almeida CAN, Dutra-de-Oliveira JE, Crott GC, et al. Effect of fortification of drinking water with iron plus ascorbic acid or with ascorbic acid alone on hemoglobin values and anthropometric indicators in preschool children in day-care centers in Southeast Brazil. Food Nutr Bull. 2005;26:259–65.
28. Beinner MA, Lamounier JA, Tomaz C. Effect of iron-fortified drinking water of daycare facilities on the hemoglobin status of young children. J Am Coll Nutr. 2005;24:107–14.
29. Lamounier JA, Capanema FD, Rocha DS, et al. Effect of drinking water fortification with iron and vitamin C in nutritional status and reducing anemia among children in day care centers of Belo Horizonte City Brazil. In: Proceedings of the micronutrient forum: consequences and control of micronutrient deficiencies: science, policy and programs—defining issues. Istanbul, Turkey, April 2007, abstract t20. p. 73.
30. Dutra de Oliveira JE, Ferreira JB, Vasconcellos VP, et al. Drinking water as an iron carrier to control anemia in preschool children in a day-care center. J Am Coll Nutr. 1994;13:198–202.
31. Arcanjo FPN, Amancio OMS, Braga JAP, et al. Randomized controlled trial of iron-fortified drinking water in preschool children. J Am Coll Nutr. 2010;29:122–9.

Chapter 11
Heme Iron as Source of Iron in Food Fortification

Javier Polo and Carmen Rodríguez

Key Points

- Heme iron concentrate is the most efficiently absorbed source of iron.
- Heme iron is naturally present in meat and fish.
- Heme iron is not influenced by other dietary components.
- Heme iron is absorbed by a specific pathway that differs from other sources of iron.
- Heme iron absorption is less affected by inhibitory substances present in the diet.
- Heme iron does not cause gastric irritation or other side effects.

Keywords Heme iron • Iron availability • Food fortification • Iron absorption • Dietary iron

Abbreviations

DMT-1	Divalent metal transporter
Fe	Iron
Hb	Hemoglobin
HCP-1	Heme carrier protein 1
HIP	Heme iron polypeptide
IS	Iron sulfate
PC	Placebo

J. Polo (✉) • C. Rodríguez
APC EUROPE, S.A. R&D Department,
Avda. Sant Julià 246-258. P.I. El Congost. E-08403, Granollers 080403, Spain
e-mail: javier.polo@ampc-europe.com; carmen.rodriguez@ampc-europe.com

V.R. Preedy et al. (eds.), *Handbook of Food Fortification and Health: From Concepts to Public Health Applications Volume 1*, Nutrition and Health, DOI 10.1007/978-1-4614-7076-2_11,

Introduction

Iron (Fe) deficiency is one of the most widely known nutritional disorders that affect an estimated two billion people worldwide [1]. It occurs when there is a negative balance between iron requirements, absorption, and losses. In developing countries iron deficiency is caused not only by an iron-deficient diet but also by low bioavailability of iron in the diet [2]. Pregnant women, infants, young children, and adolescents have higher iron requirements and are at greater risk of developing iron deficiency. Despite the numerous initiatives implemented to control iron deficiency the problem persists along with substantial health and economic costs.

Iron fortification of regular foods or condiments directed to the whole population is a sustainable and cost-effective approach to prevent and control iron deficiency; however technical challenges limit the amount of bioavailable iron sources used in food fortification [3]. Heme iron has greater bioavailability than inorganic iron because its absorption process differs [4] and it is not negatively affected by other dietary compounds [5]. Ingestion of heme iron is not associated with gastric irritation or other side effects including stomach irritation, nausea, and constipation, which are commonly associated with inorganic iron oral supplementation [6–9].

Heme is a biologically important source of dietary iron. Studies estimate that in Western societies iron derived from heme sources such as myoglobin and hemoglobin (Hb) make up two-thirds of the average person's total iron stores although it only represents one-third of the total ingested iron [10]. Several studies have evaluated fortification of heme iron in different foods using biscuits [11, 12], cookie fillings [13], weaning foods [14], flour [15], and black beans [16].

Bioavailability and Absorption Mechanism

The chemical form of iron is the main factor affecting its bioavailability. Iron is naturally present in two forms: non-heme iron and heme iron with the latter having greater bioavailability. Absorption of non-heme iron (present mainly in vegetable-based food and food supplements) is determined mainly by its luminal solubility, which diminishes as the pH of the gastric content approaches neutral. During digestion the ferric complexes are reduced to the ferrous form, which binds to soluble low molecular weight complexes. Several compounds in food such as hydrochloric, lactic, ascorbic and citric acid, fructose, sorbitol, cysteine, lysine, and histidine help stabilize iron in its soluble and more absorbable ferrous form. Conversely, other dietary compounds, such as carbonates, oxalates, phytates, phosphates, tannins, polyphenols, albumin, proteases, egg yolk, Ca, Mn, Cu, Cd, Co, and fiber inhibit iron absorption, although fiber has modest inhibitory capacity [17–20]. The major characteristics associated with heme and non-heme iron are listed in Fig. 11.1.

Heme iron is derived mainly from Hb and myoglobin in animal tissues and is at high concentration in liver. Heme iron is an important dietary source of iron because it is absorbed more efficiently than non-heme iron and it also enhances absorption of non-heme iron.

The absorption process for heme iron differs from non-heme iron; however, mechanisms that regulate the quantity of iron absorbed do not distinguish between the two forms of iron but apparently depend on body iron requirements [21].

Heme iron enters the mucosa through a different route from the absorption of non-heme iron. Therefore, it is not regulated by the divalent metal transporter (DMT-1) but instead involves interaction of the iron in the porphyrin complex with an iron receptor [22, 23]. Heme iron absorption is less regulated and ranges between 15 % in individuals with full iron reserves and 35 % in individuals with iron depletion [24]. During iron-deficient conditions heme iron absorption increases due to greater microvilli iron affinity [23] and induction of hemo-oxygenase in the membrane which breaks the porphyrin ring and releases iron for transport into cells. Iron enters the enterocyte as an intact metalloporphyrin probably by means of an endocytic vesicular system or through the action of an integrin-

NON-HEME IRON

- Absorption 1-15%
- Absorption is affected by other components in the diet
- Source: vegetables and ferrous salts
- Percentage consumed, very high (>85%)

HEME IRON

- Absorption 20-35%
- Absorption is not affected by other components in the diet
- Source: Myoglobin and hemoglobin
- Percentage consumed, very low (<15%)

Fig. 11.1 Main characteristics of heme and non-heme iron. Non-heme iron (present in plant foods), the most common dietary iron, has limited absorption because is significantly influenced by other dietary components. Heme iron, found in animal foods containing hemoglobin (Hb) and myoglobin (meat, fish, and poultry) is better absorbed since is not significantly affected by other ingredients in the diet

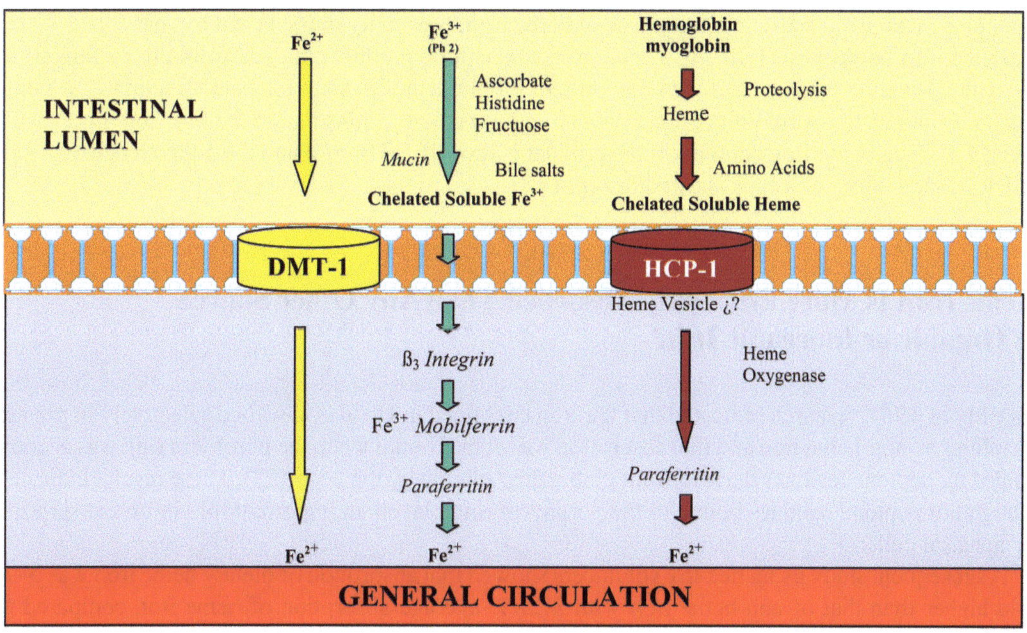

Fig. 11.2 Pathways of absorption of non-heme and heme iron (adapted from Dr. Quintero-Gutiérrez). The figure shows the different absorption processes followed by heme and non-heme iron. Ferrous iron bind to DMT-1 and is transferred into the enterocyte. Ferric iron binds chelators and is absorbed via integrin-mobilferrin pathway and further reduced by paraferritin inside the enterocyte. Heme iron is absorbed as an intact metalloprotein throughout the HCP-1 transporter. Inside the enterocyte the enzyme heme oxygenase releases ferrous iron. *DMT-1* divalent metal transporter 1; *HCP-1* heme carrier protein 1

like binding protein. Recently, a heme carrier protein 1 (HCP-1) was identified, cloned and characterized as the carrier in the apical region of the duodenum responsible for the absorption of heme iron into intestinal cells [4]. HCP-1 seems to be regulated pre- and posttranscriptionally in hypoxic and iron-deficient rats, respectively [4]. The discovery *of HCP-1* has led to a better understanding of the extensively studied mechanism by which heme iron is absorbed from the diet into the intestine. Inside the cell iron is then released as inorganic iron (Fe^{2+}) through the action of hemo-oxygenase; afterwards, the pathway for heme iron is similar to that described for inorganic iron (Fig. 11.2).

As previously described, heme iron absorption is independent of other compounds in the diet, although high concentrations of luminal calcium can reduce its absorption [7, 25].

In the excellent review of human iron absorption, the authors stated that in countries with high meat consumption, heme iron made up one-third of the iron in the diet but accounted for two-thirds of the iron absorbed by the body [26]. They attributed this difference to the preference for heme iron absorption since it is soluble at the pH of the small intestine, and to the fact that its absorption by the enterocytes is not affected adversely by dietary inhibitors in the diet as happens with inorganic iron. They also confirmed that iron reserves were balanced via transfer receptors in the basolateral membrane of the absorptive cells.

Sources of Heme Iron

Iron is a common nutrient in most foods (Table 11.1). Non-heme iron is found in vegetables, cereals, fruits, eggs, and milk products. Heme iron is found only in animal tissue products such as poultry, pork, beef, fish, or seafood products. An especially high content of heme iron is found in liver, quail, and horse meat. Fish is also a good source of heme iron, especially mussels and oysters.

Heme iron polypeptide (HIP) is a heme iron concentrate product obtained from the hydrolysis of Hb with unspecific protease and the separation of globin peptones from the heme fraction. The heme fraction contains the porphyrin complex bound to amino acid chains that make this iron more available [27]. Usually the iron content of this product is around 1.0 % iron and the equivalence of 1 g of HIP to other sources of iron is showed in Fig. 11.3.

Heme Iron Is More Efficiently Absorbed Than Any Other Source of Organic or Inorganic Iron

As early as 1967, research indicated that the iron contained in Hb was absorbed selectively in greater quantities as non-heme iron and that absorption was at maximum when the porphyrin ring was accompanied by peptone residues derived from globin degradation by the body [27]. These results indicated that globin peptone residues bound to the porphyrin ring played an important role in iron absorption by mucosal cells.

A subsequent study using healthy volunteers showed that absorption of dietary heme iron was 5–7-fold higher than that of non-heme iron with 37.3 % average absorption of heme iron compared to 5.3 % absorption for non-heme iron as a percentage of total intakes [28]. A similar study reported that heme iron absorption was 2–3.6 times higher in all types of meal and food combinations compared with the ferrous (non-heme) iron [29].

Authors of another report stated that absorption of the dietary heme iron ranged from 15 to 35 % depending on individual iron reserves, while absorption of non-heme iron ranged from 2 to 20 % depending not only on individual iron reserves but also on the presence or absence of dietary iron absorption promoters or inhibitors [30]. In a study performed in Cuba subjects were given iron-fortified food (8 mg/day, 75 % of which was heme iron) for 6 months [31]. Rate of anemia was significantly reduced for all the risk groups studied with a 295 % and 267 % reduction in the rate of anemia in children aged 1–4 years and women aged 15–59 years, respectively [31]. In another study performed in Cuba on pregnant women aged 20–30 years, the same authors identified pregnant participants with anemia (Hb < 11 g/dL) at the start of heme iron supplementation. Two study groups were formed, composed of pregnant women with and without anemia at baseline. One of the groups was given food fortified with ferrous fumarate from the time of recruitment (before the 18th week of

Table 11.1 Iron content in common foods

Food (100 g)	mg Iron	Food (100 g)	mg Iron
Meat (heme iron foods)		Flours, sugars, cereals & pasta	
Pork chops	2.50	Cacao powder	12.50
Cooked pork ham	2.30	Sugar	0.29
Pork loin	1.80	Honey	1.30
Beef filet	2.78	Potatoes starch	1.80
Beef chops	2.60	Rice	0.60
Quail	4.50	White bread	0.95
Horse meat	3.82	Toasted bread	2.20
Lamb	2.30	Cooked pasta	0.80
Chicken legs	1.80	Soy flour	12.10
Chicken breast	1.10	Vegetables	
Lamb liver	12.40	Green peas	5.00
Pork liver	22.10	Beans	6.10
Rice blood sausage	1.99	Lentils	6.90
Salami	1.30	Cooked potatoes	0.80
Pork/beef Hotdog	1.15	Egg plant	0.42
Fish (heme iron foods)		Spinach	4.10
Dried & Salted cod fish	2.50	Tomato	0.50
Cod fish	0.44	Carrot	2.10
Trout	0.69	Fruit	
Tuna	1.00	Cherries	0.35

Table 11.1 (continued)

Sardines	2.40	Orange	0.40
Mussels	5.12	Banana	0.55
Oysters	5.80	Nut	
Egg & dairy		Almonds	4.13
Whole egg	2.10	Roasted peanuts	2.32
Cow's milk 0.07% fat	0.12	Others	
Cow's milk 3.5 % fat	0.05	Coffee drink	4.13
Whey powder (11%)	1.24	Red wine	0.71
Low fat yogurt	0.06		
Blue cheese	0.66		
Parmesan cheese	1.02		

Legend: The table shows the amount of total iron in food expressed as mg/100g food. Iron from most animal sources (heme iron) is more readily absorbed than iron from plant sources of food (non-heme iron).

pregnancy) to birth. The other group received food fortified with heme iron. In the pregnant women with anemia at baseline and supplemented with heme iron, the anemia diminished progressively by time of delivery. This progressive reduction in anemia was not observed in pregnant women supplemented with dietary ferrous fumarate [31] (Table 11.2).

Eskeland et al. [32] performed a double-blinded study on pregnant women who were supplemented during the second half of pregnancy with a dietary product containing a mixture of heme and non-heme iron (27 mg Fe in total), compared with a product containing an equal quantity of iron in purely non-heme form and vitamin C, or a placebo (PC) group given no iron supplement [32]. Both iron-supplemented groups had a lower percentage of anemic women at delivery compared to the placebo group (25 % vs. 52 %); but the percentage of women with low postpartum iron reserves was reduced to 8 % in the group supplemented with heme/non-heme mixture vs. 27 % for the non-heme group and 52 % for the placebo group. These results suggest that the heme/non-heme mixture given during the second half of pregnancy improved postpartum iron status parameters.

Heme iron supplementation may improve intelligence and concentration test scores of school children from families with limited financial resources. An interesting study involving 53 school children given heme iron-supplemented biscuits for 6–8 weeks reported significantly improved intelligence and concentration test scores compared to a non-fortified control group of 55 children [33]. In another study conducted in Cuba with 6–36 month-old children diagnosed with iron-deficiency anemia and intolerant to iron salt supplements, 86 % of the cases had recovery of Hb values when their food was supplemented with 8 mg total Fe/kg/day of Trofín, a product containing heme iron and small quantities of inorganic iron [34].

A study with 215 healthy schoolchildren fed biscuits fortified with 6 % bovine Hb were associated with good iron absorption (19.7 %) and that the Hb-fortified biscuit was readily accepted, although no differences

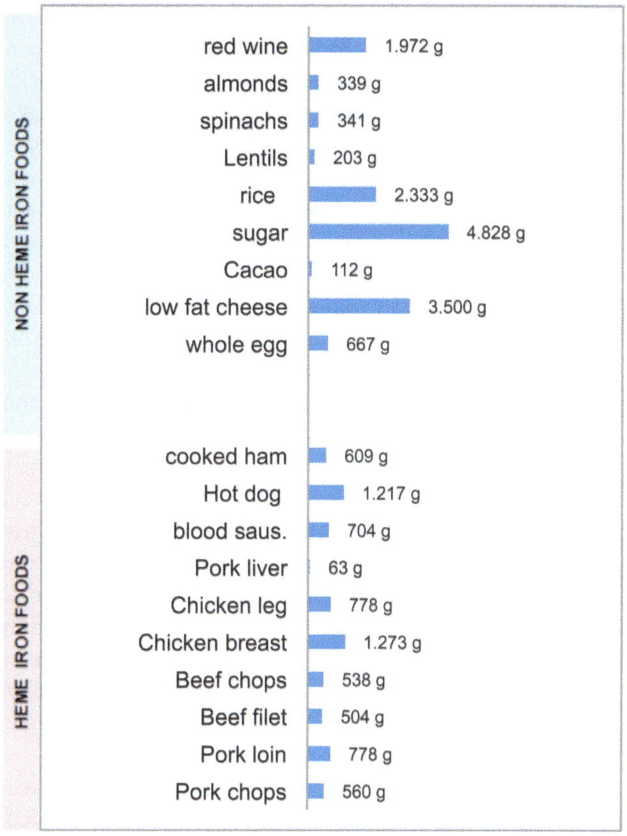

Fig. 11.3 Equivalence of 1 g of heme iron polypeptide (HIP) to other sources of iron. The table shows the equivalence in terms of iron content between 1 g of HIP obtained by enzymatic hydrolysis of Hb and a variety of common foods

Table 11.2 Effect of giving foods fortified with heme iron or ferrous fumarate to pregnant women

Women	Ferrous fumarate group				Heme iron group			
(Hb, g/L)	*N*	Baseline	3 months	Delivery	*N*	Baseline	3 months	Delivery
Control	34	11.9[a]	11.4[a]	11.7[a]	28	11.8[a]	11.0[a]	11.5[a]
Anemic	13	10.3[a]	10.7[a]	10.6[a]	12	10.4[a]	10.8[a,b]	11.2[b]

Source: Dr. Fernández

Value of Hb in pregnant women with and without anemia at baseline, 3 months pregnancy and at delivery receiving either food fortified with ferrous fumarate or heme iron

[a,b]Values in the same line with different superscript were significantly different ($P<0.05$)

were observed in serum Hb content between the control (non-fortified) and fortified groups; however, the fortified group had higher iron reserves, as measured by serum ferritin level [35]. The same research group also studied 4-month-old babies consuming a cereal formula fortified with bovine Hb and determined that the number of babies with iron-deficiency anemia at 12 months of age was significantly reduced [36]. Conversely, no differences in iron absorption was observed for infants fed baby food prepared in jars and fortified with ferrous iron sulfate (IS) or heme iron in the form of Hb [37].

A 3-year study involving approximately 1,000 Chilean schoolchildren given biscuits fortified with bovine Hb and compared with a non-supplemented control group reported significant increases in Hb and serum ferritin levels for the supplemented group, even for students who were not anemic when iron supplementation was started [12].

Studies using HIP derived from either porcine or bovine Hb have been reported. A clinical study was performed using a dietary product that contained greater than 1 % iron from a highly soluble HIP with small globin polypeptide chains [38]. The HIP product was derived from the pig Hb digested with proteolytic enzymes. Iron absorption rate in 14 healthy subjects was determined during and 3 and 6 h after one meal of a supplement containing 20 mg of HIP or a supplement containing the same quantity of iron as ferrous fumarate or a 20 mg of glucose as a placebo. Iron absorption in the HIP-supplemented group was at least 2 mg, while iron absorption in the ferrous fumarate group was less than 1 mg.

Other studies have showed that when pig Hb was hydrolyzed by an enzyme obtained from *Bacillus subtilis*, the increase in iron absorption in rats (using an in vitro chamber model system) was significantly higher than whole Hb [39, 40]. Absorption was dependent on the enzyme used and the degree of hydrolysis; it was higher when hydrolysis was performed with subtilisin vs. pepsin. Also, iron absorption was higher when the degree of hydrolysis of Hb was greater than 10 % compared with intact un-hydrolyzed Hb. These results highlighted the importance of globin peptide residues around the heme group for increasing the absorption of HIP iron.

Bovine HIP is obtained by enzymatic hydrolysis of bovine Hb and has been shown to have similar iron bioavailability as porcine HIP [41]. During a 12-week study 52 premenopausal women with moderate body iron levels received 5 mg of heme iron in two capsules per day, or 50 mg of electrolytic iron, reduced iron or ferrous sulfate in pastry products. Changes in body iron reserves were monitored by analyzing the serum transferrin/serum ferritin receptor ratio, which is the most sensitive detection method of iron reserves. Body iron (mg/kg body weight) increased with all four sources of iron when compared with a placebo group that received no iron supplements. The serum transferring/serum ferritin receptor ratio results indicated that the electrolytic and reduced iron sources were 50 % and 85 % as effective as ferrous sulfate. Although only 5 mg of heme iron was provided daily, it was 50 % as effective as 50 mg/day of ferrous sulfate.

Two studies involving female teenagers enrolled in secondary schools in the Mexican State of Morelos were done to assess serum iron status after supplementation of iron sources provided in biscuits, cookies, or chocolate bars [42, 43]. The initial study involved 112 female teenagers age 12–15 years who were distributed in three groups [42]. Group 1 ($n=35$) females included those with the highest initial serum Hb that were fed non-iron-supplemented biscuits (*Suavicremas*, a Gaufrette style cookie made by a leading bakery company). Group 2 ($n=40$) and Group 3 ($n=37$) received biscuits supplemented with either HIP or ferrous sulfate, respectively. The iron-supplemented groups each received about 7.7 mg iron/day for a total of 380 mg of iron over the 7-week study period. This daily dose was about 50 % of the recommended iron requirement for this population group. The biscuits were readily consumed by all groups. Serum ferritin results indicated decreased concentration over time for the placebo and ferrous sulfate groups, whereas the ferritin concentration of the HIP group was maintained over time. The authors suggested that HIP supplementation maintained iron reserves in teenage females. A subsequent 13-week study by the same research group involved 193 teenage (11–16 year old) females from different secondary schools [43]. In this study, Group 1 ($n=70$) consisted of subjects with higher baseline serum Hb that were given a non-iron-supplemented placebo as a choice of either a cookie or chocolate bar. Groups 2 ($n=59$) and 3 ($n=64$) consisted of subjects with lower baseline serum Hb that received either a cookie or chocolate bar supplemented with either HIP or ferrous sulfate, respectively. Both iron-supplemented groups received at total of 678 mg of iron over the 13-week study period that provided about 9.5 mg of iron/day which was about 50 % greater than the recommended daily iron intake for this population. As shown in Fig. 11.4, the placebo group maintained the highest average serum Hb over time because this group consisted of females with higher initial serum Hb levels. The ferrous sulfate groups had lower initial Hb which remained lower than the placebo group over time. By the end of the study, the HIP group had significantly higher average Hb values than the group given ferrous sulfate and was similar to the placebo group. As observed in the initial study adolescents had serum Hb levels within normal ranges for this population group, so significant increases in iron absorption were not expected.

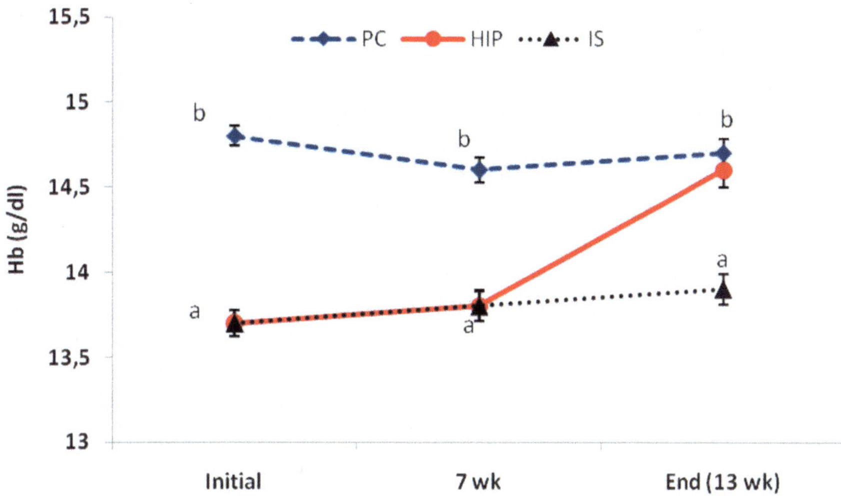

Fig. 11.4 Serum Hb of experimental group at baseline, 7 and 13 weeks of daily supplementation. The graph showed the Hb levels (g/dL) in teenage females ($n=193$, 11–16 years old) after 7 and 13 weeks of iron supplementation (9.5 mg/day) with iron sulfate (IS) or heme iron (HIP), and compared with a group that did not receive supplementation (placebo, PC)

Heme Iron Consumption Does Not Cause Nausea, Gastric Irritation, Vomiting, or Diarrhea

Two studies have reported that subjects supplemented with heme iron had less side effects such as stomach ache, constipation, nausea, or diarrhea compared to inorganic iron [6, 8]. In a comparative absorption study of iron sources both healthy and anemic pregnant women supplemented with heme iron had significantly higher iron absorption (16.1 % and 22.0 %, respectively) with less reported side effects than the groups given ferrous sulfate (4.6 % and 9.4 %, respectively) [6]. A second study reported reduced side effects and similar serum ferritin and Hb concentrations in healthy volunteers supplemented daily with a mixture of 1.2 mg Fe from porcine heme iron and 8 mg Fe from ferrous fumarate compared to a control group supplemented daily with 60 mg Fe from ferrous fumarate [8].

Fewer side effects were reported for the heme iron groups in both studies because heme iron was supplemented at lower quantities and absorbed more efficiently than inorganic iron resulting in less quantity of free ferric ion radicals in the intestinal lumen.

Absorption of the Heme Iron Is Not Affected by Other Components of the Diet

Reizenstein stated that heme iron was better absorbed in all types of meals and food combinations than ferrous (non-heme) iron [29]. Also, it was observed that cysteine given to human subjects during meals improved absorption of non-heme iron more than that of heme iron suggesting that heme iron absorption was less affected by other dietary components [44]. Absorption of non-heme iron was enhanced by the presence of heme iron in the diet, while the absorption of heme iron remained stable for all meals irrespective of the food eaten and the concentration of heme iron [45]. Dietary heme iron absorption ranged from 15 to 35 % depending on individual iron reserves, while non-heme iron absorption was from 2 to 20 % depending not only on individual iron reserves but also on the presence of dietary iron absorption promoters or inhibitors [30].

Hurrell indicated that the absorption of heme iron was not affected by inhibitor substances in the diet but that it was affected by body iron reserves [46]. It was also reported that heme iron absorption is less affected by substances in the diet than non-heme iron, indicating that heme iron absorption is determined mainly by the body iron levels and, to a very minor extent, by dietary factors [47]. However there are two exceptions; meat increases heme iron absorption and calcium inhibits it although the inhibitory effect of calcium is several orders of magnitude higher for non-heme iron.

Roughead and Hunt observed that absorption of non-heme (50 mg Fe/day from ferrous sulfate) iron diminished over a 12-week study using healthy volunteers ($n=57$) even though body iron reserves (serum ferritin) remained high [48]. However, the absorption of heme iron was stable throughout the entire supplementation period. Nevertheless other authors reported that heme iron absorption in 28–50-year-old healthy women ($n=27$) became saturated at a maximum of 2 mg of heme iron absorbed per day [49]. They suggested that saturation of heme iron absorption could be due to a protective mechanism that prevents iron overload when meat or blood consumption is high. Lastly, the 2004 European Food Safety Authority (EFSA) [7] stated that heme iron absorption was higher than inorganic iron and that regulation of heme iron absorption was not influenced by other substances in the diet but was regulated only by levels of iron already present in the body.

Guidance on Supplemental Iron Levels Suitable for Beneficial Effects

According to the National Academy of Sciences [50] the recommended daily iron intake varies by the population group, as shown in Table 11.3.

Table 11.3 Recommended daily allowance for iron by population group

	Recommended daily allowance (RDA) for iron		
Population group	Recommended individual intake (mg Fe/day)	Average estimated requirement by group (mg Fe/day)	Maximum tolerable intake (mg Fe/day)
Infants			
0–6 months	0.27		40
7–12 months	11	6.9	40
Children			
1–3 years	7	3.0	40
4–8 years	10	4.1	40
Adult males			
9–13 years	8	5.9	40
14–18 years	11	7.7	45
19 to >70 years	8	6	45
Adult females			
9–13 years	8	5.7	40
14–18 years	15	7.9	45
19–50 years	18	8.1	
50 to >70 years	8	5	45
Pregnancy			
14–50 years	27	22	45

The table shows the recommended dietary allowance or RDA for iron according to the segments of population. The RDA is defined as "the average daily intake level that is sufficient to meet the nutrient requirement of nearly all (98 %) healthy individuals"

The recommended daily allowance for iron supplementation is 1.0 g of heme iron as HIP with 1 % Fe content or 3.2 g as Hb powder (with 0.31 % Fe content) which is equivalent to *10 mg* of elemental iron. In the case of iron-fortified food, the recommended daily allowance of heme iron is a maximum fortification of 25 % of the recommended daily intake for women of childbearing age; this means the recommendation of a maximum per day of 4 mg iron in final fortified food or 0.4 g of heme iron as HIP.

The maximum tolerable intake values refer to non-heme iron intake and supplements. According to data published by EFSA 50 mg/day is considered to be the lowest observed adverse effect level (LOAEL) to avoid effects on the gastrointestinal mucosa in humans, although it specifies that this value is only applicable to non-heme iron supplements [7].

Thus the recommendation for a maximum daily intake of HIP (with an approximate iron content of 1 %) could be 2 g which is equivalent to 20 mg of elemental iron or about half of the maximum recommended iron intake for inorganic iron.

However, the acute toxicity (LD50) of HIP (1 % purity of heme iron) in rats is greater than 2,500 mg product/kg of body weight which means that the product has a very low acute toxicity (J. Polo, personal communication). This indicates that a 70 kg adult would need to consume more than 175 g of HIP/day (equivalent to 1,750 mg Fe/day) to develop acute Fe toxicity. Nevertheless, EFSA reported that acute toxicity was induced in mice after oral doses of ferrous compounds in the range 200–650 mg Fe/kg body weight with ferrous sulfate being the most toxic [7]. This means that heme iron is between 3.5 and 10 times less toxic than current sources of non-heme iron used for food supplements or food fortification.

Recommendations to the Manufacturers

Compatibility with Food

Hb or HIP powder is very dark in color (black in case of HIP) and has a characteristic taste. Water solubility of HIP is usually less than 50 %. Consequently these features of HIP should be considered before its use in food products or supplements.

The dark color of HIP may limit its use in light colored food products but it can be favorable to use in foods that naturally already have darker color, such as chocolate fillings, cocoa cream, blackberry jam, dark sausages, etc.

The use of HIP in drinks may cause significant product precipitation due to its low solubility; however the precipitated product can be resuspended by shaking the container or it can be kept in suspension through the use of hydrocolloids.

Due to its iron content (approximately 1 % in case of HIP), care should be taken when adding it to food with a high fat content to prevent potential fat oxidation and rancidity. The addition of appropriate antioxidants to avoid fat oxidation would be advisable [51]. However, in pastries and sandwich-type biscuits supplemented with HIP added to the chocolate filling and with a total fat content of 10.2 % and 6.3 %, respectively, the products did not develop rancidity when stored for 1 year in their original packs under appropriate temperature and humidity storage conditions (dry and temperature around 20–22 °C).

Compatibility with Food Preparation Process

Excellent compatibility of Hb or heme iron concentrate either alone (in capsules or tablets) or fortified in various foods (baby food in jars, biscuits, mixed with cereals, pâtés, or meat products) have been reported in the literature [14, 32–34, 36, 42].

High luminal calcium has been shown to be incompatible with heme iron. It has been observed a significant reduction in heme iron absorption in the presence of high calcium doses (300–600 mg Ca) and suggested that calcium interferes with the iron carrier through the cell membrane [25, 52].

The risk of fat oxidation and development of rancidity may increase in foods fortified with iron. Some authors studied the effectiveness of antioxidants in preventing oxidation of palm oil (commonly used in baked products) enriched with HIP (1 % purity on heme iron) and found that the addition of either 500 ppm ascorbyl palmitate or 500 ppm ascorbyl palmitate plus 300 ppm citric acid were effective to prevent oil oxidation [51].

Conditions for Use

HIP or Hb in powder form can be used directly in the formulation of a variety of food products such as chocolate fillings for pastry products, jams, baby food in jars, meat products, pâtés, sweets, dairy desserts, bread products, drinks, etc. HIP or Hb powder should be added during mixing or homogenization in order to ensure uniform distribution in the final product; likewise for liquid foods, HIP or Hb should be suspended first in water or another liquid before blending it with the other ingredients in order to ensure the final food product is homogeneous.

Conclusions

Heme iron concentrate is the most efficiently absorbed source of iron that is naturally present in meat and fish. Heme iron absorption is not influenced by other dietary components and is absorbed by a specific pathway that differs from other sources of iron. Heme iron intake is a source of iron that does not cause gastric irritation or other side effects

References

1. Benoist B, McLean E, Cogswell M, Egli I, Wojdyla D. Worldwide prevalence of anaemia 1993–2005. WHO global database on anaemia. Geneva: World Health Organization; 2008.
2. Layrisse M, García-Casal MN. Strategies for the prevention of iron deficiency through foods in the household. Nutr Rev. 1997;55:233–9.
3. Huma N, Salim-Ur-Rehman, Anjum FM, Murtaza MA, Sheikh MA. Food fortification strategy-preventing iron deficiency anemia: a review. Crit Rev Food Sci Nutr. 2007;47:259–65.
4. Shayeghi M, Latunde-Dada GO, Oakhill JS, et al. Identification of an intestinal heme transporter. Cell. 2005;122(5):789–801.
5. Uzel C, Conrad M. Absorption of heme iron. Semin Hematol. 1998;1:27–34.
6. Ekman M, Reizenstein P. Comparative absorption of ferrous and heme-iron with meals in normal and iron deficient subjects. Z Ernahrungswiss. 1993;32(1):67–70.
7. European Food Safety Authority (EFSA). Opinion of the scientific panel on dietetic products, nutrition and allergies on a request from the commission related to the tolerable upper intake of iron. EFSA J. 2004;125:1–34.
8. Frykman E, Bystrom M, Jansson U, Edberg A, Hansen T. Side effects of iron supplements in blood donors: superior tolerance of heme iron. J Lab Clin Med. 1994;123:561–4.
9. Cook JD. Diagnosis and management of iron deficiency anaemia. Best Pract Res Clin Haematol. 2005;18:319–32.
10. West AR, Oates PS. Mechanisms of heme iron absorption: current questions and controversies. World J Gastroenterol. 2008;14:4101–10.
11. Asenjo JA, Amar M, Cartagena N, King J, Hiche E, Stekel A. Use of bovine heme iron concentrate in the fortification of biscuits. J Food Sci. 1985;50:795–9.

12. Walter T, Hertrampf E, Pizarro F, et al. Effect of bovine-haemoglobin-fortified cookies on iron status of schoolchildren: a nationwide program in Chile. Am J Clin Nutr. 1993;57:190–4.
13. Quintero-Gutiérrez AG, González-Rosendo G, Arenas ML, Polo J, Rodríguez-Jerez JJ. Bioavailability of heme iron in biscuit filling using piglets as an animal model for humans. Int J Biol Sci. 2008;4(1):58–62.
14. Martínez C, López G, Ros G, Vidal ML, Abellán P. Use of heme iron concentrate in the fortification of weaning foods. J Agric Food Chem. 2000;48:2930–6.
15. Albaldawi A, Brennan CS, Alobaidy K, Alammar W, Aljumaily D. Effect of flour fortification with haem liposome on bread and bread doughs. Int J Food Sci Technol. 2005;40:825–8.
16. Schümann K, Romero-Abal ME, Mäurer A, et al. Haematological response to haem iron or ferrous sulfate mixed with refried black beans in moderately anaemic Guatemalan pre-school children. Public Health Nutr. 2005;8:572–81.
17. Brune M, Rossander-Hultén L, Hallberg L, Gleerup A, Sandberg AS. Iron absorption from bread in humans: inhibiting effects of cereal fiber, phytate and inositol phosphates with different numbers of phosphate groups. J Nutr. 1992;122(3):442–9.
18. Craig WJ. Iron status of vegetarians. Am J Clin Nutr. 1994;59(5 Suppl):1233S–7.
19. Claydesdale FM. Physicochemical determinants of iron bioavailability. Food Technol. 1983;37(10):133–8.
20. Layrisse M, García-Casal MN, Solano L, et al. Iron bioavailability in humans from breakfasts enriched with iron bis-glycine chelate, phytates and polyphenols. J Nutr. 2000;130(9):2195–9.
21. Hallberg L, Hulten L, Gramatkovsky E. Iron absorption from the whole diet in men: how effective is the regulation of iron absorption? Am J Clin Nutr. 1997;66:347–56.
22. Tenhunen R, Grasbeck R, Kouronen I, Landberg M. An intestinal receptor for heme: its partial characterization. Int J Biochem. 1980;12:713–6.
23. Roberts ST, Henderson RW, Young GP. Modulation of uptake of heme by rat small intestinal mucosa in iron deficiency. Am J Physiol. 1993;265:G712–8.
24. Finch C. Regulators of iron balance in humans. Blood. 1994;84:1697–702.
25. Hallberg L, Rossander-Hulten L, Brune M, Gleerup A. Inhibition of haem iron absorption in man by calcium. Br J Nutr. 1992;69:533–40.
26. Conrad ME, Umbreit JN. Pathways of iron absorption. Blood Cells Mol Dis. 2002;29(3):336–55.
27. Conrad ME, Benjamin BI, Williams HL, Foy AL. Human absorption of haemoglobin iron. Gastroenterology. 1967;53:5–10.
28. Björn-Rasmussen EB, Hallberg L, Isaksson B, Arvidsson B. Applications of the two-pool extrinsic tag method to measure heme and non-heme iron absorption from the whole diet. J Clin Invest. 1974;53:247–55.
29. Reizenstein P. Haemoglobin fortification of food and prevention of iron deficiency with heme iron. Acta Med Scand Suppl. 1979;629:1–47.
30. Monsen ER. Iron nutrition and absorption: dietary factors which impact iron bioavailability. J Am Diet Assoc. 1988;88(7):786–90.
31. Fernández S. Utilización del hierro hémico en alimentos para su uso en el tratamiento o prevención de anemias y deficiencias en hierro. Ph.D. Thesis. Cuba: University of Havana; 1991.
32. Eskeland B, Malterud K, Ulvik RJ, Hunskaar S. Iron supplementation in pregnancy: is less enough? A randomized, placebo-controlled trial of low-dose iron supplementation with and without heme iron. Acta Obstet Gynecol Scand. 1997;76(9):822–8.
33. Salinas-Piélago JE, Vega-Dienstmaier JM, Rojas-Oblitas M. Efecto de las galletas fortificadas con hierro heme sobre el estado intelectual en preescolares. Rev Neurol. 1998;27(157):400–4.
34. Fernández N, Gautier du Défaix H, Forrellat M, Cedré T, González R, Aznar E. Tratamiento con Trofín en niños intolerantes a las sales de hierro. Rev Cubana Hematol Inmunol Hemoter. 2000;16(2):115–21.
35. Olivares M, Hertrampf E, Pizarro F, et al. Haemoglobin-fortified biscuits: bioavailability and its effect on iron nutriture in school children. Arch Latinoam Nutr. 1990;40(2):209–20.
36. Hertrampf E, Olivares M, Pizarro F, et al. Haemoglobin fortified cereal: a source of available iron to breast-fed infants. Eur J Clin Nutr. 1990;44(11):793–8.
37. Martínez C, Fox T, Eagles J, Fairweather-Tait S. Evaluation of iron bioavailability in infant weaning foods fortified with haem concentrate. J Pediatr Gastroenterol Nutr. 1998;27(4):419–24.
38. Seligman PA, Moore GM, Schleicher RB. Clinical studies of HIP: an oral heme-iron product. Nutr Res. 2000;20(9):1279–86.
39. Vaghefi N, Nedjaoum F, Guillochon D, Bureau F, Arhan P, Bouglé D. Influence of the extent of haemoglobin hydrolysis on the digestive absorption of haem iron in rat. An in vitro study. Exp Physiol. 2000;85(4):379–85.
40. Vaghefi N, Nedjaoum F, Guillochon D, Bureau F, Arhan P, Bouglé D. Influence of the extent of haemoglobin hydrolysis on the digestive absorption of heme iron. An in vitro study. J Agric Food Chem. 2002;50:4969–73.
41. Swain JH, Johnson LK, Hunt JR. Combating iron deficiency: bioavailability of iron from two elemental iron powders and a heme iron supplement in humans. Exp Biol Meeting Abst. 2004;130.21:A155.

42. González-Rosendo G, Polo J, Rodríguez-Jerez JJ, Puga-Díaz R, Reyes-Navarrete EG, Quintero-Gutiérrez AG. Bioavailability of a heme-iron concentrate product added to chocolate biscuit filling in adolescent girls living in a rural area of México. J Food Sci. 2010;75(3):H73–8.
43. Quintero-Gutiérrez AG, Mariaca-Gaspa G, Villanueva-Sánchez J, Polo J, Rodríguez C, González-Rosendo G. Acceptability and use of heme-iron concentrate product added to chocolate biscuit filling as alternative source of high available form of iron. CyTA-J Food. 2012;10(2):112–8.
44. Martínez-Torres C, Romano E, Layrisse M. Effect of cysteine on iron absorption in man. Am J Clin Nutr. 1981;34:322–7.
45. Bezwoda WR, Bothwell TH, Charlton RW, et al. The relative dietary importance of haem and non-haem iron. S Afr Med J. 1983;64(14):552–6.
46. Bothwell TH, Baynes RD, MacFarlane BJ, MacPhail AP. Nutritional iron requirements and food iron absorption. J Intern Med. 1989;226:357–65.
47. Martínez C, Ros G, Periago MJ, López G. Biodisponibilidad del hierro de los alimentos. Arch Latinoam Nutr. 1999;49(2):106–13.
48. Roughead ZK, Hunt JR. Adaptation in iron absorption: iron supplementation reduces non-heme iron but not heme iron absorption from food. Am J Clin Nutr. 2000;72:982–9.
49. Pizarro F, Olivares M, Hertrampf E, Mazariegos DI, Arredondo M. Heme-iron absorption is saturable by heme-iron dose in women. J Nutr. 2003;133:2214–7.
50. National Academy of Sciences (NAS). Dietary reference intakes for vitamin A, vitamin K, arsenic, boron, chromium, copper, iodine, iron, manganese, molybdenum, nickel, silicon, vanadium and zinc. Washington, DC: National Academy Press; 2001.
51. Aleman M, Nuchi CD, Bou R, et al. Effectiveness of antioxidants in preventing oxidation of palm oil enriched with heme iron: a model for iron fortification in baked products. Eur J Lipid Sci Technol. 2010;112:761–9.
52. Hallberg L, Brune M, Erlandsson M, Sandberg A-S, Rossander-Hulten L. Calcium: effect of different amounts on non-heme and heme iron absorption in humans. Am J Clin Nutr. 1991;53:112–9.

Part III
Fortified Foods and Beverages

Chapter 12
Fortification of Corn Flour-Derived Products

Isaias Dichi and Lucia Helena Silva Miglioranza

Key Points

- Fortification of maize (corn) flour is common due to its wide availability.
- Corn flour-derived products can be fortified with any micronutrient or vitamin.
- The majority of studies have been performed with iron and folic acid fortification.
- Processing methods to reduce the phytate content of cereals seem to improve the efficiency of fortification more so than the use of a particular cereal grain.
- The complete degradation of phytic acid in maize increases iron absorption by up to 10 times.
- The way in which meals are prepared and the choice of appropriate combinations of foods for target groups are fundamental aspects of food fortification.
- Human studies have shown excellent results with corn flour fortified by elemental iron.
- Reports on reductions in neural tube defects prevalence after folic acid fortification of corn vary from 16 to 78 %.

Keywords Iron fortification • Phytate content • Phytic acid • Neural tube defect • Folic acid fortification

Abbreviations

ID	Iron deficiency
IDA	Iron deficiency anaemia
LPM porridge	Low-phytate maize
$Na_2FeEDTA$	Disodium ferrous ethylenediaminetetraacetate
NTD	Neural tube defect

I. Dichi, M.D., Ph.D.
Department of Internal Medicine, University of Londrina,
60, Robert Koch Avenue, Londrina-PR, Brazil

L.H.S. Miglioranza, D.Sc. (✉)
Department of Food Science and Technology, University of Londrina,
Km 380 Celso Garcia Cid Road, Londrina-PR, Brazil
e-mail: dichi@sercomtel.com.br; luciah@uel.br

V.R. Preedy et al. (eds.), *Handbook of Food Fortification and Health: From Concepts to Public Health Applications Volume 1*, Nutrition and Health, DOI 10.1007/978-1-4614-7076-2_12,

Introduction

The wide availability of maize (*Zea mays*) and corn flour (*Zea mays var. amylacea*), even in populations with poor resources, make these popular vehicles for food fortification worldwide.

Maize is a fundamental staple food in many parts of the world, particularly in Africa but also in Asia and Central and South America. For this reason, maize is among the leading commodities used in international food aid. As a percentage of overall food aid, maize ranks third after wheat and rice, ranging from 1 to 1.5 million tons, depending on the year. While maize represents between 20 and 30 % of total annual food aid shipments, this accounts for less than 2 % of the annual world trade in maize. The United States is the largest food aid donor of maize, followed by the European Union, China, and the Republic of Korea. Many African countries typically occupy the top ten positions as the recipients of food aid, although consecutive droughts in recent years led the Democratic Republic of Korea to join the world's top recipients. In Africa, several countries, including Angola, Ethiopia, Kenya, Malawi, Mozambique, United Republic of Tanzania, Uganda, Zambia, and Zimbabwe, have received large amounts of food aid in the form of maize in past years [1].

Developed and developing countries utilise almost 350 million tons of maize per year. Total maize consumption reached 800 million tons in 2009. However, consumption differs between countries. In the United States , for example, maize is used primarily to feed livestock. However, corn is a versatile grain with a wealth of other uses. It is also processed into a multitude of food and industrial products, including starches, popcorn, and corn flakes, which is the most common breakfast cereal in North America. Furthermore, corn is used to produce sweeteners, such as high fructose corn syrup; ingredients for cakes, ice cream, cookies, soda, and corn oil; and beverage and industrial alcohol, as well as ethanol.

Corn for human consumption is prepared using different methods around the world. Despite regional particularities, meals are commonly prepared from coarse or fine-milled whole maize, which is sometimes degerminated and precooked or fermented. Maize is made into a thick porridge in many cultures, including polenta in Italy, angu in Brazil, mamaliga in Romania, mush in the United States (called grits in the South), and the dish referred to as mealie pap in South Africa and sadza, nshima, and ugali in other parts of Africa. Maize is also used in place of wheat flour to make cornbread and other baked products. Masa (corn meal treated with lime water) is the main ingredient for tortillas, atole, and many other dishes of Mexican origin [2].

Of the three major cereal grains (wheat, maize, and rice), maize has the lowest concentration of protein, calcium, and niacin. The nutritive value of the grain can also increase or decrease depending upon the method by which it is processed. For instance, milling maize reduces its concentration of protein, lipids, and fibre. The nutritional disease pellagra, which is caused by a deficiency in niacin, is associated with maize-based diets in the Americas and Africa. Diets that rely heavily on corn may require the consumption of complementary foods to compensate for its deficiency in lysine, tryptophan, and vitamins [3].

The corn kernel is made up of the endosperm, the germ, the pericarp, and the tip cap. The protein concentration is highest in the germ, but the protein quality is higher in the endosperm. Since the germ proteins contain essential amino acids, maize food products without the germ are lower in protein quality compared to products made from the whole kernel [4].

Fortifying Crops

The developed world has had tremendous success in alleviating nutrient deficiencies through dietary diversification, improved public health care, food fortification, and supplementation. In developing countries, these strategies are often too expensive and difficult to sustain, especially in rural areas. Poor people from rural areas typically consume what they plant and are dependent upon a small number of staple crops for the vast majority of their nutrition. Therefore, genetic improvement of staple crops (biofortification) is the most cost-effective and sustainable solution to this global health problem [5].

Table 12.1 Corn flour-derived products fortified with micronutrient or vitamin

Product	Fortification	References
Precooked yellow and white maize flours	Ferrous fumarate, thiamine, riboflavin, niacin, vitamin A	[8]
Bread/ precooked corn flour	Iron, vitamin A, beta-carotene	[9]
Extruded blue maize meal	Calcium	[10]
Corn flakes	Iron, vitamin A, C	[11]
Tortilla	Iron, zinc	[12]
Maize meal	Iron, vitamin A	[13]
Nixtamal tortillas	Iron, zinc, folic acid, niacin, riboflavin, thiamin	[14, 15]
Corn masa flour	Folic acid	[16]
Transgenic corn	Beta-carotene, ascorbate, folate	[17]
Bakery	Lutein	[18]

Genetic biofortification can employ either conventional breeding or genetic manipulation approaches. These techniques can be used to increase, for example, calcium, magnesium, and vitamin K concentrations, in the edible portions of horticultural crops [6]. Cereal grains have low concentrations of several minerals, notably calcium, as a consequence of their physiology. Low mineral concentrations are compounded when cereal crops are grown in soils of low mineral phytoavailability and when the grain is processed [7].

Fortification of Corn Flour-Derived Products

Although corn flour-derived products can be fortified with any micronutrient or vitamin (Table 12.1), the great majority of studies have been performed with iron and folic acid fortification. The following characteristics have been proposed for choosing a proper food vehicle for fortification: (1) The food chosen as a vehicle should be consumed by the target population in sufficient quantities and with a small variability; (2) The fortified food should be stable and its physicochemical properties, such as appearance, texture, and flavour, should not change when the nutrient is added; (3) The added nutrient should be relatively bioavailable and well-tolerated; (4) Fortification of the food should not significantly increase its price; (5) Fortification should be carried out using readily available ingredients and technology and preferably at a low cost; (6) The food vehicle or vehicles selected should reach the entire population and deliver most of the calories of the diet; (7) The food vehicle should be consumed daily, but at the same time, without the risk of excessive consumption [11, 19]. The following will report on some debates on how to improve fortification in several parts of the world.

Which Iron Fortified Compound? The First Dilemma

Fortification of food with iron, when an appropriate diet is not available, is considered the best way to prevent iron deficiency (ID). However, it is challenging to find the ideal combination of an iron compound and an appropriate food vehicle [20].

It was suggested that the following order of preference should be used to choose the ideal iron compound for fortifying cereal flours: ferrous sulphate, ferrous fumarate, encapsulated ferrous sulphate or fumarate, electrolytic iron (at twice the amount of ferrous sulphate), ferric pyrophosphate (at twice the amount of ferrous sulphate), and disodium ferrous ethylenediaminetetraacetate ($Na_2FeEDTA$) [21]. Ferrous sulphate can be used in flours that are consumed shortly after they are milled. However, in

Table 12.2 Iron absorption maximisation in fortified corn derivatives

Corn product	Strategies	References
Cereal meal	Decrease the phytic acid content, ascorbic acid	[30]
Precooked corn flour bread	Iron amino acid chelate (ferrochel)	[8]
LPM porridge[a]	Genetically modified low-phytate maize, sodium iron-EDTA[b]	[31]
Maize porridge	Exogenous phytase, no milk	[32]
Tortilla	Ferrous sulphate, NaFe(III)EDTA	[33]
Whole-maize porridge	Addition of phytase, ascorbic acid, NaFeEDTA	[34]

[a]LPM—low-phytate maize
[b]EDTA—ethylenediaminetetraacetic acid

many developing countries flour remains in storage for long periods of time. Hence, elemental iron powders are used, despite their lower bioavailability [22, 23]. Elemental iron powders are the most commonly used iron fortifiers because they cause the least discolouration, flavour changes, and rancidity in food products, and are generally less expensive [20, 24]. However, many concerns about the use of elemental iron powders remain. First, there is little evidence that they have beneficial effects on iron status. Second, powdered elemental iron is water insoluble and poorly soluble in dilute acids. Therefore, the iron never completely dissolves in the gastric juice, which leads to a low and variable bioavailability, ranging from 5 to 148 % relative to the standard, ferrous sulphate. Third, large particle size powders (>149 μm or 100 mesh) interfere negatively with iron absorption [20, 24].

There are five different types of elemental iron powders used for food fortification: electrolytically reduced, hydrogen-reduced, carbon monoxide-reduced, atomised (reduced), and carbonyl iron. Studies on iron absorption measured by ^{58}Fe in ten non-anaemic female volunteers with fairly low iron stores, demonstrated that wheat flour fortified with hydrogen-reduced iron powder has an absorption efficiency comparable to well-absorbed iron (iron II ascorbate), which reinforced the current use of reduced iron powder to fortify flour in the United Kingdom [25].

Body iron stores changes were studied during 35-week with Taiwanese women to compare the efficacy of wheat-based snacks fortified with ferrous sulphate, electrolytic iron, or hydrogen-reduced elemental iron [23]. The reported findings demonstrated that electrolytic and hydrogen-reduced iron were absorbed 77 % and 49 %, respectively, compared with ferrous sulphate (12 mg Fe/day). Electrolytic iron-fortified rice cereal was also successful in Chile [26]. However, a study in Sri Lanka did not find improvements in iron status with the use of wheat flour fortified with electrolytic iron [27].

Another strategy used to increase the bioavailability of iron compounds, mainly in phytic acid-rich foods, such as corn tortillas, is through the use of $Na_2FeEDTA$ [28, 29]. It was reported the influence of $Na_2FeEDTA$ on the bioavailability of iron from ferrous fumarate and ferrous sulphate in meals of corn tortillas and black beans in Guatemala [28]. The conclusion was that $Na_2FeEDTA$ serves as an iron bioavailability enhancer with water-soluble fortification compounds (ferrous sulphate), but not with compounds soluble in dilute acid (ferrous fumarate). In Chile, the reports [29] showed similar results; they did not find an increase in elemental iron absorption using $Na_2FeEDTA$ in corn masa flour tortillas.

Strategies applied in some studies are shown in Table 12.2.

Which Cereal Must Be Fortified? The Second Dilemma

There are still doubts as to whether iron fortification of staple foods, such as iron-fortified cereals, is a useful strategy to combat ID [20, 35, 36]. There are two major disadvantages to the use of cereal products as vehicles for iron fortification. First, they contain high levels of phytic acid, a potential

Table 12.3 Epidemiologic studies on fortification of corn flour-derived products

Local	Product	Fortification	Impact	References
Venezuela	Precooked yellow and white maize and wheat flours	Ferrous fumarate	ID[a] decreased from 37 to 15 % in 1 year	[8]
Venezuela	Corn flakes compared to cereal	Hydrogen-reduced iron	Corn flakes had a higher absorption rate	[11]
USA	Corn tortillas prepared with corn fortified masa flour	3 mg/100 g hydrogen-reduced iron	Ineffective to 5–7-year-old children	[29]
South Africa	Maize-meal porridge	Beta carotene, zinc, 11 mg of ferrous fumarate	Anaemia decreased from 45 to 17 % after 6 months	[40]
Kenya	Porridge made from whole maize flour	56 mg/kg of $Na_2FeEDTA$[b]	Decreased ID and IDA[c]	[41]
Kenya	Porridge made from whole maize flour	28 mg/kg of $Na_2FeEDTA$	Decreased ID and did not decrease IDA	[41]
Zambia	Milled maize grain	Non-specified elemental iron	Anaemia decreased in 6–59 month old children by 23.4 %	[13]
Brazil	Corn flour-derived products	9.8 mg/100 g hydrogen-reduced elemental iron	ID decreased from 18.0 % to 5.6 % and IDA from 14.9 % to 1.2 % after six months	[41]

[a]ID—iron deficiency
[b]$Na_2FeEDTA$—disodium ferrous ethylenediaminetetraacetate
[c]IDA—iron deficiency anaemia

inhibitor of iron absorption. Second, cereal products are extremely sensitive to fat oxidation during storage when highly bioavailable iron compounds, such as ferrous sulphate, are used [37].

Therefore, there are concerns about using this combination in phytate-rich diets, and poorer areas of many countries, such as Brazil, where the diet is composed mostly of rice, beans, and vegetables. With these diets, it is assumed that fortifying corn flour with elemental iron would not be an ideal combination.

According to the International Consultation Group in 1982, absorption of iron is lower from maize than from other cereals [30]. However, the type of cereal grain (rice, wheat, maize, or oats) has shown little influence on iron bioavailability in infant cereals [31]. Furthermore, processing cereals to reduce the phytate content appears more important than the choice of a particular cereal grain [31]. The complete degradation of phytic acid in maize and other infant cereals increased iron absorption by up to 10 times [24].

It should be noted that reports on iron absorption were conducted with single meals under special conditions. On the other hand, studies of iron absorption enhancers and inhibitors using whole meals showed results that were far less significant than those from single meals [38, 39].

Studies of Corn Flour-Derived Product Fortification

A summary of the epidemiologic studies on fortification of corn flour-derived products is shown in Table 12.3.

Results of a fortification programme in Caracas, Venezuela with precooked yellow and white maize and wheat flours enriched with 50 and 20 mg of ferrous fumarate, respectively, were reported [8].

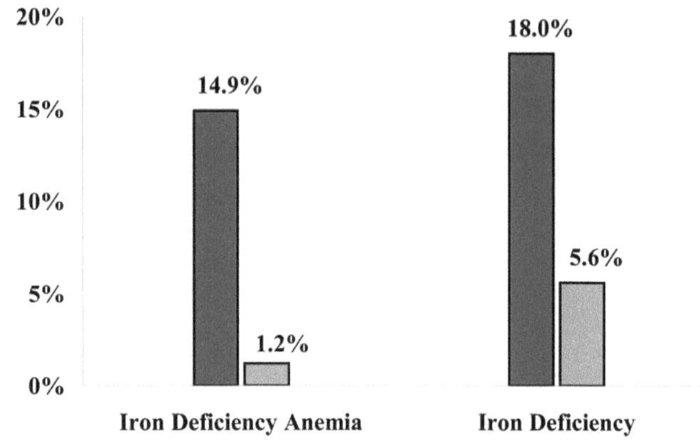

Fig. 12.1 Iron deficiency and iron deficiency anaemia prevalence in children and adolescents at the beginning of the study and following 6 months of treatment with iron fortified corn flour. *Source*: Ref. [42]. Copyright 2008 by the Cambridge University Press, reprinted with permission

After 1 year, the prevalence of ID and iron deficiency anaemia (IDA) in 307 children and adolescents from 7 to 15 years old decreased from 37 % and 19 % to 15 % and 10 %, respectively.

The reported findings in a study with hydrogen-reduced iron-fortified corn flakes [11] had a significantly higher absorption rate than cereal without iron fortification (9.27 % and 3.38 %, respectively). The iron content of the corn flakes was 3.5 mg/30 g. In addition, it was found that 3 mg/100 g of hydrogen-reduced iron powder was ineffective as a fortifier in corn tortillas prepared with corn masa flour given to 5–7-year-old children [29].

A study in 292 infants aged 6–12 months from South Africa [40] showed that low-cost, finely milled, maize-meal porridge fortified with beta carotene, zinc, and iron (11 mg of ferrous fumarate) had an intervention effect of 9.4 μg/L for serum ferritin and 9 g/L for haemoglobin concentrations after 6 months. They also reported improvements in motor development after fortification.

In a study involving 516 children 3–8 years old from Kenya, the porridge made from whole maize flour fortified with high-dose $Na_2FeEDTA$ (56 mg/kg) decreased IDA and ID prevalence, whereas low-dose $Na_2FeEDTA$ (28 mg/kg) decreased ID but not IDA prevalence [41].

Another study involving 157 children (6–59 months old), 212 adolescents (10–19 years old), and 118 women (20–49 years old) from a food aid-dependent refugee population showed that maize grain milled and fortified with elemental iron caused an increase in haemoglobin in children and adolescents, but not in women after 12 months [13]. Anaemia decreased in children by 23.4 %, but there were no significant changes in anaemia rates among adolescents and women. Adolescents did show an improvement in iron status as measured by serum transferrin receptors.

A similar evaluation was performed with 162 children and adolescents at public education centres in Londrina, Paraná (southern Brazil) who consumed corn flour-derived products fortified with reduced elemental iron (9.8 mg/100 g) [42]. After 6 months, the prevalence of ID and IDA decreased from 18.0 % and 14.9 % to 5.6 % and 1.2 %, respectively (Fig. 12.1). The authors attributed the favourable response in this study to milling and degerming methods, which decreased the phytic acid in the grain, and to sufficient doses and the small size of the reduced elemental iron.

Studies on Folic Acid Fortification of Corn Flour-Derived Products

Neural tube defects (NTDs) are congenital malformations that occur during the early stages of foetal development, leading to anencephaly, spina bifida, and encephalocele. The high cost of lifetime medical attention for patients with spina bifida and the incalculable emotional cost to their families make NTD a major public health problem. NTD are congenital malformations that can be prevented through public health measures, such as supplementation and/or food fortification with folic acid [43]. Folic acid can prevent up to 70 % of folic acid-preventable NTD when taken before and during early pregnancy [44].

Currently, more than 40 countries have implemented policies for mandatory flour fortification with folic acid. Studies on the impact of these policies have been conducted in the United States [45], Canada [46], Chile [43], Costa Rica [47], Australia [48], and South Africa [49]. In general, fortification with folic acid is performed with wheat and maize flours [50]. Reports on NTD prevalence reduction have varied from 16 % in the United States [51] to 78 % in Canada [52]. However, even within the same country, there are regional and ethnic disparities in both flour consumption and NTD rates. In Brazil, the mean household flour consumption was 144 g/day in the Southern region and 70 g/day in the North with a predictive folic acid intake of 0.217 mg in the South and 0.1 mg in the Northern region [50]. In the United States, Hispanic women have higher rates of NTD than other racial ethnic groups. Before folic acid fortification, NTD occurred in 10.34 per 10,000 births in Hispanic women, whereas non-Hispanic white women showed a rate of 7.92 per 10,000 births. NTD prevalence was reduced after fortification, but differences between the ethnic groups remained [53]. The reason for these differences was explained later by the reports [53] showing that a lower proportion of Hispanic women ingesting more than 400 μg of folic acid from fortified foods and supplements than non-Hispanic white women. It was developed a model that predicted the contribution of folic acid fortification of corn masa flour [54]. The greatest increase (16.8 %) in daily folic acid intake for Mexican Americans was found because corn masa flour is a key ingredient in many traditional Latin American foods, including corn tortillas, enchiladas, and tamales. The conclusion is that Mexican American women may need more than 400 μg of folic acid per day, the recommended dose to prevent NTD in all women of childbearing age [55]. This study reinforces the importance of fortifying products that can target specific populations. Recently, it was outlined the next steps for the fortification of corn masa flour with acid folic in order to target Hispanic women in the United States [56].

Several studies suggest that folic acid may also play a role in other diseases. In humans, folate is needed to transfer a methyl group in the conversion of homocysteine to methionine. As a result, inadequate folate intake leads to elevated homocysteine concentrations, which have been associated with an increased risk for cardiovascular diseases [57, 58].

However, concerns have also been reported about the potential undesirable effects of high folic acid levels, such as masking vitamin B12 deficiency, which can cause an exacerbation of neurologic effects and cognitive decline [59, 60].

Studies on Other Micronutrients and Calcium Fortification of Corn Flour-Derived Products

Some studies from Mexico have demonstrated that corn flour can also be fortified with other micronutrients, such as zinc, copper, vitamin B1, vitamin B2, and calcium [19, 61, 62]. Corn fortification is an important consideration within Mexico because corn tortillas are the most widely consumed staple food. These studies together highlight the possibility of fortifying with micronutrients other than iron and folic acid in populations with multiple deficiencies.

Conclusions

In attempts to choose the right staple foods to eliminate undernutrition or "hidden hunger," cereal-based products are frequently used. Notably, maize or corn-derived products are often considered for this proposal because maize is one of the most cultivated, highly available crops worldwide.

Several studies have shown the effectiveness of maize fortification programmes that combine grain processing technology to minimise nutrient losses and reduce anti-nutrition factors with fortifiers that have greater bioavailability. The stability of micronutrients and the concentration to be added are important factors to be considered for the success of fortification programmes.

The way that meals are prepared as well as the appropriate combination of foods for target groups are also fundamental.

For underdeveloped regions where populations are difficult to reach through fortification, biofortification programmes where crops are bred to improve their micronutrient profiles are another potential option.

Finally, food fortification should be considered a preventive food-based approach to improve micronutrient status of populations over time; it can be used in conjunction with other interventions to reduce vitamin and mineral deficiencies as an integrated public health policy. The main goal is still to find the most cost-effective and sustainable solutions to this global health problem.

References

1. FAO Food and Agriculture Organization of the United Nations. Maize: international market profile. Available at http://www.fao.org/es/esc/common/ecg/54/en/MaizeProfile.pdf. Accessed 15 July 2011.
2. BRITANNICA online Encyclopedia. Available at http://www.britannica.com/EBchecked/topic/137741/corn. Accessed 18 July 2011.
3. FAO Food and Agriculture Organization of the United Nations. Human nutrition in the developing world. Available at http://www.fao.org/DOCREP/W0073e/w0073e00.htm. Accessed 15 July 2011.
4. Dickerson GW. Nutritional analysis of New Mexico blue corn and dent corn kernels. Available at http://aces.nmsu.edu/pubs/_h/h-233.pdf, 2003. Accessed 18 July 2011.
5. Hoekenga OA, Lung'aho MG, Tako E, et al. Iron biofortification of maize grain. Plant Genet Resour. 2001;9:327–9.
6. White PJ, Broadley MR. Biofortification of crops with seven mineral elements often lacking in human diets—iron, zinc, copper, calcium, magnesium, selenium and iodine. New Phytol. 2009;182:49–84.
7. Broadley MR, White PJ. Eats roots and leaves. Can edible horticultural crops address dietary calcium, magnesium and potassium deficiencies? Proc Nutr Soc. 2010;69:601–12.
8. Layrisse M, Chaves JF, Mendez-Castellano H, et al. Early response to the effect of iron fortification in the Venezuelan population. Am J Clin Nutr. 1996;64:903–7.
9. Layrisse M, Garcia-Casal MN, Solano L, et al. New property of vitamin A and beta-carotene on human iron absorption: effect on phytate and polyphenols as inhibitors of iron absorption. Arch Latinoam Nutr. 2000;50:243–8.
10. Zazueta-Morales JJ, Martinez-Bustos F, Jacobo-Valenzuela N, et al. Effect of the addition of calcium hydroxide on some characteristics of extruded products from blue maize (Zea mays L) using response surface methodology. J Sci Food Agric. 2001;81:1379–86.
11. Garcia-Casal MN, Layrisse M, Pena-Rosas JP, et al. Iron absorption from elemental iron-fortified corn flakes in humans. Role of vitamins A and C. Nutr Rev. 2003;23:451–63.
12. Tovar LR, Larios-Saldana A. Iron and zinc fortification of corn tortilla made either at the household or at industrial scale. Int J Vitam Nutr Res. 2005;75:142–8.
13. Seal A, Kafwembe E, Kassim IAR, et al. Maize meal fortification is associated with improved vitamin A and iron status in adolescents and reduced childhood anaemia in a food aid-dependent refugee population. Public Health Nutr. 2008;11:720–8.
14. Burton KE, Steele FM, Jefferies L, et al. Effect of micronutrient fortification on nutritional and other properties of nixtamal tortillas. Cereal Chem. 2008;85:70–5.
15. Dunn ML, Serna-Saldivar SO, Sanchez-Hernandez D, et al. Commercial evaluation of a continuous micronutrient fortification process for nixtamal tortillas. Cereal Chem. 2008;85:746–52.

16. Hamner HC, Mulinare J, Cogswell ME, et al. Predicted contribution of folic acid fortification of corn masa flour to the usual folic acid intake for the US population: National Health and Nutrition Examination Survey 2001–2004. Am J Clin Nutr. 2009;89:305–15.
17. Naqvi S, Zhu C, Farre G, Ramessar K, et al. Transgenic multivitamin corn through biofortification of endosperm with three vitamins representing three distinct metabolic pathways. Proc Natl Acad Sci U S A. 2009;106:7762–7.
18. Abdel-Aal EM, Young JC, Akhtar H, et al. Stability of lutein in wholegrain bakery products naturally high in lutein or fortified with free lutein. J Agric Food Chem. 2010;58:10109–17.
19. Rosado JL. Zinc and copper: proposed fortification levels and recommended zinc compounds. J Nutr. 2003;133(Suppl):2985S–9.
20. Hurrell RF. Fortification: overcoming technical and practical barriers. J Nutr. 2002;132(Suppl):806S–12.
21. Zimmermann MB, Hurrell RF. Nutrition iron deficiency. Lancet. 2007;370:511–20.
22. Hurrell RF, Bothwell T, Cook JD, et al. The usefulness of elemental iron for cereal flour fortification: a SUSTAIN Task Force report. Sharing United States technology to aid in the improvement of nutrition. Nutr Rev. 2002;60:391–406.
23. Zimmermann MB, Winichagoon P, Gowachirapant S, et al. Comparison of the efficacy of wheat-based snacks fortified with ferrous sulfate, electrolytic iron, or hydrogen-reduced elemental iron: randomized, double-blind, controlled trial in Thai women. Am J Clin Nutr. 2005;82:1276–82.
24. Hurrell RF. How to ensure adequate iron absorption from iron-fortified food. Nutr Rev. 2002;60(Suppl):S7–15.
25. Roe MA, Fairwheather-Tait SJ. High bioavailability of reduced iron added to UK flour (letter). Lancet. 1999;353:1938–9.
26. Walter T, Dallman PR, Pizarro F, et al. Effectiveness of iron-fortified infant cereal in prevention of iron deficiency anemia. Pediatrics. 1993;91:976–82.
27. Nestel P, Nalubola R, Sivakaneshan R, et al. The use of iron-fortified wheat flour to reduce anemia among the estate population in Sri Lanka. Int J Vitam Nutr Res. 2004;74:35–51.
28. Davidson L, Dimitriou T, Boy E, et al. Iron bioavailability from iron-fortified Guatemalan meals based on corn tortillas and black bean paste. Am J Clin Nutr. 2002;75:533–9.
29. Walter T, Pizarro F, Boy E, et al. The poor bioavailability of elemental iron in corn masa flour is not affected by disodium EDTA. J Nutr. 2004;134:380–3.
30. International Nutritional Anemic Consultive Group. The effects of cereals and legumes on iron availability. Washington, DC: Nutrition Foundation; 1982.
31. Cook JD, Reddy MB, Burri J, et al. The influence of different cereal grains on iron absorption from infant cereal foods. Am J Clin Nutr. 1997;65:964–9.
32. Mendoza C, Viteri FE, Lönnerdal B, et al. Absorption of iron from unmodified maize and genetically altered, low-phytate maize fortified with ferrous sulfate or sodium iron EDTA. Am J Clin Nutr. 2001;73:80–5.
33. Hurrell RF, Reddy MB, Juillerat M-A, et al. Degradation of phytic acid in cereal porridges improves iron absorption by human subjects. Am J Clin Nutr. 2003;77:1213–9.
34. Hernandez M, Sousa V, Villalpando S, et al. Cooking and Fe fortification have different effects on Fe bioavailability of bread and tortillas. J Am Coll Nutr. 2006;25:20–5.
35. Troesch B, Egli I, Zeder C, et al. Optimization of a phytase-containing micronutrient powder with low amounts of highly bioavailable iron for in-home fortification of complementary foods. Am J Clin Nutr. 2009;89:539–44.
36. Hallberg L. Advantages and disadvantages of an iron-rich diet. Eur J Clin Nutr. 2002;56(Suppl):S12–8.
37. Hurrell R. Preventing iron deficiency through food fortification. Nutr Rev. 1997;55:210–22.
38. Cook JD, Dassenko SA, Lynch SR. Assessment of the role of nonheme-iron availability in iron balance. Am J Clin Nutr. 1991;54:717–22.
39. Cook JD, Reddy MB. Effect of ascorbic acid intake on nonheme-iron absorption from a complete diet. Am J Clin Nutr. 2001;73:93–8.
40. Faber M, Kvalsvig JD, Lombard CL, et al. Effect of a fortified maize-meal porridge on anemia, micronutrient status, and motor development of infants. Am J Clin Nutr. 2005;82:1032–9.
41. Andangò PEA, Osendarp SJM, Ayah R, et al. Efficacy of iron-fortified whole maize flour on iron status of schoolchildren in Kenya: a randomized controlled trial. Lancet. 2007;369:1799–806.
42. Miglioranza LHS, Breganó JW, Dichi I, et al. Effectiveness of fortification of corn flour-derived products with hydrogen-reduced elemental iron on iron-deficiency anaemia in children and adolescents in southern Brazil. Public Health Nutr. 2009;12:244–9.
43. Hertrampf E, Cortés F. Folic acid fortification of wheat flour: Chile. Nutr Rev. 2004;62(6 Pt 2):S44–8.
44. Berry RJ, Li Z, Erickson JD, et al. Prevention of neural-tube defects with folic acid in China. China-U.S. collaborative project for neural tube defect prevention. N Engl J Med. 1999;341:1485–90.
45. Honein MA, Paulossi LJ, Mathews TJ, et al. Impact of fortification of the US food supply on the occurrence of neural tube defects. JAMA. 2001;285:2981–6.
46. Ray JG, Meier C, Vermeulen MJ, et al. Association of neural tube defects and folic acid food fortification in Canada. Lancet. 2002;360:2047–8.

47. Chen LT, Rivera MA. The Costa Rica experience: reduction of neural tube defects following food fortification programs. Nutr Rev. 2004;62:S40–3.
48. Bower C, Eades S, Payne J, et al. Trends in neural tube defects in Western Australia in indigenous and non-indigenous populations. Paediatr Perinat Epidemiol. 2004;18:277–80.
49. Steyn NP, Wolmarans P, Nel JH, et al. National fortification of staple foods can make a significant contribution to micronutrient intake of South African adults. Public Health Nutr. 2008;11:307–13.
50. Santos LMP, Pereira MZ. The effect of folic acid fortification on the reduction of neural tube defects. Cad Saude Publica. 2007;23:17–24.
51. Williams LJ, Mai CT, Edmonds LD, et al. Prevalence of spina bifida and anencephaly during the transition to mandatory folic acid fortification in the United States. Teratology. 2002;66:33–9.
52. Liu S, West R, Randell E, Longerich L, O'Connor KS, Scott H, et al. Comprehensive evaluation of food fortification with folic acid for the primary prevention of neural tube defects. BMC Pregnancy Childbirth. 2004;4:20.
53. Williams LJ, Rasmussen SA, Flores A, et al. Decline in the prevalence of spina bifid and anencephaly by race/ethnicity: 1995–2002. Pediatrics. 2005;116:580–6.
54. Hammer HC, Mulinare J, Cogswell ME, et al. Predicted contribution of folic acid fortification of corn masa flour to the usual folic acid intake for the US population: National Health and Nutrition Examination Survey, 2001-224. Am J Clin Nutr. 2009;89:305–15.
55. CDC. Recommendations for the use of folic acid to reduce the number of cases of spina bifida and other neural tube defects. MMWR. 1992;41:1–7.
56. Fleischman AR, Oinuma M. Fortification of corn masa flour with folic acid in the Unites States. Am J Public Health. 2011;101:1360–4.
57. Wald DS, Law M, Morris JK. Homocysteine and cardiovascular disease: evidence on causality from a meta-analysis. BMJ. 2002;325:1202–8.
58. Forman JP, Rimm EB, Stampfer MJ, et al. Folate intake and the risk of incident hypertension among U.S. women. JAMA. 2005;293:320–9.
59. Hirch S, Maza P, Barrera G, et al. The Chilean flour folic acid fortification program reduces serum homocysteine levels and masks vitamin B-12 deficiency in elderly people. J Nutr. 2002;132:289–91.
60. Morris MS, Jacques PF, Rosenberg IH, et al. Folate and vitamin B12 status in relation to anemia, macrocytosis, and cognitive impairment in older American in the age of folic acid fortification. Am J Clin Nutr. 2007;85:193–200.
61. Rosado JL, Cassís L, Solano L, et al. Nutrient addition to corn masa flour: effect of corn flour stability, nutrient loss, and acceptability of fortified corn tortillas. Food Nutr Bull. 2005;26:266–72.
62. Rosado JL, Díaz M, Rosas A, et al. Calcium absorption from corn tortilla is relatively high and is dependent upon calcium content and liming in Mexican women. J Nutr. 2005;135:2578–81.

Chapter 13
Fortified Margarine and Fat Spreads

Isabelle Sioen

Key Points

- Margarine is an interesting and effective food vehicle to be fortified with lipid soluble compounds.
- Many European member states currently require the mandatory addition of vitamins A and D to margarine and fat spreads.
- Vitamin D fortified margarine is an important contributor to vitamin D intake, however, in most countries the vitamin D intake is below the dietary recommendations for the major part of the population.
- Omega-3 fortified margarine is an important food product within the gamma of omega-3 fortified foods. It helps to increase the intake of omega-3 fatty acids; however, other strategies will still be needed to increase the population's intake of omega-3 fatty acids in the long term.
- Plant sterol enriched margarines can help in the reduction of cardiovascular risk; however, the efficacy in comparison to prescription drugs is still debatable.
- Fortification of margarine with iodine is tested and seems promising to help in the reduction of the worldwide problem of iodine deficiency.
- Margarines fortified with different antioxidants can help to increase the blood levels of these antioxidants.

Keywords Margarine • Fat spread • Vitamin A • Vitamin D • n-3 LC PUFA • Plant sterols • Plant stanols • Iodine • Antioxidants

Abbreviations

AA	Arachidonic acid
CVD	Cardiovascular diseases
DHA	Docosahexaenoic acid

I. Sioen, Ph.D., M.Sc.
Department of Public Health, Ghent University,
UZ-2 Blok A, De Pintelaan 185 9000, Ghent, Belgium

Research Foundation—Flanders, Brussels, Belgium
e-mail: Isabelle.Sioen@UGent.be

V.R. Preedy et al. (eds.), *Handbook of Food Fortification and Health: From Concepts to Public Health Applications Volume 1*, Nutrition and Health, DOI 10.1007/978-1-4614-7076-2_13,

DPA	Docosapentaenoic acid
EPA	Eicosapentaenoic acid
HDL	High-density lipoprotein
IMACE	International Margarine Association of the Countries of Europe
LA	Linoleic acid
LC	Long chain
LDL	Low-density lipoprotein
LNA	a-Linolenic acid
n-3 PUFA	Omega-3 poly-unsaturated fatty acids
n-6 PUFA	Omega-6 poly-unsaturated fatty acids
PUFA	Poly-unsaturated fatty acids
RE	Retinol-equivalent
SCF	Scientific Committee on Food

Introduction: Margarine and Fat Spreads: Definition and History

Under European Union directives, margarine is defined as a water-in-oil emulsion derived from vegetable/animal fats, with a fat content of at least 80 % but less than 90 %, that remains solid at a temperature of 20 °C and is suitable as spread. Margarines may not have a milk fat content of more than 3 % [1]. When the fat percentage of the fat spread does not lie between 80 an 90 %, the name of the product changes. This is summarized in Table 13.1.

Margarine was discovered in 1869 by Hippolyte Mège Mouriès, a French food research chemist, in response to Emperor Louis Napoleon III of France who offered a prize to anyone who could make a satisfactory substitute for butter (Fig. 13.1). It is not entirely clear whether the primary aim was the betterment of the working classes or economics in the food supply to the French army. In a laboratory, Mège Mouriès solidified purified fat, after which the resulting substance was pressed in a thin cloth that formed stearine and discharged oil. This oil formed the basis of the butter substitute. He called the substance oleomargarine, the name of which became shortened to the trade name "margarine." Mège Mouriés patented the concept in 1869 and expanded his initial manufacturing operation from France but had little commercial success. In 1871, he sold the patent to the Dutch company Jurgens, now part of Unilever [2, 3].

In the early days margarine contained two types of fat—a large proportion of animal fat and a small proportion of vegetable fat. Time passing, the small vegetable element increased. There were two stages in that process. First, by improving the process of refining vegetable oils, use could be made of a greater variety of liquid oils and a higher proportion of solid vegetable fats. Secondly, through the

Table 13.1 Name of the fat spread depending on the fat percentage [1, 2]

	% of fat
Margarine	80–90
Fat spread *x*%	>62 to <80
Three-quarter-fat margarine or reduced-fat margarine	60–62
Fat spread *x*%	>41 to <60
Half-fat margarine, low-fat margarine, light margarine, or minarine	39–41

This table gives the name of the fat spread in function of the fat percentage that the product contains

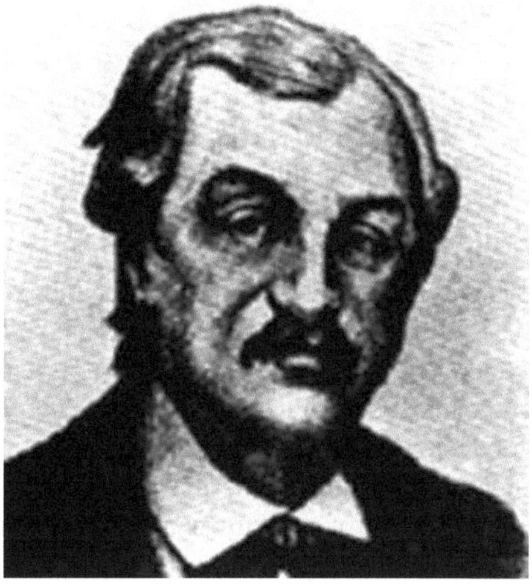

Fig. 13.1 Hippolyte Mège Mouriès who discovered margarine. This figure shows a portrait of Hippolyte Mège Mouriès, a French food research chemist that discovered margarine in 1869

development of processes for turning liquid oils into solid fats on a commercial scale, use could be made of larger quantities of liquid vegetable oils [3].

At these days, the market share of margarine and other fat spreads has overtaken that of butter. It is consumed as a spread, but it is also used in the preparation of many other foods (e.g., pan frying of foods) as well as an ingredient in many processed foods (cookies, cakes, etc.). Modern margarines can be made from any of a wide variety of animal or vegetable fats. Most countries in the European Union produce lower fat spreads as an alternative to margarine and butter.

Margarine is an interesting and effective food vehicle to be fortified with lipid soluble compounds. The first compounds that will be described in this chapter are vitamin A and D. Next, omega-3 enrichment of margarines and other fat spreads will be discussed as well as the importance of this enriched margarine in the overall gamma of omega-3 enriched food items. One of the aims of the omega-3 enrichment of margarine is to help in the prevention of cardiovascular diseases (CVD). With the same goal, also enrichment of foods (inclusive margarines) with plant sterols became a common practice and this will be illustrated in the next part of this chapter. After that, some other less common enrichments of margarines that are described in literature will be discussed, i.e., iodine fortification and antioxidant fortification. Next, a section will describe guidance on safe levels to be added for vitamin A and D, omega-3 fatty acids, and plant sterols.

Vitamin A and D Fortification of Margarine and Fat Spreads

Many European member states currently require the mandatory addition of vitamins A and D to margarine and fat spreads for reasons of public health. Voluntary fortification of margarine with vitamins had been practiced by manufacturers since 1925, but in 1940 with the advent of the war, certain governments took action to safeguard the nutritional status of their populations by making the addition of vitamin A and D compulsory. This mandatory fortification was justified in the view that margarine was being used to replace butter in the dietary pattern [1, 4]. Indeed, if margarine had not been fortified there was evidence that a large proportion of the population, particularly children, were at risk of deficiencies. Vitamin A and D were added at that time to equate to the levels found in butter [4].

Vitamin A

In the 1980s, it was shown that vitamin A capsule distribution reduces child mortality rates by as much as 30 % [5]. This was very relevant for developing countries with high child mortality rates. Since then, politicians and public health specialists have become more sensitized to eradicating vitamin A deficiency as part of child survival strategies [6]. The three main intervention approaches to control vitamin A deficiency are dietary behavioral change through communications strategies, periodic supplementation with high dose capsules and fortification [7].

Krause et al. investigated the vitamin A intake from food sources, not including breast milk, for 55 children (mean age 20.8 months) from two poor communities of Guatemala City [7]. They found that more than 90 % of total vitamin A intake from non-breast milk food sources was derived from only ten food items. Over half came from three fortified foods, of which one was fortified margarine. These results showed that fortified foods including margarine make an important contribution towards vitamin A intake in this sample of poor urban Guatemalan toddlers [7].

In the Philippines, an intervention study was conducted assessing the effects of consuming a highly hydrogenated, vitamin A fortified margarine not requiring refrigeration on the vitamin A status of preschool children. They performed a double-masked randomized community trial, including 296 and 285 children (3–6 years of age) in the vitamin A fortified and non-fortified (control) margarine groups, respectively [8]. The results of the study showed that the consumption of vitamin A fortified margarine significantly improved the vitamin A status of preschool Filipino children [8].

Vitamin D

Vitamin D is an important determinant of bone health at all ages [9]. Vitamin D increases the absorption of calcium and phosphate from the gastro-intestinal tract for the mineralisation of the skeleton. In utero and during childhood, vitamin D deficiency can cause growth retardation and skeletal deformities and is associated with an increased risk of hip fracture later in life [9–11]. In addition to its role to bone health, vitamin D has also been reported as a relevant factor in decreasing the risk of many chronic illnesses including common cancers, and autoimmune, infectious and CVD [10].

Concerning vitamin D intake via food in most Western diets, fortified foods are the major sources of vitamin D, of which fortified margarine is an important one [12]. For example for Belgian pre-school children and adolescents, the major source of vitamin D intake is fortified margarine, however, for both populations the current vitamin D intake is far below the current dietary recommendations [13, 14]. The same conclusion was drawn in a Finnish study, investigating the effect of the mandatory vitamin D fortification of fluid milks and margarines (since 2003) in Finland. This fortification was inadequate to prevent vitamin D insufficiency in adolescent females in Finland [15], as well as in other subgroups of the Finnish population [16, 17]. The authors concluded that new innovative and feasible ways of improving vitamin D nutrition are urged [15–17].

The Hoorn study in the Netherlands evaluated potentially modifiable determinants of vitamin D status in an older population, in a cross-sectional study from a population-based cohort including 538 white Dutch men and women aged 60–87 years. They found that regular use of fortified margarine products was inversely associated with vitamin D deficiency, together with fatty fish products and vitamin D containing supplements. As other studies, they also concluded that it is difficult to achieve adequate vitamin D status through increasing intakes because few foods are vitamin D fortified and the amounts of vitamin D in supplements are low [18].

Also the US and Canadian populations are largely dependent on fortified foods and dietary supplements to meet their needs of vitamin D, because foods naturally rich in vitamin D are limited.

Fluid milk and breakfast cereals are the predominant vehicles for vitamin D in the United States, whereas Canada fortifies fluid milk and margarine with vitamin D. So the same conclusions counts for these populations, i.e., that current US/Canadian fortification practices are not effective in preventing hypovitaminosis D, particularly among vulnerable populations during the winter [17].

Omega-3 Enrichment of Margarine and Fat Spreads

The group of poly-unsaturated fatty acids (PUFAs) is divided into two groups: omega-3 (n-3) and omega-6 (n-6) poly-unsaturated fatty acids (PUFA), differing in the position where the first double C-bound is located. Two PUFAs are called "essential fatty acids" since they cannot be synthesized in the human body and are vital for physiological integrity. Therefore, they must be obtained from the diet. One is linoleic acid (LA, C18:2n-6) and belongs to the n-6 family. The other one is α-linolenic acid (LNA, C18:3n-3) belonging to the n-3 family. These essential parent compounds can be converted in the human body to long-chain (LC) fatty acids, but humans cannot interconvert n-3 and n-6 fatty acids [19]. LA can be converted to arachidonic acid (AA, C20:4n-6) and further on to longer chain derivates, and LNA to eicosapentaenoic acid (EPA, C20:5n-3) in a first step and docosahexaenoic acid (DHA) (C22:6n-3) in a next step. This conversion is summarized in Fig. 13.2.

There is a growing body of evidence demonstrating that the regular consumption of n-3 PUFA is associated with significant health benefits in the prevention of CVD [20]. In the meantime, there are considerable indications that the current intake of n-3 PUFA via the Western diet is too low [21–27].

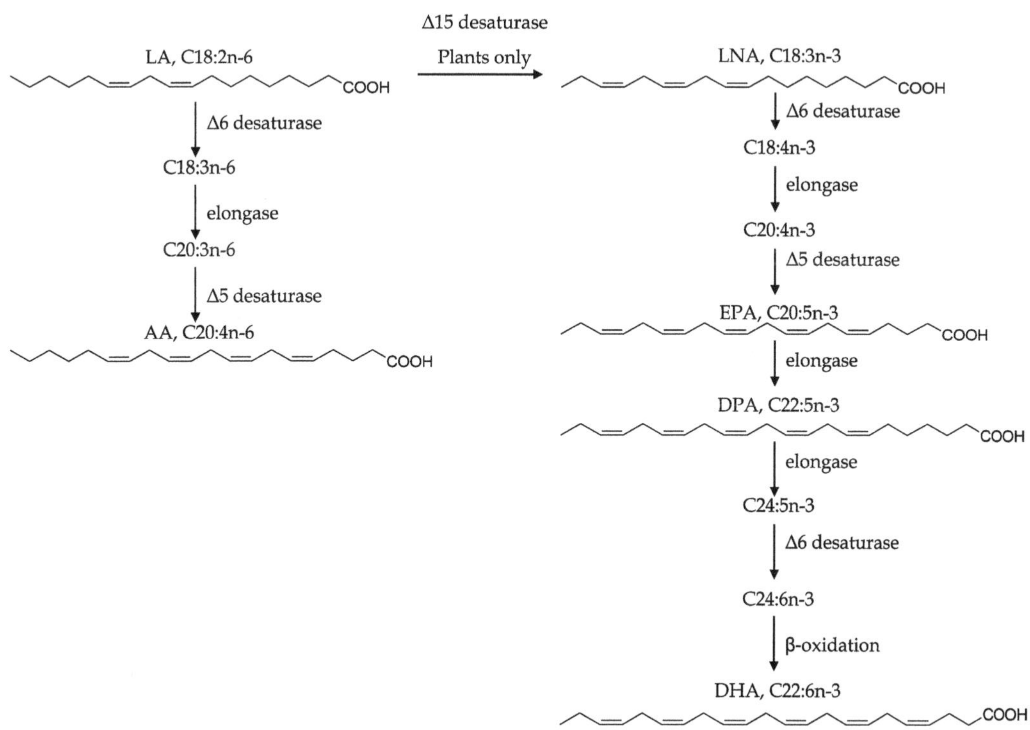

Fig. 13.2 Desaturation and elongation of n-6 and n-3 PUFAs (based on Din et al. [49]). This figure shows how the conversion of linoleic acid (LA) and α-linolenic acid (LNA) to longer chain fatty acids happens. *AA* arachidonic acid; *EPA* eicosapentaenoic acid; *DPA* docosapentaenoic acid; *DHA* docosahexaenoic acid

A possible solution to increase the n-3 PUFA intake is to increase the fatty fish consumption, the most important natural source of long-chain (LC) n-3 PUFA (EPA and DHA). However, it is not likely that we will all start eating fish on a daily basis just because the n-3 PUFA are beneficial to health. If everyone in the world starts consuming even 2–3 servings of fish per week, the supply of fish will run out very quickly [28]. An alternative strategy for enhancing n-3 PUFA intake may be to provide a wide range of commercial food products and ingredients fortified with n-3 PUFA, which can be incorporated in an existing diet. Many of these food items are currently available, among others n-3 fortified margarine. Metcalf et al. assessed the effects of providing a wide range of foodstuffs containing n-3 PUFA, occurring naturally or from fortification, on intake and blood and tissue proportions of n-3 PUFA in 16 healthy males living in Australia [29]. Based on the health beneficial changes in the fatty acid pattern in the blood of the participants, they concluded that incorporating fish oil into a range of novel commercial foods provides the opportunity for wider public consumption of n-3 PUFA with their associated health benefits [29].

Recently, Molendi-Coste et al. [30] evaluated the fatty acid profile in collective catering in relation to the current dietary recommendations for fatty acids. They found that n-3 PUFA content in lunches provided by municipal catering and in in-hospital menus were slightly below recommended intakes. In the latter, n-3 PUFA enriched margarine contributed for 50 % to daily intakes, showing the importance of this enriched food item in the overall food consumption pattern when considering n-3 PUFA intake. They concluded that that meeting n-3 PUFA nutritional recommendation remains challenging for collective catering [30].

Also a Belgian study, assessing the influence of n-3 PUFA enriched products on the n-3 LC PUFA intake for Flemish women of reproductive age, showed that a big gap remains between the EPA and DHA intake and the recommendation for these fatty acids [31]. Of all the n-3 PUFA enriched foods on the Flemish market, enriched margarines and cooking fat are most frequently consumed by young women, again illustrating the importance of enriched margarine. Nevertheless, the authors concluded that other strategies will be needed to increase the EPA and DHA intake in the long term. A possible suggestions that is formulated by the authors is that combination of regular fish consumption (twice a week) with important contribution of fatty fish species, in combination with regular consumption of margarine enriched with EPA and DHA, can be advised to achieve the recommendation for LC n-3 PUFA intake [32].

Plant Sterol Fortification of Margarine and Fat Spreads

Already back in the 50s, the cholesterol lowering effect of phytosterols, phytosterol esters, phytostanols and/or phytostanol esters—in this chapter referred to by the term "plant sterols"—was described [33]. Based on this health beneficial characteristic, food industries started to add plant sterols to food products [34]. These food products were meant to help people with an increased cholesterol level by a diet-based approach. Based on scientific evidence, it is generally accepted that the consumption of 1–3 g plant sterols per day lowers low-density lipoproteins (LDL) blood cholesterol by 5–15 %, without having a negative effect on high-density lipoproteins (HDL) cholesterol level [33–36].

Food enriched with plant sterols are novel foods that cannot be placed on the European market without permission of the European Commission. Moreover, the necessary labeling of foods and food ingredients with added plant sterols is described in detail in the Commission Regulation (EC) No. 608/2004. Some aspects of this regulation are summarized in Table 13.2.

In 2006, a Dutch study studied the effectiveness of customary use of plant sterol enriched margarines on blood cholesterol in free-living conditions with data from the Dutch Doetinchem cohort [37]. The authors characterized the beneficial effect of the plant sterol enriched margarine, used under customary

Table 13.2 Aspects of necessary labeling and special provisions for the presentations of foods with added plant sterols according to the Commission Regulation (EC) No. 608/2004

Aspects of necessary labeling of foods and food ingredients with added plant sterols
1. Clear indication that the food contains added plant sterols
2. Declaration of amount of plant sterols per 100 g of food
3. Statement that the food is exclusively for people who want to lower their blood cholesterol levels
4. Statement that patients on cholesterol lowering medication should consume such foods only under medical supervision
5. Statement that the food is not nutritionally appropriate for pregnant and breast feeding women and children under the age of 5 years
6. Statement that the food should be part of a balanced diet, including regular consumption of fruits and vegetables to help maintain carotenoids levels
7. Statement that consumption of more than 3 g/day of added plant sterols should be avoided
8. Requirement to define a portion and to indicate the amount of plant sterols in a portion
Special provisions for the presentation of foods with added plant sterols
1. They have to be presented in such a manner that they may be easily divided into portions containing either max 1 g (three portions/day) or max 3 g of plant sterols (one portion/day)
2. A container of beverages may not contain more than 3 g of plant sterols
3. Certain foods have to be packed as single portions

This table gives all aspects of necessary labeling and special provision for the presentation of foods with added plant sterols

conditions as a stabilization of cholesterol levels. This was the first report to find a modest beneficial effect on blood cholesterol level under customary conditions [37].

In Belgium, a market inventory was performed to have an indication of the different plant sterol enriched food items and supplements as well as their plant sterol concentration available on the Belgian market. Fat spreads, yoghurt drinks, and cheese spreads were found, being enriched with plant sterols. Moreover, a questionnaire was developed to investigate the consumption of plant sterol enriched foods and supplements in Belgium. Within the group of people who consumed plant sterol enriched food items, it was found that plant sterol enriched margarines and other fat spreads contributed most (65.4 %) to the overall plant sterol intake, followed by yoghurt drinks (33.4 %) and cheese spread (1.2 %). Within the group of people who consumed plant sterol enriched food items, more than half of them (56 %) consumed plant sterol enriched spreads on a daily basis. The Belgian adults' mean plant sterol intake due to the consumption of the enriched products was 1.51 ± 1.42 g/day [38]. However, within the group of consumers, 50 % had a plant sterol intake lower than or equal to 1 g/day, which can be considered as a suboptimal dose to reach the aimed LDL-cholesterol lowering effect. In contrast, 16.4 % of the consumers had a plant sterol intake above 3 g/day, even 7.8 % had an intake above 4 g/day. The consumers that exceed the intake of 3 g/day use all but one plant sterol enriched fat spread. Some of them combine it with other plant sterol enriched food products. The results of these Belgian adults can be compared with the results of an Irish study, focusing on the consumers of plant sterol enriched food products [39]. This study collected data by means of an interview-assisted questionnaire in order to calculate the plant sterol intake and to characterize the consumer group. In the Irish study, 23 % of the consumers had an intake above 3 g/day, compared to 16 % of the Flemish consumers. Plant sterol intake data via the consumption of plant sterol enriched food products can be compared for both the Flemish and the Irish population in Table 13.3. The data in this table are only valid for the consumers of plant sterol enriched products and not for the overall population.

In 2011, the results of a prospective, randomized, placebo-controlled study were published, in which 50 mildly hypercholesterolaemic subjects were randomized to Mediterranean diet, a spread containing plant stanol esters (2 g/day) or a placebo spread. The aim was to compare the effects of the Mediterranean diet and plant stanol esters on vascular risk factors and estimated CVD (eCVD) risk. They concluded that

Table 13.3 Comparison of the plant sterol intake via enriched food products for the Flemish (this study) and Irish [39] adults

		Plant sterol intake (g/day)						
	Country	Mean	Standard deviation	Minimum	Percentile 90	Percentile 95	Percentile 97.5	Maximum
All consumers	Belgium	1.51	1.42	0.01	3.46	4.20	5.07	6.80
	Ireland	2.45	1.46	0.21	4.41	5.48	6.61	9.84
Men	Belgium	1.77	1.65	0.01	4.17	5.06	6.51	6.80
	Ireland	2.71	1.50	0.25	4.61	5.91	6.91	8.90
Women	Belgium	1.32	1.22	0.03	3.21	3.83	4.55	5.20
	Ireland	2.29	1.41	0.21	3.97	5.25	6.34	9.84

This table shows data on the intake of plant sterols (mean and standard deviation, as well as minimum intake and maximum intake and different percentiles of the intake distribution) for consumers of plant sterol enriched food products, living in Belgium or Ireland. Moreover, the data are also shown separately for men and women in both countries

the consumption of plant stanol esters by moderately hypercholesterolaemic patients may be a useful option to reduce eCVD risk in those who do not adopt a Mediterranean diet [40].

However, very recently, Doggrell published a review in order to answer the question whether lowering LDL cholesterol with margarine containing plant sterols is still relevant in 2011. She concludes that prescription drugs have a much greater ability to lower LDL cholesterol than the plant sterol esters, and at the same time increase levels of HDL cholesterol and decrease levels of triglycerides, whereas plant sterols do not. She states that many of the claims made in the present advertising of plant sterols are exaggerated and are not backed up with good evidence. Doggrell concludes that, except in borderline normo/hypercholesterolemia, prescription drugs should be preferred to plant sterols for lowering LDL cholesterol [41]. Also Eussen et al. stated that in daily medical practice, general practitioners and pharmacists should urge subjects not to take plant sterol enriched functional foods as replacement for their prescribed medication [42]. They concluded this after assessing the influence of the use of plant sterol enriched functional foods on adherence to statin therapy among patients initiating treatment.

Based on the current available evidence about plant sterol enriched food items, it can be stated that the efficacy is still debatable.

Other Fortifications of Margarine and Fat Spreads

Iodine Fortification

Insufficient iodine intake is a common problem all over the world. Currently, the correction of iodine intake with iodized salt is a methods used at international scale. However, it does not meet the needs of all categories of the population. Recently, the incorporation of iodine in lipids was investigated, first of all in sunflower oil. This iodized sunflower oil was used for the manufacture of iodized margarine in order to fortify this product with iodine. Physicochemical indices of iodized margarine did not differ from the characteristics of the product without iodine. The author concluded that lipids represent an important vehicle for food fortification with iodine and that daily consumption of 30–50 g iodized margarine, with a content of 1 μg iodine per gram product would contribute in part to eradicate iodine deficiency [43].

Antioxidant Fortification

As was previously described for n-3 PUFA and plant sterols, also antioxidants may be effective in reducing the risk of CVD. Synergistic effects may occur between different antioxidants because of differences in lipophilicity. Van het Hof et al. [44] investigated the effect of consumption of moderate doses of a combination of antioxidants, incorporated into a habitually used food product, on the body's antioxidant status and on parameters of oxidative damage to lipids was assessed. A full-fat margarine, fortified with 31 mg/day vitamin E, 121 mg/day vitamin C, 2.7 mg/day α-carotene and 5.3 mg/day β-carotene, was used as vehicle to supply the antioxidants. Volunteers consumed during the 4 weeks either 15 g/day of this antioxidant fortified margarine or an ordinary margarine. Fasting blood samples were taken before and at the end of the study. Based on the study results, the authors concluded that consumption of moderate doses of vitamin E, vitamin C, α-carotene, and β-carotene, supplied in a full-fat margarine and consumed as part of a normal diet, effectively increases the blood levels of these antioxidants [44].

Guidance on Safe Levels to Be Added

Vitamin A and D

The International Margarine Association of the Countries of Europe (IMACE) published in 2004 a Code of Practice on vitamin A & D fortification of margarines and fat spreads [4]. This Code of Practice is based on scientific risk assessment and concerns the addition of vitamin A and D to margarines and fat spreads which will be delivered as such to the ultimate consumer. The Scientific Committee on Food (SCF) has set the tolerable upper intake levels for vitamin A and D at 3,000 μg retinol-equivalent (RE) per day and 50 μg/day, respectively [45, 46]. A review by the SCF on reference intakes has lead to the reference values of 800 μg vitamin A and 5 μg vitamin D per day [47]. Based on these data IMACE concluded that 800 μg vitamin A per 100 g end product and 7.5–10 μg vitamin D per 100 g end product can be safely incorporated in margarine and fat spread whilst being nutritionally relevant. The Code demonstrates that fortified margarines and fat spreads can be consumed at similar intake levels within a diversified diet and will even help to improve the public health situation within the European Community. The issues on safety concerning margarine and fat spread fortification are limited, since the carrier is self-limitative: the risk of overconsumption of this food item is very small [4]. The chemical substances that can be used as sources of vitamin A and D are summarized in Table 13.4.

Omega-3 Fatty Acids

IMACE recommends that margarine and fat spreads must contain a minimum of 3 g LNA per 100 g and/or 300 mg LC n-3 PUFA per 100 g in order to substantially improve the intake of these fatty acids. As a result, a reasonable daily intake of 20 g of margarine or fat spread would provide 0.6 g LNA and 60 mg of LC n-3 PUFA [2], which can partially help in reaching the dietary recommendations for these fatty acids.

Plant Sterols

The SCF conducted a safety assessment of the use of plant sterols in margarine and fat spreads. Based on this assessment, the Committee concluded that the use of plant sterols in fat spreads at a maximum level corresponding to 8 % free plant sterols is safe for human use. The Committee is also of the opinion that the β-carotene lowering effect of plant sterols should be communicated to the consumer, together with appropriate dietary advice regarding the regular consumption of fruits and vegetables [48].

Table 13.4 Chemical substances that can be used as sources of vitamin A and D [4]

Vitamin A	Vitamin D
Retinyl-acetate	Ergocalciferol (vitamin D2)
Retinyl-palmitate	Cholecalciferol (vitamin D3)
Retinol	
Beta-carotene of mixed carotenes with provitamin A activity	

This table shows the chemical substances that can be used to fortify margarine and fat spreads with vitamin A and/or vitamin D

Recommendations

Fortification of margarine and fat spreads with vitamin A, vitamin D, and omega-3 fatty acids is shown to help increase the intake of these beneficial nutrients of which the current populations intake is generally low compared to the recommendations. Therefore, it can be recommended that these fortifications should be further stimulated in the future. Concerning the fortification of margarine and fat spreads with plant sterols, more research will be needed in the future to evaluate the efficacy of this fortifications in the view of public health.

Conclusion

Margarine and fat spreads are an interesting and effective food vehicle to be fortified with lipid soluble compounds. At the same time, it is a food item that is regularly consumed in small amounts. Since it is used as a replacement of butter—naturally rich in vitamin A and D—many European Member States currently require the mandatory addition of vitamin A and D to margarine and fat spreads in order to help to improve the public health situation within the European Community. Besides these two vitamins, margarine and fat spread are used as a carrier for fortification with omega-3 fatty acids and plant sterols, both in the framework of reduction of the risk for CVD. Omega-3 fortified margarine helps to increase the population's intake of omega-3 fatty acids, however, beside this other strategies are still needed to increase the intake of omega-3 fatty acids in the long term. Concerning plant sterol enriched margarines, the efficacy of these products in helping to reduce cardiovascular risk, is still debatable comparing to prescription drugs. It can be concluded that margarine and fat spreads are very interesting products for fortification with fat soluble compounds, however, they only partially help to increase the intake of beneficial nutrients and need to be combined with other healthy strategies.

Acknowledgments Isabelle Sioen is financially supported by the Research Foundation—Flanders (Grant no: 1.2.683.11.N.00).

References

1. European Commission. Council Regulation (EC) No 2991/94 of 5 December 1994 laying down standards for spreadable fats. Report No.: 31994R2991; 1994.
2. IMACE. Website of the International Margarine Association of the Countries of Europe. Available at: URL: http://www.imace.org/. Accessed 30 Sept 2011.
3. Unilever. How it all started. Available at URL: http://www.unilever.co.uk. Accessed 30 Sept 2011.
4. IMACE. Code of practice on vitamin A & D fortification of margarines and fat spreads; Available at: URL: http://www.imace.org/. Accessed 30 Sept 2011.
5. Labbe KA, Beaton GH, Martorell R, et al. Reduction of mortality in young-children after vitamin-A supplementation—combined analysis of 8 field trials. Am J Epidemiol. 1993;138(8):617.
6. West KP, Howard GR, Sommer A. Vitamin-A and infection—public-health implications. Annu Rev Nutr. 1989;9:63–86.
7. Krause VM, Delisle H, Solomons NW. Fortified foods contribute one half of recommended vitamin a intake in poor urban Guatemalan toddlers. J Nutr. 1998;128(5):860–4.
8. Solon FS, Solon MS, Mehansho H, et al. Evaluation of the effect of vitamin A-fortified margarine on the vitamin A status of preschool Filipino children. Eur J Clin Nutr. 1996;50(11):720–3.
9. Schoenmakers I, Goldberg GR, Prentice A. Abundant sunshine and vitamin D deficiency. Br J Nutr. 2008;99(6):1171–3.
10. Holick MF, Vitamin D. Deficiency. N Engl J Med. 2007;357(3):266–81.

11. Cashman KD. Vitamin D, in childhood and adolescence. Postgrad Med J. 2007;83(978):230–5.
12. Picciano MF, Vitamin D. Status and health. Crit Rev Food Sci Nutr. 2010;50:24–5.
13. Huybrechts I, Lin Y, De KW, et al. Dietary sources and sociodemographic and economic factors affecting vitamin D and calcium intakes in Flemish preschoolers. Eur J Clin Nutr. 2011;65(9):1039–47.
14. Sioen I, Matthys C, De Backer G, Van Camp J, De Henauw S. Importance of seafood as nutrient source in the diet of Belgian adolescents. J Hum Nutr Diet. 2007;20(6):580–9.
15. Lehtonen-Veromaa M, Mottonen T, Leino A, Heinonen OJ, Rautava E, Viikari J. Prospective study on food fortification with vitamin D among adolescent females in Finland: minor effects. Br J Nutr. 2008;100(2):418–23.
16. Hirvonen T, Sinkko H, Valsta L, Hannila ML, Pietinen P. Development of a model for optimal food fortification: vitamin D among adults in Finland. Eur J Nutr. 2007;46(5):264–70.
17. Rasanen M, Kronberg-Kippila C, Ahonen S, et al. Intake of vitamin D by Finnish children aged 3 months to 3 years in relation to sociodemographic factors. Eur J Clin Nutr. 2006;60(11):1317–22.
18. van Dam RM, Snijder MB, Dekker JM, et al. Potentially modifiable determinants of vitamin D status in an older population in the Netherlands: the Hoorn Study. Am J Clin Nutr. 2007;85(3):755–61.
19. Ruxton CHS, Calder PC, Reed SC, Simpson MJA. The impact of long-chain n-3 polyunsaturated fatty acids on human health. Nutr Res Rev. 2005;18(1):113–29.
20. Deckelbaum RJ, Akabas SR. n-3 Fatty acids and cardiovascular disease: navigating toward recommendations. Am J Clin Nutr. 2006;84(1):1–2.
21. Loosemore ED, Judge MP, Lammi-Keefe CJ. Dietary intake of essential and long-chain polyunsaturated fatty acids in pregnancy. Lipids. 2004;39(5):421–4.
22. Sioen IA, Pynaert I, Matthys C, De Backer G, Van Camp J, De Henauw S. Dietary intakes and food sources of fatty acids for Belgian women, focused on n-6 and n-3 polyunsaturated fatty acids. Lipids. 2006;41(5):415–22.
23. Sioen I, Huybrechts I, Verbeke W, Camp JV, Henauw SD. n-6 and n-3 PUFA intakes of pre-school children in Flanders, Belgium. Br J Nutr. 2007;98(4):819–25.
24. Sioen I, Hacquebard M, Hick G, et al. Effect of ALA-enriched food supply on cardiovascular risk factors in males. Lipids. 2009;44(7):603–11.
25. Astorg P, Arnault N, Czernichow S, Noisette N, Galan P, Hercberg S. Dietary intakes and food sources of n-6 and n-3 PUFA in French adult men and women. Lipids. 2004;39(6):527–35.
26. Howe P, Meyer B, Record S, Baghurst K. Dietary intake of long-chain [omega]-3 polyunsaturated fatty acids: contribution of meat sources. Nutrition. 2006;22(1):47–53.
27. Meyer BJ, Mann NJ, Lewis JL, Milligan GC, Sinclair AJ, Howe PRC. Dietary intakes and food sources of omega-6 and omega-3 polyunsaturated fatty acids. Lipids. 2003;38(4):391–8.
28. Garg ML, Wood LG, Singh H, Moughan PJ. Means of delivering recommended levels of long chain n-3 polyunsaturated fatty acids in human diets. J Food Sci. 2006;71(5):R66–71.
29. Metcalf RG, James MJ, Mantzioris E, Cleland LG. A practical approach to increasing intakes of n-3 polyunsaturated fatty acids: use of novel foods enriched with n-3 fats. Eur J Clin Nutr. 2003;57(12):1605–12.
30. Molendi-Coste O, Legry V, Leclercq IA. Are n-3 PUFA dietary recommendations met in in-hospital and school catering? Acta Gastroenterol Belg. 2011;74(2):281–8.
31. Sioen I, Devroe J, Inghels D, Terwecoren R, De Henauw S. The influence of n-3 PUFA supplements and n-3 PUFA enriched foods on the n-3 LC PUFA intake of Flemish women. Lipids. 2010;45(4):313–20.
32. Sioen I, De Henauw S, Verbeke W, Verdonck F, Willems JL, Van Camp J. Fish consumption is a safe solution to increase the intake of long-chain n-3 fatty acids. Public Health Nutr. 2008;11(11):1107–16.
33. Ostlund RE. Phytosterols in human nutrition. Annu Rev Nutr. 2002;22:533–49.
34. EFSA. Consumption of foods and beverages with added plant sterols in the European Union. EFSA J. 2008;133:1–21.
35. Katan MB, Grundy SM, Jones P, Law M, Miettinen T, Paoletti R. Efficacy and safety of plant stanols and sterols in the management of blood cholesterol levels. Mayo Clin Proc. 2003;78(8):965–78.
36. Caswell H, Denny A, Lunn J. Plant sterol and stanol esters. Nutr Bull. 2008;33:368–73.
37. Wolfs M, de Jong N, Ocke MC, Verhagen H, Verschuren WMM. Effectiveness of customary use of phytosterol/-stanol enriched margarines on blood cholesterol lowering. Food Chem Toxicol. 2006;44(10):1682–8.
38. Sioen I, Matthys C, Huybrechts I, Van Camp J, De Henauw S. Consumption of plant sterols in Belgium: consumption patterns of plant sterol-enriched foods in Flanders, Belgium. Br J Nutr. 2011;105(6):911–8.
39. Hearty A, Duffy E, Joyce J, O'Connor C, Gibney MJ. Phytosterol-enriched products on the Irish market: examination of intake and consumption patterns. Public Health Nutr. 2009;12(1):51–8.
40. Athyros VG, Kakafika AI, Papageorgiou AA, et al. Effect of a plant stanol ester-containing spread, placebo spread, or Mediterranean diet on estimated cardiovascular risk and lipid, inflammatory and haemostatic factors. Nutr Metab Cardiovasc Dis. 2011;21(3):213–21.
41. Doggrell SA. Lowering LDL, cholesterol with margarine containing plant stanol/sterol esters: is it still relevant in 2011? Complement Ther Med. 2011;19(1):37–46.

42. Eussen SRBM, Bouvy ML, Rompelberg CJM, et al. Influence of the use of functional foods enriched with phytosterols/-stanols on adherence to statin therapy. Pharmacoepidemiol Drug Saf. 2011;20(8):830–7.
43. Pop F. Evolution of some physicochemical parameters of iodine fortified sunflower oil and margarine. Int J Food Sci Technol. 2010;45(2):327–33.
44. Hof KHVH, Tijburg LBM, de Boer HSM, Wiseman SA, Weststrate JA. Antioxidant fortified margarine increases the antioxidant status. Eur J Clin Nutr. 1998;52(4):292–9.
45. SCF. Opinion of the Scientific Committee on Food on the tolerable upper intake levels of preformed vitamin A (retinol and retinyl esters). Report No.: SCF/CS/NU/UPPLEV/24 Final; 26 Sep 2002.
46. SCF. Opinion of the Scientific Committee on Food on the tolerable upper intake levels of vitamin D. Report No.: SCF/CS/NUT/UPPLEV/38 Final; 4 Dec 2002.
47. SCF. Opinion of the Scientific Committee on Food on the revision of reference values for nutrition labeling. Report No.: SCF/CS/NUT/GEN/18 Final; 5 Mar 2003.
48. SCF. Opinion of the Scientific Committee on Food on a request for the safety assessment of the use of phytosterol esters in yellow fat spreads. Report No.: SCF/CS/NF/DOS/1 Final; 6 Apr 2000.
49. Din JN, Newby DE, Flapan AD. Science, medicine, and the future—omega 3 fatty acids and cardiovascular disease—fishing for a natural treatment. Br Med J. 2004;328(7430):30–5.

Chapter 14
Commercial Conjugated Linoleic Acid (CLA) Fortified Dairy Products

Luis Miguel Rodríguez-Alcalá, Antonia Villar-Tajadura, Manuela Juarez, and Javier Fontecha

Key Points

- CLA is mainly found in food products from ruminants such as dairy products.
- The most abundant isomer is rumenic acid (RA; C18:2 *cis* 9, *trans* 11) accounting 75–90 % of total CLA in milk fat related with several biological effects as anticarcinogenic, antiaterogenic, antioxidative, and immune system stimulation activities.
- The CLA activity on body fat reduction has been described in humans associated to C18:2 *trans* 10, *cis* 12 isomer.
- Possible adverse effects of CLA isomers when either synthetic CLA oils are used in high concentrations or when long-term CLA intakes, remain still unclear.
- 3 g/day of CLA dosage has been extrapolated from animal studies to exert positive biological effects.
- Some strategies to increase CLA content in dairy products are (1) PUFA supplementation of ruminant diet, (2) CLA-producing bacteria, or (3) addition/substitution milkfat with synthetic CLA oils.
- Further investigations are required to know the biological mechanisms of the CLA activity, to develop efficient strategies of administration, and to solve possible safety issues in human health.

Keywords Conjugated linoleic acid • CLA isomers • Dairy products • Milkfat • Functional foods • Probiotic bacteria

Abbreviations

BMI	Body mass index
CLA	Conjugated linoleic acid
CVD	Cardiovascular diseases
EFSA	European Food Safety Authority
GRAS	Generally recognized as safe
LA	Linoleic acid (C18:2 *cis* 9, *cis* 12)

L.M. Rodríguez-Alcalá, Ph.D. • A. Villar-Tajadura, Ph.D. • M. Juarez, Ph.D. • J. Fontecha, Ph.D. (✉)
Department of Bioactivity and Food Analysis, Group of Lipids, Instituto de Investigación en Ciencias de la Alimentación (CIAL; CSIC-UAM), Nicolás Cabrera, 9, Campus Universidad Autónoma de Madrid, Madrid, Spain 28049
e-mail: j.fontecha@csic.es

V.R. Preedy et al. (eds.), *Handbook of Food Fortification and Health: From Concepts to Public Health Applications Volume 1*, Nutrition and Health, DOI 10.1007/978-1-4614-7076-2_14,

MUFA	Monounsaturated fatty acid
PUFA	Polyunsaturated fatty acid
RA	Rumenic acid (C18:2 *cis* 9, *trans* 11)
SFA	Saturated fatty acid
TAG	Triacylglycerol
TVA	*trans* vaccenic acid (C18:1 *trans* 11)

Introduction

Conjugated linoleic acid (CLA) is a mixture of positional and geometric conjugated isomers of the essential linoleic fatty acid (LA, C18:2 *cis* 9, *cis* 12) characterized by the presence of double bonds from 6 to 14 position (6–8; 7–9; 8–10; 9–11; 10–12; 11–13; 12–14) and four conformations (*cis, trans; trans, cis; trans, trans, and cis, cis*) yielding 28 possible isomers [1]. The CLA is mainly found in food products from ruminants such as dairy products (0.34–1.07 g/100 g fat) [2] and beef (0.12–0.68 g/100 g fat) [3], because it is produced as an intermediate in the biohydrogenation pathway by ruminal bacteria (Fig. 14.1). The most abundant isomers (Table 14.1) are rumenic acid (RA; C18:2 *cis* 9, *trans* 11) accounting 75–90 % of total CLA in milk fat and C18:2 *trans* 7, *cis* 9 with 3–16 % [4]. Many research works had investigated the biological effects of RA reporting anticarcinogenic [10], antiaterogenic [11], antioxidative [12], and stimulation of the immune system [13]. Reduction of body fat [14] (antiobesity activity) has been associated with the C18:2 *trans* 10, *cis* 12 isomer mainly present in CLA synthetic oils. In the current market there are available rich CLA oils with a concentration of 80 g CLA/100 g oil with a 1:1 mixture of the two major isomers C18:2 *cis* 9, *trans* 11 and C18:2 *trans* 10, *cis* 12 and other minor isomers consisting of all *cis*/*trans* isomers of C18:2 9,11; 10,12 and 11,13 [15]. Various methods are available to produce synthetic CLA oil but alkaline isomerization of linoleic acid is the most common method [16] (Fig. 14.2).

Biological Activities of CLA

From initial studies showing the CLA anticarcinogenic effects as inhibited epithelial tumors in animals [10], a high number of research works have been performed in the determination of their biological and physiological properties (Table 14.2.). The available information on the effects of the CLA isomer RA in cancer cell metabolism together with its antiproliferative and apoptotic activities [17] place CLA as an interesting compound in cancer therapy naturally present in food. CLA investigations have been mostly carried out either in growing cancer cells or in animal models with CLA synthetic mixtures or using meat extracts [18]. There are only few studies accomplished in humans using dairy products as source of CLA and some of them have found positive effects in the incidence of breast and colorectal cancer in women [19]. However other studies reporting the presence of CLA in adipose tissue and serum, concluded that there are inconsistent anticancer evidences [20]. The isomer C18:2 *trans* 10, *cis* 12, has achieved a great relevance since it has been reported to promote weight loss [14] although it could also incite increase in glycemia and plasma insulin resistance [21].

Tricon et al. [22] had showed that incorporation of the individual isomers RA and C18:2 *trans* 10, *cis* 12 or mixtures, into the diet of healthy volunteers affects positively plasma lipid levels leading to a significant reduction of the total cholesterol and triacylglycerides (TAG) concentrations mainly associated to RA while C18:2 *trans* 10, *cis* 12 appears not to enhance the beneficial effects of weight loss on cardiovascular disease risk markers.

Recent studies in obese and overweight children (6–10 year old) consuming CLA-enriched chocolate milk (3–4.2 g/day) reported attenuation in the BMI increase but did not improve plasma lipids or

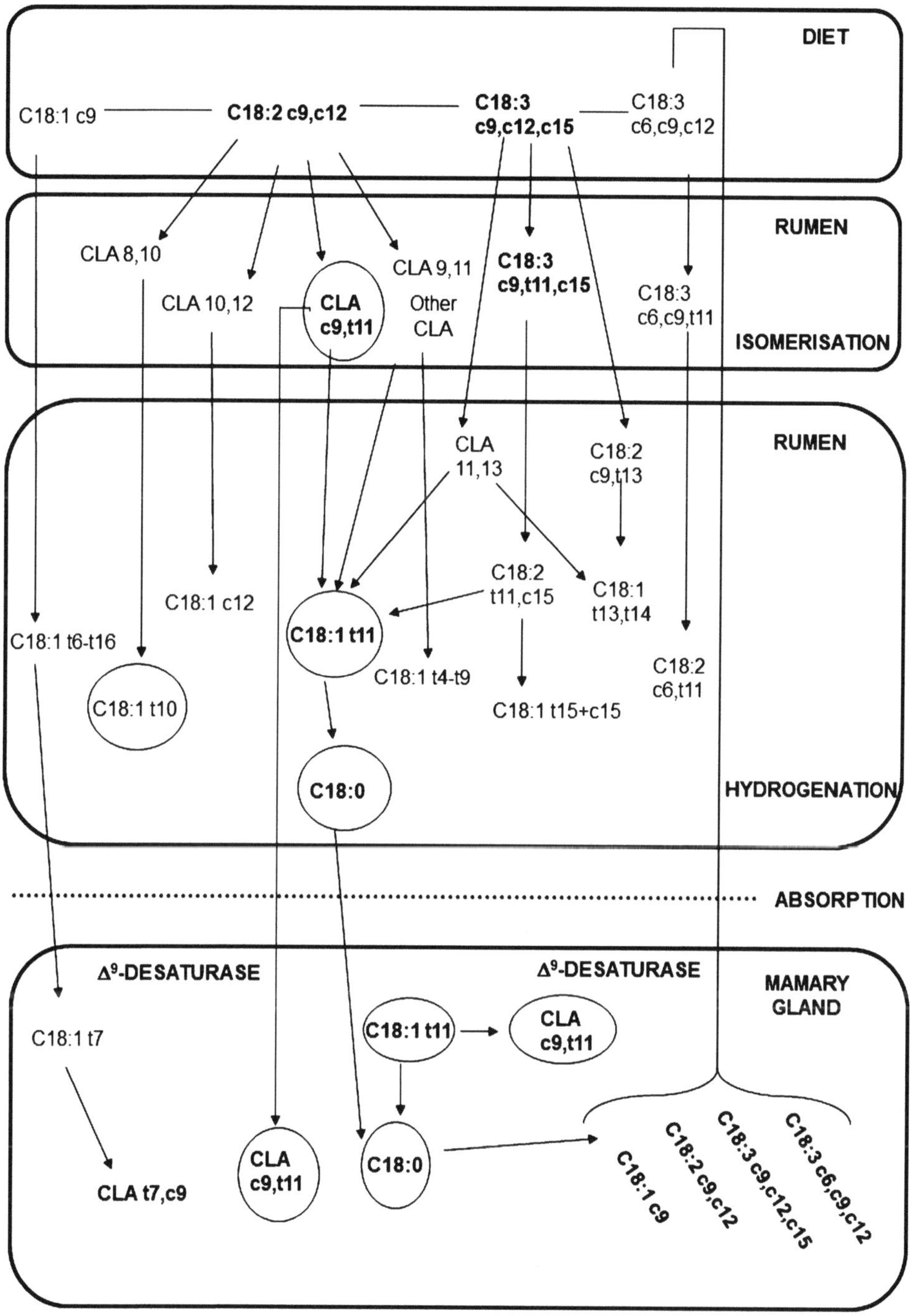

Fig. 14.1 Biohydrogenation pathways in rumen and Δ9-desaturase activity in mammary gland [4–7]

glucose and showed decreased HDL cholesterol level [23]. It has been suggested that these compounds can regulate expression of nuclear receptors PPAR and the enzyme cascade related to the lipid metabolism being even useful in therapies for type II diabetes [24]. About the biological activity of other CLA isomers, the C18:2 *cis* 9 *cis* 11 has been shown to be a blocking agent of estrogen signaling in

Table 14.1 Range distribution (minimum and maximum) of CLA isomers in cow's, sheep's, and goat's milk (g/100 CLA)

Isomers	Cow	Sheep	Goat
trans, trans			
12, 14	1.5–2.6	1.3–3.5	0.2–0.5
11, 13	2.6–4.6	1.2–5.1	0.7–1.5
10, 12	1.0–1.5	1.2–1.8	0.5–1.4
9, 11	2.3–3.5	1.1–2.0	1.7–2.6
8, 10	0.4–0.9	1.0–1.4	0.5–0.8
7, 9	0.9–1.1	0.5–0.6	0.4–0.6
cis, trans/trans, cis			
11, 13	2.0–7.5	0.8–4.2	0.3–0.8
10, 12	0.7–1.8	0.3–0.4	0.6–0.8
9, 11	76.7–80.7	76.5–82.4	81.8–85.9
7, 9	1.9–5.8	3.3–9.7	6.6–8.0
Total CLA			
	0.5–1.0	0.56–0.97	0.32–1.17
Total fat (g/100 mL)			
	3.6	5.8	3.7

Adapted from Luna et al. [8, 45] and Park et al. [9]

human breast cancer cells in vitro assays [25]. Other studies have reported a potent inhibitory effect of C18:2 *trans* 9 *trans* 11 on the growth of human colon cancer cells [26] as well as antiproliferative and pro-apoptotic effects on bovine endothelial cells [27]. On the other hand some research works involving human studies do not demonstrate a clear association between the consumption of CLA and positive biological effects. It could be related to several factors such as very high doses of synthetic CLA used, metabolic differences associated with the species, and if the effect is produced by a single CLA compound or mixtures [28].

The multiple physiologic effects reported for CLA could be the result of multiple interactions of the biologically active CLA isomers with numerous metabolic signaling pathways. Therefore, further studies are needed in this field, which demands more evidences to define the beneficial and the detrimental effects of each individual CLA isomer.

CLA Safety Dosage and Functional Foods: Recommendations

It has been estimated that the average daily intake of CLA in the Western diet is 100–200 mg/person [29] and its ingestion is decreasing due to the tendency to reduce whole milk, butter, and meat consumption.

Ip et al. [30] calculated that 0.1 % dietary CLA, the amount that prevented breast cancer in rats, would be equivalent to a daily intake of 3.5 g for humans. Similarly, CLA supplementation in overweight subjects after weight loss seems to aid the regain of fat-free mass at experimental doses of 1.8 and 3.6 g/day [31]. Nevertheless, the extrapolation of CLA effects observed in animals to the human situation should be made with caution. Studies focused in the CLA safety performed in humans using high CLA content oils or mixtures of the isomers RA and C18:2 *trans* 10, *cis* 12 concluded that consumption of 6 g/day for 1 year [32] and 3 g/day during 2 years [33] has no adverse effects on the consumer health, which has prompted the FDA to confer the GRAS status to these oils at 1.5 g/day [34]. However the EFSA Panel on Dietetic Products, Nutrition and Allergies has recently concluded that although CLA consumption does not appear to have adverse effects on insulin sensitivity, blood glucose control, or liver function for up to 6 months, and that observed effects on blood lipids are unlikely to have an impact on CVD risk, long-term effects of CLA intake have not been adequately addressed in

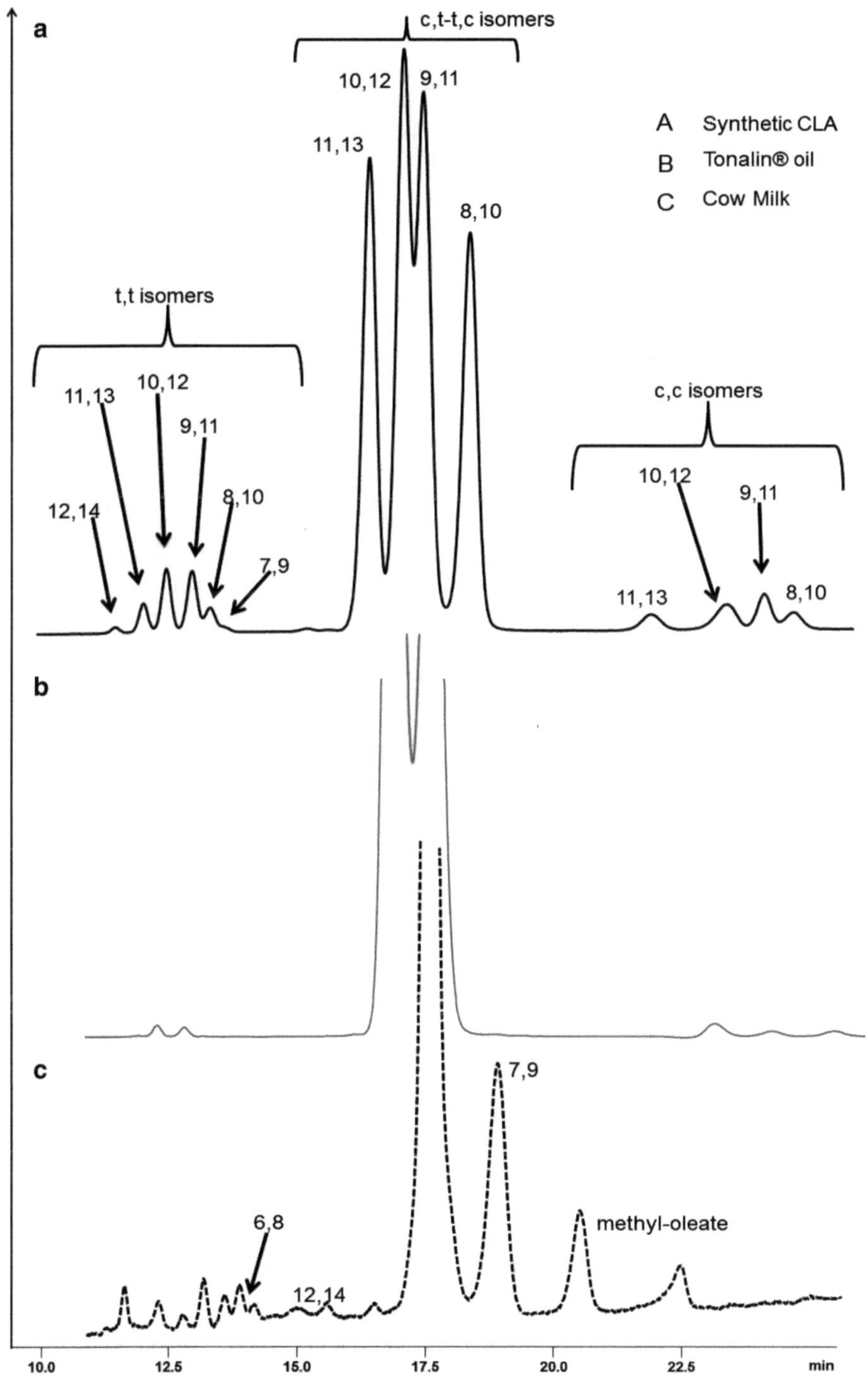

Fig. 14.2 CLA isomer distribution in synthetic mixture (Nu-Chek Prep), enriched CLA oil (Tonalin), and cows milkfat by HPLC-Ag^{+}

humans [35]. It reflects the existence of an intense debate about the safety of CLA intake in humans. Therefore several studies showed that even at the proposed safe doses, oxidative stress, increases in LDL/HDL and total cholesterol/HDL ratio, hepatotoxicity, and insulin resistance addressing the isomer C18:2 *trans* 10, *cis* 12 could occur [22, 36–38].

Table 14.2 Documented effects of conjugated linoleic acid

Effects	Subject	Isomers	Study
Anticarcinogenic	In vitro	RA, *trans* 9, *trans* 11, *trans* 11, *trans* 13	Degen et al. Cell Biol. L. 2011; 1811(12):1070–1080
	Animal models	RA/*trans* 10, *cis* 12	Tiam, M. et al. Mol. Nutr. Food Res. 2011;55(2):268–277
	Human	RA (Meat, dairy products)	Larsson et al. Am. J. Clin. Nutr. 2005; 82(4):894–900
Inmune system modulator	In vitro	RA/*trans* 10, *cis* 12	Stachowska et al. Int J Food Sci Nutr. 2012;63(1):30–35
	Animal models	RA/*trans* 10, *cis* 12	Selga et al. BMC Genomics. 2011;12
	Humans	RA/*trans* 10, *cis* 12	Turpeinen et al. Br. J. Nutr. 2008;100(1):112–119
Antiarterioesclerotic	Animal models	RA/*trans* 10, *cis* 12	Mitchell and McLeod. BBA-Mol. Cell Biol. L. 2005;1734(3):269–276
	Humans	RA	Tricon et al. Am. J. Clin. Nutr. 2004;80(3): 614-620; Tholstrup et al. J. Nut. 2008;138(8):1445–1451
Bone mineralization	In vitro	RA/*trans* 10, *cis* 12	Platt and El-Sohemy. J. Nutr. Biochem. 2009;20(12):956–964
	Animal models	RA/*trans* 10, *cis* 12	Rahman et al. J. Cell. Physiol. 2011;226(9):2406–2414
	Humans	RA/*trans* 10, *cis* 12	Brownbill et al. J. Am. Coll. Nutr. 2005;24(3):177–181
Antidiabetic	Animal models	*trans* 10, *cis* 12	Li et al. J Food Biochem. 2011;35(6):1593–1602
Body mass modification	Animal models	*trans* 10, *cis* 12	Ribot et al. Br. J. Nutr. 2007;97(6):1074–1082
	Humans	RA/*trans* 10, *cis* 12	Schoeller et al. Appl. Physiol., Nutr., Metab. 2009;34(5):975–978
Plasmatic insulin resistance	Animal models	RA/*trans* 10, *cis* 12	Zhou et al. Growth Horm. IGF Res. 2008;18:361–368
	Humans	RA/*trans* 10, *cis* 12	Ahren et al. Eur. J. Clin Nutr. 2009;63(6):778–786
Antihypertensive	Animal models	RA/*trans* 10, *cis* 12	Park et al. J. Funct. Foods. 2010;2(1):54–59
	Humans	RA/*trans* 10, *cis* 12	Zhao et al. Am. J. Hypertens. 2009;22(6):680–686

RA; rumenic acid C18:2 *cis* 9, *trans* 11
trans 10, *cis* 12: C18:2 *trans* 10, *cis* 12
trans 9, *trans* 11: C18:2 *trans* 9, *trans* 11

A good way to raise the CLA content in the diet, without radical changes of eating habits, seems to be the enrichment of frequent and common consumed food products with CLA supplements. Dairy products enriched with synthetic CLA oil are now commercially available in some countries (Fig. 14.3), and considerable interest of the CLA composition and stability of these preparations have been reported [15].

Strategies for Increasing the Content of CLA in Dairy Products

Nowadays milk has lower contents of unsaturated fatty acids and CLA than 30 years ago due to that dairy management systems have changed from predominantly grazing to confine feeding systems based largely on maize silage and concentrates for high milk producing cows. But as milk fat is the major natural dietary source of CLA in the human diet, over the last years there has been great interest in developing strategies to obtain naturally CLA enriched dairy products with heath beneficial effects.

Nutritional modification of ruminant diet has received considerable attention due to its major influence on the substantial variations of milk FA profile and CLA content. The key objective has

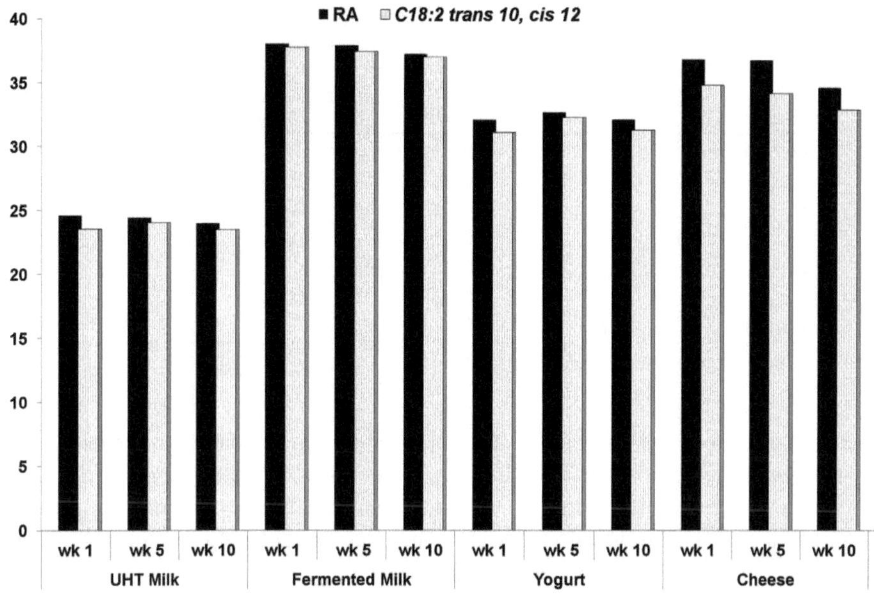

Fig. 14.3 Concentration (g FA/100 fat) and stability of RA and C18:2 *trans* 10, *cis* 12 in commercial CLA enriched dairy products from the Spanish market, after 10 weeks of refrigerated storage

usually been to reduce saturated fatty acid (SFA) concentration and to increase monounsaturated (MUFA) and polyunsaturated fatty acid (PUFA) concentrations in milk, specially enhancing the content of some unsaturated fatty acids like n-3 FA and CLA.

The CLA content of milk depends on ruminal production of CLA and 18:1 *trans* 11 (*trans* vaccenic acid, TVA) and the activity of Δ9 desaturase in mammary gland [39]. The importance of TVA lies in its role as a precursor of RA that not only occurs in the bovine mammary gland but also in human and other animal tissues [40].

Animal feeding strategies for CLA enrichment of milk have been reviewed, and diets with seed/oil supplements rich in PUFA that provide lipid substrates for the production of RA and TVA have proved to be effective [5, 41]. In addition to enhancing CLA content, the dietary changes also result in milk fat containing a lower proportion of SFA and greater amounts of MUFA and PUFA.

Plant oils from different oilseeds differ widely in their FA profile and cause major changes in the composition of milk fat. Dietary oil treatments (peanut oil, high in oleic acid; sunflower oil, high in linoleic acid; linseed oil and flaxseed, high in alpha-linolenic acid) have been shown to exert different degrees of enrichment of milk fat with CLA [42, 43] and have been successfully tested in cow and ovine cattle's [44, 45]. With soybean, canola, sunflower, or flax oils the CLA content can reach values higher than 2 % [46] although fish oil supplement is more effective at enhancing milk fat CLA content than are plant oils [47]. However, the alterations in the ruminal ecosystem can lead to an increase in the synthesis of C18:1 *trans* 10 undesirable from the point of view of human health [48]. Studies carried out in cow and sheep milk showed that extruded to linseed leads increments in the CLA and TVA concentration up to threefold and C18:1 distributions similar to that in non-supplemented animals or pasture feeding [49, 50] (Table 14.3.).

On the other hand, some studies have confirmed that range-fed animals or those grazing solely on pastures have a higher content of CLA in their milk than do those raised on grains and forage, largely due to a more favorable rumen pH [51], despite the inherent production inefficiencies. Recently Smit et al. [52] provided a very clear evidence of a substantial health benefit from consuming high CLA content milk from grass-fed ruminants. This study showed that higher content of RA in adipose tissue

Table 14.3 Effect of extruded linseed supplementation to the ewes diet (A: 6 g/100 DM; B: 12 g/100 DM) in the CLA concentration (g/100 total FA) of milk

		Extruded linseed dose	
Isomers	Control	A	B
cis 9, *trans* 11	0.79	1.32	1.85
trans 9, *cis* 11	0.02	0.01	0.02
trans 10, *cis* 12	0.01	0.01	0.01
trans 11, *cis* 13	0.02	0.09	0.18
trans 12, *trans* 14	0.01	0.02	0.02
trans 11, *trans* 13	0.02	0.05	0.06
trans, trans 8, 10/9, 11/10, 12	0.02	0.02	0.02

Adapted from Gomez-Cortes et al. [49]

is associated with a reduced risk of nonfatal acute myocardial infarction (heart attack) in Costa Rica consumers. However, the authors indicate that it is uncertain whether an increase in CLA in dairy products will have beneficial effects that would counterbalance the adverse effects of saturated fat. However, Warensjo et al. [53] conclude that milk consumption does not raise the risk of a first heart attack, despite the significant increase in saturated fat intake.

CLA-Producing Bacteria

The presence of CLA compounds in dairy products is partly due to the isomerization and biohydrogenation of linoleic and linolenic acids that take place in the rumen; these processes are performed by ruminal bacteria [54] (Fig. 14.4).

Such observation has raised the hypothesis that other microorganisms may also be able to produce CLA. This hypothesis and the fact that several fermented dairy products contain higher levels of CLA than non-fermented counterparts could make the possibility of producing fermented dairy products with high levels of CLA.

Over the last years, several works have described that different bacteria of the Lactobacillus and Bifidobacterium genera are able to produce CLA isomers in culture media when free fatty acids as LA, TVA, ricinoleic acid or oils as safflower, rich in LA, or castor oil, high in ricinoleic were added [59, 60]. A possible reason of the bacteria ability to transform LA to CLA would be a detoxification mechanism [61].

Puniya et al. [62] reported that *L. brevis* isolated from ruminal fluid produced 10 mg CLA/g fat in skim milk using 0.25 % of sunflower oil as source of LA, while *L. lactis* with 1 % sunflower oil produced 9.2 mg CLA/g fat. When probiotic bacteria *L. acidophilus* or *B. animalis* were used jointly with a yogurt starter culture (*S. thermophilus* and *L. delbreckii ssp. bulgaricus*) and fructo-oligosaccharides in whole milk (3 % fat) 6 mg CLA/g fat was produced [63]. Recent studies also pointed out that bifidobacteria and lactic bacteria were able to produce 40–50 mg CLA/g fat in skim milk when 1 mg/mL of free LA as substrate was added [64]. Gorissen and collaborators have observed that the strains *Bifidobacterium breve* and *Bifidobacterium bifidum* are the most efficient CLA producers among the range of strains tested [65].

Other possible alternative to increase CLA dose in human diet by using microorganism is the establishment of probiotic cultures in the gastrointestinal tract. In fact, a research group has demonstrated that oral administration of a *B. breve* strain, with ability to produce CLA, can modify the fatty acid composition of the host (mice and pigs), including significantly elevated concentrations of RA and n-3 fatty acids in liver and adipose tissue [66]. Furthermore, a recent study has verified that a gene (encoding for LA isomerase) expressed in an intestinal microbe can influence the fatty acid composition of host fat [67].

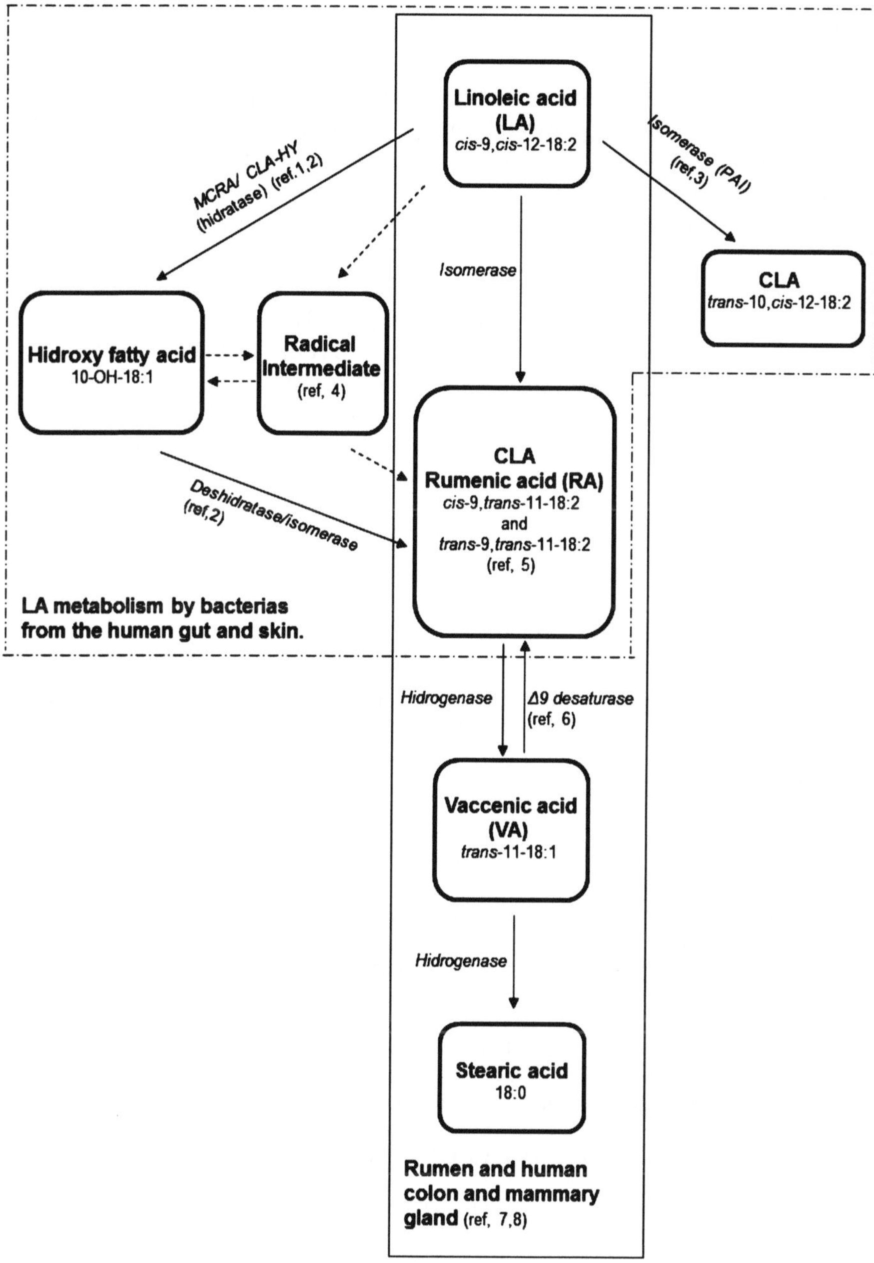

Fig. 14.4 CLA production pathways by lactic acid bacteria and bioconversion of TVA in human tissues [55–58]. *MCRA* myosin reactive antigen; *CLA-HY* CLA-hydroxy fatty acid; *PAI Propionibacterium acnes* polyunsaturated fatty acid isomerase

The identification of CLA producer bifidobacteria is of great importance because in addition to the beneficial effects of produced CLA, these microorganisms may confer other health benefits such as improvement of immune function and reduction of gastrointestinal disturbances [68].

Although probiotic bacteria with high CLA-producing abilities could further increase the CLA content of fermented dairy products (fermented milk, yogurt, and cheese) to our knowledge there is no availability of commercial dairy products including CLA producer microorganism during the fermentation process.

Conclusion

Several studies suggest that CLA isomers mainly RA is a potentially functional ingredient due to its bioactivity and recognized safety. However there is contradictory information about the possible effects of some of the CLA isomers when high concentrations of synthetic CLA oil are used or after a long-term intake. Even more, the lack of knowledge about the mechanisms of action of these isomers avoids the utilization of appropriate dosage to assure their action. Therefore more research studies in these aspects are needed.

Some strategies have demonstrated the possibility to increase the CLA concentration in dairy products as (1) the supplementation of ruminant feeding with high PUFAs sources oils or seeds (decreasing also the SFAs and increasing other healthy fatty acids as TVA or n-3 FA) or (2) by fermentation with CLA producer bacteria or (3) addition/substitution of milk fat with synthetic CLA oils. Nevertheless, further investigations are required to establish the contributions about the biological mechanisms of the CLA activity either to develop efficient strategies of administration or to solve possible safety issues in human health. Documentation of the different CLA isomers activity also provides a long-needed approach to investigating a numerous compounds on intermediary human metabolism.

References

1. Roach JAG, Mossoba MM, Yurawecz MP, et al. Chromatographic separation and identification of conjugated linoleic acid isomers. Anal Chim Acta. 2002;465(1–2):207–26.
2. Schmid A, Collomb M, Sieber R, et al. Conjugated linoleic acid in meat and meat products: a review. Meat Sci. 2006;73(1):29–41.
3. Fritsche J, Rickert R, Steinhart H, et al. Conjugated linoleic acid (CLA) isomers: formation, analysis, amounts in foods, and dietary intake. Fett Lipid. 1999;101(8):272–6.
4. Collomb M, Schmid A, Sieber R, et al. Conjugated linoleic acids in milk fat: variation and physiological effects. Int Dairy J. 2006;16(11):1347–61.
5. Chilliard Y, Glasser F, Ferlay A, et al. Diet, rumen biohydrogenation and nutritional quality of cow and goat milk fat. Eur J Lipid Sci Technol. 2007;109(8):828–55.
6. Jenkins TC, McGuire MA. Major advances in nutrition: impact on milk composition. J Dairy Sci. 2006;89(4): 1302–10.
7. Wallace RJ, McKain N, Shingfield KJ, et al. Isomers of conjugated linoleic acids are synthesized via different mechanisms in ruminal digesta and bacteria. J Lipid Res. 2007;48(10):2247–54.
8. Gómez-Cortés P. Efecto de la suplementación de la dieta ovina con distintas fuentes lipídicas sobre el perfil de ácidos grasos de la leche. E-prints Complutense: Facultad de Ciencias Químicas, Departamento de Química Física I, Universidad Complutense de Madrid; 2010.
9. Park YW, Juárez M, Ramos M, et al. Physico-chemical characteristics of goat and sheep milk. Small Rumin Res. 2007;68(1–2):88–113.
10. Ha YL, Grimm NK, Pariza MW. Anticarcinogens from fried ground beef: heat-altered derivatives of linoleic acid. Carcinogenesis. 1987;8(12):1881–7.
11. Tanaka K. Occurrence of conjugated linoleic acid in ruminant products and its physiological functions. Anim Sci J. 2005;76(4):291–303.
12. Hur SJ, Park GB, Joo ST. Biological activities of conjugated linoleic acid (CLA) and effects of CLA on animal products. Livest Sci. 2007;110(3):221–9.
13. O'Shea M, Bassaganya-Riera J, Mohede ICM. Immunomodulatory properties of conjugated linoleic acid. Am J Clin Nutr. 2004;79(6):1199S–206.
14. Park Y, Pariza MW. Mechanisms of body fat modulation by conjugated linoleic acid (CLA). Food Res Int. 2007;40(3):311–23.
15. Rodriguez-Alcala LM, Fontecha J. Hot topic: fatty acid and conjugated linoleic acid (CLA) isomer composition of commercial CLA-fortified dairy products: evaluation after processing and storage. J Dairy Sci. 2007;90(5): 2083–90.
16. Villeneuve P, Lago R, Barouh N, et al. Production of conjugated linoleic acid isomers by dehydration and isomerization of castor bean oil. J Am Oil Chem Soc. 2005;82(4):261–9.

17. Ochoa JJ, Farquharson AJ, Grant I, et al. Conjugated linoleic acids (CLAs) decrease prostate cancer cell proliferation: different molecular mechanisms for cis-9, trans-11 and trans-10, cis-12 isomers. Carcinogenesis. 2004;25(7): 1185–91.
18. de la Torre A, Debiton E, Juaneda P, et al. Beef conjugated linoleic acid isomers reduce human cancer cell growth even when associated with other beef fatty acids. Br J Nutr. 2006;95(2):346–52.
19. Larsson SC, Bergkvist L, Wolk A. High-fat dairy food and conjugated linoleic acid intakes in relation to colorectal cancer incidence in the Swedish Mammography Cohort. Am J Clin Nutr. 2005;82(4):894–900.
20. Chajés V, Lavillonniére F, Maillard V, et al. Conjugated linoleic acid content in breast adipose tissue of breast cancer patients and the risk of metastasis. Nutr Cancer. 2003;45(1):17–23.
21. Risérus U, Arner P, Brismar K, et al. Treatment with dietary trans10cis12 conjugated linoleic acid causes isomer-specific insulin resistance in obese men with the metabolic syndrome. Diabetes Care. 2002;25(9):1516–21.
22. Tricon S, Burdge GC, Jones EL, et al. Effects of dairy products naturally enriched with cis-9, trans-11 conjugated linoleic acid on the blood lipid profile in healthy middle-aged men. Am J Clin Nutr. 2006;83(4):744–53.
23. Racine NM, Watras AC, Carrel AL, et al. Effect of conjugated linoleic acid on body fat accretion in overweight or obese children. Am J Clin Nutr. 2010;91(5):1157–64.
24. Belury MA, Kavanaugh CJ, Liu K-L. Conjugated linoleic acid modulates phorbol ester-induced PPAR-[delta] and K-FABP mRNA expression in mouse skin. Nutr Res. 2007;27(1):48–55.
25. Tanmahasamut P, Liu J, Hendry LB, et al. Conjugated linoleic acid blocks estrogen signaling in human breast cancer cells. J Nutr. 2004;134(3):674–80.
26. Coakley M, Johnson MC, McGrath E, et al. Intestinal bifidobacteria that produce trans-9, trans-11 conjugated linoleic acid: a fatty acid with antiproliferative activity against human colon SW480 and HT-29 cancer cells, vol. 56. Philadelphia, PA: ETATS-UNIS: Taylor & Francis; 2006.
27. Lai K-L, Torres-Duarte A, Vanderhoek J. 9-trans, 11-trans-CLA: antiproliferative and proapoptotic effects on bovine endothelial cells. Lipids. 2005;40(11):1107–16.
28. Benjamin S, Spener F. Conjugated linoleic acids as functional food: an insight into their health benefits. Nutr Metab (Lond). 2009;6:36.
29. Ritzenthaler KL, McGuire MK, Falen R, et al. Stimation of conjugated linoleic acid intake by written dietary assessment methodologies underestimates actual intake evaluated by food duplicate methodology. J Nutr. 2001;131(5):1548–54.
30. Ip C, Singh M, Thompson HJ, et al. Conjugated linoleic acid suppresses mammary carcinogenesis and proliferative activity of the mammary gland in the rat. Cancer Res. 1994;54(5):1212–5.
31. Kamphuis MMJW, Lejeune MPGM, Saris WHM, et al. The effect of conjugated linoleic acid supplementation after weight loss on body weight regain, body composition, and resting metabolic rate in overweight subjects. Int J Obes Relat Metab Disord. 2003;27(7):840–7.
32. Larsen TM, Toubro S, Gudmundsen O, et al. Conjugated linoleic acid supplementation for 1 y does not prevent weight or body fat regain. Am J Clin Nutr. 2006;83(3):606–12.
33. Gaullier J-M, Halse J, Hoye K, et al. Supplementation with conjugated linoleic acid for 24 months is well tolerated by and reduces body fat mass in healthy, overweight humans. J Nutr. 2005;135(4):778–84.
34. Food and Drug Administration (FDA). GRASS notice for conjugates linoleic acid (CLA)-rich oil for use in certain foods. GRAS Notice No. GRN 000153. 2004.
35. EFSA Panel on Dietetic Products NaAN. Scientific opinion on the safety of "conjugated linoleic acid (CLA)-rich oil" (Tonalin® TG 80) as a novel food ingredient. EFSA J. 2010;8(5):1600.
36. Silveira MB, Carraro R, Monereo S, et al. Conjugated linoleic acid (CLA) and obesity. Public Health Nutr. 2007;10(10 A):1181–6.
37. Tricon S, Burdge GC, Kew S, et al. Opposing effects of cis-9, trans-11 and trans-10, cis-12 conjugated linoleic acid on blood lipids in healthy humans. Am J Clin Nutr. 2004;80(3):614–20.
38. Ramos R, Mascarenhas J, Duarte P, et al. Conjugated linoleic acid-induced toxic hepatitis: first case report. Dig Dis Sci. 2009;54(5):1141–3.
39. Palmquist DL, Lock AL, Shingfield KJ, et al. Biosynthesis of conjugated linoleic acid in ruminants and humans. In: Steve LT, editor. Advances in food and nutrition research, vol. 50. San Diego, California: Academic; 2005. p. 179–217.
40. Mosley EE, McGuire MK, Williams JE, et al. Cis-9, trans-11 conjugated linoleic acid is synthesized from vaccenic acid in lactating women. J Nutr. 2006;136(9):2297–301.
41. Morand-Fehr P, Fedele V, Decandia M, et al. Influence of farming and feeding systems on composition and quality of goat and sheep milk. Small Rumin Res. 2007;68(1–2):20–34.
42. Collomb M, Sieber R, Buetikofer U. CLA isomers in milk fat from cows fed diets with high levels of unsaturated fatty acids. Lipids. 2004;39(4):355–64.
43. Dhiman TR, Satter LD, Pariza MW, et al. Conjugated linoleic acid (CLA) content of milk from cows offered diets rich in linoleic and linolenic acid. J Dairy Sci. 2000;83(5):1016–27.

44. Khanal RC. Factors affecting conjugated linoleic acid (CLA) content in milk, meat, and egg: a review. Pak J Nutr. 2004;3(2):82.
45. Luna P, Fontecha J, Juarez M, et al. Conjugated linoleic acid in ewe milk fat. J Dairy Res. 2005;72(4):415–24.
46. Gómez-Cortés P, Frutos P, Mantecón AR, et al. Milk production, conjugated linoleic acid content, and in vitro ruminal fermentation in response to high levels of soybean oil in dairy ewe diet. J Dairy Sci. 2008;91(4):1560–9.
47. Chouinard PY, Corneau L, Butler WR, et al. Effect of dietary lipid source on conjugated linoleic acid concentrations in milk fat. J Dairy Sci. 2001;84(3):680–90.
48. Anadón A, Martínez-Larrañaga MR, Martínez MA, et al. Acute oral safety study of dairy fat rich in trans-10 C18:1 versus vaccenic plus conjugated linoleic acid in rats. Food Chem Toxicol. 2010;48(2):591–8.
49. Gómez-Cortés P, Bach A, Luna P, et al. Effects of extruded linseed supplementation on n-3 fatty acids and conjugated linoleic acid in milk and cheese from ewes. J Dairy Sci. 2009;92(9):4122–34.
50. Fuentes MC, Calsamiglia S, Sanchez C, et al. Effect of extruded linseed on productive and reproductive performance of lactating dairy cows. Livest Sci. 2008;113(2–3):144–54.
51. Bauman DE, Mather IH, Wall RJ, et al. Major advances associated with the biosynthesis of milk. J Dairy Sci. 2006;89(4):1235–43.
52. Smit LA, Baylin A, Campos H. Conjugated linoleic acid in adipose tissue and risk of myocardial infarction. Am J Clin Nutr. 2010;92(1):34–40.
53. Warensjö E, Jansson JH, Cederholm T, et al. Biomarkers of milk fat and the risk of myocardial infarction in men and women: a prospective, matched case-control study. Am J Clin Nutr. 2010;92(1):194–202.
54. Bauman DE, Griinari JM. Nutritional regulation of milk fat synthesis. Annu Rev Nutr. 2003;23:203–27.
55. Howard FAC, Henderson C. Hydrogenation of polyunsaturated fatty acids by human colonic bacteria. Lett Appl Microbiol. 1999;29(3):193–6.
56. Jiang J, Björck L, Fondén R. Production of conjugated linoleic acid by dairy starter cultures. J Appl Microbiol. 1998;85(1):95–102.
57. Kishino S, Park S-B, Takeuchi M, et al. Novel multi-component enzyme machinery in lactic acid bacteria catalyzing CC double bond migration useful for conjugated fatty acid synthesis. Biochem Biophys Res Commun. 2011;416(1–2):188–93.
58. Liavonchanka A, Hornung E, Feussner I, et al. Structure and mechanism of the Propionibacterium acnes polyunsaturated fatty acid isomerase. Proc Natl Acad Sci U S A. 2006;103(8):2576–81.
59. Van Nieuwenhove CP, Oliszewski R, Gonzalez SN, et al. Influence of bacteria used as adjunct culture and sunflower oil addition on conjugated linoleic acid content in buffalo cheese. Food Res Int. 2007;40(5):559–64.
60. Alonso L, Cuesta EP, Gilliland SE. Production of free conjugated linoleic acid by Lactobacillus acidophilus and Lactobacillus casei of human intestinal origin. J Dairy Sci. 2003;86(6):1941–6.
61. Adamczak M, Bornscheuer UT, Bednarski W. Properties and biotechnological methods to produce lipids containing conjugated linoleic acid. Eur J Lipid Sci Technol. 2008;110(6):491–504.
62. Puniya AK, Chaitanya S, Tyagi AK, et al. Conjugated linoleic acid producing potential of lactobacilli isolated from the rumen of cattle. J Ind Microbiol Biotechnol. 2008;35(11):1223–8.
63. Akalin AS, Tokusoglu O, Gonc S, et al. Occurrence of conjugated linoleic acid in probiotic yoghurts supplemented with fructooligosaccharide. Int Dairy J. 2007;17(9):1089–95.
64. Rodríguez-Alcalá LM, Braga T, Malcata FX, et al. Quantitative and qualitative determination of CLA produced by Bifidobacterium and lactic acid bacteria by combining spectrophotometric and Ag+-HPLC techniques. Food Chem. 2011;125:1373–8.
65. Gorissen L, Raes K, Weckx S, et al. Production of conjugated linoleic acid and conjugated linolenic acid isomers by Bifidobacterium species. Appl Microbiol Biotechnol. 2010;87(6):2257–66.
66. Wall R, Ross RP, Shanahan F, et al. Metabolic activity of the enteric microbiota influences the fatty acid composition of murine and porcine liver and adipose tissues. Am J Clin Nutr. 2009;89(5):1393–401.
67. Rosberg-Cody E, Stanton C, O'Mahony L, et al. Recombinant lactobacilli expressing linoleic acid isomerase can modulate the fatty acid composition of host adipose tissue in mice. Microbiology. 2011;157(2):609–15.
68. Park HG, Heo W, Kim SB, et al. Production of conjugated linoleic acid (CLA) by Bifidobacterium breve LMC520 and its compatibility with CLA-producing rumen bacteria. J Agric Food Chem. 2010;59(3):984–8.

Chapter 15
Calcium-Fortified Soymilk

Pattavara Pathomrungsiyounggul, Michael J. Lewis, and Alistair S. Grandison

Key Points

- Natural soymilk has a low content of calcium and is often supplemented with calcium to levels found in cow's milk.
- It is possible to supplement with a wide variety of calcium salts. These will have different solubilities and different effects on the properties of the soymilk.
- Soymilk is subjected to pasteurisation or sterilisation processes to ensure that it is safe and has a long shelf life.
- The main problem arising from addition of soluble calcium salts is that they will reduce heat stability. This becomes a problem if addition results in a decrease in pH and an increase in ionic calcium.
- Stabilising salts such as disodium hydrogen phosphate and tri-sodium citrate are useful for improving heat stability of calcium-fortified soymilk.
- Calcium salts with low solubility such as calcium carbonate and calcium phosphate can also be added. One advantage is that they do not change pH and ionic calcium to the same extent as addition of soluble salts. One disadvantage results from their insolubility.
- How these different combinations of calcium salts and stabilising salts affect properties such as particle size and viscosity are discussed in this review.
- It is worthwhile measuring pH and ionic calcium of fortified beverages to gain a better understanding of their effects on the physical properties and sensory characteristics of soymilk.

Keywords Calcium-fortified soymilk • Calcium salt • Chelating agent • Pasteurisation • Sterilisation

P. Pathomrungsiyounggul, Ph.D. (✉)
Division of Food Engineering, Chiang Mai University, 155 Moo 2, Liebklongchonpratan Road, Tambon Maehea, Amphur Muang, Chiang Mai 50100, Thailand
e-mail: patavara@chiangmai.ac.th

M.J. Lewis • A.S. Grandison
Department of Food and Nutritional Sciences, The University of Reading, Reading, UK

V.R. Preedy et al. (eds.), *Handbook of Food Fortification and Health: From Concepts to Public Health Applications Volume 1*, Nutrition and Health, DOI 10.1007/978-1-4614-7076-2_15,

Abbreviations

$[Ca^{2+}]$	Calcium ion concentration
Ca	Calcium
CFSM	Calcium-fortified soymilk

Introduction

Soymilk is a traditional drink of Chinese origin. Recently a calcium-fortified soymilk (CFSM) has been developed as a functional beverage. The consumption of soy protein is claimed to result in a lower risk of some chronic diseases (including cardiovascular disease, cancer and osteoporosis) and alleviation of menopausal symptoms. Thus, CFSM has been consumed increasingly by European and North American consumers, with a large growth in sales.

The choice of appropriate calcium (Ca) salts for fortification of soymilk is a challenge for the beverage industry. Depending on the form of salt used, the addition of Ca to soymilk is likely to have a major impact on the palatability and stability of the final product. Enhancement of palatability and stability of the CFSM by addition of chelating agents has been investigated.

With the development of pasteurisation, sterilisation and ultra high temperature, microbial quality and safety are now no longer problems for manufacturers in CFSM production. Their main challenge is how to develop beverages that meet consumer demands (i.e. high Ca bioavailability, satisfactory flavour and texture), as well as having good heat stability. Thus, this review concentrates on the chemical, physical and sensory characteristics of CFSM. The effects of Ca ion and pH on viscosity and particle diameter of CFSM will be discussed.

Calcium-Fortified Soymilk

Soymilk has been commonly consumed by the Chinese for several centuries [1] and nowadays it is increasingly popular in Western countries. This is attributed to the health benefits of soy protein consumption, such as cholesterol reduction and lower risk of heart disease and cancer [2]. A comparison of nutrient contents of soymilk and skim milk shows that soymilk contains a satisfactory level of protein, carbohydrate, potassium, sodium, iron, riboflavin and niacin, but it provides much less Ca. There are 25 and 122 mg Ca/100 g in soymilk and skim milk, respectively [3].

As we know, Ca is a vital mineral for the structure of bones and teeth as well as in metabolic regulation. Consumption of foods deficient in Ca may be the cause of osteoporosis in later life and insufficient Ca within the body can lead to health problems and disease because Ca is essential for muscle contraction, neurotransmitter secretion, digestion and blood coagulation [4]. Thus, CFSM has been produced commercially in many countries for consumers who are aware of the need to consume food rich in Ca. Also, it is a good Ca source as a beverage for people who are allergic to milk and avoid milk consumption, such as lacto-vegetarians and lactose-intolerant people [5].

Calcium Salts

Calcium salts approved for food fortification in Europe and the USA are divided into two groups, i.e. the inorganic salts such as Ca carbonate, Ca chloride and triCa phosphate and the organic salts such as Ca citrate, Ca gluconate, Ca lactate and Ca lactogluconate. Solubility, Ca content, taste, bioavailability and cost are the main factors which influence the selection of the appropriate salt for

Table 15.1 Summary of fortification of Ca salts, addition of chelating agents and total Ca contents in soymilk

Calcium salt	Chelating agent	Total Ca content	References
Ca citrate 15 mM Ca and triCa phosphate 10 mM Ca	–	Top[a] 0.53 g/100 g Bottom 1.40 g/100 g (on dry basis)	[10]
Ca citrate 20 mM Ca and triCa phosphate 5 mM Ca	–	Top 0.52 g/100 g Bottom 1.20 g/100 g (on dry basis)	[10]
TriCa phosphate 25 mM Ca	–	Top 0.22 g/100 g Bottom 1.30 g/100 g (on dry basis)	[10]
Ca chloride 0.416 % (w/v)	Sodium tripolyphosphate 0.75 % (w/v)	121.7 mg/100 mL	[12]
Ca lactate 0.45 % (w/v)	Trisodium citrate 0.4 % (w/v)	74.7 mg/100 mL	[14]
Ca gluconate 1.3 % (w/v)	Sodium hexametaphosphate 1.0–1.2 % (w/v)	139–145 mg/100 mL	[15]
Ca lactogluconate 1.55 % (w/w)	Potassium citrate 1.25 % (w/w)	200 mg/100 g	[16]
Ca carbonate, 0.1 % Ca (w/v)	Potassium citrate 0.3 % (w/v)	133 mg/100 mL	[8]
TriCa phosphate, 0.1 % Ca (w/v)	Potassium citrate 0.3 % (w/v)	137 mg/100 mL	[8]
TriCa phosphate	Tripotassium citrate	120 mg/100 mL	[5]
TriCa phosphate	Tripotassium citrate and tripotassium phosphate	123 mg/100 mL	[5]
Ca chloride 25.0 mM Ca	0.9 % Sodium hexameta-phosphate	111 mg/100 g	[11]

[a]Top and bottom = the concentration of total Ca in the top and bottom of container, respectively

fortifying a soy drink [5]. It was pointed out [5] that organic Ca salts are more interesting than inorganic Ca salts for fortifying soymilk because of their higher bioavailability, even though they are more expensive. The producers should therefore use organic Ca salts if they are concerned about the nutritional value of the product rather than its price.

Table 15.1 presents Ca salts which have been studied to fortify soymilk. One of the most used Ca salts is Ca carbonate which is possibly the most cost-effective inorganic Ca salt because it contains a high percentage of mineral Ca (40 %) [6]. One undesirable effect of Ca carbonate, i.e. potential chalky mouth-feel leading to astringency or bitter taste in the beverage, can be masked with potassium citrate and carrageenan [7]. This Ca salt is slightly soluble in soymilk but its solubility is increased in soymilk containing potassium citrate and carrageenan [8].

TriCa phosphate has high Ca content and poor solubility. However, the reported finding [8] shows that addition of potassium citrate and carrageenan results in a higher solubility in soymilk and triCa phosphate-fortified soymilk has satisfactory sensory attributes. Unfortunately, triCa phosphate-fortified soymilks have a slightly lower Ca bioavailability than cow's milk [8, 9]. A research team [10] succeeded in producing triCa phosphate-fortified soymilk without addition of chelating agent and the product was high in Ca (Table 15.1), without undesirable flavour or chalkiness.

Calcium chloride contains high Ca content (36 %) and has a high solubility but its use is limited due to its imparting bitterness and saltiness [5]. Arising from its excellent solubility, soymilk with added Ca chloride (25 mM Ca) coagulated [11]. To formulate Ca chloride-fortified soymilk containing comparable Ca levels to cow's milk, a chelating agent must be added to prevent the coagulation of soy proteins [11, 12]. It was claimed [12] that Ca chloride and sodium tripolyphosphate were the preferable Ca salt and chelating agent combination required for making stable CFSM.

Among the organic Ca salts, Ca citrate provided satisfactory properties, high bioavailability and a more neutral taste profile, at a reasonable cost for fortification of soymilk [5]. An additional advantage was that Ca citrate was absorbed, regardless of gastric acid, resulting in people having low gastric acid secretion being able to consume it [13]. Since it is slightly soluble, Ca citrate-fortified soymilk, containing as much as 120 mg Ca/100 mL (30 mM), with no added chelating agent could be produced [5].

Calcium lactate must be used with a chelating agent in order to produce CFSM. The amount of Ca lactate and a chelating agent required to produce Ca lactate-fortified soymilk is presented in Table 15.1 but it provided only about 60 % of the Ca in cow's milk [14].

Calcium gluconate contains less Ca (9 % Ca) but it could be used with soymilk because it has little effect on the taste of food and a high Ca bioavailability [5]. Calcium gluconate-fortified soymilk with satisfactory heat stability has been developed [15].

Calcium lactogluconate is a highly bioavailable organic Ca source and provides a neutral taste [5]. It is very soluble. As a result, addition of 1.55 % Ca lactogluconate (w/w) caused coagulation of soymilk [16]. However, the coagulation was overcome by adding a chelating agent such as sodium hexametaphosphate or potassium citrate [16].

Chelating Agents

Chelating agents can form soluble complexes with alkaline earth ions; therefore, they have been used in the production of CFSM prepared from highly soluble Ca salts. To understand how chelating agents inhibit coagulation in CFSM, the mechanisms of coagulation must be known. These mechanisms have been described as follows [17]: On addition of Ca salt to soymilk which contains denatured protein, Ca ions dissociate and bind to negatively charged acidic amino acid residues of denatured protein molecules. This leads to protein molecules approaching each other sufficiently to form a coagulated soy curd because of (1) reduction of electrostatic repulsion between protein molecules, (2) formation of the –SH/S–S interchange reaction and (3) hydrophobic interactions between the molecules. Owing to interactions between chelating agents and Ca ions, ionic Ca concentrations in CFSM are reduced [11, 18]. Thus Ca ion levels become insufficient to promote coagulation of protein.

Chelating agents employed in formulated CFSM are trisodium citrate, potassium citrate, sodium tripolyphosphate and sodium hexametaphosphate and their appropriate concentrations are presented in Table 15.1. Another effective chelating agent was disodium hydrogen orthophosphate at 1 % w/w [18].

Calcium-Fortified Soymilk Production

The general method for producing CFSM is firstly to make soymilk, followed by addition of the Ca salt and other ingredients. However, there are differences between methods such as raw materials, operational steps in soymilk manufacture and temperature of mixing. Soymilk can be manufactured from soybean or soy protein isolate. One example of procedures to produce a heat stable CFSM is illustrated in Fig. 15.1. Sugar, from 2 to 7 % (weight/volume) can be added to soymilk to sweeten the product [8, 12, 14]. More information for production of CFSM can be found in other studies [10, 15, 19].

Chemical and Physical Properties and Shelf-Life of CFSM

Chemical Properties

Proximate Analysis

Information on proximate composition of CFSM has been less widely reported, compared to soymilk, although one would not expect there to be substantial differences. Calcium lactogluconate-fortified soymilk contained approximately: water 84.6 %, protein 5.2 %, carbohydrate 6.8 %, fat 1.8 % and ash 1.6 % [16]. Another study [10] reported that pasteurised CFSMs contained protein 28.4–29.4 g/100 g (on dry basis). Proximate composition of several CFSMs is available in the database of the US Department of Agriculture [3].

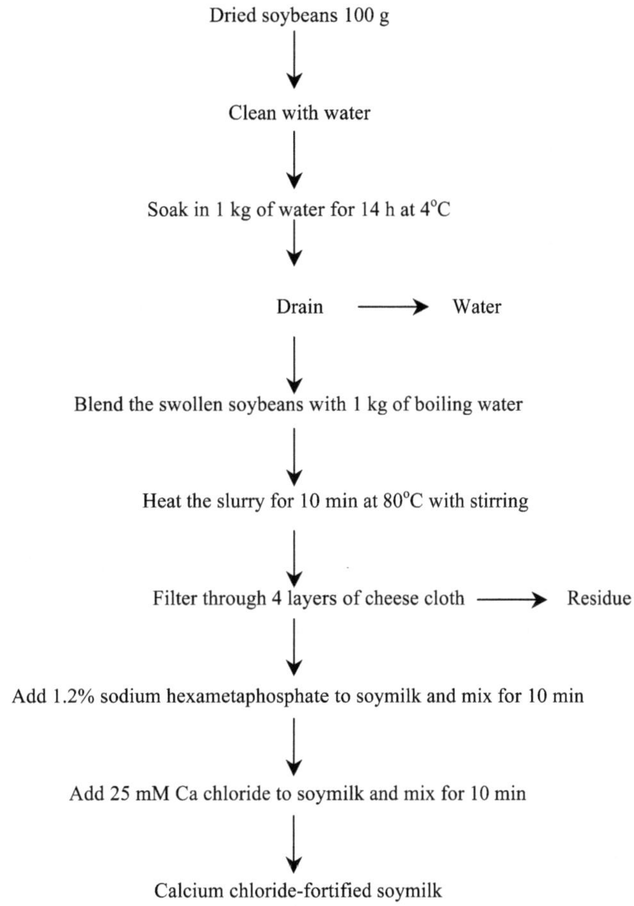

Fig. 15.1 Flow diagram for preparation of Ca chloride-fortified soymilk (from Pathomrungsiyounggul et al. [11], with permission)

Isoflavones

Soy isoflavones such as daidzein, glycitein and genistein, which are believed to confer health benefits related to the lower risk of heart disease, have been found in soymilk [20]. Total isoflavones in soymilk have been reported to be 182 μg/g on a wet weight basis [21]. Hot grinding of soybeans leads to a greater extraction of isoflavones into soymilk, compared to cold grinding but direct and indirect ultra high temperature treatment do not significantly influence the level of isoflavones [22]. Little information about isoflavones in CFSM is available. One study [9] reported that a serving (240 mL) of CFSMs contained 30.6 mg total isoflavones, which was equivalent to 127 μg/mL. Owing to their health benefits, the effects of Ca salts, chelating agent and methods for CFSM production on isoflavone levels in CFSM may warrant further study.

Total Ca

The total Ca of CFSMs has been successfully increased to a similar level to that of cow's milk (~120 mg/100 g) or higher, as summarised in Table 15.1. Total Ca consists of bound Ca and unbound Ca. It has been established that Ca ions are bound to protein and phytic acid in soymilk [23, 24]. In some cases CFSMs only reached a total Ca level of 60 % of that in cow's milk, for example, when

14 mM Ca of Ca lactate was added to soymilk; but it was still double the level of total Ca in human milk [14]. Total Ca of CFSMs was tested in samples taken from the top and bottom of the containers in some cases, and these were found not to be equal; the top section contained a lower amount [10], as presented in Table 15.1, presumably due to sedimentation of Ca-rich material. This suggests that the drink must be shaken well before consumption and also when samples are taken for analysis.

Calcium Bioavailability

There are two methods, in vitro and in vivo, for determination of Ca bioavailability. The in vitro method was chosen for CFSM because it is quicker, less complicated and cheaper [8]. The in vivo method reflects true bioavailability, but it is complicated, time-consuming and costly [9].

In a study [8] using an in vitro method that involved a simulated human gastrointestinal digestion followed by measurement of dialysable Ca, it was shown that Ca bioavailability followed the order: Ca carbonate-fortified soymilk > cow's milk > triCa phosphate-fortified soymilk [8]. The authors [8] also found that addition of carrageenan significantly reduced Ca bioavailability of triCa phosphate-fortified soymilk.

The Ca absorption from CFSMs and cow's milk was studied [9] in young women and the results showed that Ca bioavailability from Ca carbonate-fortified soymilk was similar to that of cow's milk, but both beverages had significantly higher Ca bioavailability than triCa phosphate-fortified soymilk.

The bioavailability of other CFSMs should be evaluated to ensure that they are a good source of Ca.

Calcium Ion Concentration ([Ca^{2+}])

Until recently there have been few reports on ionic Ca measurement in soymilk; however, several recent studies have provided more information. An unfortified soymilk was reported to contain a [Ca^{2+}] of 0.22 mM after pasteurisation [25]. This is much lower than mammalian milks, i.e. 1.43–2.50 mM in cows' milk at different stages of lactation [26].

The more soluble the Ca salt, the more Ca ions are liberated in solution and are available for reaction [7]. When freely soluble Ca salts, such as Ca gluconate and Ca lactate, were added, [Ca^{2+}] in soymilk increased significantly [25]. Similar results were found for adding Ca chloride as shown in Table 15.2. However, adding Ca carbonate and Ca citrate gave only a slight increase in [Ca^{2+}] in soymilk [25]. Coagulation generally occurs when [Ca^{2+}] in soymilk reaches approximately 0.40 mM [11].

Non-coagulated CFSMs contained much less [Ca^{2+}] than cow's milk [11, 25]. It has been found that Ca ions are better absorbed intestinally than Ca complexes, and it is frequently assumed that Ca is absorbed only in the form of dissolved Ca ions [27]. The low [Ca^{2+}] found in CFSM might on first appearance seem to provide only a small amount of Ca for nutritional purpose. However their Ca complexes may change after ingestion. One study [4] suggests that gastric acid in the stomach and intestine increases [Ca^{2+}] leading to greater Ca absorption.

Adding chelating agents clearly reduces [Ca^{2+}], as illustrated in Tables 15.2 and 15.3. The rate of [Ca^{2+}] reduction depends on the chelating agent (Table 15.3). Calcium ions were also reduced when stabilisers such as Ca-D-saccharic acid were added [15]. Adjustment of pH of CFSM was another contributing factor; increasing pH resulted in a lowering of [Ca^{2+}] [11]. There were insignificant changes of [Ca^{2+}] due to pasteurisation of CFSM (Table 15.3).

Phosphorus

Phosphorus is just as important as Ca for bone structure. As expected, the phosphorus content of Ca carbonate-fortified soymilk was the same as in soymilk (53 mg/100 mL) but phosphorus content in

Table 15.2 Effect of Ca chloride and sodium hexametaphosphate on [Ca^{2+}] (mM) of soymilk after pasteurisation

Sodium hexametaphosphate (%)	Added Ca chloride (mM Ca)		
	12.50	18.75	25.00
0	1.88±0.08 d(a)*	4.17±0.39 d(b)*	7.66±0.38 e(c)*
0.3	0.28±0.05 c(a)	0.89±0.13 c(b)*	1.96±0.19 d(c)*
0.5	0.20±0.07 bc(a)	0.41±0.06 b(b)*	0.99±0.10 c(c)*
0.7	0.17±0.04 ab(a)	0.33±0.05 ab(b)	0.59±0.04 b(c)*
0.9	0.09±0.02 a(a)	0.25±0.03 ab(b)	0.38±0.05 ab(c)
1.2	<0.02	0.05±0.02 a(a)	0.18±0.01 a(b)

[a]Means ± standard deviation in the same column followed by the same letter are not significantly different ($P>0.05$)
[(a)]Means ± standard deviation in the same row followed by the same letter are not significantly different ($P>0.05$)
*Coagulated after pasteurisation (from Pathomrungsiyounggul et al. [11], with permission)

Table 15.3 The [Ca^{2+}] (mM) of soymilks fortified with 25 mM Ca chloride

Chelating agent		[Ca^{2+}] (mM)	
Type	% (w/w)	Before pasteurisation	After pasteurisation
Sodium hexametaphosphate	0 (control)	8.55±0.17 c*	8.38±0.38 c*
	0.5	0.82±0.14 b	0.91±0.15 b*
	1.0	0.37±0.06 a	0.38±0.06 a
Disodium hydrogen orthophosphate	0 (control)	8.55±0.17 c*	8.38±0.38 c*
	0.5	1.11±0.17 b	0.78±0.13 b
	1.0	0.32±0.05 a	0.28±0.05 a
Trisodium citrate	0 (control)	8.55±0.17 c*	8.38±0.38 c*
	0.5	1.53±0.20 b*	1.51±0.18 b*
	1.0	0.50±0.06 a	0.50±0.06 a
Disodium ethylenediamine tetraacetic acid	0 (control)	8.55±0.17 c*	8.38±0.38 c*
	0.5	3.76±0.26 b*	3.75±0.21 b*
	1.0	1.25±0.23 a*	1.21±0.20 a*

No significant effect of pasteurisation on [Ca^{2+}] of samples (from Pathomrungsiyounggul et al. [18], with permission)
Means ± standard deviation of samples using the same type of chelating agent followed by the same letter are not significantly different ($P>0.05$)
*Sample showed coagulation

triCa phosphate-fortified soymilk increased to 109 mg/100 mL [8]. The latter CFSM, containing a higher phosphorus level, should be of more interest to the consumer.

pH

Generally, the pH of soymilk is slightly acidic and variations have been found among published reports. For example, pH has been reported as 6.48 [15], 6.60–6.62 [28] and 6.73 [11]. The pH is affected by soybean variety, soybean genotypes, location and year of growing, extraction methods and storage time of soymilk [28–30]. Soymilk pH decreases with increasing storage time of soybeans as well as their water activity [31], and the temperature and relative humidity of storage [32]. Soymilk pH reflects the freshness of soybeans and greatly influences soymilk coagulation, i.e. soymilk made from soybeans kept for a longer time, had a lower pH and coagulated with a lower amount of Ca chloride [31]. Thus manufacturers must control the quality of soybeans and soymilk pH in order to produce a CFSM of uniform quality.

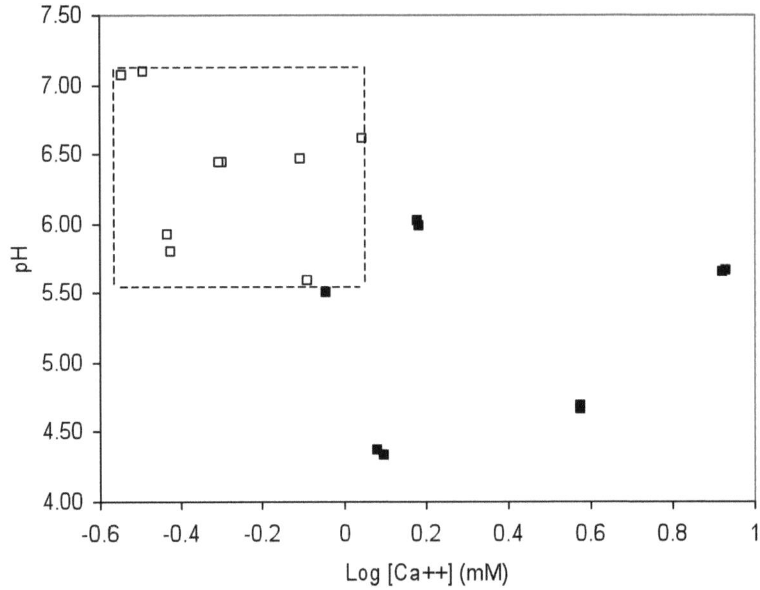

Fig. 15.2 Relationship between log of [Ca^{2+}] (log [Ca^{2+}]) and pH of CFSM (*open square* non-coagulated and *filled square* coagulated sample) (from Pathomrungsiyounggul et al. [18], with permission)

Addition of many Ca salts reduces the pH of soymilk. Those are Ca gluconate, Ca chloride, Ca acetate, Ca lactate, Ca sulphate, triCa phosphate, Ca citrate and Ca lactogluconate [10, 11, 16, 24, 25, 32–34]. An initial coagulation in soymilk occurred at about pH 6.0 regardless of the type of salt used [35]. It was found [33] that Ca citrate addition did not coagulate soymilk although it reduced pH to 5.57. The main cause of pH reduction in soymilk is that hydrogen ions are liberated when added Ca binds to phytate and protein [24]. Calcium carbonate increased significantly soymilk pH and as a result it did not coagulate soymilk [25].

Ideally, producers must adjust the pH of CFSM close to the pH of soymilk prior to its fortification. Some authors [12, 15] maintained pH of CFSMs between 6.70 and 6.85. Also, pasteurised CFSMs having pH slightly above 7.0 have been produced [10]. Chelating agents affect pH of CFSM. Addition of potassium citrate [16], trisodium citrate and disodium hydrogen orthophosphate [18] progressively increased the pH of CFSM but disodium ethylenediamine tetraacetic acid reduced pH of CFSM [18]. Sodium hexametaphosphate sometimes decreased and sometimes increased pH of CFSM. It caused a progressive reduction in pH in Ca lactogluconate-fortified soymilk [16]. Addition of 0.3 % sodium hexametaphosphate increased pH of soymilk with 12.5 mM added Ca chloride but decreased pH of soymilk with 25 mM added Ca chloride [11].

Pasteurisation did not affect pH of CFSM when trisodium citrate and disodium ethylenediamine tetraacetic acid were used as chelating agent but decreased pH when phosphate-based agents (sodium hexametaphosphate and disodium hydrogen orthophosphate) were used [18].

Storage time is another factor influencing soymilk pH. Pasteurised soymilks stored at ambient temperature (29 °C) and refrigerated temperature (10 °C) showed a reduction in pH [28]. In the case of sterilised CFSMs, there was little reduction in pH over 6 months' storage at 1 °C [10].

A relationship between pH and [Ca^{2+}] was observed [11] demonstrating that pH of CFSM decreased when [Ca^{2+}] increased. To fortify soymilk without coagulation, its pH needs to be maintained within the ranges 5.6–7.1 and [Ca^{2+}] should be 0.28–1.12 mM (i.e. log [Ca^{2+}] –0.55 and 0.05 mM) as illustrated in Fig. 15.2.

Physical Properties

Colour

Despite its importance, colour has been little studied in CFSM. Hunter L^*, a^* and b^* values of soymilk were 82.7, - 2.2 and 14.7, respectively [36]. It has been shown [8] that addition of Ca did not change the colour of soymilk when tested by Munsell™ colour book and observed by panellists. The effects of heat treatment and storage conditions, which normally affect the colour of foods, may warrant further study in CFSM.

Viscosity

Viscosity of CFSM is very important for acceptance of the product. Pasteurised CFSMs having satisfactory sensory tests had a viscosity of 5.7 cP when triCa phosphate was used and 4.9 cP when triCa phosphate and Ca citrate were used together [10]. Another study [25] found that soymilks fortified by Ca carbonate, triCa phosphate or Ca citrate had a viscosity of about 2 cP after pasteurisation, similar to that of unfortified soymilk. A sterilised Ca citrate-fortified soymilk had initial viscosity 7.1 cP and its viscosity reduced to 6.7 cP when it was stored at 1 °C for 6 months [10]. The flow behaviour index suggested that sterilised Ca citrate-fortified soymilk was pseudoplastic [10]. Moreover, the same authors [10] studied viscosity of triCa phosphate-fortified soymilk and soymilk fortified with Ca citrate plus triCa phosphate, which were sterilised and stored for 6 months, and found that viscosity decreased marginally during storage.

Addition of Ca lactate [14], Ca lactogluconate [16] and Ca chloride [11] increased soymilk viscosity. Fortifying these Ca salts in soymilk in order to reach the same Ca level as cow's milk produced an unacceptable viscosity. Trisodium citrate [14, 18], sodium hexametaphosphate [11, 16, 18], potassium citrate [16] and disodium hydrogen orthophosphate [18] showed a clear reduction in viscosity of CFSMs. However, disodium ethylenediamine tetraacetic acid increased viscosity [18]. Thus, not all types of chelating agents can be used in the formulation of stable CFSMs.

The results [14] showed that higher trisodium citrate concentration decreased the viscosity of sterilised Ca lactate-fortified soymilk but trisodium citrate, when used at 0.2 % and higher, did not greatly alter the viscosity of the samples because they were beyond the concentration required to prevent coagulation of CFSM. The same trend was found for other chelating agents. The viscosity of CFSMs became stable when sodium hexametaphosphate and potassium citrate were ≥1.0 % w/w and ≥0.65 % w/w, respectively [16]. The initial concentration of sodium hexametaphosphate required to stabilise the kinematic viscosity of CFSM was dependent on concentration of added Ca. It was found to be 0.5, 0.9 and 0.9 % sodium hexametaphosphate for soymilk with added 12.50, 18.75 and 25 mM Ca, respectively [11].

Generally, pasteurisation increased the absolute viscosity of CFSMs containing sodium hexametaphosphate, disodium hydrogen orthophosphate and trisodium citrate, although this was not statistically significant [18].

It was found [14] that when Ca lactate and trisodium citrate were added together before homogenisation, they might interact, reducing the availability of trisodium citrate to decrease viscosity of soymilk. Hence a suitable procedure to make a low viscosity CFSM was to add Ca lactate followed by homogenising and finally adding trisodium citrate.

Particle Size

Particle size influences the mouth-feel of drinks. Bovine milk provides a better mouth-feel than cereal milk because bovine milk is creamier, while cereal milk is watery. Therefore to produce cereal milk

Table 15.4 Effect of Ca and sodium hexametaphosphate on mean particle diameter (nm) of pasteurised soymilk

Sodium hexametaphosphate (%)	Added Ca chloride (mM Ca)		
	12.50	18.75	25.00
0	>1,000*	>1,000*	>1,000*
0.3	717.1 ±131.2 b	>1,000*	>1,000*
0.5	460.6±24.5 a	>1,000*	>1,000*
0.7	423.5±12.4 a(a)	498.7±44.1 b(b)	>1,000*
0.9	379.9±21.6 a(a)	438.3±10.9 a(b)	556.2±34.1 b(c)
1.2	406.6±25.0 a(a)	404.0±9.0 a(a)	438.0±42.6 a(a)

[a]Means ± standard deviation in the same column followed by the same letter are not significantly different ($P>0.05$).
[(a)]Means ± standard deviation in the same row followed by the same letter are not significantly different ($P>0.05$).
*Coagulated after pasteurisation (from Pathomrungsiyounggul et al. [11], with permission)

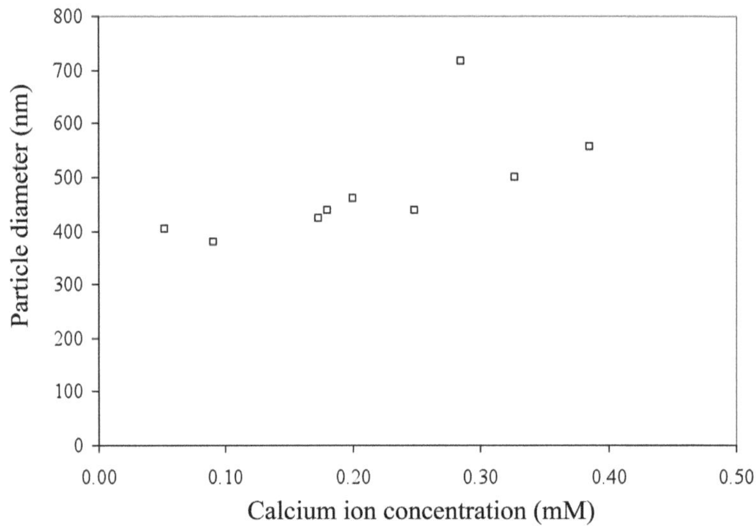

Fig. 15.3 Relationship between [Ca^{2+}] and particle diameter in Ca chloride-fortified soymilk which did not coagulate (from Pathomrungsiyounggul et al. [11], with permission)

with favourable mouth-feel, its particle diameter should be 400–500 nm [37]. A commercial bovine milk and a commercial CFSM had mean particle diameters of 450 and 420 nm, respectively, and they both exhibited creaming [38]. The particle diameters of soymilk fortified by Ca carbonate, triCa phosphate and Ca citrate were 327, 358 and 451 nm, respectively [25].

A literature report [39] explained that when adding Ca to soymilk, the protein particles (80 nm) first combine with the oil globules (350 nm), and then the bound globules aggregate with each other. As a result, the particle size of soymilk becomes larger and eventually coagulates. These results are presented in Table 15.4. It is assumed that in coagulated soy protein the oil globule is coated with three layers of proteins: oleosin, particulate proteins and soluble proteins [39]. Addition of some chelating agents reduced particle size of CFSM [18]. A significant reduction in particle size of CFSM due to addition of sodium hexametaphosphate is presented in Table 15.4. Figure 15.3 shows how particle size increased as [Ca^{2+}] increased in Ca chloride-fortified soymilk.

Shelf-Life of CFSM

The shelf-life of soymilk depends on the raw materials, processing conditions and type of packaging used. For example, pasteurised, sterilised and ultra high temperature treated soymilk should have a shelf-life of 1 week under refrigerated storage, at least 2 years without refrigeration and 6–8 months without refrigeration, respectively [1]. Little information is available on the shelf-life of CFSM. Pasteurised CFSMs were judged to be acceptable in flavour and chalkiness by panellists after 10 days' storage at 1 °C [10]. A pasteurised CFSM had a refrigerated shelf-life of approximately 3 weeks [12]. The sterilised Ca citrate-fortified soymilk still had acceptable sensory characteristics after 6 months' storage at room temperature or 1 °C [10]. Most of the other studies in CFSM did not investigate shelf-life of CFSMs, but focused on their physical and chemical properties [8, 11, 14–16, 18, 25, 38] and nutritional status [8, 9]. More research on shelf-life of CFSM may be useful.

Guidance on Safe Levels

The addition of Ca salts as discussed in this review in order to raise total Ca in soymilk to that of cow's milk (~120 mg/100 g) should pose no harm to humans at the concentrations recommended. The awareness should be focused on usage of chelating agents. Since chelating agents can react with a variety of metal ions, they may bind not only Ca ion but also other ions in CFSM. Hence the effect of chelating agent on ions of other important minerals, such as magnesium and iron, may need to be studied to ensure that the CFSM dose not have any undesirable effects on human health.

Recommendations

To produce CFSM requires considerable care and a good understanding of the interactions caused by Ca ions, pH, soy proteins and chelating agents, and their effects on chemical and physical properties, and to the sensory quality of the drink. The [Ca^{2+}] is an important property which governs the coagulation behaviour in soymilk and is hence a very useful indicator for investigating the effect of ingredients and processes on the quality of this healthy drink. It is vital that the products should be stable throughout storage and the Ca should be effectively dispersed within the soymilk.

Conclusions

This review concludes that, while scientific studies on the preparation and properties of CFSM are limited, it is possible to prepare a satisfactory product with similar Ca levels to cows' milk, by the addition of Ca salts to soymilk, in conjunction with appropriate chelating agents. Assuming that the production methods are appropriate, the organoleptic and physicochemical properties of these products should be acceptable to the consumer, and the products should offer similar nutritional availability of Ca to that of cows' milk.

References

1. Liu K. Soybeans: chemistry, technology, and utilization. New York: Chapman & Hall; 1999.
2. Omoni A, Aluko RE. Soy foods and their benefits: potential mechanisms of action. Nutr Rev. 2005;63:272–83.
3. US Department of Agriculture. National nutrient database for standard reference release 24. http://ndb.nal.usda.gov/ndb/foods/list. Accessed 10 Feb 2012.
4. Theobald HE. Dietary calcium and health. Nutr Bull. 2005;30:237–77.
5. Gerstner G. Feasibility of calcium fortification in dairy and soy drinks. Food Mark Technol. 2005;18:10–4.
6. Wade MA. Calcium: the chosen form. Prepared Food. 2004;173(5):61–7.
7. Gerstner G. How to fortify beverages with calcium. Drink Tech Market. 2003;7:8–11.
8. Chaiwanon P, Puwastien P, Nitithamyong A, Sirichakwal PP. Calcium fortification in soybean milk and in vitro bioavailability. J Food Compos Anal. 2000;13:319–27.
9. Zhao Y, Martin BR, Weaver CM. Calcium bioavailability of calcium carbonate fortified soymilk is equivalent to cow's milk in young women. J Nutr. 2005;135:2379–82.
10. Weingartner KE, Nelson AI, Erdman JWJ. Effects of calcium addition on stability and sensory properties of soy beverage. J Food Sci. 1983;48:256–7; 263.
11. Pathomrungsiyounggul P, Grandison AS, Lewis MJ. Effects of calcium chloride and sodium hexametaphosphate on certain chemical and physical properties of soymilk. J Food Sci. 2007;72:E428–34.
12. Zemel MB, Shelef LA. Calcium fortified soy milk. European Patent. Applicant number 85309154.4; 1986.
13. Goldscher RL, Edelstein S. Calcium citrate: a revised look at calcium fortification. Food Technol. 1996;50:96–8.
14. Prabharaksa C, Olek AC, Steinkraus KH. Enrichment of soybean milk with calcium. Acta Biotechnol. 1989;9:9–16.
15. Rasyid F, Hansen PMT. Stabilization of soy milk fortified with calcium gluconate. Food Hydrocoll. 1991;4:415–22.
16. Yazici F, Alvarez VB, Mangino ME, Hansen PMT. Formulation and processing of a heat stable calcium-fortified soy milk. J Food Sci. 1997;62:535–8.
17. Kohyama K, Sano Y, Doi E. Rheological characteristics and gelation mechanism of tofu (soybean curd). J Agric Food Chem. 1995;43:1808–12.
18. Pathomrungsiyounggul P, Grandison AS, Lewis MJ. Effects of calcium-chelating agents and pasteurisation on certain properties of calcium-fortified soymilk. Food Chem. 2010;118:808–14.
19. Hirotsuka M, Taniguchi H, Narita H, Kito M. Calcium fortification of soy milk with calcium-lecithin liposome system. J Food Sci. 1984;49:1111–2, 1127.
20. Kao TH, Lu YF, Hsieh HC, Chen BH. Stability of isoflavone glucosides during processing of soymilk and tofu. Food Res Int. 2004;37:891–900.
21. Prabhakaran MP, Perera CO, Valiyaveettil S. Effect of different coagulants on the isoflavone levels and physical properties of prepared from tofu. Food Chem. 2006;99:492–9.
22. Prabhakaran MP, Perera CO. Effect of extraction methods and UHT treatment conditions on the level of isoflavones during soymilk manufacture. Food Chem. 2006;99:231–7.
23. Saio K, Koyama E, Yamazaki S, Watanabe T. Protein-calcium-phytic acid relationships in soybean: part III: effect of phytic acid on coagulative reaction in tofu-making. Agric Biol Chem. 1969;33:36–42.
24. Ono T, Katho S, Mothizuki K. Influences of calcium and pH on protein solubility in soybean milk. Biosci Biotech Biochem. 1993;57:24–8.
25. Pathomrungsiyounggul P, Grandison AS, Lewis MJ. Effect of calcium carbonate, calcium citrate, tricalcium phosphate, calcium gluconate and calcium lactate on some physicochemical properties of soymilk. Int J Food Sci Technol. 2010;45:2234–40.
26. Lin MJ, Lewis MJ, Grandison AS. Measurement of ionic calcium in milk. Int J Dairy Technol. 2006;59:192–9.
27. Gerstner G. How can we get more calcium? Int Food Ingred. 2003;3:24–6.
28. Iwuoha CI, Umunnakwe KE. Chemical, physical and sensory characteristics of soymilk as affected by processing method, temperature and duration of storage. Food Chem. 1997;59:373–9.
29. Lim BT, DeMan JM, DeMan L, Buzzell RI. Yield and quality of tofu as affected by soybean and soymilk characteristics. calcium sulfate coagulant. J Food Sci. 1990;55:1088–92.
30. Poysa V, Woodrow L. Stability of soybean seed composition and its effect on soymilk and tofu yield and quality. Food Res Int. 2002;35:337–45.
31. Liu ZS, Chang SKC. Optimal coagulant concentration, soymilk and tofu quality as affected by a short-term model storage of proto soybeans. J Food Process Preserv. 2008;32:39–59.
32. Kong F, Chang SKC, Liu Z, Wilson LA. Changes of soybean quality during storage as related to soymilk and tofu making. J Food Sci. 2008;73:S134–43.
33. Kamel BS, deMan JM. Composition and properties of bean curd made from Ontario soybeans. Can Inst Food Sci Technol J. 1982;15:273–6.

34. Shun-Tang G, Ono T, Mikami M. Incorporation of soy milk lipid into protein coagulum by addition of calcium chloride. J Agric Food Chem. 1999;47:901–5.
35. Lu JY, Carter E, Chung RA. Use of calcium salts for soybean curd preparation. J Food Sci. 1980;45:32–4.
36. Lakshmanan R, Lamballerie MD, Jung S. Effect of soybean-to-water ratio and pH on pressurized soymilk properties. J Food Sci. 2006;71:E384–91.
37. Saeseaw S, Shiowatana J, Siripinyanond A. Sedimentation field-flow fraction: size characterization of food materials. Food Res Int. 2005;38:777–86.
38. Durand A, Franks GV, Hosken RW. Particle sizes and stability of UHT bovine, cereal and grain milks. Food Hydrocoll. 2003;17:671–8.
39. Ono T. Soy (soya) cheeses. In: Caballero B, Trugo LC, Finglas PM, editors. Encyclopedia of food science and nutrition. London: Academic; 2003. p. 5398–402.

Chapter 16
The Stability of Water-Soluble Vitamins and Issues in the Fortification of Foods

Lan T.T. Bui, Darryl M. Small, and Ross Coad

Key Points

- Vitamin stability is not readily predictable as it is often determined by multiple factors acting within the food matrix.
- Staple foods including grains are often used as vehicles for fortification as they are consumed frequently and in sufficient quantity by the target population to ensure a high likelihood of consumption of the desired amount of fortificant.
- Rice is a staple food for more than half the world's population and offers a largely untapped potential for fortification.
- Modern processing and fortification techniques are likely to result in greatly improved accessibility to fortified rice.
- The vitamin contents of commercially available noodles are highly variable.
- The stability of B-group vitamins added as fortificants to three types of noodles prepared under experimental conditions varied among the types.
- In these studies, overall losses were high and typically more than half of the added vitamin was lost upon cooking.
- Folic acid was the most stable of the vitamins and these noodle products represent suitable vehicles for enhancing dietary intakes of this nutrient.
- Further investigation into the B-group vitamins is warranted regarding ways to enhance stability, particularly where alkaline conditions contribute to losses of riboflavin and thiamin.

Keywords Asian noodles • B-group vitamins • Cereal grain foods • Fortification • Folate • Vitamin stability • Vitamin analysis • Vitamin retention

L.T.T. Bui, BSc. FoodTech (Hons), PhD. (✉) • R. Coad, BAppSc, MBA
Human Protection and Performance Division, Defence Science and Technology Organisation,
76 George Street, Scottsdale, TAS 7260, Australia
e-mail: Lan.bui@dsto.defence.gov.au; rosscoad@hotmail.com

D.M. Small, BScAgr (Hons), PhD
School of Applied Sciences, RMIT University, La Trobe Street, GPO Box 2476V,
Melbourne, VIC 3001, Australia
e-mail: small.darryl@gmail.com

V.R. Preedy et al. (eds.), *Handbook of Food Fortification and Health: From Concepts to Public Health Applications Volume 1*, Nutrition and Health, DOI 10.1007/978-1-4614-7076-2_16,

Introduction

Vitamins are organic compounds, essential for normal metabolism. The human body cannot manufacture vitamins, with two exceptions: niacin, which can be synthesised from dietary tryptophan, and vitamin D, which can be synthesised when the skin is exposed to sunlight. However, dietary sources of niacin and vitamin D remain important as, depending on the amount of dietary tryptophan and level of exposure to sunlight, the amount synthesised may be insufficient to meet the needs of the body.

Vitamins, or their precursors, are required in small amounts regularly from the diet. Vitamins are classified as being either fat-soluble vitamins—which are not discussed here—and those that are water soluble, comprising ascorbic acid (vitamin C) and the B group: thiamin (B1), riboflavin (B2), niacin (B3), pantothenic acid (B5), B6 (pyridoxine, pyridoxal, pyridoxamine), biotin (B7), folate (B9) and cobalamin (B12). These vitamins are not generally stored in the body, except for folate and B12, found in the liver, and ascorbic acid occurring in many body tissues.

When vitamin intakes would otherwise be too low—possible reasons include naturally low levels, processing losses, poor access to good nutrition, special needs—it may be appropriate to provide vitamins in supplements or through fortification. Some water-soluble vitamins are far more important as fortificants than others: fortification of cereal staples with thiamin, riboflavin, niacin and/or folate is performed either on a voluntary or mandatory basis in most countries around the world. Incorporation of ascorbic acid is also permitted in most countries and this is also commonly used as an antioxidant.

Stability of the Vitamins

In general, vitamin losses can occur at any stage from harvest up to the moment of consumption. One of the characteristics of the water-soluble vitamins is their instability during food preparation, processing and storage. The physical characteristics and stability of added B-group vitamins are summarised in Table 16.1. Susceptibilities vary among the vitamins but causes of losses include leaching into water during cleaning and cooking, thermal effects associated with food processing, storage or preparation, light stimulated degradation, oxidation and other chemical reactions due to pH conditions and other food components. Stability is not readily predictable as it is often determined by multiple factors acting within the food matrix.

Losses during preparation and processing will be covered in more detail later in the context of selected foods. Removing one or more of the reactants may control losses due to degradation reactions that proceed during storage. Careful consideration of ingredients, water activity, food matrix, headspace and packaging materials may lead to longer term retention of naturally present or added vitamins. In a recent study, losses of added vitamins during 2 years storage at 30 °C were not significant in fortified freeze dried meals that had been nitrogen flushed then vacuum packed in a high barrier foil laminate material [2].

The use of specialised processing and packaging techniques may be appropriate and warranted for some special purpose foods, but large scale fortification programmes intended to achieve public health outcomes require more economical approaches and generally operate on shorter shelf lives. These programmes look to fortify foods that are used frequently and in sufficient quantity by the target population to ensure a high likelihood of consumption of the desired amount of fortificant. Staple foods, particularly grains, are therefore often used as vehicles for fortification.

Table 16.1 Vitamin B fortificants: physical characteristics and stability

Vitamin	Fortificant compound	Physical characteristics	Stability
Thiamin (B1)	Thiamin hydrochloride	More soluble in water than the mononitrate form White or almost white	Both forms are stable to oxygen in the absence of light and moisture but are unstable in the presence of sulfites
	Thiamin mononitrate	White or almost white	Losses during leavening and baking are estimated to be 15–20 % Available in a coated form. The mononitrate is preferred for dry products
Riboflavin (B2)	Riboflavin	Relatively water insoluble Yellow	Very unstable in light Rapid loss from milk on exposure to light but stable in white bread
	Sodium salt of riboflavin 5′-phosphate	Soluble in water Yellow	
Niacin	Niacin (nicotinic acid)	Soluble in alkali, sparingly soluble in water White	Very stable to oxygen, heat and light, both in the dry state and in aqueous solution
	Niacinamide (nicotinamide)	Water soluble White	
Pyridoxine (B6)	Pyridoxine hydrochloride	White or almost white	Stable in oxygen and heat, but relatively sensitive to UV light Available in a coated form
Folic acid (B9)	Pteroyl monoglutamic acid	Sparingly soluble in water, soluble in dilute acid and alkali Yellow-orange	Moderately stable to heat. Stable in solution at neutral pH but increasingly unstable at higher or lower pH Unstable in UV light
Vitamin B12 (cobalamin)	Cyanocobalamin	Pure vitamin B12 is sparingly soluble in water; the diluted forms are however completely soluble Dark red, often supplied diluted on a carrier (0.1 %)	Relatively stable to oxygen and heat in neutral and acid solution, but unstable in alkali and strong acids, in strong light, and in alkaline solutions at >100 °C

With permission from [1]

Cereal Grain Foods as Staple Foods

World grain production for 2009 included 819 million metric tonnes (mmt) of maize (corn), 686 mmt of wheat and 685 mmt of rice [3]. In some countries maize is an important human food crop; however, in most developed countries around 80 % is used as livestock feed [4]. Global consumption of maize as a human food ranks behind that of wheat and rice. The maize used in developing countries for human consumption is used to some extent as milled grain, for example as polenta, but most is used in processed forms including corn syrup.

Increasingly, fortification of maize has been demonstrated to be beneficial and is practised in Latin American countries and sub-Saharan Africa, where it is a staple food [5–7]. Fortification of corn masa flour has also been proposed as a public health measure aimed at Hispanics in the United States of America [8, 9]. Global guidelines for the fortification of wheat and maize flours have been published [10].

Table 16.2 Losses of thiamin during cooking of pasta and noodle products

Product	Thiamin content (mg/kg)[a]	Thiamin loss (%)[b]	References
Spaghetti	1.09	58	[11]
Asian white salted noodles[c] (4 brands)	1.36 (0.76–1.55)	61.7 (46.1–69.1)	[12]
Asian yellow alkaline noodles[c] (5 brands)	0.64 (0.28–1.76)	49.9 (27.3–62.5)	
Asian instant noodles[c] (5 brands)	1.06 (0.66–1.55)	71.4 (66.3–80.1)	
Spaghetti	9.3–13.7	41.9–56.1	[13]
Egg noodles	10.0–12.9	43.4–57.9	
Macaroni	9.9–11.1	30.6–65.7	
Spaghetti	9.4–14.0	46 (43–48)	[14]
Egg noodles	9.0–11.5	42 (10–55)	
Macaroni	8.1–10.9	43 (37–50)	
Noodles, eggs enriched	11.3±0.60	30.7	[15]
Noodles, eggs, spinach enriched	10.9±0.65	38.2	
Noodles, Japanese, soba	4.8±0.17	34.8	
Noodles, Japanese, somen	1.0±0.04	48.4	
Spaghetti, enriched	8.91±0.35	29.8	
Spaghetti, protein-fortified	11.9±0.59	47.8	
Spaghetti, whole-wheat	4.9±0.34	40.6	

Table compiled from published data (references cited)
[a]Thiamin contents are expressed in units of mg/kg in the product as purchased and average of values are presented where different brands were analysed or as mean value ± sd where possible for individual samples
[b]Thiamin loss values are expressed as the percentage loss from dried to cooked product with allowance for changes in moisture during cooking
[c]Cooking times were those recommended on product labels—no times were provided for the alkaline noodles so the optimum cooking times were determined and used

Wheat is a staple food on a global basis and owing to its higher protein content than maize and rice, it is a primary source of vegetable protein. The grain is typically milled to provide white flour, despite the increasing interest in wholegrain foods in developed countries, along with the mounting evidence that higher extraction rates provide a diversity of advantages to health and well-being. However, the milling of grain to produce white flour provides flours having excellent processing characteristics and the resultant products have appearance and texture which is appealing to consumers. Whilst wheat grain is typically regarded as a good source of a number of important micronutrients, it has long been recognised that these are concentrated in the outer layers, which are removed during milling. As a further example of losses of B-group vitamins in cereal products, thiamin data for the cooking of noodles and pasta are presented in Table 16.2. Despite the indications of low rates of retention, it is of concern that foods formulated using wheat flour have been and continue to be regarded as suitable vehicles for fortification, partly reflecting their status as staples.

Vitamins and Asian Noodle Products

In a major investigation of Asian wheat flour noodles the amounts of selected vitamins have been studied along with an evaluation of vitamin retention, the influence of processing and storage parameters and potential for fortification. These studies have focussed on thiamin, riboflavin, folates, and vitamin B6 with particular emphasis upon three commonly identified styles of Asian wheat flour noodles. These were selected as they have traditionally been popular in many Asian countries.

The history of noodles can be traced back 4,000 years to northwestern China [16]. Currently, in many Asian countries, 20–50 % of total wheat flour consumption is in the form of noodles [17].

In China, the world's largest producer and consumer of wheat, 40 % of wheat flour is consumed as noodles. The instant forms of noodles, which were introduced to the Japanese market in 1958 [18], have been a major growth product around the world and continue to increase in popularity [17].

Although there was probably a common origin of European pasta products and Asian noodles, there are strong reasons for a thorough investigation of Asian noodles. Firstly, the species of wheat are different: noodles are made from finely milled "bread" or common wheat (*Triticum aestivum*) representing 90–95 % of world wheat production, whereas pasta is typically prepared from semolina, which is a coarse and "gritty" product from milling of durum wheat (*T. durum*). Secondly, the commercial preparation of pasta involves an extrusion process, whereas Asian noodles are prepared by repeated sheeting and cutting of a dough. Our recent investigations have shown quite varied retention of different vitamins with losses as high as 97 % in one case.

Vitamins in Commercial Asian Noodles

A range of noodle samples, representing the traditional white salted, yellow alkaline and instant noodles, were purchased and analysed to determine the levels of folate, thiamin, riboflavin and vitamin B6. Samples were selected to include as many different countries as practically possible. This was partly to incorporate variations in factors such as the geographic and genetic origins of wheat used, the organoleptic preferences of the consumers, the ingredient formulations as well as the processing conditions applied during manufacture [12, 19].

In preliminary studies it was found that the levels of vitamin B6 and riboflavin in wheat flours and commercial samples of noodles were relatively low. Therefore, more detailed studies of commercial noodle samples were restricted to analysis of folate [19] and thiamin [12]. For these, samples were analysed for pH and vitamin content both before and after cooking. The findings were that:

- The measured pH values generally confirmed those expected for each sample (Table 16.3). However the appearance and pH of some samples were not consistent with the listing of ingredients declared in the labelling and packaging of the product. The vitamin content results were interpreted in relation to the measured pH values of the samples.
- The pH values of yellow alkaline noodles varied widely. The appearance of some products may have resulted from the presence of undeclared colorants.
- Considerable variation was observed in the levels of each of the vitamins in the noodles. For total folate the range was 53–393 μg/kg and for thiamin 0.11–1.76 mg/kg (dry weight basis).
- Overall, yellow alkaline noodles with high pH values had lower thiamin and higher total folate contents than the other styles of noodles.
- Interpreting the data for the commercial products was difficult because the results indicated that some of the noodles might have been made from fortified flours.

Table 16.3 The pH values of Asian wheat flour noodles

Noodle style	pH of noodles prepared traditionally[a]	Incorporation of alkaline salts (%)[b]	pH of commercial products[c]
White salted	5.9	0	3.9–5.9 (11)
Yellow alkaline	10.6	1.0	7.9–10.4 (8)
Instant	7.6	0.1	6.1–8.2 (14)

Table compiled from unpublished and published data (references cited).

[a]Mean values for samples prepared under laboratory conditions using sodium carbonate at the incorporation rates shown.

[b]Values expressed relative to a flour weight of 100 %.

[c]Samples selected to include a wide range of origins and values in parentheses indicate number of different brands analysed [12, 19].

- When the influence of cooking was investigated there appeared to be no clear pattern or trend although significant losses were observed in virtually all samples evaluate.

From the results for commercial noodle samples, it was difficult to draw conclusions regarding the factors which might have been responsible for the observed vitamin contents. It is likely that the results were ultimately due to the combination of a number of factors. The extent of flour fortification was unclear, as was the influence of other ingredients. Although limited in number, the results for flours reported in related studies also indicate quite wide variations in vitamin contents [20]. Some of the relevant factors may be the environment, genetic variability or milling parameters, or a combination of these.

Laboratory Investigation of Noodle Retention and Fortification

In order to further investigate the factors determining vitamin contents and stability in these products, the three styles of Asian noodles were prepared in the laboratory under controlled conditions. Procedures for the preparation of each style of noodle were selected to reflect formulations and processes widely used in commercial manufacture. However, it must be recognised that noodle preparation practices vary considerably among different countries, regions within countries and even among individual manufacturers.

Noodles were made from commercial flours and in many of the experiments the formulation included vitamin added as a fortificant. The primary purposes were to assess the effects of ingredients and processing conditions, the relative importance of processing and cooking as contributors to losses of the vitamins, along with storage, and the potential of particular styles of noodles to act as vehicles for fortification.

In order to provide a clear understanding of the losses, samples representing noodles at each stage of processing were analysed and the results are presented in Table 16.4 as cumulative values. The overall

Table 16.4 Comparison of cumulative losses of B-group vitamins during processing and cooking of three styles of Asian noodles

Noodle style and processing stage		B6 %	Riboflavin %	Folate %	Thiamin %
White salted					
Flour →	Dough	21.7	8.6	1.3	0.0
	↓				
	Dried	21.7	27.1	1.3	1.0
	↓				
	Cooked	57.3	52.9	41.3	44.2
Yellow alkaline					
Flour →	Dough	20.3	11.9	0.93	25.4
	↓				
	Dried	20.3	36.4	1.55	91.4
	↓				
	Cooked	62.2	71.1	40.9	96.7
Instant					
Flour →	Dough	21.7	11.3	0.94	4.9
	↓				
	Steamed	23.1	13.9	20.3	8.1
	↓				
	Fried	42.7	38.4	31.9	24.0
	↓				
	Cooked	65.7	51.6	43.4	67.8

Cumulative relative losses compared to vitamin levels in the ingredient formulation. Table compiled from published data [21–24].

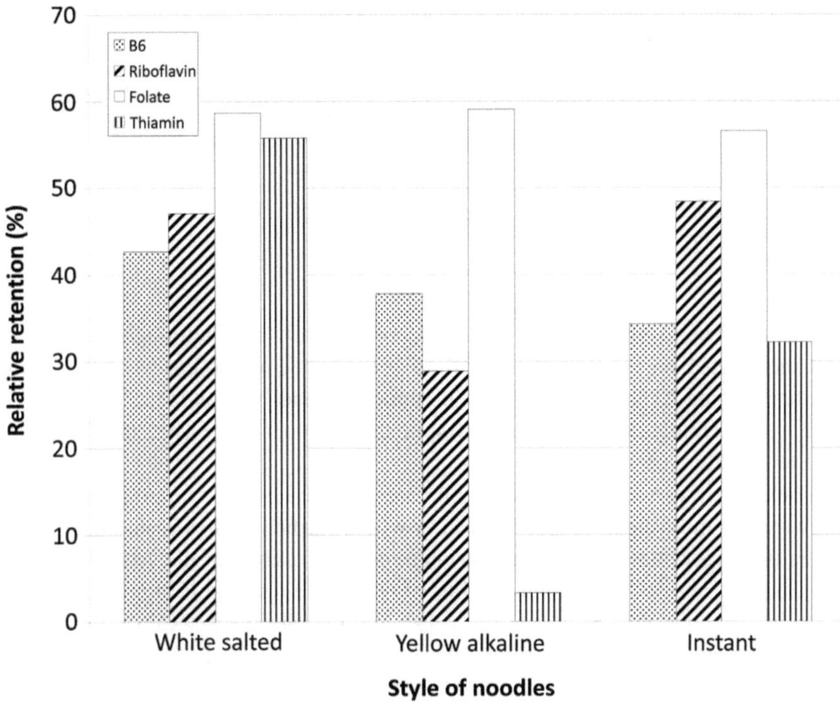

Fig. 16.1 Retention of B-group vitamins in three styles of Asian noodles. Values compare levels remaining in the processed product, after preparation for consumption, to that in the initial formulation. Compiled from published data [21–24]

losses of all of the vitamins are high in each of the styles of Asian noodles (Fig. 16.1). The vitamin demonstrating the greatest stability is folate for which the losses were essentially the same in all three styles. The overall losses for B6 were higher but again similar for each style and the highest losses were for riboflavin and thiamin in yellow alkaline noodles. The data shows that not only were all total losses high, in most cases there were significant losses during cooking. However there are quite different patterns when cooking and processing are compared. In some cases there was virtually no loss during noodle processing (folate in white salted and yellow alkaline as well as thiamin in white salted). In contrast there were very high losses of thiamin in yellow alkaline noodles during processing.

When the cumulative losses are compared, further differences in the patterns are highlighted. Firstly, the losses during dough mixing are surprisingly high in some cases. Thus 20 % of B6 is lost in mixing of all styles and for yellow alkaline noodles both riboflavin and thiamin were lost at this stage. The latter observations can be explained by the relatively high pH of the yellow alkaline noodles and the known instability of both riboflavin and thiamin under these conditions. The similar level of losses for B6 for each of the styles indicates that pH is not the primary factor and the findings for B6 during dough mixing cannot be readily explained from the known characteristics of this vitamin.

White salted and yellow alkaline noodles are often dried after preparation and for this step vitamin losses were typically low. However, the results for riboflavin were relatively high for both styles of noodles [22]. This indicates that pH was not the primary reason for the losses of riboflavin; the temperature of 40 °C, together with the moisture present in the dough, may have been sufficiently high to have an effect on riboflavin. The same effect was not observed for thiamin which was stable during the drying of white salted noodles whereas the very high loss of thiamin in yellow alkaline noodles is attributed to pH (Table 16.3). These results are consistent with the relatively low thiamin contents found in commercial samples which had the higher pH values.

The losses in the vitamins at each stage of processing for instant noodles do not show a strong response to pH except in the case of thiamin where overall losses were intermediate between those of

Table 16.5 Main factors influencing loss of B-group vitamins in Asian noodles

Vitamin	Factors causing losses
Vitamin B6	Losses during dough mixing and during high temperature treatments. Not influenced by pH.
Riboflavin	Some losses on dough mixing, significant losses on drying at 40 °C. Losses during high temperature treatments. Each of these loss effects is increased at high pH.
Folate	Only affected by high temperatures, pH has little effect.
Thiamin	Losses at any stage where high pH or high temperature applies.

Unpublished data

the other two styles. The losses during steaming were generally low, although the time period was 2 min. This is unexpected, particularly as the boiling of each style of noodles was associated with high losses. The folate loss of 20 % is quite high and cannot be readily explained. The losses during the deep-frying of instant noodles were also high, despite the short period of 45 s, and these are attributed to the use of a temperature of 150 °C.

Although some analyses were carried out to investigate the levels of vitamins which had leached into cooking water, in most cases the levels were low and further studies would be required to fully explore the relative importance of leaching and chemical degradation of the vitamins lost from Asian noodles [21]. Cooking of dried processed noodles of each style resulted in significant losses for each of the vitamins in dried noodles. In the case of folate and thiamin these results largely confirm those found for commercial noodles [19]. When samples of noodles were cooked for varying times, including for periods well beyond the optimum point, the thiamin content continued to decline. Ideally noodles should be cooked for periods as short as possible to minimise the losses. Further analyses for thiamin showed additional losses upon extended storage of dried noodles were minimal [20].

Many of the results reported from the current study are consistent with existing knowledge. However, the pattern for folate provides an interesting comparison with published information [19]. Typically folates are regarded as relatively unstable under most conditions known to adversely affect retention of vitamin compounds in foods. It has also been reported that different forms of folate vary in stability characteristics [25]. The findings here for Asian noodles highlight the difficulties in using previous findings for the prediction of vitamin stability and demonstrate that direct studies of specific products under laboratory conditions can have considerable value.

The primary conclusions from these studies of noodle processing are that the overall losses of each vitamin are high, the patterns of loss are different for individual vitamins and these relate to the style of Asian noodles. The investigation of laboratory noodles also shows that different factors cause losses for each of the four B-group vitamins. The specific factors identified are summarised in Table 16.5.

If Asian noodles were to be fortified with the B-group vitamins studied here, the relatively high losses of the vitamins would require the addition of substantial overages for each of the vitamins and for each of the styles of noodles. In the cases of thiamin and riboflavin in yellow alkaline noodles, as well as B6 in all styles, fortification may not be practical unless some means can be found to enhance the stability of the vitamin during manufacture of these products.

The recent studies have concentrated on wheat noodles. Whilst there is now a strong scientific basis for understanding the retention of some of the water-soluble vitamins in noodles made from wheat flours, it cannot be assumed that similar results would be obtained for the various forms of noodles for which the formulation is based upon other starch-rich ingredients [26] including mung bean starch, tapioca, and rice flour.

It would also be of value to extend this work to other flour and cereal grain foods. Preliminary data from our laboratory (Table 16.6) shows that the use of niacin as a fortificant for instant noodles is effective as retention is high. In contrast, ascorbic acid is less stable during processing of this product. Microencapsulation may provide a means of enhancing retention of fortificants and recently the use of hydrocolloids for protection of ascorbic acid has been described [27].

Table 16.6 Retention of fortificants during processing of instant noodles

Fortificant	Dough following mixing	Dried product
Ascorbic acid	93	63
Nicotinic acid	100	93

Percent retention with respect to the vitamin present in the formulation including the added fortificant, with adjustment for changes in moisture contents. Unpublished data.

Fortification of Rice

Rice is another of the major food staples, the most important food crop of the developing world and the staple food of more than half of the world's population [28]. Grains of rice are usually milled to remove the outer layer, thereby improving ease of cooking and palatability. This has the same effect as the milling of wheat and other grains: loss of most of the vitamins and minerals. In contrast to wheat however, rice is predominantly used as a grain rather than being milled to a flour.

The large size of the particles (the rice grain) as it is commonly used, the fact that washing often occurs prior to cooking and the use of excess water for cooking and subsequent loss of soluble components when the water is discarded, are all issues in the effectiveness of attempts to fortify rice. Early approaches relied on dusting the grains with the fortificants, but this was ineffective. Fortification of rice has also been relatively limited as the techniques used with other grain staples—addition to the grain flour—are not directly applicable to rice.

Four main rice fortification techniques have been identified [29]. Two of the processes—hot extrusion and cold extrusion—are based on addition of fortificant to rice flour dough followed by extrusion to produce simulated rice grains. These techniques overcome the difficulty of adding fortificant to whole grains of rice but the end product can be used in a similar manner to polished rice. The third process involves coating grains of rice with the fortificant by spraying with a fortificant mixture. A variation on this is to soak the grains in a fortificant solution at an elevated temperature. The fourth process—the oldest—is to dust rice grains with a powder form of fortificant. The first three processes produce a rice-premix for blending with retail rice whereas the fourth applies a micronutrient-premix directly to rice.

Fortification of cold extruded rice with thiamin, folic acid and other micronutrients has been evaluated to determine stability of the vitamins during storage. The most successful in a series of studies [30–32] achieved in excess of 70 % retention of folic acid and minimal losses of thiamin following storage for 9 months at 40 °C and 60 % relative humidity. Cracked rice was sprayed with a fortificant mixture; thiamin losses of 25 % were observed following 90 days storage at 40 °C and folic acid losses of 20 % after processing and 12 % during storage were also observed [33].

Losses during processing are significant, although useful levels may be retained. Rice fortified with thiamin, riboflavin, niacin, biotin, pantothenic acid and pyridoxine using spraying and soaking techniques retained on average in excess of 53 % of these vitamins [34] while retention of cobalamin was lower.

Cost is an issue in the fortification of rice. Whilst fortification using hot and cold extrusion techniques minimises vitamin losses when consumers wash the grains, the cost is increased considerably. Recent attention has focused on enhancements to techniques for the fortification of rice grains and the development of rice varieties—bio-fortified rice—with high levels of some vitamins. The potential for rice fortification to enhance the health of millions of consumers in developing countries has scarcely been tapped. Critical factors will be development of industry capability and experience, reductions in cost, integration into the supply chain and development of supporting legislation. Drivers are likely to include pressure from local, national and global humanitarian organisations, health and nutrition bodies, politicians and community leaders.

Other Considerations in Fortification of Foods

The military can also play a role in developing market and industry acceptance and capacity for new products, including fortified foods. In the USA in 1942 the Army decided it would purchase only fortified flour, thereby promoting public support for fortified flour. This action also encouraged compliance by manufacturers with demands by nutritionists for fortification of flour and bread as a public health measure. In developing nations, manufacturers might be encouraged to fortify if military purchasers demand fortified products [35].

It should be recognised however, that on a global scale, there are quite divergent underlying philosophies and outcomes regarding the fortification of foods. Whereas fortification of selected foods has been practised since the 1940s in the US and UK, many countries have been very hesitant to adopt either mandatory specifications or voluntary practices. Thus, for example, it was not until some 20 years ago that limited thiamin fortification was mandated in Australia when the Australian Food Standards Code was amended to require that bread-making flour contain not less than 6.4 mg/kg of thiamin. As this exceeded the natural levels, fortification was necessary to ensure that the legal requirement would be met. In the UK, flour must contain not less than 0.24 mg thiamin/100 g of flour and not less than 1.60 mg nicotinic acid or nicotinamide per 100 g of flour [36].

A total of 59 countries mandate fortification of flour with folate [37]. Although fortification of flour with folate is mandatory in North and South American countries, it is not mandatory in any country in the European Union [38]. Voluntary addition has been permitted in the United Kingdom since the mid 1980s, Australia since 1995 and New Zealand since 1996. It has been mandated in USA and Canada since 1998 and Australia since 2009 for selected staple foods.

The differing approaches around the world towards compulsory incorporation of folic acid have been associated with quite acrimonious debate. This, and earlier debates about thiamin fortification, has reflected a variety of reasons but especially concerns regarding excessive intakes and potential adverse health effects. With the introduction of folate fortification in many countries, there has been strong recognition of the need to monitor the efficacy measured as levels of folate in the blood as well as broader influences on community health [39]. In the case of folic acid, although regarded as a B-group vitamin, it is thought that reserves sufficient for 1 month of body requirements can be stored in the liver. This leads to concerns that storage of excess folate might be associated with adverse health implications. A further specific area for consideration is the imbalances that might ensue following fortification. In the case of folates it is known that, along with the adequacy of intakes, the interaction with vitamin B12 is also very important, but not fully understood [40].

The introduction of mandatory folate fortification in Australia expressed the requirement that bread-making flour contain no less than 2 mg/kg and no more than 3 mg/kg of folic acid, thereby specifying a minimum and maximum level of incorporation. For the industry involved, ensuring a uniform degree of fortification involving such a small amount of addition is very difficult. Compounding this, from an analytical perspective there are serious implications because of the relatively narrow range within which fortification was required, along with the small amounts requiring measurement and the difficulties of achieving the level of precision implied by such a regulatory requirement.

Analytical Challenges in Fortification

This is an area that is readily overlooked and some of the issues in the analysis of foods to determine the levels of naturally occurring and added vitamins include:

- Internationally accepted standard procedures are available for many analyses, however quite a few of these rely on earlier techniques and further standardisation is both ongoing and warranted
- The relatively low levels of vitamins in many food ingredients and products, even following fortification, inevitably contributes to the difficulties faced by the analyst

- The rapid development of instrumental analysis in recent decades, particularly with HPLC and increasing availability of a range of detection systems
- The critical importance of selecting extraction procedures which minimise or eliminate losses due to instability of the target analyte
- The increasing availability of purified enzymes with reduced levels of "side activities" has facilitated the effective extraction of vitamins from complex food matrices
- The presence of vitamer and provitamin forms of many of the vitamins of interest. These often have varying stabilities while presenting specific analytical problems. The predominant forms of a particular vitamin may vary widely between different foods including those regarded as staples
- In the case of fortificants, in at least some jurisdictions regulatory requirements restrict the number of permitted forms of a vitamin to one or a very limited number. Despite this it is important that each form is measured in fortification and retention studies
- It is imperative that analysis procedures are systematically validated. The significance of ensuring that extraction conditions have been optimised for particular foods is emphasised

As examples of some of these issues, from research on folates and folic acid, it has been demonstrated that optimisation of the trienzyme extraction approach to treatment of samples should be carefully adapted to the analysis of particular food products and that one method does not necessarily apply for all [41, 42]. This has been confirmed in recent work on Asian noodles [43] and for instrumental analyses of folic acid fortificant the use of the standard addition approach was required to overcome matrix effects during analysis [44, 45]. These findings emphasise the difficulties when a standard method requires adaptation to different food matrices and inter-laboratory inconsistencies in folate results might be attributed to modifications of standard published methods of analysis [46, 47].

Guidance on Levels to Be Added

Comprehensive studies of vitamin retention and fortification of Asian wheat flour noodles have demonstrated wide variation in the efficacy of fortification with the B-group vitamins. Manufacturers need to take into account the specific characteristics of the noodles, including the pH and heating profiles for processing and subsequent preparation by the consumer. In addition the recent investigations emphasise the different retention properties of individual vitamins. Therefore, the addition of niacin does not require allowance for significant losses, whereas for folic acid and pyridoxine the incorporation of overages into formulations is indicated (approximately 40 % and 60 % respectively). The strong effect of pH upon thiamin and riboflavin retention requires careful consideration and for some products the high losses minimise the usefulness of fortification unless reformulation or additional strategies for protection can also be utilised.

Conclusions

Increasingly, the significance of close attention to the analysis has been highlighted for individual vitamers, provitamins and the vitamins generally. A large amount of data has been published on the extraction and analysis of the folates and folic acid, along with the other vitamins which have been studied recently in Asian noodles products. The adaptation and validation of procedures for particular food products is very important. Whilst advances in instrumental techniques are providing more rapid and sensitive analyses, obtaining useful data is strongly dependent on the application of extraction procedures that are effective and minimise losses during sample handling and preparation.

A further series of cautionary lessons from recent research include the wide range of retention values that can be found for samples that appear to represent a particular style of noodles.

Recommendations

Further investigation into the B-group vitamins is warranted regarding ways to enhance stability, particularly where alkaline conditions contribute to losses of riboflavin and thiamin.

Care needs to be exercised if assumptions are being made that similar patterns might be expected for different vitamins or for products prepared using different ingredient formulations and processing steps. It is hoped that increased emphasis on caution in these areas may contribute to enhanced intakes of vitamins and thereby to health and well-being globally.

References

1. Allen L, de Benoist B, Dary O, Hurrell R. Guidelines on food fortification with micronutrients. Geneva: World Health Organisation and Food and Agricultural Organization of the United Nations; 2006. p. 127.
2. Bui L, Coad R. Suitability of a freeze dried product as a vehicle for vitamin fortification of military ration packs: a preliminary study. DSTO-TN-0983. Canberra: Defence Science and Technology Organisation, Department of Defence; 2011.
3. Food and Agriculture Organization of the United Nations (FAO). Food and agricultural commodities production. http://faostat.fao.org/site/339/default.aspx. Accessed 11 Sept 2011.
4. Bayer Cropscience Global. Corn/maize. http://compendium.bayercropscience.com/bayer/cropscience/cropcompendium/bcscropcomp.nsf/id/EN_CornMaize. Accessed 11 Sept 2011.
5. Orioli IM, do Nascimento RL, López-Camelo JS, Castilla EE. Effects of folic acid fortification on spina bifida prevalence in Brazil. Birth Defects Res A Clin Mol Teratol. 2011;91(9):831–5.
6. Nesamvuni AE, Vorster HH, Margetts BM, Kruger A. Fortification of maize meal improved the nutritional status of 1-3-year-old African children. Public Health Nutr. 2005;8(5):461–7.
7. Faber M, Kvalsvig JD, Lombard CJ, Benade AJS. Effect of fortified maize-meal porridge on anaemia, micronutrient status, and motor development of infants. Am J Clin Nutr. 2005;82(5):1032–9.
8. Hamner CH, Mulinare J, Cogswell ME, et al. Predicted contribution of folic acid fortification of corn masa flour to the usual folic acid intake for the US population: National Health and Nutrition Examination Survey 2001–2004. Am J Clin Nutr. 2009;89:305–15.
9. Fleischman AR, Oinuma M. Fortification of corn masa flour with folic acid in the U.S. Am J Public Health. 2011;101:1360–4.
10. Berry RJ, Bailey L, Mulinare J, Bower C. Fortification of flour with folic acid. In: Serdula M, Peña-Rosas JP, Maberly GF, Parvanta I, editors. Flour fortification with iron, folic acid, vitamin B12, vitamin A, and zinc: proceedings of the second technical workshop on wheat flour fortification. Food Nutr Bull. 2010;31(1):S32–5.
11. Watanabe E, Ciacco CF. Influence of processing and cooking on the retention of thiamin, riboflavin and niacin in spaghetti. Food Chem. 1990;36(3):223–31.
12. Bui LTT, Small DM. The contribution of Asian noodles to dietary thiamine intakes: a study of commercial dried products. J Food Compos Anal. 2007;20(7):575–83.
13. Ranhotra GS, Gelroth JA, Novak FA, Bock MA. Losses of enrichment vitamins during the cooking of pasta products. Nutr Rep Int. 1983;28(2):423–6.
14. Ranhotra GS, Gelroth JA, Novak FA, Matthews RH. Retention of selected B vitamins in cooked pasta products. Cereal Chem. 1985;62(6):476–7.
15. USDA ARS. USDA nutrient database for standard reference, release 23, 2010. Nutrient data laboratory home page. http://www.nal.usda.gov/fnic/foodcomp. Accessed 19 Sept 2011.
16. Lu H, Yang X, Ye M, et al. Culinary archaeology: Millet noodles in late Neolithic China. Nature. 2005;437:967–8.
17. Hou GG. Asian noodles: science, technology, and processing. Hoboken, NJ: Wiley; 2010. p. ix–xii.
18. Fu BX. Asian noodles: history, classification, raw materials, and processing. Food Res Int. 2008;41:888–902.
19. Bui LTT, Small DM. Folates in Asian noodles: II. A comparison of commercial samples and the impact of cooking. J Food Sci. 2007;72(5):C283–7.
20. Bui LTT, Small DM. The impact of flours and product storage on the thiamin content of Asian noodles. LWT Food Sci Technol. 2008;41(2):262–9.
21. Bui LTT, Small DM. The stability of pyridoxine hydrochloride used as a fortificant in Asian wheat flour noodles. Food Chem. 2012;130(4):841–6.
22. Bui LTT, Small DM. Riboflavin in Asian noodles: the impact of processing, storage and the efficacy of fortification of three product styles. Food Chem. 2009;114(4):1477–83.

23. Bui LTT, Small DM. Folates in Asian noodles: III Fortification, impact of processing, and enhancement of folate intakes. J Food Sci. 2007;72(5):C288–93.
24. Bui LTT, Small DM. The influence of formulation and processing on stability of thiamin in three styles of Asian noodles. Food Chem. 2007;102(4):1394–9.
25. Eitenmiller RR, Landen WO. Folate. In: Vitamin analysis for the health and food sciences. New York: CRC Press; 1999. p. 411–66.
26. Collado LS, Corke H. Starch. In: Wrigley CW, Corke H, Walker CE, editors. The encyclopedia of grain science. Oxford, UK: Elsevier Academic Press; 2004. p. 293–304.
27. Wijaya M, Small DM, Bui L. Microencapsulation of ascorbic acid for enhanced long-term retention during storage. DSTO-TR-2504. Canberra: Defence Science and Technology Organisation, Department of Defence; 2011.
28. International Rice Research Institute. Rice fact sheets: rice basics. http://irri.org/about-rice/rice-facts/rice-basics. Accessed 1 Sept 2011.
29. Alavi S, Bugusu B, Cramer G, et al. Rice fortification in developing countries: a critical review of the technical and economic feasibility. Washington, DC: Academy for Educational Development; 2008. p. 13–26.
30. Li Y, Diosady L, Jankowski S. Effect of iron compounds on the storage stability of multiple-fortified Ultra Rice®. Int J Food Sci Technol. 2008;43:423–9.
31. Li Y, Diosady L, Jankowski S. Folic acid stability in the presence of various formulation components including iron compounds in fortified extruded Ultra Rice® over prolonged storage at 40°C and 60% relative humidity (RH). Int J Food Sci Technol. 2011;46:379–85.
32. Li Y, Diosady L, Jankowski S. Stability of vitamin B1 in Ultra Rice® in the presence of encapsulated ferrous fumarate. Int J Food Sci Nutr. 2008;59(1):24–33.
33. Porasuphatana S, Chavasit V, Vasinrapee S, Suthutvoravut U, Hurrell RF. Production and shelf stability of multiple-fortified quick-cooking rice as a complementary food. J Food Sci. 2008;73(7):S359–66.
34. Kyritsi A, Tzia C, Karathanos VT. Vitamin fortified rice grain using spraying and soaking methods. LWT Food Sci Technol. 2011;44(1):312–20.
35. Bishai D, Nalubola R. The history of food fortification in the United States: its relevance for current fortification efforts in developing countries. Econ Develop Cult Chan. 2002;51(1):37–53.
36. The National Archives: legislation.gov.uk. Bread and Flour Regulations 1998. http://www.legislation.gov.uk. Accessed 26 June 2011.
37. Flour Fortification Initiative (FFI). Map of global progress: fortification status September 2011. http://www.sph.emory.edu/wheatflour//globalmap.php. Accessed 11 Sept 2011.
38. Oakley GP, Tulchinsky TH. Folic acid and vitamin B12 fortification of flour: a global basic food security requirement. Public Health Rev. 2010;32(1):284–95.
39. Rader JI, Yetley EA. Nationwide folate fortification has complex ramifications and requires careful monitoring over time. Arch Intern Med. 2002;162(5):608–9.
40. Halsted CH. Perspectives on obesity and sweeteners, folic acid fortification and vitamin D requirements. Fam Pract. 2008;25:i44–9.
41. Hyun TH, Tamura T. Trienzyme extraction in combination with microbiologic assay in food folate analysis: an updated review. Exp Biol Med. 2005;230:444–54.
42. Cho S, Choi Y, Lee J, Eitenmiller RR. Optimization of enzyme extractions for total folate in cereals using response surface methodology. J Agric Food Chem. 2010;58:10781–6.
43. Bui LTT, Small DM. Folates in Asian noodles: I. Microbiological analysis and the use of enzyme treatments. J Food Sci. 2007;72(5):C276–82.
44. Hau Fung Cheung R, Morrison PD, Small DM, Marriott PJ. Investigation of folic acid stability in fortified instant noodles by use of capillary electrophoresis and reversed-phase high performance liquid chromatography. J Chromatogr A. 2008;1213(1):93–9.
45. Hau Fung Cheung R, Hughes JG, Marriott PJ, Small DM. Investigation of folic acid stability in fortified instant Asian noodles by use of capillary electrophoresis. Food Chem. 2009;112:507–14.
46. Koontz JL, Phillips KM, Wunderlich KM, et al. Comparison of total folate concentrations in foods determined by microbiological assay at several experienced U.S. commercial laboratories. J AOAC Int. 2005;88:805–13.
47. Puwastien P, Pinprapaia N, Judprasonga K, Tamura T. International inter-laboratory analyses of food folate. J Food Compos Anal. 2005;18:387–97.

Chapter 17
Fortification of Milk with Mineral Elements

Elvan Ocak and Rajkumar Rajendram

Key Points

- Milk is one of the most nutritious foods available. It contains minerals and trace elements in significant quantities.
- Milk fortification is a public health measure that addresses inadequate micronutrient intake, without affecting dietary patterns.
- Commonly, milk is fortified with minerals such as calcium, iron, zinc, iodine and selenium.
- Whilst these elements are essential, they can be toxic in large doses.
- When large amounts of minerals are added to dairy products, the quality of these products may be adversely affected.

Keywords Fortification • Minerals • Milk • Dairy • Calcium • Zinc • Selenium

Abbreviations

Ca	Calcium
Cl	Chlorine
CPP	Casein phosphopeptide
Cu	Copper
Fe	Iron
Se	Selenium
SO_4	Sulphate
Zn	Zinc

E. Ocak (✉)
Department of Food Engineering, Yuzuncu Yil University, 65080 Van, Turkey
e-mail: elvanocak@yyu.edu.tr

R. Rajendram A.K.C. B.Sc. (Hons), M.B.B.S. (dist)
Departments of General Medicine and Intensive Care, John Radcliffe Hospital, Oxford, Oxfordshire OX3 9DU, UK

Division of Diabetes & Nutritional Sciences, School of Medicine, King's College London, Franklin-Wilkins Building 150 Stamford Street, London SE1 8WA, UK
e-mail: rajkumarrajendram@doctors.org.uk

V.R. Preedy et al. (eds.), *Handbook of Food Fortification and Health: From Concepts to Public Health Applications Volume 1*, Nutrition and Health, DOI 10.1007/978-1-4614-7076-2_17,

Introduction

Micronutrient malnutrition is a significant public health issue. It affects billions of people worldwide, in both developing and developed countries. Mineral ions are involved in many physiological processes, including the regulation of enzyme activity and the maintenance of pH, osmotic pressure and electrical stability of cell membranes [1, 2]. Deficiency of these ions causes serious health problems. As a poignant example of this global phenomenon, it is estimated that over two billion people are at risk of iron deficiency worldwide [3]. Adverse effects on the health of these individuals ranges from exhaustion, to impaired cognition and increased susceptibility to infection [4]. Besides significantly reducing quality of life, the complications of micronutrient malnutrition can cause significant mortality; 0.8 million deaths each year are related to iron deficiency [5]. The high morbidity and mortality of micronutrient malnutrition has important economic sequelae, including the loss of individual and government income and financial stability.

There are several potential solutions including promotion of dietary change (requiring education, advice and incentives), dietary supplementation and fortification of food. Educational interventions are, in theory, the ideal solution. However, changing dietary habits on the population level is challenging [3], and may have poor efficacy, at least in the short term [6]. Dietary supplementation is a rapid and cost-effective solution for individuals at risk of deficiency, that also limits overdose in those with adequate dietary intake. However, supplements may have adverse side effects and compliance may be poor. Food fortification is another potential solution. This involves enrichment of food with nutrients to greater concentrations than those naturally present [7]. Food fortification has increased recently, as it has been recognised that fortification is a public health intervention for nutritional deficiencies, which has a wider and more sustained impact than supplementation. Although not without limitations, food fortification is an important intervention to treat micronutrient malnutrition, which should be used in combination with promotion of dietary change and dietary supplements.

Milk is widely consumed; thus, the fortification of milk and milk products could provide vital nutrition to a large proportion of the world's populace. Milk is a natural highly nutritious food that contains all ten essential amino acids, as well as fats, and important minerals and vitamins. However, milk has low concentrations of some important vitamins and minerals including iron [8]. Increasing the quantity of some of these micronutrients could improve dietary balance and health in malnourished individuals. The micronutrient composition and fortification of milk and milk products is therefore an important public health issue and is discussed in detail below.

Minerals in Milk and Dairy Products

Milk contains significant quantities of important micronutrients (Table 17.1). However, the concentrations vary according to environmental factors as well as the nutritional status, stage of lactation and genetic make-up of the source animal [9].

The most abundant element in milk is calcium, with a typical concentration of 120 mg/100 g. Phosphorous, potassium, magnesium and sodium are also present. Very low levels of important trace elements including zinc, iron, copper, iodine, fluorine and selenium are also present [10].

Other dairy products have different micronutrient compositions. Cheese, for example, is an excellent source of calcium and phosphorous, but also contains higher quantities of zinc, iodine and selenium than natural milk (see Table 17.2). Micronutrients also vary according to type of cheese; some have high concentrations of potassium (100–200 mg/100 g cheese), and the sodium content in 100 g of cheese can vary from 30 mg to 1 g. Most types of cheese contain less magnesium than milk, with concentrations varying from 10 to 50 mg per 100 g [10].

Table 17.1 Concentrations of minerals and trace elements in milk [10]

	Pasteurised milk			Sterilised milk			UHT milk		
Milk	Whole	Semi-skimmed	Skimmed	Whole	Semi-skimmed	Skimmed	Whole	Semi-skimmed	Skimmed
Calcium (mg/100 g)	120	114	125	119	114	125	120	114	120
Sodium (mg/100 g)	45	46	50	45	46	52	45	48	50
Phosphorus (mg/100 g)	87	85	89	90	85	89	86	85	89
Chloride (mg/100 g)	102	101	100	106	101	100	110	101	100
Potassium (mg/100 g)	148	166	170	150	166	180	150	166	170
Magnesium (mg/100 g)	10	10	10	10	10	12	10	11	11
Iodine (μg/100 g)	7.3	11	12	7	11	12	8	11	12

Table 17.2 Concentration of minerals and trace elements in cheese [10]

Cheese	Camembert (45 %)	Munster	Cantal	Roquefort	French Emmental	Soft goat cheese	Cream cheese	Processed cheese (45 %)
Calcium (mg/100 g)	400	430	800	600	1,000	160	118	300
Sodium (mg/100 g)	642	930	940	1,600	300	564	36	587
Magnesium (mg/100 g)	18	23	25	27	43	23	10	22
Phosphorus (mg/100 g)	310	320	500	430	746	216	113	756
Chloride (mg/100 g)	926	1,286	928	2,530	463	ND	ND	721
Potassium (mg/100 g)	110	130	136	120	103	132	130	143
Zinc (mg/100 g)	2.8	3.9	3	3	5	1	ND	8
Selenium (μg/100 g)	5	4.3	5.4	7	7	ND	ND	7
Iodine (μg/100 g)	21	30	21	50	32	60	10	25

Table 17.3 Concentration of minerals and trace elements in yoghurt and fermented milk [10]

Yoghurt & fermented milk	Yoghurt of whole milk	Yoghurt of semi-skimmed milk	Fermented milk	Drink yoghurt of semi-skimmed milk with fruits, sugar	Yoghurt of whole milk with fruits, sugar	Yoghurt of goat's milk, semi-skimmed milk	Yoghurt of ewe's milk
Calcium (mg/100 g)	161	142	144	111	110	112	150
Sodium (mg/100 g)	68	53	61	35	43	36	150
Magnesium (mg/100 g)	11	13	13	10	12	13	16
Phosphorus (mg/100 g)	95	98	105	82	80	103	140
Potassium (mg/100 g)	217	176	182	116	140	159	190
Iodine (μg/100 g)	15	20	20	11	15	ND	ND

Table 17.4 Concentration of minerals and trace elements of butter and cream [10]

Butter and cream (mg/100 g)	Butter	Cream	Low fat cream
Calcium	15	73	98
Sodium	9	27	40
Potassium	12	101	128

Cream and butter are poor sources of micronutrients (see Table 17.3). Fermented milks, however, are a good source of a range of nutrients including calcium, phosphorus, potassium, zinc and magnesium (see Table 17.4).

The Advent of Dairy Fortification

Rickets is caused by vitamin D deficiency in childhood, which results in inadequate bone mineralisation. Vitamin D deficiency in childhood affects the development of bones which leads to their softening and deformation resulting in characteristic complications such as bowed legs and stunted growth [11]. In 1932, the dairy industry started to fortify milk with vitamin D to address the high prevalence of rickets at the time [12]. Vitamin D supplementation increases the bioavailability of calcium, regulates phosphate levels and increases bone mineralisation, preventing and treating Rickets [8].

Vitamin A deficiency causes visual impairment, blindness and increased risk of infection and mortality. Although whole milk is an excellent source of Vitamin A, skimmed and semi-skimmed milk contain low concentrations of the fat soluble nutrient [13]. Fortification of these products was, therefore, introduced in the 1940s. Since then, the dairy fortification industry has grown rapidly. The trends for fortification with different nutrients vary according to the nutritional requirements of the population. This is affected by changes in diet, lifestyle and population demographics. For example ageing populations have different requirement compared to younger populations or higher consumers of 'fast foods'.

Principles of Fortification

There are four key principles of food fortification [14].

1. The demand for the food should be constant and unaffected by fortification.
2. Fortification should not adversely affect the odour, texture, taste or appearance of the food.
3. The nutrient should be absorbed by the body resulting in an increase in bioavailability.
4. There should be a demonstrable positive effect on the consumer's health of adding the nutrient.

Level of Fortification

The fortification of milk depends on several factors. These include the levels of milk consumption and the nutritional requirements of the target population; the effect of added nutrients on the functional or sensory (odour, flavour and colour) characteristics of milk; and the stability of the nutrients during the processing and storage of milk [15].

Fortification levels should be monitored at factory, retail and household levels. If transportation results in a long delay between production and consumption, regular monitoring at intermediate levels (distributor and wholesaler) may be required to provide more rapid feedback and to indicate whether the fortified product has retained adequate fortificant levels [16].

Enrichment of food products with various cations can improve the functional, technological and nutritional properties of these foods. However, it is important to note that whilst these elements are essential, they can be toxic in excess. Fortification of dairy products by rapid addition of large amounts of minerals can cause several adverse technological problems.

Philippe et al. reported that metals, when present in milk and milk products, can lead to spoilage by accelerating the development of oily, tallow, fishy or putrid smells and tastes in addition to their specific metallic taste [17]. Some metals may also increase loss of vitamin C. Studies on the effects of different cations on the physico-chemical characteristics of casein micelles also demonstrated that the hydrophobicity of casein micelles decreased after addition of ferric iron and copper [17].

The effect of mineral fortification of milk on the production and texture of yoghurt was described by Ocak and Köse [1], who studied the properties of yoghurt fortified with copper (Cu), iron (Fe) and zinc (Zn). The presence of Cu and Zn inhibited the fermenting activity of a yoghurt starter culture. The incubation time of yoghurt produced from milk fortified with Cu and Zn was longer than that of the controls and yoghurt produced from milk fortified with Fe.

Increased $FeCl_2$ concentration (1) increased clotting time, (2) increased aggregation time and (3) decreased curd firmness. Increasing $FeCl_3$ concentration slightly increases clotting time, increases aggregation time and slightly decreases curd firmness [18].

Technology

The technology required to fortify milk is simple. All the minerals and vitamins that can be added to milk are available in dry powder form. As several nutrients are generally added to milk, fortificants are ideally added as a premix; a homogenous mixture of desired amount of fortificants (vitamins and minerals) concentrated in a small amount of the food to be fortified. Premixes ensure the addition of correct amounts and uniform homogenisation of the micronutrients in the final product [15].

Three types of mineral compounds have been used for mineral fortification of milk and milk products.

1. Mineral salts (soluble)
2. Elemental minerals
3. Mineral protein complexes

Mineral salts are most commonly used. These salts, which have two oxidation states (e.g. Fe^{+2}, Fe^{+3}, Zn^{+2}, Zn^{+3}), are completely soluble in water and in milk.

Elemental minerals (e.g. elemental iron) are obtained by reduction with hydrogen or carbon monoxide, by electrolysis or by the carbonyl process. These compounds are powders with varying particle size and are poorly soluble or insoluble in water and are chemically inert. As this form of mineral is insoluble in neutral liquids, it can only be used to fortify solid dehydrated food [18].

Mineral protein (e.g. casein and whey proteins) or phosphopeptides (Casein phosphopeptide (CPP)) complexes include, for example, CPPs–Zn complexes and also iron bound to amino acids such as phosphoserine, aspartate and glutamate [17–19]. The preparation of iron can also vary. Thus, $FeSO_4$ microencapsulated with lecithin has the same bioavailability as $FeSO_4$ but has the advantage of being coated with phospholipid membrane. Similarly, lipid microcapsules of $FeSO_4$, alone or with ascorbic acid, have been developed to fortify cheese and other foods with a high moisture content [18].

Mineral Stability

The success of a fortification program depends on a number of factors, including the stability of micronutrients added the food. Prior to selecting the fortificant(s), it is important to consider the factors affecting fortificant stability [16].

Minerals are, in general, less sensitive than vitamins to physical and chemical factors. Nevertheless, they are reactive in nature and must be selected after considering possible interactions with milk proteins, potential adverse effects on the sensory properties of milk and the bioavailability of the mineral form. Minerals are changed or lost on exposure to heat, air or light. It has been reported that copper shifts from casein to fat after heating, whereas iron added to bovine milk does not change its distribution after pasteurisation. It has also been reported that gastrointestinal iron loss is increased in infants fed heat-treated milk [20]. So manufacturers ensure optimum intake of minerals from infant formula by fortification with essential trace elements at supraphysiological levels (i.e. levels higher than those occurring in natural human milk) to compensate for reduced bioavailability and losses during processing and storage [21]. Minerals such as copper, iron and zinc are also affected by moisture, and may react with other food components such as proteins and carbohydrates [16]. For example calcium may react with protein, particularly when foods are heat processed resulting in sedimentation and gelation. The heat stability of milk depends on the type of calcium salt used and the type of milk [22].

Calcium

Calcium is an essential nutrient required for critical biological functions such as nerve conduction, muscle contraction, mitosis, blood coagulation, structural support of the skeleton, activation of enzyme reactions and stimulation of hormone secretions [23, 24]. A great deal of scientific literature shows that high dietary calcium intake and its bioavailability are associated with the reduced risk of osteoporosis, hypertension, colon cancer, kidney stones, stroke, obesity, polycystic ovary syndrome, lead absorption and premenstrual syndrome [22–25].

Milk and dairy products are the best natural sources of calcium. Cows' milk contains an average of 1.20 g calcium per litre. Most of the calcium in milk is colloidal as a caseinate–phosphate complex and is readily released during digestion in vivo; hence, its potential bioavailability is high [22].

There are many factors that influence calcium bioavailability. Both exogenous and endogenous factors influence calcium bioavailability. Level of calcium intake, vitamin D status, phytates, oxalates, lipids, type of salts, phosphopeptides and other proteins, lactose, phosphorus and caffeine are among the exogenous factors influencing the intestinal calcium absorption [9, 23, 26, 27].

Calcium in milk is more easily absorbed by the intestine than calcium from the vegetables and cereals. Phytates (present in cereals, bean and pulses), oxalates (present in leafy vegetables), long-chain saturated fatty acids and dietary fibre can reduce the bioavailability of calcium by forming insoluble calcium complexes [22, 25]. For this reason, dairy products such as ice cream, yoghurt and cheese are an excellent source of dietary calcium and are ideal vehicles for calcium supplements and can meet nutritional requirements in a single serving [28, 29].

Several commercial calcium salts have been used for calcium fortification of dairy products (Table 17.5). Calcium salts used for supplementation in dairy industry include [22, 27, 30]:

- Inorganic salts such as calcium carbonate, calcium chloride and calcium phosphate
- Calcium from animal or vegetable origin, such as milk calcium (comprised mainly of calcium phosphate) and seaweed calcium (comprised mainly of calcium carbonate)
- Organic salts such as tricalcium citrate, calcium lactate, calcium lactate gluconate and calcium gluconate

The selection of the appropriate calcium source for a specific application is usually based on consideration of the gastronomic and physico-chemical properties of the product such as solubility, calcium content, taste and bioavailability. However, economic constraints are also important [27].

Depending on the form of salt used, calcium fortification can affect the colour, texture, stability, flavour and processing characteristics of dairy products [22, 31, 32]. Singh et al. [22], studied the heat stability and calcium bioavailability of calcium-fortified milk and found that fortification of milk with calcium lactate or gluconate and stabilised with disodium phosphate improved its sensory acceptance, calcium bioavailability and heat stability. Singh et al. suggested that heat stability of milk can be affected by the type of calcium salt used and the final processing step for adjustment of pH [22]. Singh and Muthukumarappan also reported that calcium in fruit yoghurt can be increased up to 50 mg calcium per 100 mL by addition of calcium lactate without any negative influence on the organoleptic properties [25].

The challenge for dairy product manufacturers is to provide products with high calcium content and good taste. As a result, micronised tricalcium citrate has replaced inorganic and organic salts for the fortification of dairy products. An important explanation from the technological standpoint is that

Table 17.5 Calcium fortified dairy products

Fortified product	Ca salt	Ca content	Claim	Ref.
Milk	Ca chloride dihydrate, Ca lactate tetrahydrate, Ca gluconate monohydrate, Ca carbonate	50–75–100 mg/100 mL	Sensory quality, heat stability and in vivo absorbability	[22]
Soy milk	Ca chloride	25 mM	Investigate (Ca^{2+}), pH, absolute viscosity, particle diameter and dry sediment content of Ca-fortified soy milk incorporating SHMP, DSHP, TSC or EDTA-Na_2, before and after pasteurisation	[33]
Reconstituted skim milk powder	Ca carbonate, phosphate, lactate and citrate	0.15, 0.18 and 0.24 % (wt/wt)	The effect of calcium fortification on the heat stability of reconstituted skim milk powder	[31]
Fruit yoghurt	Ca lactate pentahydrate	25–50–75–100 mg/100 mL	The effect of calcium enrichment of yogurt on its sensory characteristics and various physical and rheological properties, viz. WHC, flow behaviour, thixotropy and loss tangent values	[25]
Yoghurt	Ca lactate, Ca gluconate	400–600–800 mg/100 g (Ca lactate) 600–800–1,000 mg (Ca gluconate)	Investigate the changes in chemical, microbiological and organoleptic properties of yoghurts fortified	[29]
Cheese	Ca chloride	0.02–0.03–0.05 %	Effect of calcium addition on yield of cheese manufactured	[34]
Low fat yoghurt	Tricalcium citrate	180 mg/100 g		[27]
Evaporated milk	Ca carbonate	169 mg/100 g		
Whole milk	Ca gluconate monohydrate	166 mg/100 g	The milk promotes healthy bones and teeth, growth and repair, vision and skin, release of energy, healthy blood and nervous system and pregnancy	

especially in the milk matrix, a highly dispersible calcium salt has advantages over highly soluble alternatives. Of the organic salts with high bioavailability and more neutral taste profiles, tricalcium citrate (21 % calcium) is clearly one of the most economic options for calcium fortification and is currently the first choice for milk products [27].

Zinc

Zinc is one of the most important essential trace metals of human nutrition. Signs of zinc deficiency in humans were first described in the 1960s [35]. After zinc was shown to be an essential micronutrient, there was an explosion of research into the role of zinc in human health. In the last years zinc deficiency has become a global problem affecting developed and developing countries [36].

Most of the zinc (85 %) is found in skimmed milk whilst about is 15 % of the zinc is in the fat in natural milk. Whilst zinc fortification increases the content of zinc in milk, the ratio of zinc bound to the whey increases [1].

Table 17.6 Key points about zinc

Biological function	Zinc is required for catalytic activity of >300 enzymes [35, 37] DNA and RNA synthesis [9, 38] Structural role in bone matrix [9] Antioxidant [36, 39] Synthesis of GH and somatomedin-c [40] Cellular division [36] Vitamin A metabolism [36] Insulin storage and release [36, 37] Immune building [37, 41] Injury healing [52]
Deficiency consequences	Growth retardation, hypogonadism, intercurrent infections, altered immune response, increased abortion risk, complications during delivery, neural tube defects of foetus, delayed wound healing, abnormal dark adaptation, oligospermia [36] Osteoporosis, increased susceptibility to diabetes, cancer, Alzheimer and Wilson disease, rheumatic disease, especially rheumatoid arthritis, stunted growth, anorexia [35, 39] Weight loss, early death [40] Diarrhoea, age-related macular degeneration, upper respiratory infection (URI) and human immunodeficiency virus (HIV) [39] Taste and appetite [42]
Prevention of deficiency	RDAs (and AIs) set by the Food and Nutrition Board for zinc (mg/day) are: infants age 0–0.5 year, 2 (AI) and age 0.5–1 year, 3; children age 1–3 years, 3 and age 4–8 years, 5; males age 9–13 years, 8, and age ≥14 years, 11; females age 9–13 years, 8, age 14–18 years, 9, age ≥19 years, 8, pregnant age ≤18 years, 12, and age ≥19 years, 11, lactating age ≤18 years, 13, and age ≥19 years, 12 [35]
Zinc bioavailability enhancers	Protein, histidine, lactose, peptides (CPPs) [19, 43]
Zinc bioavailability inhibitors	Phytate, casein, iron, calcium, copper [19]
Absorption	In the small intestine [39]

Foods consumed in large quantities such as milk, which are considered ideal carriers of food fortificants, naturally have a very low zinc content. As nutritional causes of zinc deficiency are most important worldwide and food fortification is an effective and economic strategy to prevent nutritional deficiencies, fortification of milk with zinc could be the key to treatment of zinc deficiency [36].

Despite large daily consumption of dairy products, the low zinc content of milk means that intake of natural dairy products cannot provide sufficient zinc to meet the recommended dietary requirements for adults and adolescents (8 mg/day). The fortification and enrichment of milk, cheese, dried cow's milk or beverages with zinc has been investigated [38, 44].

Several zinc compounds are available for fortification including zinc sulphate, zinc oxide, zinc acetate, zinc chloride [38, 45]. Of these, zinc oxide and zinc sulphate are least expensive and most commonly used by the food industry. Zinc sulphate should theoretically provide more reliable absorption than zinc oxide because of its greater solubility, but is more expensive [45].

Abd-Rabou et al. [38], who studied the properties of Edam cheese fortified by dietary zinc salts, observed that all score's properties of Edam cheese samples were increased generally during ripening period. The high remarked scores for cheeses fortified with zinc salts indicated that they were perceived to be more tasty, with better flavour intensity, body and texture, colour and appearance. Abd-Rabou et al. suggested that the addition of zinc acetate or zinc chloride improved the organoleptic properties of Edam cheese and accelerated its ripening process [38] (Table 17.6).

Selenium

Selenium (Se) is a trace mineral that was only relatively recently shown to have an essential role in human health. Chemically, it is classed as a metalloid, with properties of both metals and non-metals [21, 46]. The revised 1989 Recommended Dietary Allowances (RDAs) [47] for selenium, stated in micrograms, are as follows:

- 10 for infants under 6 months
- 15 for infants 6–12 months
- 20 for children 1–6 years
- 30 for children 7–10 years
- 40 for males 11–14
- 45 for females 11–14
- 50 for both sexes 15–18
- 70 for males over 19
- 55 for females over 19
- 65 for pregnant women
- 75 during lactation

Milk and dairy products are poor sources of Se. Selenium concentration in milk is directly affected by levels in the food chain and, hence, reflects the food habits and the geochemical environment. Se concentration in cow's milk can vary as much as 2–1,270 $\mu g\ L^{-1}$ depending on the availability of this element in the food and geographical area [48].

Several forms of Se occur in the typical human diet. Selenium is usually present in animal foods and plants as selenoproteins containing seleno-amino acids, for example selenocysteine and selenomethionine, and inorganic species, for example Se (IV) and Se (VI) [49, 50]. Owing to the different concentrations of these nutrients, and other substances that modify their absorption, there is much interest in the significance of micronutrient supplies, within the quest for improvement of new foods. The nutritional bioavailability and toxicity of Se depend on the concentration and chemical form of Se ingested [49].

Some studies have investigated fortification of milk, cheese, brine, whole milk powder and infant formula powder or fermented milk with Se [21, 46, 48, 51]. Alzate et al. reported [50] that fermentation of Se-enriched milk is an interesting way to increasing the human intake of organic compounds of Se for many reasons. Milk is usually present in traditional meals, it is consumed regularly in moderate amounts, it is affordable and it already supplies the body with a significant amount of Se, at least 50 % of the RDA.

The effect of Se and Zn fortification on the quality of Turkish white cheese was reported by Gulbas and Saldamlı [46]. They assessed the chemical composition and sensory properties of cheese on the 1st and 60th day of the ripening period. The appearance and taste scores of cheeses produced by fortification of cheese milk were better than those of cheeses produced by the fortification of brine solution. However, fortification with brine solution resulted in better texture and body scores. Gulbas and Saldamlı also suggested that Se recovery was highest when fortificants were added to the brine solution [46] (Table 17.7).

Recommendations

Mineral fortification of dairy products must be carefully controlled to ensure the desired level of fortificants in the final products and avoid toxicity. Just as mineral deficiencies can cause complications, excessive mineral intake also has side effects. For example, too much calcium can cause renal disease.

Table 17.7 Key points about selenium

Biological function	Se is an integral part of glutathione peroxidase (GSH-Px), an enzyme involved in cellular protection against oxidative damage and iodothyronine 5-deiodinase, an enzyme involved in thyroid metabolism [21, 52, 53]
	Se has an active role in several metabolic pathways and may also be a modulator in inflammatory and immune responses. Se may be relevant in the emergence of viral mutations [21, 52]
	Se may reduce the incidence of some cancers [46, 47, 49, 52]
Consequences of deficiency	A high incidence of Keshan disease (a juvenile cardiomyopathy) and Kaschin–Beck disease (osteoarthritis) [21, 47]
	Growth abnormalities and generalised muscle diseases, including muscular dystrophy [47]
	Infertility [49]
Absorption	Se is absorbed through intestines and stored in the liver, kidneys and muscles [54]

Mineral fortification often does not affect the sensory or physico-chemical properties of the dairy product. However, some fortificants can cause unacceptable changes in colour, flavour or texture of dairy products. The long time and high cost required to develop new combinations of suitable minerals fortificant preparations and dairy products must be offset by the use of better fortification system and fortification methods.

Conclusions

Micronutrient malnutrition is a global phenomenon that affects both developing and industrialised countries, with serious health and economic implications. Food fortification has been recognised as an important, continuous, self-sustaining strategy to improve the health and nutrition status of millions of people.

Dairy products are inexpensive and consumed in moderate amounts and so are an obvious vehicle for dietary mineral fortification. Milk is, therefore, fortified with minerals such as Ca, Fe, Zn and Se.

Fortification of milk products is beneficial to consumers and provides opportunities for marketing for the dairy product industry. The consumer benefits from healthy products that provide alternatives sources of micronutrients to meet their nutrient requirements. The dairy industry benefits from the development of fortified products that are tasty and appealing and can be advertised as having high mineral contents.

However, food fortification cannot prevent micronutrient deficiency if:

1. The target population have little or no access to the fortified food
2. Micronutrient deficiency is too severe
3. Co-incident infection increases the metabolic demand for micronutrients

References

1. Ocak E, Köse Ş. The effects of fortifying milk with of Cu, Fe and Zn minerals on the production and texture of yoghurt. J Food Agr Environ. 2010;8:122–5.
2. Achanta K, Aryana KJ, Boeneke CA. Fat free plain set yogurts fortified with various minerals. LWT—Food Sci Technol. 2007;40:424–9.
3. Fletcher RJ, Bell IP, Lambert JP. Public health aspects of food fortification: a question of balance. Proc Nutr Soc. 2004;63:605–14.

4. Childs F, Aukett A, Darbyshire P, et al. Dietary education and iron deficiency anaemia in the inner city. Arch Dis Child. 1997;76:144–7.
5. Allen L, de Benoist B, Dary O, Hurrell R, editors. Guidelines on food fortification with micronutrients. The World Health Organisation & Food and Agricultural Organization of the United Nations. 2006. http://www.who.int/nutrition/publications/micronutrients/GFF_Part_1_en.pdf. Accessed 28 June 2012.
6. Huch R, Schaefer R. Iron deficiency and iron deficiency anemia: a pocket atlas special. Stuttgart: Georg Thieme; 2006. p. 35.
7. Fortification of food with micronutrients: the role and position of FAO. http://www.ceecis.org/iodine/01_global/01_pl/01_01_other_fao.pdf. Accessed 15 Oct 2011.
8. McCollum EV. Is there need for the fortification of milk? Am J Public Health Nations Health. 1942;32:80–4.
9. Cashman KD. Milk minerals (including trace elements) and bone health. Int Dairy J. 2006;16:1389–98.
10. International Dairy Federation. Minerals in milk and milk products. IDF. http://www.idfdairynutrition.org. Accessed 21 July 2011.
11. Porth CM. Essentials of pathophysiology: concepts of altered health states. 3rd ed. Philadelphia, PA: Lippincott Williams & Wilkins; 2010. p. 1135–6.
12. Institute of Medicine, Food and Nutrition Board. Dietary reference intakes for calcium and vitamin D. Washington, DC: National Academy Press; 2010.
13. Rinzler CA. The new complete book of food. 2nd ed. New York, NY: Infobase; 2010. p. 233.
14. Haylock SJ. Fortification of consumer milk products. Bulletin of the International Dairy Federation (375). Brussels: IDF; 2002. p. 111–5.
15. United States Agency for International Development (US AID), DSM Nutritional Products Ltd. Fortification basics: milk. Arlington,VA : Opportunities for Micronutrient Interventions; 1997. http://www.nutritionimprovement.com/fortification.html. Accessed 18 July 2011.
16. United States Agency for International Development (US AID), DSM Nutritional Products Ltd. Fortification basics: stability. Arlington, VA: Opportunities for Micronutrient Interventions; 1998. http://www.nutritionimprovement.com/fortification.html. Accessed 18 July 2011.
17. Philippe M, Le Graët Y, Gaucheron F. The effect of different cations on the physicochemical characteristics of casein micelles. Food Chem. 2005;90:673–83.
18. Gaucheron F. Iron fortification in dairy industry. Trends Food Sci Technol. 2000;11:403–9.
19. Miquel E, Farre R. Effects and future trends of casein phosphopeptides on zinc bioavailability. Trends Food Sci Technol. 2007;18:139–43.
20. Mata L, Sanchez L, Puyol P, et al. Changes in the distribution of cadmium and lead in human and bovine milk induced by heating or freezing. J Food Prot. 1996;59:46–50.
21. Foster LH, Chaplin MF, Sumar S. The effect of heat treatment on instrinsic and fortified selenium levels in cow's milk. Food Chem. 1998;62:21–5.
22. Singh G, Arora S, Sharma GS, et al. Heat stability and calcium bioavailability of calcium-fortified milk. LWT- Food Sci Technol. 2007;40:625–31.
23. DiRienzo D. Whey products, milk minerals and dairy calcium. Am J Clin Nutr. 2000;71:1166–9.
24. Perales S, Barbera R, Lagarda MJ, et al. Fortification of milk with calcium: effect on calcium bioavailability and interactions with iron and zinc. J Agric Food Chem. 2006;54:4901–6.
25. Singh G, Muthukumarappan K. Influence of calcium fortification on sensory, physical and rheological characteristics of fruit yogurt. LWT- Food Sci Technol. 2008;41:1145–52.
26. Recker RR, Bammi A, Barger-Lux J, et al. Calcium absorbability from milk products, an imitation milk, and calcium carbonate. Am J Clin Nutr. 1988;47:93–5.
27. Münchbach M, Gerstner G. Calcium fortification in dairy products. Food Market Technol. 2010:4–8.
28. Van Der Hee RM, Miret S, Slettenaar M, et al. Calcium absorption from fortified ice cream formulations compared with calcium absorption from milk. J Am Diet Assoc. 2009;109:830–5.
29. Pirkul T, Temiz A, Erdem YK. Fortification of yoghurt with calcium salts and its effect on starter microorganisms and yoghurt quality. Int Dairy J. 1997;7:547–52.
30. Gerstner G. Dairy products: the calcium challenge. Int Food Ingredients. 2002;3:45–8.
31. Vyas HK, Tong PS. Impact of source and level of calcium fortification on the heat stability of reconstituted skim milk powder. J Dairy Sci. 2004;87:1177–80.
32. Williams RPW, D'ath L, Augustin MA. Production of calcium-fortified milk powders using soluble calcium salts. Lait. 2005;85:369–81.
33. Pathomrungsiyounggul P, Lewis MJ, Grandison AS. Effects of calcium-chelating agents and pasteurisation on certain properties of calcium-fortified soy milk. Food Chem. 2010;118:808–14.
34. Ustunol Z, Hicks CL. Effect of calcium addition on yield of cheese manufactured with Endothia parasitica protease. J Dairy Sci. 1990;73:17–25.
35. Nielsen FH. Trace mineral deficiencies. In: Berdanier CD, Duryer J, Feldmen EB, editors. Handbook of nutrition and food. 2nd ed. Boca Raton: Taylor & Francis; 2008:159–76.

36. Salgueiro MJ, Zubillaga MB, Lysionek AE, et al. Zinc as an essential micronutrient: a review. Nutr Res. 2000;20:737–55.
37. Özrenk E, Akyüz N. The pollution levels of heavy metals and the content of some minerals of cows' milk produce in Van province. Ph.D. Thesis, Institute of Science, Yuzuncu Yil University, Van, Turkey; 2002. p. 76.
38. Abd-Rabou NS, Zaghloul AH, Seleet FL, et al. Properties of Edam cheese fortified by dietary zinc salts. J Am Sci. 2010;6:441–6.
39. Saper RB, Rash R. Zinc: an essential micronutrient. Am Fam Physician. 2009;79:768–72.
40. Salgueiro MJ, Zubillaga MB, Lysionek AE, et al. The role of zinc in the growth and development of children. Nutrition. 2002;18:510–9.
41. Shelke K, Feder D. Heavy metal: iron and zinc fortification. http://www.foodprocessing.com/articles/2006/019.html. Accessed 15 Sept 2011.
42. Torrejón CS, Castillo-Durán C, Hertrampf ED, et al. Zinc and iron in Chilean children fed fortified milk provided by the Complementary National Food Program. Nutrition. 2004;20:177–80.
43. Pabón ML, Lönnerdal B. Bioavailability of zinc and its binding to casein in milks and formulas. J Trace Elem Med Biol. 2000;14:146–53.
44. Ruz M, Codoceo J, Inostroza J, et al. Zinc absorption from a micronutrient-fortified dried cow's milk used in the Chilean National Complementary Food Program. Nutr Res. 2005;25:1043–8.
45. Importance of zinc for human health. International Association of Infant Food Manufacturers. http://www.ifm.net/industry/zinc3.htm. Accessed 29 July 2011.
46. Gulbas Yalcintas S, Saldamlı I. The effect of selenium and zinc fortification on the quality of Turkish white cheese. Int J Food Sci Nutr. 2005;56:141–6.
47. Nutrition. http://www.drkrider.com/Topics/Nutrition/Selenium.htm. Accessed 23 Sept 2011.
48. Aleixo PC, Nóbrega JA. Direct determination of iron and selenium in bovine milk by graphite furnace atomic absorption spectrometry. Food Chem. 2003;83:457–62.
49. Muniz-Naveiro O, Dominguez-González R, Bermejo-Barrera A, et al. Study of the bioavailability of selenium in cows' milk after a supplementation of cow feed with different forms of selenium. Anal Bioanal Chem. 2006;385:189–96.
50. Rooke JA, Flockhart JF, Sparks NH. The potential for increasing the concentrations of micro-nutrients relevant to human nutrition in meat, milk and eggs. J Agric Sci. 2010;148:603–14.
51. Alzate A, Pérez-Conde MC, Gutiérrez AM, et al. Selenium-enriched fermented milk: a suitable dairy product to improve selenium intake in humans. Int Dairy J. 2010;20:761–9.
52. Van Dael P, Davidsson L, Munoz-Box R, et al. Selenium absorption and retention from a selenite- or selenate-fortified milk-based formula in men measured by a stable-isotope technique. Br J Nutr. 2001;85:157–63.
53. Milner JA, Sherman L, Picciano MF. Distribution of selenium in human milk. Am J Clin Nutr. 1987;45:617–24.
54. Therapeutic nutrition based upon biochemical individuality. http://orthomolecular.org/nutrients/micronutrients.shtml. Accessed 20 Sept 2011.

Chapter 18
Iodine Nutrition: Salt Fortification with Iodine

Izzeldin S. Hussein

Key Points

- Healthy humans require iodine, an essential component of the thyroid hormones, thyroxin, and triiodothyronine.
- Fortification of foods that are commonly consumed by the population at risk has been demonstrated to be a viable and cost-effective food-based strategy for the control of IDD and micronutrient deficiencies.
- The correction of iodine deficiency has to be achieved by supplying iodine from an external source, fortification or by periodic supplementation of deficient populations with iodine.
- Correction of iodine deficiency is associated with a risk of a temporary increased incidence of hyperthyroidism because of hormone production in the enlarged and structurally changed thyroid gland, which has been transformed due to a long period of iodine deficiency.
- The recommended minimum daily requirement of iodine varies from 150 to 250 μg. Continuous monitoring of iodine levels is one of the best and simplest ways of monitoring the entire IDD elimination program when salt iodization is the intervention strategy. Frequent testing of iodine levels at iodization plants and periodically at intermediate points in the distribution network, retail outlets and the household level has been characteristic of countries with successful programs.

Keywords Salt • Iodine • Fortification • IDD • Universal • Iodization • Indicators • Elimination • Fortification • Micronutrients

Abbreviations

ICCIDD	International Council for Control of Iodine Deficiency Disorders
IDD	Iodine deficiency disorders
KIO_3	Potassium iodate
NaCl	Sodium chloride
PPM	Parts per million

I.S. Hussein, B.Sc., M.Sc., M.B.A., Ph.D (✉)
Research Centre (ICCIDD) MENA and Gulf Region, International Council for Control of Iodine Deficiency Disorders, P.O. Box 1087, 133, Region 01 Al Khuwair, Oman
e-mail: izzeldin.alsharief@gmail.com; shigla50@hotmail.com

V.R. Preedy et al. (eds.), *Handbook of Food Fortification and Health: From Concepts to Public Health Applications Volume 1*, Nutrition and Health, DOI 10.1007/978-1-4614-7076-2_18,

TGR	Total goiter rate
TSH	Thyroid stimulating hormone
UIE	Urinary iodine excretion
UNICEF	United Nations Children's Fund
USI	Universal salt iodization
WHO	World Health Organization

Introduction

Iodine deficiency, through its effects on the developing brain, has condemned millions of people to a life of few prospects and continued underdevelopment. On a worldwide basis, iodine deficiency is the single most important preventable cause of brain damage. Prevention of the determinant effects of inadequate intake of iodine is of immense importance to global development. People living in areas affected by severe iodine deficiency may have an intelligence quotient (IQ) of up to 13.5 points below that of those from comparable communities in areas where there is no iodine deficiency. This mental deficiency has an immediate effect on child learning capacity, women is health, the quality of life in communities, and economic productivity.

Iodization of salt of common food used by the vast majority of the population is a proven intervention and all countries must ensure that all salt for human consumption is adequately iodized. This chapter has validated new indicators with public health significance. In fact major contributors to this chapter came from a variety of disciplines, including laboratory science, engineering, medicine, public health, Law and legislations, and nutrition and epidemiology. This variety of backgrounds indicates the complexity and diversity required in national programs to address iodine deficiency disorders (IDD). The chapter in addition to the above provides information on new requirements for pregnant and lactating women, which results in an increased median urinary iodine concentration to define a public health problem in pregnant women. This chapter also provides the revised programmatic criteria to assess the elimination of Iodine Deficiency.

Salt Iodization is currently the most widely used strategy to control and eliminate IDD. However the public should be made aware of the impact of increased salt intake on health. This chapter emphasis on process, in particular those related to the monitoring of iodized salt at production and it use in the population level. The chapter although intended primarily for academician, public health, and students, but it will mainly help the Nutritionist and national Nutrition and micronutrition program managers and policy makers to establish a solid prevention and control of one of the immense important program to global development.

I hope the information provided in this chapter will be of benefit for all those interested in the prevention of micronutrient deficiencies in general and that it will contribute to the international goal of prevention and elimination of Iodine Deficiency (IDD) in particular.

Salt as Vehicle for Micronutrients

The control of micronutrient malnutrition, presently occupies the attention of nutrition and public health workers throughout the developing world [1]. Notably the prevention of the detrimental effects of inadequate intake of three micronutrients—iodine, vitamin A and iron—is of immense importance to global development.

Fortification of foods that are commonly consumed by the population at risk has been demonstrated to be a viable and cost-effective food-based strategy for the control of micronutrient deficiencies.

Table 18.1 Spectrum of iodine deficiency disorders

Fetus	Abortion, stillbirths, congenital anomalies, increased prenatal and infant mortality, neurologic cretinism (mental deficiency, deaf autism, spastic dysplasia, and squint), hypothyroid cretinism, psychomotor defects
Neonate	Neonate goiter, neonatal hypothyroidism
Child and adolescent	Goiter, juvenile hypothyroidism, impaired mental function and retarded physical development, overt or subclinical hypothyroidism
Adult	Goiter and its complications, hypothyroidism, endemic mental retardation, decreased fertility rate, impaired mental function, and iodine-induced hyperthyroidism
All ages	Goiter, hyperthyroidism, impaired mental function, increased susceptibility to nuclear radiation

Source: Hetzel (1993)

Since humans universally consume salt in small fairly constant amount daily, it is an ideal vehicle to deliver physiological amounts of micronutrients like iodine to the population in large. Iodization of salt (USI) has been practiced successfully in several countries for over 95 years.

Iodine Deficiency Disorders

Healthy humans require iodine, an essential component of the thyroid hormones, thyroxin, and triiodothyronine. Failure to have adequate iodine leads to insufficient production of these hormones, which affects different parts of the body, particularly muscle, heart, liver, kidney, and the development of the brain. Inadequate hormone production adversely affects the tissue, resulting in the disease status known collectively as "Iodine deficiency disorders" or IDD. These consequences include (a) mental retardation, (b) other defects in the development of the nervous system, (c) goiter—enlarged thyroid, (d) physical sluggishness, and economic stagnation. The most devastating of these consequences are on the developing human brain [2]. Unlike nutrients such as iron, calcium, or vitamins, iodine does not occur naturally in specific foods; rather, it is present in the soil and is ingested through food grown in that soil.

Clinical and Subclinical Manifestation

An iodine-deficient diet causes a wide spectrum of illnesses (Table 18.1). The healthy adult human body contains 15–20 mg of iodine of which about 70–80 % is in the thyroid gland. The pool of iodine is concentrated mainly in the thyroid [3]. However, in response to prolonged iodine deficiency, the thyroid gland can increase about fivefold to the size of football, a condition recognized as goiter [4].

Nomenclature and Biochemistry of Iodine

Iodine stems from the Greek (*iodes* "violet"). It is a chemical element that has the symbol (I) and atomic number (53). Naturally occurring iodine is a single isotope with 74 neutrons. Bernard Courtois discovered iodine in 1811 [5].

Elemental iodine can be prepared by oxidizing iodides with chlorine:

$$^{2}I^{-} + Cl_2 \rightarrow I_2 + ^{2}Cl^{-}$$

or with manganese dioxide in acid solution:

$$^{2}I^{-} + {}^{4}H^{+} + MnO_2 \rightarrow I_2 + {}^{2}H_2O + Mn_2^{+}$$

Iodine is reduced to hydroiodic acid by hydrogen sulphide:

$I^2 + H_2S \rightarrow {}^{2}HI + S\downarrow$ or by hydrazine:

$^{2}I_2 + N_2H_4 \rightarrow {}^{4}HI + N_2$

Iodine is oxidized to iodate by nitric acid:

$$I_2 + {}^{10}HNO_3 \rightarrow {}^{2}HIO_3 + {}^{10}NO_2 + {}^{4}H_2O$$

or by chlorates:

$$I_2 + {}^{2}ClO_3^{-} \rightarrow {}^{2}IO_3^{-} + Cl_2$$

Biological Functions

All biologic actions of iodide are attributed to the thyroid hormones. The major thyroid hormone secreted by the thyroid gland is T4 (tetra-iodo-thyronine). T4 in circulation is taken up by the cells and is de-iodinated by the enzyme 5′ prime-mono-de iodinase in the cytoplasm to convert it into tri-iodo-thyronine (T3), the active form of thyroid hormone. T3 traverses to the nucleus and binds to the nuclear receptor. All the biologic actions of T3 are mediated through the binding to the nuclear receptor, which controls the transcription of a particular gene to bring about the synthesis of a specific protein [3].

The physiologic actions of thyroid hormones can be summarized as growth and development and control of metabolic processes in the body. Thyroid hormones play a major role in the growth and development of brain and central nervous systems in humans from the 15th week of gestation to age 3 years. If iodine deficiency exists during this period that leading to thyroid hormone deficiency, the consequence is derangement in the development of brain and central nervous system. These derangements are irreversible, the most serious form being that of cretinism [6].

Iodine and Pregnancy

Iodine at 150 μg/day for adolescents and adults is justified by the fact that it corresponds to the daily urinary excretion of iodine and to the iodine content of food in non-endemic areas (areas where iodine intake is adequate). It also provides the iodine intake necessary to maintain the plasma iodide level above the critical limit of 0.10 μg/dl, which is the average level likely to be associated with the onset of goiter [7]. The iodine requirement during pregnancy is increased to provide for the needs of the fetus and to compensate for the increased loss of iodine in the urine resulting from an increased renal clearance of iodine during pregnancy [8]. These requirements have been derived from studies of thyroid function during pregnancy and in the neonate under conditions of moderate iodine deficiency. The World Health Organization (WHO) and United Nations Children's Fund (UNICEF) and the International Council for Control of Iodine Deficiency Disorders (ICCIDD) technical consultation proposed to increase the current Food and Agriculture Organization (FAO) and the WHO recommended nutrient intake for iodine during pregnancy from 200 to 250 μg per day (Table 18.2).

Table 18.2 Recommended dosage of daily and annual iodine supplementation

Population group	Daily dosage of iodine supplement (μg/day)	Single annual dose of iodized oil supplement (μg/year)
Pregnant women	250	400
Lactating women	250	400
Women of reproductive age (15–49 years)	150	400
Children <2 years[a]	90	200

Source: Indicators for assessing iodine deficiency disorders and their control through salt iodization, WHO (2007)
[a]These figures for iodine supplements are given in situations where complementary food fortified with iodine is not available, in which case iodine supplementation is required for children of 7–24 months of age

Table 18.3 Properties of pure sodium chloride

Molecular weight—NaCl	58.4428
Atomic weight—Na	22.989768 (39.337 %)
Atomic weight—Cl	35.4527 (60.663 %)
Eutectic composition	23.31 % NaCl
Freezing point of eutectic mixture	−21.12 °C (−6.016 °F)
Crystal form	Isometric, cubic
Color	Clear to white
Index of refraction	1.5442
Density or specific gravity	2.165 (135 lb/ft^3)
Bulk density, approximate (dry, ASTM D 632 gradation)	1.154 (72 lb/ft^3)
Critical humidity at 20 °C (68 °F)	75.3 %
pH of aqueous solution	Neutral

Rationale and the Public Health Imperative of Permanent Elimination of Iodine Deficiency Disorders

Iodine deficiency thus results mainly from geological rather than social and economic conditions. It cannot be eliminated by changing diet habits or by eating specific kinds of foods grown in the same area. Rather the correction has to be achieved by supplying iodine from an external source, fortification or by periodic supplementation of deficient populations with iodine. While both strategies are effective, the iodization of salt is the common, long termed sustainable solution that will ensure that iodine reaches the entire population and is ingested on a regular basis. In specific areas that iodized salt will not reach soon, iodized oil supplementation is something recommended as a short-term intervention.

The Salt

Common salt, or sodium chloride, is the chemical compound (NaCl). Salt occurs naturally in many parts of the world as the mineral halite and as mixed evaporites in salt lakes. Seawater containing lots of salt is one of the best sources of this natural nutrient. It has an average of 2.6 % NaCl (by weight), or 26 million metric tons per cubic kilometer (Table 18.3).

The Salt and Human Health

Sodium chloride, more commonly known as salt, represents an essential element of life, being one of the elements the human body cannot do without. A certain amount of salt must be incorporated into our daily diet, not only because it is very rapidly eliminated by our bodies and also because it enhances the taste of our food, but above all because the recognition of salty taste by the body triggers the production of the saliva and gastric juices, both essential for food digestion. In addition, the presence of sodium and chloride is essential in the digestive processes, since they are both present in the gastric juices, in the saliva, in the pancreatic juice and in the bile. The sodium and the chloride act then at different levels, along the digestive track, since sodium contributes to the absorption of glucides, while chloride, in the form of hydrochloric acid, is essential for the digestion of solids. The consumption of sodium is on an average about 3 g a day in the United State of America, corresponding to the ingestion of 7–8 g of salt [8].

The kidneys regulate the sodium balance. They are able to quickly adjust the sodium balance, when the quantity of salt varies between 1 and 16 g a day. Under these conditions, there are no variations in the extra-cellular volume or in body weight. With quantities of salt higher than 16 g a day, kidney adjustment requires 3–5 days, during which time an increase in the extra-cellular volume and in body weight is evident. After this period of time, the two values stabilize themselves to the new acquired levels. Sodium chloride is present for 2/3 in the extra-cellular liquids and for 1/3 it is primarily fixed within the bones. Every imbalance in the extra-cellular hydration is connected to anomalies in the presence of sodium (that is, of salt).

The relationship between salt and blood pressure was previously considered in 1994 by the Committee on Medical Aspects of Food and Nutrition Policy (COMA) as part of their report on *Nutritional Aspects of Cardiovascular Disease*. COMA recommended a reduction in the average intake of salt by the adult population from 9 to 6 g per day [9].

Evidence suggests that obesity coupled with a lack of exercise is an important factor involved in the development of high blood pressure. However, there is much stronger evidence to suggest that salt intake is related to the development of hypertension, and in particular the rise in blood pressure with age [10], and that potassium intake has the opposite effect and may, in certain circumstances, partially offset the effects of a high salt intake [11].

Salt Iodization: Rationale

In many developing countries, where iodine deficiency is most severe, the population is largely dependent on subsistence food. Their diet is typically based on one or two cereals, tubers or pulses as the staple. Over the past 70 years, in the effort to introduce iodine regularly into the daily diet, several foods have been considered as possible vehicles. These include salt, bread, sweets, milk, sugar, and water. Among these salt has become the most commonly accepted owing to a variety of reasons.

- Salt is one of the few commodities that come close to being universally consumed by almost all sections of a community irrespective of economic level. It is consumed approximately the same level throughout the year in a given region by all normal adults. Thus, a micronutrient like iodine when introduced through salt will be administered to each individual at a uniform dosage throughout the year.
- A major portion of salt produced in the world is from sea water. Sea water contains iodine in addition to salt. However, when sea water evaporates, much of the iodine either remains in solution or is lost by evaporation. Only a small portion of the iodine is retained in the salt. Iodization, therefore, restores a natural constituent of sea salt.
- The addition of iodine to salt (usually as potassium or sodium iodide or iodate) does not impart any color, taste, or odor to the salt. In fact iodized salt is indistinguishable from unionized salt.

Table 18.4 Typical chemical analysis of different types of salt on dry basis

Type of salt	NaCl	Mg	Ca	SO_4	Insoluble
Pure evaporated salt vacuum	99.95	0.0001	0.002	0.04	Trace
Vacuum salt	99.70	0.01	0.01	0.2	Trace
Refined salt	99.0	0.05	0.06	0.2	0.02–0.3
Solar salt	96–99	0.01–0.17	0.04–0.3	0.11–2.0	0.05–0.6
Rock salt	90–99	0.01–0.17	0.04–1.1	0.2–1.3	0–5

Table 18.5 Physical properties of iodine compounds

Name	Chemical formula	Iodine	Solubility in water				
			0 °C	20 °C	30 °C	40 °C	60 °C
Iodine	I_2	100			0.3	0.4	0.6
Potassium iodide	KI	76.5	1,280	1,440	1,520	1,600	1,760
Potassium iodate	KIO_3	59.5	47.3	81.3	117	128	185
Sodium iodide	$NaI{\cdot}2H_2O$	85.0	1,590	1,790	1,900	2,050	2,570
Sodium iodate	$NaIO_3$	64.0		25.0	90.0	150	210

Salt Quality and Refining Technology

The physical characteristics and chemical composition of salt vary widely, depending upon the composition of the raw material and the manufacturing process. Salt for iodization should be at least 98 % NaCl by weight, and less than 0, 2 % calcium, 0, 1 % magnesium, 0, 5 % sulphate, 0, 5 % insoluble, and 3 % moisture (Table 18.4).

Processes for Refining Salt

Refined salt is very pure (NaCl 99.0 %), dry and white with uniform grain size (0.3–1.0 mm). Refined salt could be with or without additives such as

- Anticaking agents: such as potassium or sodium ferrocyanide in the range (5–15 ppm)
- Free flowing agents: such as magnesium carbonate, calcium silicate, sodium silico-aluminate, and tricalcium phosphate, at a level of 1–2 %
- Iodizing agents: such as potassium iodide or iodate at level of 15–40 mg/kg

Choice and Dosage of Iodine Compound for Salt Iodization

The term iodine usually refers to the chemical element in a general sense without specifying its chemical form, but it is also used to denote the form (I_2). Occasionally salt or another vehicle is described as "iodated" when potassium iodate (KIO_3) is added, or as "iodinated" when iodine (I_2) is added to a vehicle such as water. Iodine is normally introduced as the iodide or iodate of potassium or sodium (Table 18.5).

The Iodine Content of Salt

The recommended minimum daily requirement of iodine varies from 150 to 250 µg. Numerous factors influence the selection of an appropriate level for a given population, including: (a) per capita

Table 18.6 Sample calculation for fixing the level of iodization with KIO_3, in salt

Assume that the per capita daily requirement of iodine is 200 μg
Assume that the per capita salt consumption is 10 g per day
Level of iodine required in salt is 200 μg per 10 g (1 g = 1 million μg) or 20 ppm
Level of iodine required = 20 × 1.685 ppm KIO_3 = 33.7 ppm KIO_3
The World Health, UNICEF and ICCIDD (2007) recommended the levels at 15–40 mg/kg iodine at the production level

consumption of salt in a region; (b) the degree of IDD; (c) transit loses; and shelf life. Per capita consumption of salt in different countries varies over a wide range, from about 3–15 g per day.

Discussions and regulations about iodine levels in salt must clearly specify whether they refer to total content of iodine alone or to content of iodine compound (KIO_3 or KI). From the example above, 20 ppm as iodine is the same as 33.7 ppm KIO_3 or 26 ppm as KI. In general it is recommended that the level be expressed as content of iodine alone.

A sample calculation for fixing the level of iodization of salt with potassium iodate could be as shown in (Table 18.6).

WHO/UNICEF/ICCIDD recommends [12] that, in typical circumstances, where the iodine lost from salt is 20 % from production site to household, and 20 % is lost during cooking before consumption, and average salt intake is 10 g per person per day, iodine concentration in salt at the point of production should be within the range of 20–40 mg of iodine per kg of salt (i.e., 20–40 ppm of iodine) in order to provide 150 μg of iodine per person per day [13]. In countries where iodized salt is used in processed foods, the iodine content in salt should be closer to the lower end of this range and vice versa. The iodine should preferably be added as potassium iodate. Under these circumstances, median urinary iodine levels are expected to vary from 100 to 199 μg/L.

Quality Control and Monitoring of Salt Iodine Levels

Monitoring the level of iodine in the salt is important in several respects:

1. To ensure that salt manufactured or imported into a country meets specifications—a legal requirement
2. To ensure that salt which reaches the consumer contains iodine to ensure prevention of IDD physiological requirement
3. To ensure sustainability of the program and any deviation from prescribed levels should be reported at once and action taken
4. Continuous monitoring of iodine levels is one of the best and simplest ways of monitoring the entire IDD elimination program when salt iodization is the intervention strategy

Methods of Measuring Iodine in Salt

Two techniques for measuring iodine levels in salt can be used:

1. Standard titration method
   This method is used when great accuracy of the iodine level is required. A given amount of salt is treated with concentrated Sulfuric Acid, which liberates iodine. The free iodine is titrated with sodium thiosulphate, using starch as indicator.

Table 18.7 Criteria for assessing adequacy of salt iodization program

Process indicator	Criterion of adequacy
Factory level	
Percent of food grade salt claimed to be iodized	100 %
Percent of food grade salt effectively iodized	>90 %
Adequacy of internal monitoring process	>90 %
Adequacy of external monitoring process*	10–12 monthly checks per producer per year. Corrective action systematically taken within 3 h in 90 % of cases, following the lot quality assurance methodology
District and consumer level	
Percent of monitoring sites with adequately iodized salt	Adequate in 90 % of samples
(a) Households (or schools) (b) district headquarters (including major markets)	90 % or more
Adequacy of monitoring process**	

Source: Joint WHO/UNICEF/ICCIDD Consultation on Indicators for IDD Control

*Corrective action systematically taken within three hours in 90 % of cases, following the lot quality assurance methodology

**Monitoring undertaken in 90 % of districts in each province, at household and retail level

2. Rapid Test Kits
   These consist of bottles of starch solution (stabilized) of which one drop is placed on the salt. The intensity of the blue color that develops indicates the approximate iodine level. A single ampoule of reagent (10 mL) will allow about 80–100 tests.

The Procedure for Monitoring Iodine Levels in Salt

Factory Level

The manufacturer should conduct its own monitoring at hourly intervals during the production, preferably by titration in a lab or at least with a testing kit (Rapid Test Kits) that shows some sensitivity to color change. External monitoring of production level quality control should be done by government officials to substantiate the accuracy of the manufacturer's records.

Distributor and Wholesale Level

The major distributors should be sensitized and provided with rapid test kits to check the presence of iodine in the salt before it is released for retail sale. Regular monitoring at 3-monthly intervals is advisable.

Consumer Level

The overall responsibility for quality control peripherally, inside the country, should be vested in the Ministry of Health through its Primary Health Care Department (PHD), and regional/provincial and district health departments in particular; the public health inspectors or nurses at the district level (Table 18.7).

Table 18.8 Label for iodized salt packets/bags

Iodized salt
1. Name of the manufacturer: ______________________
2. Month/year of manufacture: _______ Batch no. ________
3. Iodizing agent: potassium iodate/potassium iodide
4. Iodine content: ____________________ ppm
5. Date of expiration: ______________ (12 months from the date of manufacture)
6. Net weight: _____________ kg
7. Price: _____________/bags
Caution: Store in a cool and dry place

Table 18.9 Methodology for determination of the national salt iodization program

Status of salt iodization program	Recommended action
Nonexistent	Analysis of salt production and distribution. Analysis should include a survey of the extent and severity of the problems, and identification of the best point for iodization. Based on these data, an implementation program can be drawn up
Existent but needing substantial modification	The salt production, distribution and consumption patterns should be reviewed to identify the bottlenecks that hamper successful implementation of control programs
Existent but needing strengthening	The program should be periodically reviewed to ensure its tempo is maintained. In order to eliminate iodine deficiency permanently, iodization of salt and its distribution should become an integral part of a salt production and distribution system that will run on its own momentum after an initial period of support and monitoring
Existent and effective	Periodic monitoring of iodine levels at the production and consumption level

Packaging, Storage, and Distribution of Iodized Salt

The retention of iodine in salt depends on the iodine compound used, the type of packaging, the exposure of the package to prevailing climatic conditions, and the period of time between iodization and consumption.

Since salt is hygroscopic at relative humidity above 76 %, iodized salt that is improperly packed and transported over long distances under humid conditions attracts moisture and becomes wet, carrying the iodate to the bottom of the bag. At humidity lower than 76 %, salt can release surface moisture, and this also may result in some iodine loss. If the bag is porous, the iodine compound can leak so that little or no iodine is left in the salt by the time it reaches the consumer. It is important that each bag should be marked with the following legend to identify the contents for monitoring purposes (Table 18.8).

Salt Situation Analysis

The first step in a salt situation analysis would be to prepare a list of the major producers or importers, production/import/export statistics, and information regarding salt quality, packaging, pack sizes, transport and storage, retail marketing practices, prices and household consumption. These data need to be updated according to the country situation periodically, e.g., every 2 years.

The methodology for a salt situation analysis will depend upon the status of the salt iodization program in the country. The steps to be taken for different situations are summarized in Table 18.9.

Universal Salt Iodization Program

National personnel, aided as necessary by technical assistance from international agencies and experts, should design specific actions to increase the coverage and effectiveness of the salt iodization programs in their countries, specifically in the following areas:

(a) Undertake a detailed salt situation analysis and draw up a plan for integration of iodization in the salt production system that will ensure that all salt for human and animal consumption is adequately iodized.
(b) Develop a communications strategy that will focus on increased recognition for IDD in general and goiter in particular as disorders of serious magnitude, increasing awareness of preventability through iodized salt and emphasizing the product attributes of iodized salt.
(c) Conduct an initial review of existing legislation and legal frameworks (for example food standards, public health acts and food adulteration acts) to establish the most appropriate regulatory framework for compulsory salt iodization. Based on this, an order, standard or regulation requiring all salt for human and animal consumption to be iodized will need to be issued. This can be supported later with a law.
(d) Prepare a detailed plan for universal salt iodization (USI) and the facilities and actions required to achieve it.
(e) Establish a procurement and installation plan for the iodization equipment and the training necessary for its operation and maintenance.
(f) Establish quality control procedures, the number of random visits by inspectors to salt producing units, and the number of internal quality control checks required. Establish a procedure for checking salt quality at retail and household levels. Specify action to be taken in the event of noncompliance with regulations.
(g) Promote public education, political support and appropriate commercial means to improve the distribution and consumption of iodized salt and to ensure that the supply is regular and uninterrupted.
(h) Enact laws requiring all salt to be iodized. Provide continuing support for producers for a period sufficiently long to enable them to comply with the

Characteristics of Effective Salt Iodization Programs

While salt iodization is technically a straight forward process, its sustained large-scale implementation calls for changes within political, administrative, technical, and socio-cultural spheres. Some countries have been moderately successful in this process, but others have been struggling for many years to establish effective programs. Available country experiences indicate certain key issues have a bearing on the success of national programs:

(a) Policy support
Several health and nutrition programs compete for priority action by policy makers. Raising high level awareness of the problem and the effectiveness of its control within a short period through salt iodization has been an important factor in generating political will to support serious control and monitoring efforts. Awareness has been created by assessing and making available epidemiological information regarding IDD prevalence and the meaning of the data to high level politicians and bureaucrats.
(b) Multiple sectors in the planning of Salt iodization programs
While the responsibility for initiating, coordinating and monitoring an IDD control program rests primarily with the health sector, it's planning and implementation calls for active involvement of

Table 18.10 Iodine requirements for animals

Class of animal	Class of animal total diet (ppm)	Salt consumption (kg/year)	Iodine content required in salt (ppm)
Swine	0.14	4.1	28
Beef cattle	0.2–2.0	10	40–400
Dairy cattle	0.25–0.5	24.3	50–100
Horses	0.1	10.9	20
Sheep	0.1–0.8	4.1	20–160
Goats	0.15–0.8	4–8	30–240
Poultry	0.3–0.4	0.2	120–160

other sectors like industry, trade, planning, transport, legislators, communicators, and educators, to implement and integrate iodization into the salt production and distribution system.

(c) Monitoring of iodine levels in salt
Frequent testing of iodine levels at iodization plants and periodically at intermediate points in the distribution network, retail outlets, and the household level has been characteristic of countries with successful programs. Ecuador and Brazil [14] sampled salt on a weekly basis at production plants during the early phases of the fortification program in order to detect variability in iodine levels quickly and take corrective action. Bhutan has developed a systematic monitoring and reporting system for iodine at the levels of production, distribution, and consumption. The reports are reviewed centrally every month and corrective initiated when required. Another useful exercise is the involvement of other sectors like NGOs, voluntary organizations, and schools in monitoring the salt, using the low cost field test kits. This helps increase awareness and community participation.

Iodized Salt for Animal Consumption

It is now well appreciated that the IDD are a major public health problem in the world affecting large populations in over 110 countries with nearly 1.6 billion people at risk. What is not well known is the severe effect of iodine deficiency on animals.

Farm animals share with humans the risk of iodine deficiency at all stages of growth and development, from conception to physical performance. Salt is the predominant vehicle for providing supplemental iodine for farm animals. Iodine may be incorporated into the salt, mineral mixture, or concentrate feeds. For grazing animals in some inaccessible parts of the world iodized salt blocks are air dropped.

Iodine Levels in Salt for Animals

In the developed countries there is a range of trace mineralized salt preparations that caters to each variety of livestock and poultry. In these trace mineralized salts, typical levels for livestock are 70–80 ppm iodine. The farmer usually buys one type of salt from the market for his livestock as well as for his family. Estimates of iodine levels in salt are presented for different animals in Table 18.10, showing a wide range from 30 to 400 ppm. As an approximation, if the level of iodine in the salt is at least 20 ppm at the consumer level, this will ensure minimum requirements for many domestic animals. However, if special categories like cattle and sheep continue to demonstrate consequences of iodine deficiency, then additional iodine supplementation may be required through cattle feeds or other sources. There is no apparent risk of toxicity for any class of animals even if salt containing levels of iodine of more than 200 ppm is fed to any class of animals.

Legislation and Enforcement

Enforcement of the regulation has proved critical to ensuring the quality of iodized salt. None iodized salt, when identified by inspectors, is confiscated or destroyed. In some countries, legal sanctions in the form of fines and newspaper publication of noncompliant brand names are used to enforce quality control [14].

For most developing countries, an effective salt iodization program needs to be supported by effective legislation. The law should specifically address the following requirements:

1. Mandatory salt iodization at a level to be determined by the public health authorities of each country
2. Applicability of the measure to all salt that is produced, imported, or marketed in the country for human and animal consumption
3. The law can specify the type, quality, and amount of iodine compound to be added, the levels of production/port of import, distribution and consumption or can leave these details to enabling regulations by a designated government unit, frequently the Ministry of Health; the latter approach offers the flexibility of responding promptly to changes in salt consumption or other factors without passing new legislation (Tables 18.11, 18.12, 18.13, and 18.14)

Table 18.11 General framework for iodized salt monitoring system

Decision level	What information is needed	Who manages the information	What monitoring activities are done	What responses may be needed
Private sector responsibilities				
Factory	Is the iodine content in salt adequate when produced and packaged? Are factory standards being met? Does the label reflect the salt iodine content in bags?	Factory owner Plant manager Plant operator	Internal quality assurance Facilitate external inspection by regulatory agency Visual inspection of equipment	Make adjustments to iodization process Modify packaging, labeling, storage or procurement procedures
Wholesaler/ traders	Is iodized salt being procured? Is the iodine content at the level claimed? Is the iodized salt affordable? Is the iodized salt being purchased	Traders Salt wholesalers	Rapid testing of iodine levels in the salt Visual check on salt quality	Ensure that traders transport iodized salt only Improve storage practices at wholesale site Ensure the concept of first in first out
Retailer	Is iodized salt being supplied Is iodine content at the level claimed? Is iodized salt affordable?	Shopkeepers		Rapid testing of iodine levels in the salt?
Government responsibilities				
National	Is iodized salt available to all areas of the country? Is iodine level in salt adequate upon import and production?	National IDD committee Minister of health Program managers	External quality control of imported or domestic salt Inspection of internal quality assurance record Monitor proportion of households using adequately iodized salt	Develop legislation Provide technical support for production and monitoring of iodized salt Support social marketing efforts

(continued)

Table 18.11 (continued)

Decision level	What information is needed	Who manages the information	What monitoring activities are done	What responses may be needed
Community/household responsibilities				
Community/ household/ school	Is iodine level adequate in salt being consumed? Is iodized salt more expensive than noniodized salt? Is iodized salt labeling adequate	Community groups Household members School teachers	Inspect packet label Rapid testing of salt kits	Demand retailer to st ock only iodized salt Involve community leaders in efforts to ensure availability and quality of iodized salt

Table 18.12 Criteria for assessing iodine nutrition based on median urinary iodine concentrations in school children. Indicators and guidance for save level

Median urinary iodine (μg/L)	Iodine intake	Iodine nutrition
<20	Insufficient	Severe iodine deficiency
20–49	Insufficient	Moderate iodine deficiency
50–99	Insufficient	Mild iodine deficiency
100–199	Adequate	Optimal
200–299	Above requirement	Likely to provide adequate intake for pregnant/lactating women, but may pose a slight risk of more than adequate intake in the overall population
<300	Excessive	Risk of adverse health consequences (iodine-induced hyperthyroidism, autoimmune thyroid disease)

Source: Assessment of iodine deficiency disorders and monitoring their elimination. Guideline for program managers, WHO/UNICEF, Third edition, 2007

Table 18.13 Criteria for assessing iodine nutrition based on the median or range in urinary iodine concentrations of pregnant women[a]

Population group	Median urinary iodine intake concentration (μg/L)	Iodine intake
Pregnant women	<150	Insufficient
	150–249	Adequate
	250–499	Above requirements
	<500	Excessive[b]

[a]For lactating women and children <2 years of age a median urinary iodine concentration of 100 μg/L can be used to define adequate iodine intake, but no other categories of iodine intake are defined. Although lactating women have the same requirement as pregnant women, the median urinary iodine is lower because iodine is excreted in breast milk
[b]The term "excessive" means in excess of the amount required to prevent and control iodine deficiency

Table 18.14 Recommended dosages of daily and annual iodine supplementation [3]

Single annual dose of iodized oil supplement (mg/year)	Daily dose of iodine supplement	Population group
400	250	Pregnant women
400	250	Lactating women
400	150	Women of reproductive age (15–49 year)
200	90	Children <2 years[a,b]

[a]For children 0–6 months of age, iodine supplementation should be given through breast milk. This implies that the child is exclusively breastfed and that the lactating mother received iodine supplementation as indicated above
[b]These figures for iodine supplements are given in situations where complementary food fortified with iodine is not available, in which case iodine supplementation is required for children of 7–24 months of age

Indicators of the Universal Salt Iodization Assessment

The indicators to assess the iodization (USI) and progress of elimination are divided into three main groups:

1. *Process indicators*: Indicators to monitor and evaluate the salt iodization process. These indicators reflect monitoring salt iodine content at the production/importation site and at the household level.
2. *Impact indicators*: Indicators to assess iodine status and to monitor and evaluate the impact of salt iodization on the population. Median urinary iodine is the main indicator to be used to assess iodine status of a population. Goiter assessment by palpation or by ultrasound may be useful in assessing thyroid function.
3. *Sustainability indicators*: Indicators to assess whether iodine deficiency has been successfully eliminated and to judge whether achievements can be sustained and maintained for the decades to come. This involves a combination of median urinary iodine levels in the population, availability of adequately iodized salt at the household level, and a set of programmatic indicators which are regarded as evidence of sustainability.

Conclusion

USI involves the iodization of all human and livestock salt, including salt used in the food industry. Adequate iodization of all salt will deliver iodine in the required quantities to the population on a continuous and self-sustaining basis.

Between 1994 and 2006, the number of countries that carried out a urinary iodine national survey increased to 94, and survey data on iodine deficiency now covers 91.1 % of the world population. There is still no data for 63 countries, which together represent 8.9 % of the world population.

Out of the 130 countries with estimates based on surveys at both the national and subnational level estimates, there are only 47 countries where IDD still remains as a public health problem, compared to 54 in 2004 and 126 in 1993. Iodine intake (reflected by the median urinary iodine concentration) in the other 83 countries is as follows: “adequate” [15] or “above recommended nutrient intakes” [16] in 76 countries; and “excessive”; in 7 countries. About 31 % (1,900.9 million) of the world’s population is estimated to have insufficient iodine intakes. It is currently estimated that 70 % of households throughout the world have access to (and use) iodized salt [17].

Iodine supplementation should be implemented to prevent and treat iodine deficiency disorders; fortification should be maintained at a safe level (15–40 ppm). Levels that are more than adequate (median urinary iodine excretion, 200–299 μg/L) or excessive (median urinary iodine excretion, >500 μg/L) may not be safe, especially for susceptible populations with either potential autoimmune thyroid diseases or iodine deficiency. Supplementation programs should be tailored to the particular region. No iodine supplementation should be provided for regions in which iodine intake is sufficient, whereas salt in regions in which iodine intake is deficient should be supplemented with iodine according to the degree of iodine deficiency. Therefore, there is an urgent need for a regulatory mechanism during the process of iodine fortification [18], and at the point of entry of iodized salt, as well as the mode of delivery.

Recommendations

Previously deficient populations are particularly at risk of developing iodine-induced hyperthyroidism if levels of intake are excessive. Optimal iodine intake is therefore important, but due to poor quality control at the production level and the high levels of fortification required by some governments' legislation, which specifies up to 2.5 times of the WHO recommendation, there is now a risk that population which were previously severely deficient in iodine now consuming excess iodine. It is recommended to obtain more extensive baseline data on the prevalence, geographic distribution, knowledge, attitudes and practices relating to iodine deficiency and its elimination. The aim should be to provide a strategy that ensures optimal control of iodine supplementation levels to those in need, together with effective monitoring for efficacy and safety.

It is further recommended that academicians, governments and developing agencies need to:

- Conduct a nation-wide public health education program to promote community awareness of the importance of the use of iodized salt and the hazardous effects of inappropriate iodine intake. This should be directed mainly at the rural community and achieved through educational and social marketing campaigns.
- Introduce iodine deficiency control and prevention in education curricula at all levels.
- Introduce proper monitoring systems for the salt iodization program. The systems should have a systematic approach for supervision and regular monitoring of salt at production sites, retail shops and households and at the schools level.
- Encourage research institutions to study the pattern of iodized salt and the impact of food rich in iodine in population.
- Encourage rectifying the environment by spraying and or injecting iodine into the soil.
- Continued and strong government commitment and motivation, with appropriate annual budgetary allocations to maintain the process, are essential to eliminate IDD.
- The salt industry should have the capacity to implement effective iodization, in particular with regard to compliance with the regulations and monitoring of quality assurance.
- Monitoring systems should be in place to ensure specified salt iodine content, and should be coordinated with effective regulation and enforcement.
- Small-scale producers need to be included in this process to ensure that their products are also brought up to standard and that they deliver the right amount of iodine to the population. This is often best achieved by the formation of cooperatives working with a common distributor or any other business models that reduce the need for many small iodization units.
- The contribution of iodine from salt used in the food industry should be considered and monitored in the IDD elimination effort.

References

1. Calloway DH. Food and micronutrient relationships. Working paper 1. Washington, DC: International Food Policy Research Institute; 1995.
2. Dunn JT. What's happening to our iodine. J Clin Endocrinol Metab. 1998;83:3398–400.
3. Hetzel BS. Iodine deficiency disorders (IDD) and their eradication. Lancet. 1983;2:1126–7.
4. Delong F. The disorders induced by iodine deficiency. Thyroid. 1994;1:107–28.
5. Cotton FA, Wilkinson G. Advanced inorganic chemistry. 2nd ed. New York, NY: Interscience; 1966. p. 894–902.
6. Delange F, de Benoist B, Alnwick D. Risks of iodine-induced hyperthyroidism after correction of iodine deficiency by iodized salt. Thyroid. 1999;9:545–56.
7. Wayne EJ, Koutras DA, Alexander WD. Clinical aspects of iodine metabolism. Oxford: Blackwell; 1964. p. 1–303.
8. The consumption of sodium is on average. http://www.slatworks.us/salt info/si_Salt AndGoodHealth.asp
9. Antonios TF, Mac Gregor GA. Salt—more adverse effects. Lancet. 1996;348(9022):250–1.
10. Mac Gregor GA. Nutrition and blood pressure. Nutr Metab Cardiovasc Dis. 1999;9:6–15.
11. He FJ, Mac Gregor GA. Fortnightly review: beneficial effects of potassium. Br Med J. 2001;323:497–501.
12. WHO, ICCIDD, UNICEF. Iodine levels in salt and guidelines for monitoring their adequacy and effectiveness. Geneva: World Health Organization; 1996. WHO/NUT/96.13.

13. Allen L et al., editors. Guidelines on food fortification with micronutrients. Geneva: World Health Organization and Food and Agricultural Organization of the United Nations; 2006.
14. Nathan R. Food fortification legislation and enforcement manual. Program against micronutrients malnutrition. Atlanta, GA: Emory University of Public Health; 1994.
15. Bleichrodt N, Born MA. A meta-analysis of research on iodine and its relationship to cognitive development. In: Stanbury J, editor. The damaged brain of iodine deficiency: cognitive, behavioral, neuromotor, and educative aspects. New York, NY: Cognizant Communication Corporation; 1994. p. 195–200.
16. UNICEF–WHO Joint Committee on Health Policy. World summit for children—mid decade goal: iodine deficiency disorders. Geneva: United Nations Children's Fund, World Health Organization; 1994. JCHPSS/94/2.7.
17. UNICEF. The state of the world's children 2007: women and children—the double dividend of gender equality. New York, NY: United Nations Children's Fund; 2006.
18. Izzeldin H, Hussein IS. UAE market may hamper universal salt iodization, effects of mandatory iodization on the iodine content of retailer and household. In: 8th Salt symposium, 2000;1:999–1110.

Chapter 19
Iodine Fortification and Hyperthyroidism

Charlotte Cerqueira, Torben Jørgensen, Allan Carlé, Nils Knudsen, Lars Ovesen, Inge Bülow Pedersen, Hans Perrild, and Peter Laurberg

Key Points

- The relation between iodine intake and risk of disease is complex and even small changes in iodine intake may have a large impact on the occurrence of thyroid disease.
- Severe iodine deficiency (ID) is a preventable cause of irreversible brain damage. Correction of severe ID is therefore crucial.
- Mild-to-moderate ID may be associated with a risk of intellectual impairment, but the most tangible effect is a high occurrence of goitre (enlargement of the thyroid gland) and hyperthyroidism, especially in the elderly.
- Correction of ID is associated with a risk of a temporary increased incidence of hyperthyroidism because of hormone production in the enlarged and structurally changed thyroid gland, which has been transformed due to a long period of ID.
- When the transition phase has passed, iodine fortification prevents a significant number of cases with hyperthyroidism and goitre.
- The iodine intake should not exceed the normal range—and it may be that the intake should only be increased to the lower level of the normal range—because of the risk of hypothyroidism associated with a high iodine intake.
- Iodine content and iodine nutrition has to be continuously monitored and evaluated to make sure that the iodine intake in the population stays within the optimal range.
- Monitoring of thyroid disease when implementing iodine fortification programs is of the essence, both of short-term and long-term effects. Effects of introducing iodine fortification cannot be evaluated when the baseline status of thyroid epidemiology is not known.

C. Cerqueira, M.D., Ph.D. (✉) • T. Jørgensen, M.D., M.Sc.
Research Centre for Prevention and Health, Glostrup University Hospital,
Ndr. Ringvej 57 Building 84/85, Glostrup 2600, Denmark
e-mail: charlotte.cerqueira@regionh.dk; torben.joergensen@regionh.dk

A. Carlé, M.D., Ph.D. • I.B. Pedersen, M.D., Ph.D. • P. Laurberg M.D., M.Sc.
Department of Endocrinology, Aalborg University Hospital, Sdr. Skovvej 15, Aalborg 9000, Denmark
e-mail: i.bulow@rn.dk; peter.laurberg@rn.dk; alc@rn.dk

N. Knudsen, M.D., Ph.D., M.Sc. • H. Perrild, M.D.
Department of Endocrinology and Gastroenterology, Bispebjerg University Hospital,
Bispebjerg Bakke 23, Copenhagen 2400, Denmark
e-mail: nknu0001@bbh.regionh.dk; hper0001@bbh.regionh.dk

L. Ovesen M.D.
Department of Gastroenterology, Slagelse Hospital, Ingemannsvej 18, Slagelse 4200, Denmark
e-mail: lov@regionsjaelland.dk

V.R. Preedy et al. (eds.), *Handbook of Food Fortification and Health: From Concepts to Public Health Applications Volume 1*, Nutrition and Health, DOI 10.1007/978-1-4614-7076-2_19,

Keywords Iodine • Fortification • Hyperthyroidism • Public health • Iodine intake

Abbreviations

DanThyr	The Danish Investigation of Iodine Intake and Thyroid Diseases
ICCIDD	The International Council for the Control of Iodine Deficiency Disorders
ID	Iodine deficiency
IDD	Iodine deficiency disorders
IIH	Iodine-induced hyperthyroidism
UNICEF	United Nations Children's Fund
WHO	The World Health Organization

Introduction

Iodine is a necessary substrate for the synthesis of thyroid hormones, which are involved in the regulation of almost all metabolic processes in the human body. In the adult, a sufficient production of thyroid hormone is essential to sustain health. In the offspring, a sufficient production is vital for normal development and growth and the most critical stage of iodine requirement is during fetal stage and early childhood.

Severe iodine deficiency (ID) may cause severe enlargement of the thyroid gland (goitre) and too little production of thyroid hormones (hypothyroidism), which is associated with a decreased fertility rate, increased infant mortality, and even developmental brain disorders [1, 2]. In recent years there is growing concern that not only severe but also mild ID may affect fetal growth and development, with risk of neuropsychological deficits [3, 4].

Mild-to-moderate ID, however, is mainly linked to thyroid enlargement with the gradual development of multifocal autonomous growth and function and a risk of subsequent overproduction of thyroid hormones (hyperthyroidism).

Iodine fortification of salt is an effective strategy to prevent iodine deficiency disorders (IDD). However, excessive iodine intake may also cause an increased risk of disease with an increased occurrence of hypothyroidism [5] and goitre. To make matters even more complicated, an increase in the iodine intake in a population is associated with temporary risks in the transition phase, mainly of iodine-induced hyperthyroidism (IIH). Due to the complex relation between iodine intake and risk of disease, which will be addressed in the following sections, iodine fortification programs have to be carefully planned, cautiously put into practice, and closely monitored.

Iodine Deficiency and Hyperthyroidism

The occurrence of thyroid disorders in a population depends among other factors on the iodine intake [6]. Iodine nutrition in populations may be assessed by measuring urinary iodine excretion and classified according to the criteria outlined by international organizations [7] shown in Table 19.1. Epidemiological studies have demonstrated that even small differences in the iodine intake have large effects on the occurrence of disease. Comparing the incidence of hyperthyroidism in East-Jutland in Denmark with a low average iodine intake (moderate ID) to the incidence in Iceland with a relatively high iodine intake, several differences were found [8]. As illustrated in Fig. 19.1, hyperthyroidism

Table 19.1 Classification of iodine nutrition based on median urinary iodine excretion (μg/L) according to WHO/UNICEF/ICCIDD

Severe iodine deficiency	<20
Moderate iodine deficiency	20–49
Mild iodine deficiency	50–99
Optimal iodine intake	100–199
More than adequate iodine intake	200–299
Excessive iodine intake	>300

Iodine nutrition in populations may be assessed by measuring urinary iodine excretion and classified according to the criteria outlined by the World Health Organization (WHO), the United Nations Children's Fund (UNICEF), and the International Council for the Control of Iodine Deficiency Disorders (ICCIDD) [7]

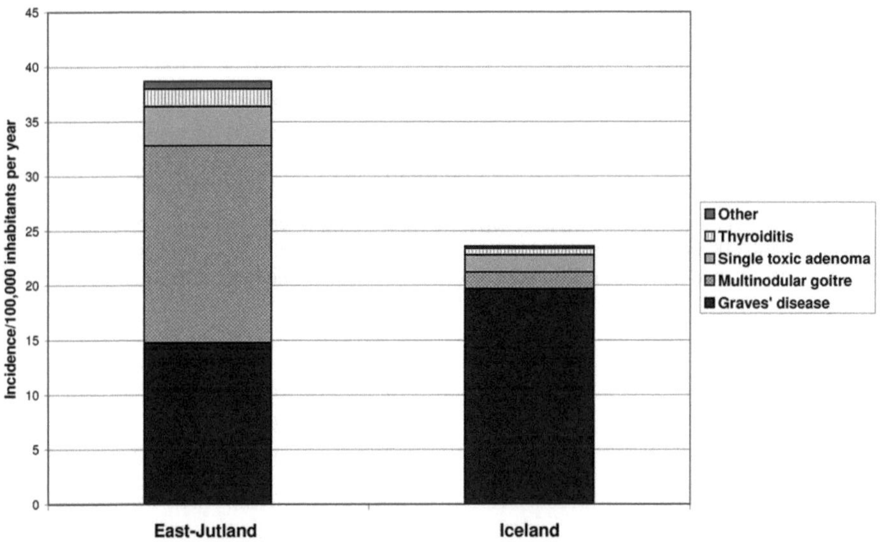

Fig. 19.1 Incidence and aetiology of hyperthyroidism in areas of different iodine intake. Incidence of hyperthyroidism per 100,000 inhabitants per year and the relative contribution of different types of thyroid disease to the incidence in East-Jutland, Denmark with low iodine intake (iodine excretion 50–60 μg/day) and Iceland with a relatively high iodine intake (300–350 μg/day). Copyright 1991, Wiley. Adapted with permission from Laurberg et al. [8]

was more common in East-Jutland than in Iceland. This was mainly due to a much higher incidence of multinodular toxic goitre. Multinodular toxic goitre is a condition that evolves from simple multinodular goitre, which is very frequent in iodine-deficient populations [9]. A subset of these nodules often function autonomously [10]—without the normal feed-back regulation of hormone production—and over time turn the simple multinodular goitre into a toxic multinodular goitre. Thus, especially in older individuals with a longstanding multinodular goitre, the thyroid may become overactive with an overproduction of thyroid hormone and development of hyperthyroidism [11, 12].

By contrast, the incidence of Graves' disease, which is an autoimmune thyroid disease caused by activating antibodies stimulating thyroid hormone production, was significantly higher in the area with relatively high iodine intake (Iceland) than in the iodine-deficient area (East-Jutland) (Fig. 19.1). This difference was most evident in the younger age groups, in which hyperthyroidism was more than twice as common in Iceland as in East-Jutland.

A similar pattern of differences has been found when studying thyroid epidemiology in areas in Denmark with even smaller differences in iodine intake (mild vs. moderate ID). In Fig. 19.2 it is illustrated that the incidence rate of hyperthyroidism was much higher in the population with moderate

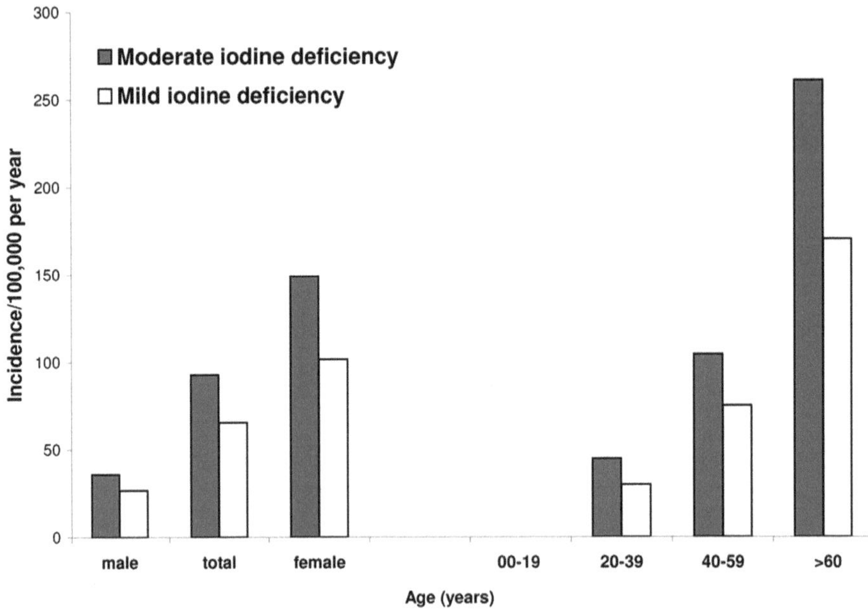

Fig. 19.2 Incidence of hyperthyroidism in areas of different iodine intake according to age group and sex. Incidence of hyperthyroidism per 100,000 inhabitants per year in two areas in Denmark; in Aalborg with moderate iodine deficiency (ID) (*filled squares*) and in Copenhagen, Denmark with mild ID (*open squares*). Copyright 2002, The Endocrine Society. Data with permission from Bülow Pedersen et al. [11]

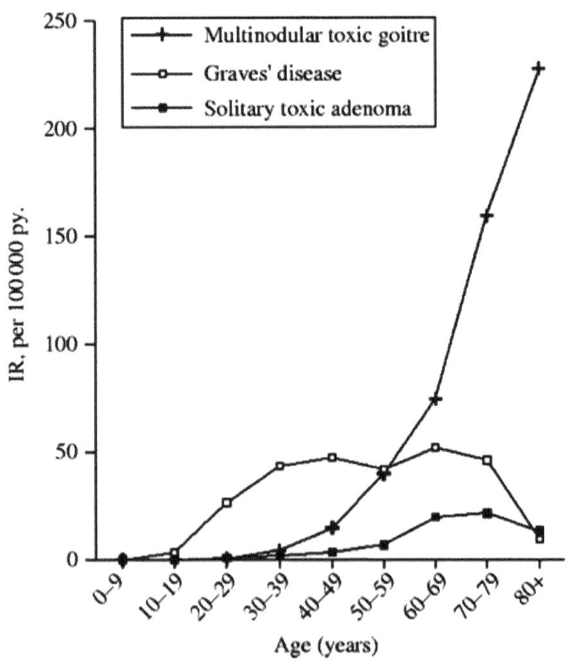

Fig. 19.3 Age-specific incidence rates of the most common subtypes of hyperthyroidism. Age-specific incidence rates (IR) of the three most common nosological types of hyperthyroidism in Denmark (Graves' disease, multinodular toxic goitre, and solitary toxic adenoma). Data with permission from Carlé et al. [12]

ID than in the population with only mild ID [11]; the two populations being otherwise comparable. After having classified patients into various subtypes of hyperthyroidism, multinodular toxic goitre was 87 % more frequent in the population living in the most iodine-deficient region, with an increasing incidence with age (Fig. 19.3) [12]. The incidence of Graves' disease, on the other hand, was similar in the two regions.

Increasing Population Intake of Iodine: Risk of Iodine-Induced Hyperthyroidism

When increasing the iodine intake in a population from deficient to sufficient, a period of transition in thyroid epidemiology will take place, before a new steady state is reached. This is much dependent on the high prevalence of thyroid tissue abnormalities in the population caused by longstanding ID, all of which are not fully reversible. In the early phase after the introduction of iodine fortification, an increase in the occurrence of hyperthyroidism is often observed—iodine-induced hyperthyroidism IIH [13]. A major mechanism behind this phenomenon is probably "feeding" of autonomous thyroid nodules with extra substrate for thyroid hormone production. Another mechanism involved may be the development of hyperthyroidism due to Graves' disease. Graves' disease appears to be highly dependent on genetic disposition [14], but a high iodine intake may have a permissive effect and lead to an earlier development of disease [8]. It is at present unknown if the appearance of Graves' disease at a younger age when the iodine intake is relatively high is caused by enhancement of the autoimmune abnormality of Graves' disease—or if the mechanism is that of "unmasking" of disease, when more substrate is present for thyroid hormone synthesis.

The risk of inducing hyperthyroidism, when iodine is given to persons with an existing goitre, has been known for many decades. In 1821 Dr. Coindet published "Nouvelles Recherches sur les effets de l'iode, et sur les precautions à suivre dans le traitement du goitre par ce nouveau remède" [15] (translation: "New research on the effects of iodine, and the precautions to be followed in the treatment of goitre by this new remedy"), where he cautioned about the use of iodine because of possible side effects. As can also be seen from the publication by Coindet, treatment of goitre by the use of iodine has been performed for many years and is still advocated by some physicians. The main value of iodine, however, is not treatment of goitre but rather prevention of goitre—the most apparent sign of ID. Iodization of salt for the nationwide eradication of IDD in populations is not a new concept, and it is among the most simple and least expensive measures to prevent nutrient disorders. In the US and in Switzerland, iodization of salt was introduced in 1920s, and has thus been practised for nearly a century.

The reports on IIH in the early phases following introduction of iodization programs are many [13], some even reporting fatal outcome. In these reports IIH has been demonstrated in the first 1–10 years with a frequency depending on prior iodine intake, the magnitude of change, and the methods used for ascertainment [16]. Most of the reports, however, are based on studies of patients referred to clinics and hospital departments in developing countries, or from small-size surveys of treated patients. Moreover, some of the studies were conducted more than a century ago when the first programs were initiated. An epidemic of IIH thoroughly investigated occurred in Tasmania in the 1960s. In Tasmania, iodine fortification of bread was introduced in 1966. However, the iodine intake in the population increased more than expected from the iodine added to bread in the iodization program because of the simultaneous introduction of the use of iodophor disinfectants in the dairy industry, leading to a concurrent increased supply of iodine from milk products. In the first 4 years following the introduction of the iodization program in Tasmania, there was more than a doubling in the number of patients referred to hospitals because of hyperthyroidism. Most patients were in older age groups and had toxic nodular goitre [17]. The epidemic of hyperthyroidism in Tasmania lasted 10–15 years, after which the incidence decreased and has persisted at a level somewhat below the pre-fortification level. In Switzerland, a similar pattern was reported when the amount of iodine added to salt was increased in 1980 from 7.5 to 15 mg iodine per kg salt [18]. In the first year following the increased iodine intake, the number of hyperthyroid patients referred to hospital showed a temporary increase of about 27 %. However, the initial increase was followed by a subsequent decrease in the number of hyperthyroid patients, primarily due to fewer patients developing multinodular toxic goitre under iodine-sufficient conditions.

The potentially fatal nature of IIH [19, 20] places an increased importance on adequate monitoring of the iodine status of populations and on early detection of IIH.

Hyperthyroidism Following Iodine Fortification: A Danish Perspective

Iodine fortification of salt was initiated in Denmark because of mild-to-moderate ID. The aim was to raise the iodine intake of the average Dane by around 50 μg/day. In 1998, a voluntary iodine fortification program was initiated, adding iodine to all salt manufactured in Denmark. The voluntary program, however, turned out to be less efficient than expected. Thus, in 2000 the program was made mandatory, adding iodine to household salt and salt used for the commercial production of bread.

As recommended by the World Health Organization (WHO), the United Nations Children's Fund (UNICEF), and the International Council for the Control of Iodine Deficiency Disorders (ICCIDD) [7] the iodization of salt in Denmark was followed by an ambitious and carefully planned monitoring program, The Danish Investigation of Iodine Intake and Thyroid Diseases (DanThyr) [21]. The main aim of the program was to monitor the effect of the iodization, but also to study risk factors and epidemiology of thyroid disease. The DanThyr monitoring program consists of four main parts, as depicted in Fig. 19.4.

The DanThyr studies have demonstrated that Denmark has changed from being a mild-to-moderately iodine-deficient nation before the introduction of iodization, to currently being an iodine-sufficient (or near-sufficient) population [22]. And the slight increase in iodine intake has had a clearly measurable impact on the frequency of thyroid disease, including hyperthyroidism.

The incidence of hyperthyroidism was monitored in different ways in the DanThyr-studies. One was from prospective identification of all individuals, who had a thyroid blood test done showing biochemical hyperthyroidism, living in two areas of Denmark—one with mild ID (Copenhagen) and

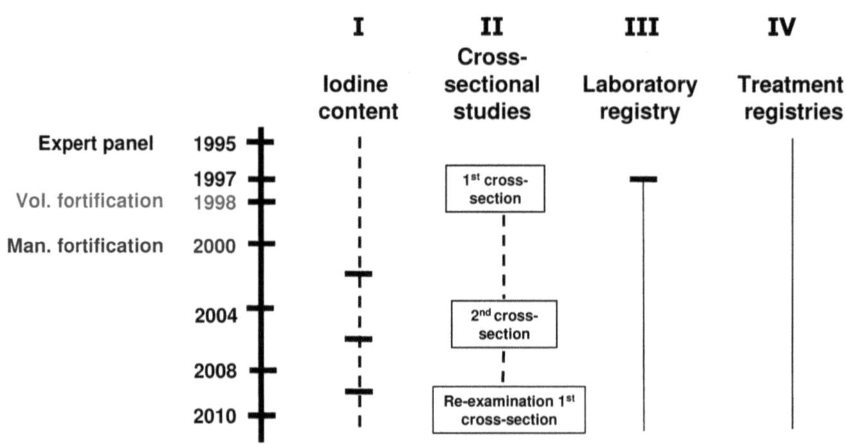

Fig. 19.4 Overview of The Danish Investigation of Iodine Intake and Thyroid Diseases (DanThyr), the monitoring program of the Danish iodine fortification program. Overview of the DanThyr monitoring program of the Danish iodine fortification program. Voluntary (vol.) iodine fortification of salt was initiated in 1998. Because of less than expected efficiency of the voluntary program the program was made mandatory (man.) in 2000. The program consist of four main parts: (I) Measurements of the iodine content in salt products and bread. (II) Cross-sectional studies performed before and after the introduction of iodization of salt (4,649 participants in the first cross-section, 3,570 in the second cross-section) in two areas of Denmark; in Aalborg with moderate ID and Copenhagen with mild ID. (III) Registration with subsequent validation of new cases of biochemical hypo- and hyperthyroidism from laboratory results of thyroid function tests in the same two areas. (IV) Analyses of data from existing nationwide registers of treatment for thyroid disease (unpublished)

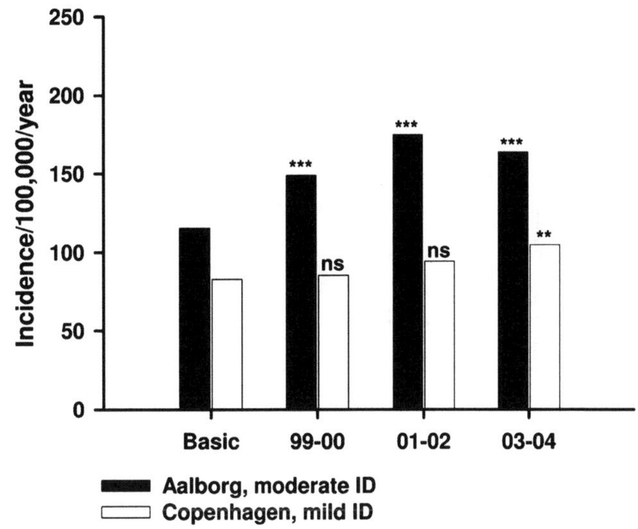

Fig. 19.5 Incidence rates of hyperthyroidism before and following the introduction of iodine fortification of salt in Denmark. The sex-specific incidence rates of hyperthyroidism before (basic) and in the first 6 years of iodine fortification of salt in Denmark. Statistical significance compared with baseline (*$p<0.05$; **$p<0.01$; ***$p<0.001$). Copyright 2006, The Endocrine Society. Data with permission from Bülow Pedersen et al. [23]

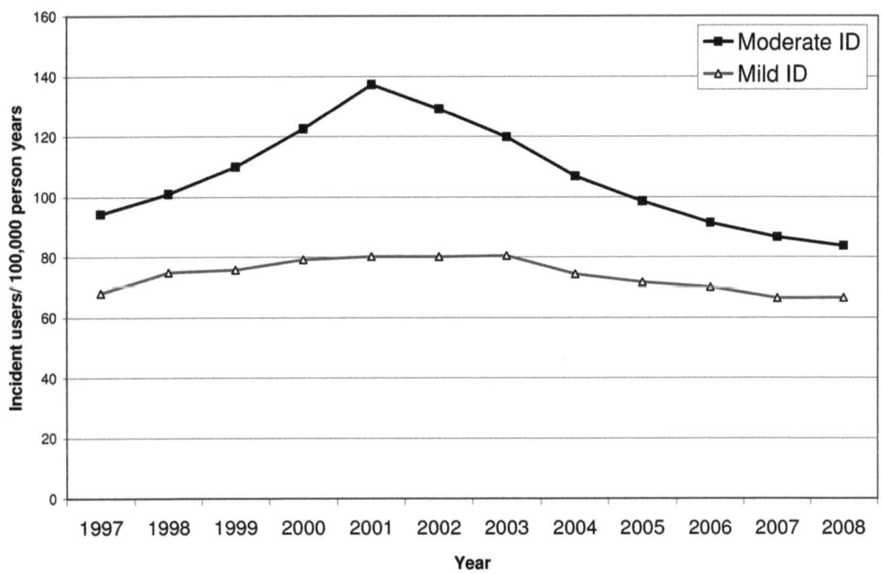

Fig. 19.6 Incident users of antithyroid medication before and following the introduction of iodine fortification of salt in Denmark. The rates were adjusted to the age- and sex-composition of the Danish population in year 2000. The annual number of new users of antithyroid medication per 100,000 persons per year in Western Denmark with moderate ID and Eastern Denmark with mild ID. Copyright 2009, The Endocrine Society. Data with permission from Cerqueira et al. [24]

the other with moderate ID (Aalborg) [23]. New disease was verified by contact to the physician requesting the thyroid function test. Another method was from identification of persons having a first-time prescription of antithyroid drugs in the entire Danish population (population around 5.4 million people) and analyzing the data separating the persons in two groups—those living in the Western part with moderate ID before the iodization program, and those living in Eastern Denmark with only mild ID [24]. Both methods for estimating the incidence of hyperthyroidism showed an increased incidence in the first years following the introduction of iodine fortification, as illustrated in Figs. 19.5 and 19.6. The most pronounced increase in the occurrence of hyperthyroidism after the

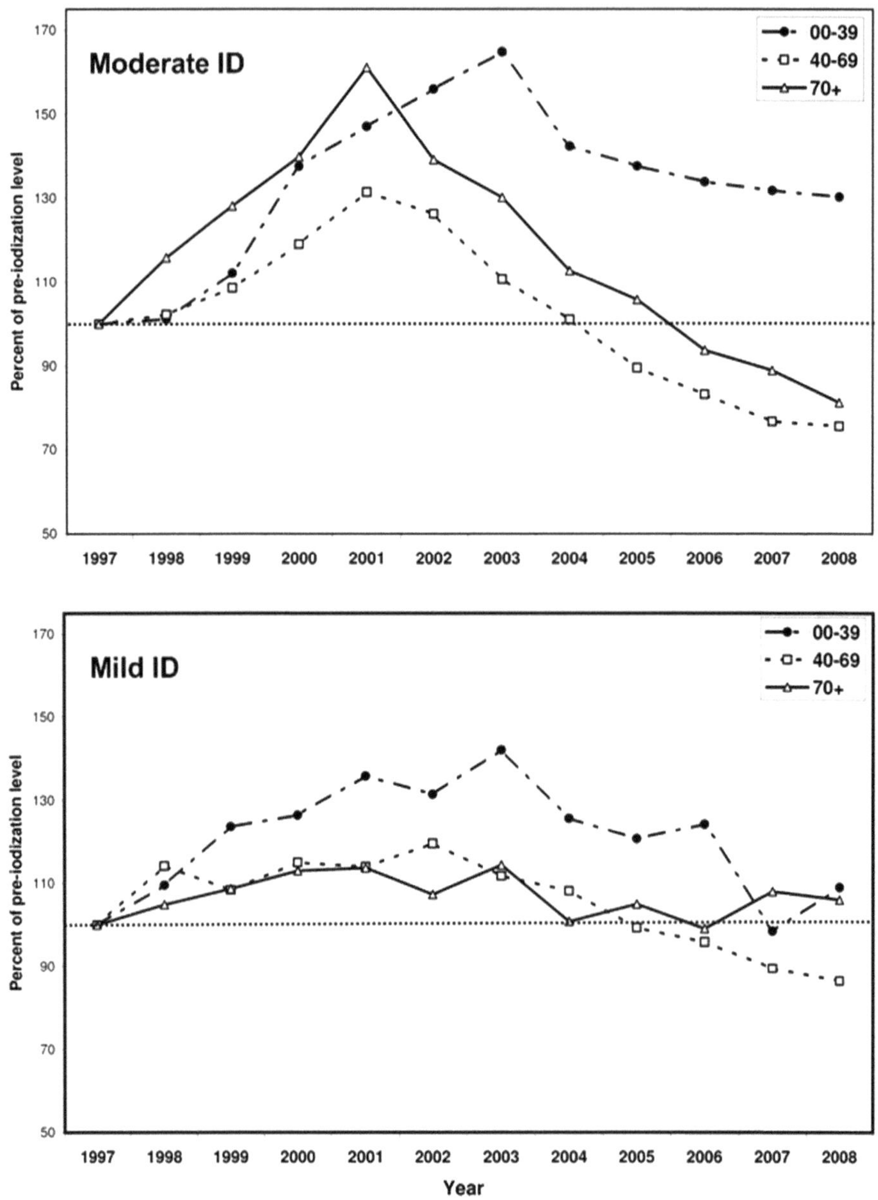

Fig. 19.7 Relative changes in incidence rates of users of antithyroid medication. Relative changes in incidence rates of users of antithyroid medication in three age groups (0–39, 40–69, 70+ years of age) in Western Denmark with moderate ID and Eastern Denmark with mild ID. The rates were compared to the rate in 1997, the year before iodization of salt was introduced. The Endocrine Society. Data with permission from Cerqueira et al. [24]

increased iodine intake was observed in the area that was moderately iodine deficient. The increase was transient and the incidence of hyperthyroidism is now back to, or even below, the level before the iodization program was initiated (Fig. 19.6). Looking at the development in different age groups (Fig. 19.7), most persons affected were in the oldest age group in the moderately deficient area. A large relative increase was also observed in people below 40 years of age, where hyperthyroidism is presumably dominated by Graves' disease. However, the absolute number of people affected in the

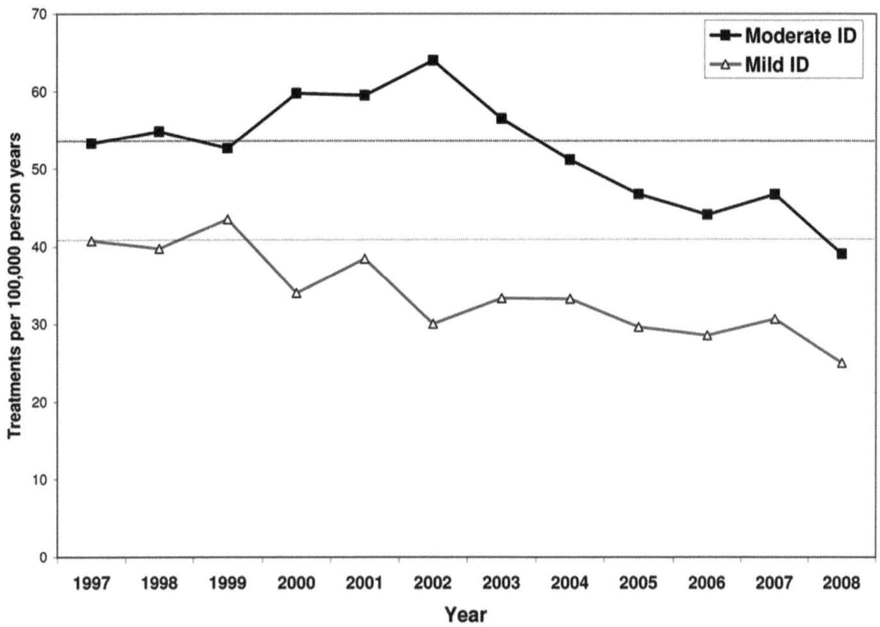

Fig. 19.8 Annual rates of radioiodine treatments for benign thyroid disease. Annual rates of radioiodine treatments of benign thyroid disease per 100,000 person years in Western Denmark with moderate ID and Eastern Denmark with mild ID. The rate in 1997 (the year before the introduction of iodization of salt) has been marked by a broken line for easier comparison. Data with permission from Cerqueira et al. [25]

younger age groups was much lower. The prescription of antithyroid drugs in the young groups is now decreasing again, suggesting that the mechanism behind the increase was earlier development of disease and not an autoimmunogenic effect of the increased iodine intake. However, it is too early to give a final conclusion.

Treatment of hyperthyroidism includes radioiodine therapy and surgery and the number of these activities has therefore been monitored in the DanThyr studies. In Fig. 19.8 the development in the number of radioiodine treatments for benign thyroid disease is illustrated, showing, once more, the temporary increase of treatment activity in the region with the higher degree of ID before the introduction of iodine fortification [25]. Notably, in Denmark radioiodine therapy is also used for treatment of benign nontoxic goitre [26, 27]. The number of thyroid operations, on the other hand, was very stable in the studied period (Fig. 19.9) [25], even though a smaller percentage of the population has an enlarged thyroid gland when evaluated by ultrasound after the introduction of iodine fortification [28]. It may be that we have to wait for the generations born under conditions of iodine sufficiency to grow up, before the full beneficial effect of introducing iodine fortification in Denmark become apparent.

Valuable knowledge has come from the DanThyr studies—both on the epidemiology of thyroid disorders in mild-to-moderate ID, and on the effects of an increase in iodine intake on thyroid epidemiology, but also on how to monitor fortification programs in general. No single optimal study design exists to monitor the effect of initiating iodine fortification. Combining several study designs, however, as done in the DanThyr monitoring program, provides us with valuable information to add to the current knowledge on the effect of iodine fortification on public health. Knowledge which can be used in the planning of future programs of fortified foods. DanThyr may be regarded as a model project for the monitoring of such programs.

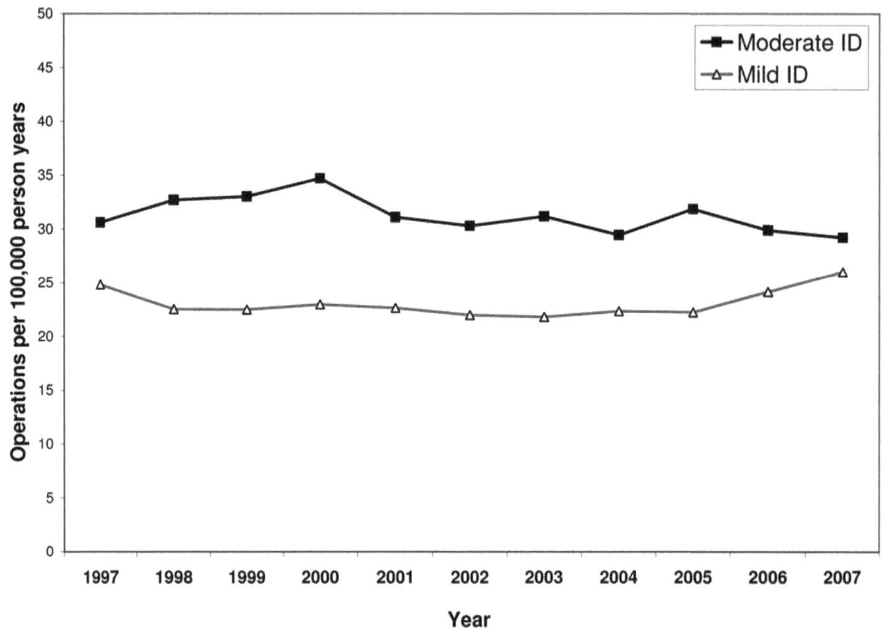

Fig. 19.9 Annual rates of operations for benign thyroid disease. Annual rates of surgery performed for benign thyroid disease in Western Denmark with moderate ID and Eastern Denmark with mild ID. Data with permission from Cerqueira et al. [25]

Guidance on Safe Levels

As described in the above sections, the relation between iodine intake and risk of disease is complex and even small changes may have a significant impact on thyroid epidemiology. Still, the severity of the IDD, especially the risk of intellectual impairment, makes it crucial to take action. Mandatory programs of iodine fortification of salt are efficient in reaching almost every individual in a population. However, the optimal range seems to be narrow, with increasing risk of disease when the iodine intake exceeds the recommended level, and thus iodine should only be added to salt at the minimum level necessary. Iodine excess is less of a health problem than ID, but it is unnecessary and avoidable. Moreover, a cautious approach is recommended to avoid any sudden increments of iodine, triggering IIH.

Recommendations

Iodine fortification programs should be carefully planned. When ID has been confirmed, the strategy for prevention should be decided. Often dietary advice by public health campaigns is not sufficient and food fortification programs are needed. The optimal fortification program will reach every person in the population by food consumed in fairly constant amounts. Thus, thorough knowledge on dietary habits has to be gathered in advance in order to choose the right vehicle and to set the right concentration of iodine to be added. A cautious approach is recommended, adding only the minimal amount of iodine needed to avoid as many cases of IIH as possible.

Before the actual fortification program is implemented a careful investigation of the pre-fortification level of thyroid disorders is recommended. Without baseline studies the evaluation of the effects of the intervention is impossible.

After the successful implementation of iodine fortification continued focus on monitoring its effects is necessary. This should include continuous evaluation of thyroid epidemiology, iodine intake, and dietary habits and form the basis for adjustments of the program if necessary.

Conclusions

ID remains a major public health problem, not only keeping individuals from reaching and attaining their full intellectual potential but also causing a high prevalence of disease, such as goitre and hyperthyroidism. However, even small changes in iodine intake have a large impact on the occurrence of thyroid disorders and the range of the optimal level seems to be narrow. If iodine intake becomes excessive the risk of disease increases, mainly of hypothyroidism. Moreover, correction of ID is followed by a time period of several years with risk of IIH, which seems to be largely unavoidable, even with a cautious approach. When past this transition phase, iodine fortification prevents many cases of goitre and hyperthyroidism. The full beneficial effect of introducing iodine fortification may only be apparent in the generations born under iodine-sufficient conditions.

References

1. Delange F. Iodine deficiency as a cause of brain damage. Postgrad Med J. 2001;77:217–20.
2. Zimmermann MB, Jooste PL, Pandav CS. Iodine-deficiency disorders. Lancet. 2008;372:1251–62.
3. Berbel P, Mestre JL, Santamaria A, et al. Delayed neurobehavioral development in children born to pregnant women with mild hypothyroxinemia during the first month of gestation: the importance of early iodine supplementation. Thyroid. 2009;19:511–9.
4. Vermiglio F, Lo PV, Moleti M, et al. Attention deficit and hyperactivity disorders in the offspring of mothers exposed to mild-moderate iodine deficiency: a possible novel iodine deficiency disorder in developed countries. J Clin Endocrinol Metab. 2004;89:6054–60.
5. Teng X, Shan Z, Chen Y, et al. More than adequate iodine intake may increase subclinical hypothyroidism and autoimmune thyroiditis: a cross-sectional study based on two Chinese communities with different iodine intake levels. Eur J Endocrinol. 2011;164:943–50.
6. Hetzel BS, Dunn JT. The iodine deficiency disorders: their nature and prevention. Annu Rev Nutr. 1989;9:21–38.
7. World Health Organization, The United Nations Children's Fund, International Council for the Control of Iodine Deficiency Disorders. Assessment of iodine deficiency disorders and monitoring their elimination. 3rd ed. Geneva: World Health Organization; 2008.
8. Laurberg P, Pedersen KM, Vestergaard H, Sigurdsson G. High incidence of multinodular toxic goitre in the elderly population in a low iodine intake area vs. high incidence of Graves' disease in the young in a high iodine intake area: comparative surveys of thyrotoxicosis epidemiology in East-Jutland Denmark and Iceland. J Intern Med. 1991;229:415–20.
9. Knudsen N, Bulow I, Jorgensen T, Laurberg P, Ovesen L, Perrild H. Goitre prevalence and thyroid abnormalities at ultrasonography: a comparative epidemiological study in two regions with slightly different iodine status. Clin Endocrinol (Oxf). 2000;53:479–85.
10. Tonacchera M, Chiovato L, Pinchera A, et al. Hyperfunctioning thyroid nodules in toxic multinodular goiter share activating thyrotropin receptor mutations with solitary toxic adenoma. J Clin Endocrinol Metab. 1998;83:492–8.
11. Bulow Pedersen I, Knudsen N, Jorgensen T, Perrild H, Ovesen L, Laurberg P. Large differences in incidences of overt hyper- and hypothyroidism associated with a small difference in iodine intake: a prospective comparative register-based population survey. J Clin Endocrinol Metab. 2002;87:4462–9.
12. Carle A, Pedersen IB, Knudsen N, et al. Epidemiology of subtypes of hyperthyroidism in Denmark: a population-based study. Eur J Endocrinol. 2011;164:801–9.
13. Stanbury JB, Ermans AE, Bourdoux P, et al. Iodine-induced hyperthyroidism: occurrence and epidemiology. Thyroid. 1998;8:83–100.
14. Brix TH, Kyvik KO, Christensen K, Hegedus L. Evidence for a major role of heredity in Graves' disease: a population-based study of two Danish twin cohorts. J Clin Endocrinol Metab. 2001;86:930–4.

15. Coindet JF. Nouvelles Recherches sur les effets de l'iode, et sur les precautions à suivre dans le traitement du goitre par ce nouveau remède. Ann Chim Phys. 1821;16:252–66.
16. Delange F, Lecomte P. Iodine supplementation: benefits outweigh risks. Drug Saf. 2000;22:89–95.
17. Connolly RJ, Vidor GI, Stewart JC. Increase in thyrotoxicosis in endemic goitre area after iodation of bread. Lancet. 1970;1:500–2.
18. Baltisberger BL, Minder CE, Burgi H. Decrease of incidence of toxic nodular goitre in a region of Switzerland after full correction of mild iodine deficiency. Eur J Endocrinol. 1995;132:546–9.
19. Todd CH, Allain T, Gomo ZA, Hasler JA, Ndiweni M, Oken E. Increase in thyrotoxicosis associated with iodine supplements in Zimbabwe. Lancet. 1995;346:1563–4.
20. Dunn JT, Semigran MJ, Delange F. The prevention and management of iodine-induced hyperthyroidism and its cardiac features. Thyroid. 1998;8:101–6.
21. Laurberg P, Jorgensen T, Perrild H, et al. The Danish investigation on iodine intake and thyroid disease, DanThyr: status and perspectives. Eur J Endocrinol. 2006;155:219–28.
22. Rasmussen LB, Carle A, Jorgensen T, et al. Iodine intake before and after mandatory iodization in Denmark: results from the Danish Investigation of Iodine Intake and Thyroid Diseases (DanThyr) study. Br J Nutr. 2008;100:166–73.
23. Bulow Pedersen I, Laurberg P, Knudsen N, et al. Increase in incidence of hyperthyroidism predominantly occurs in young people after iodine fortification of salt in Denmark. J Clin Endocrinol Metab. 2006;91:3830–4.
24. Cerqueira C, Knudsen N, Ovesen L, et al. Association of iodine fortification with incident use of antithyroid medication-a Danish nationwide study. J Clin Endocrinol Metab. 2009;94:2400–5.
25. Cerqueira C, Knudsen N, Ovesen L, et al. Nationwide trends in surgery and radioiodine treatment for benign thyroid disease during iodization of salt. Eur J Endocrinol. 2010;162:755–62.
26. Bonnema SJ, Bennedbaek FN, Wiersinga WM, Hegedus L. Management of the nontoxic multinodular goitre: a European questionnaire study. Clin Endocrinol (Oxf). 2000;53:5–12.
27. Nygaard B, Hegedus L, Gervil M, Hjalgrim H, Soe-Jensen P, Hansen JM. Radioiodine treatment of multinodular non-toxic goitre. BMJ. 1993;307:828–32.
28. Vejbjerg P, Knudsen N, Perrild H, et al. Effect of a mandatory iodization program on thyroid gland volume based on individuals' age, gender, and preceding severity of dietary iodine deficiency: a prospective, population-based study. J Clin Endocrinol Metab. 2007;92:1397–401.

Chapter 20
Lentils (*Lens culinaris* L.) as a Source of Dietary Selenium

Dil Thavarajah, Pushparajah Thavarajah, and Gerald F. Combs Jr.

Key Points

- Lentil (*Lens culinaris* L.) is an excellent medium-energy source of protein and several micronutrients including selenium.
- Lentils produced on high-Se soils contain appreciable amounts of Se, mostly as selenomethionine; consumption of 50–100 g of lentils can satisfy daily Se requirements.
- Lentils can be enriched in Se through conventional plant breeding and Se-fertilization. Se-biofortification of staple foods may be a sustainable solution to address Se deficiency.

Keywords Lentils • Selenium • Selenomethionine • Biofortification • Se fertilizer

Abbreviations

Fe	Iron
HPLC-ICP-MS	High performance liquid chromatography inductively coupled plasma mass spectrometry
N	Nitrogen
RDA	Recommended daily allowance
Se	Selenium
SeCys	Selenocystein
SeMet	Selenomethionine
XAS	X-ray absorption spectroscopy
Zn	Zinc

D. Thavarajah, B.Sc., M.Sc., Ph.D. (✉)
School of Food Systems, North Dakota State University, Dept. 7640, 223 Harris Hall, P.O. Box 6050, Fargo, ND 58108-6050, USA
e-mail: dilrukshi.thavarajah@ndsu.edu

P. Thavarajah, Ph.D., M.B.A.
School of Food Systems, North Dakota State University, 208 Harris Hall, Dept. 7640, P.O. Box 6050, Fargo, ND 58108-6050, USA
e-mail: pushparajah.thavaraj@ndsu.edu

G.F. Combs Jr, B.S., M.S., Ph.D.
Grand Forks Human Nutrition Research Center, ARS/USDA, 2420 2nd Avenue N, Grand Forks, ND 58202-9034, USA
e-mail: gerald.combs@ars.usda.gov

V.R. Preedy et al. (eds.), *Handbook of Food Fortification and Health: From Concepts to Public Health Applications Volume 1*, Nutrition and Health, DOI 10.1007/978-1-4614-7076-2_20,

Introduction

Selenium (Se) is an essential nutrient for humans and animals. Its nutritional functions are discharged by a group of proteins that contain Se in the form of selenocystein (SeCys), which is synthesized by the cotranslational addition of inorganic selenide to tRNA-bound serine [1]. The human selenoproteome consists of 25 selenoproteins [2], including four glutathione peroxidases, which catalyze the reduction of hydroperoxides [3]; three thioredoxin reductases, which are NADPH-dependent flavoenzymes that function in intracellular redox regulation [4]; three iodothyronine 5′-deiodinases, which catalyze the removal of iodine from the thyroid hormones (T_4, T_3); and selenoproteins P (the major transport form) [5], W (in muscle) [6], and R (methionine sulfoxide reductase) [7]. Because many selenoproteins have antioxidant functions, Se is regarded as important in metabolic protection from cellular-oxidative stress.

Two human diseases have been associated with severe endemic Se deficiency: Keshan disease (a cardiomyopathy) and Kashin-Beck disease (an osteoarthropathy). Each occurs in areas of central and northeastern China and eastern Russia in mountainous areas where soil Se levels are very low (<125 μg/kg) and locally produced grains generally contain <40 μg Se/kg. In these areas, the blood Se levels of residents are typically <25 ng/mL. Because Keshan disease is also associated with cardiophilic RNA-viruses, Se deficiency may also increase risks for other diseases with viral etiologies. As many as 100 million people worldwide may be Se-deficient, mainly due to low concentrations of Se in commonly eaten foods [8–10].

Epidemiological studies indicate Se status is inversely associated with cancer risk, and Se-intervention reduces cancer risk through several cellular and metabolic mechanisms in studies with a wide variety of animal tumor models [11, 12]. Supranutritional intakes of Se (ca. 300 μg/day) have been shown to reduce the risk of several types of cancer [13]. Thus, Se-enriched foods may be an effective and sustainable means of increasing Se intakes to support good general health as well as reduce cancer risk. Novel, food-based approaches for increasing Se intakes are needed to support healthful Se nutrition, especially in resource-poor countries with limited access to nutritional supplements. Biofortification of lentils with Se constitutes such an approach.

Lentil (*Lens culinaris* L.) is a nutritious grain legume with relatively high protein content (ca. 20–30 %) and moderate energy content (ca. 4.2 kcal/g). Lentil is grown in many countries and is a staple component of diets in Asia and the Middle East as well as vegetarian diets around the world. The Se content of lentil reflects the Se content of the soils in which it is grown. Accordingly, lentils grown on low-Se soils have 22–180 μg Se per g, while lentils grown on the relatively high-Se soils of western Canada, North Dakota, and the USA have 672–1,200 μg Se per g [14] (unpublished data). Such high-Se lentils can supply daily Se needs at the daily consumption rate of 50–100 g. Because lentils can be sourced from high-Se areas, bred for their capacity to retain Se, and produced using Se-fertilization, they can be used to address Se deficiency in lentil consuming countries.

This chapter presents recent results on the Se-enrichment of lentils and implications of the lentil model to other pulses.

Introduction to Lentils

Pulses, including lentil, pea (*Pisum sativum* L.), and chickpea (*Cicer arietinum* L.), are high-protein, medium-energy legume crops that are staple foods for millions of people around the world. Lentil is a traditional crop grown mostly in low-rainfall and dryland cropping systems in rotation with cereals, wheat (*Triticum* sp.), and rice (*Oryza sativa* L.). Lentils were first grown 8,500 years ago in the Near East; their cultivation has since extended to the Mediterranean, Asia, Europe, and the Western

Table 20.1 Market classes of lentils grown in North America (adapted from Thavarajah et al. [14]; personal communication with Drs. Vandenberg and McPhee)

Market class	Genotype	Seed wt. (mg)	Major consuming countries
Extra small red	CDC Robin	<30	Bangladesh, Pakistan, Egypt
	CDC Rosetown		
	CDC Imperial		
Small red	CDC Impact	30–50	England, Middle East, Sri Lanka, India, Pakistan
	CDC Redberry		
	CDC Imax		
	CDC Impala		
	CDC Maxim		
	CDC Rouleau		
	CDC Blaze		
Large red	CDC KR-1	>55	USA, Dubai, Sri Lanka
	RedChief		
Small green	CDC Milestone	30–40	Italy, Morocco, Greece, Mexico
	CDC Viceroy		
	Eston		
Medium green	CDC Impress	50–60	Latin America, Europe
	CDC Richlea		
	CDC Meteor		
Large green	CDC Greenland	>65	Spain, Turkey, Iran, Germany, Algeria
	CDC Improve		
	CDC Plato		
	CDC Sedley		
	Laird		
	Riveland		
	CDC Grandora		
	CDC Sovereign		
	CDC Glamis		
Spanish brown	Pardina	30–40	Spain, South America
French green	CDC LeMay	30–40	France

Hemisphere, including Canada and the USA. Current annual world lentil production is approximately four million MT, more than 85 % of which occurs in five regions: south Asia (India, Nepal, and Bangladesh, 32 %), western Canada (29 %), Turkey and northern Syria (18 %), Australia (4 %), and the Midwestern USA (North and South Dakota, Eastern Montana) (3 %) [15]. Canada and the USA are the major lentil producing and exporting countries. North American lentils encompassing several market classes are supplied to more than 100 countries (Table 20.1).

Lentils were introduced to the USA and Canada in the early 1900s; however, agronomic improvement did not begin until the early 1980s. Over the last 40 years, global lentil production has increased by 6.8 % annually [16], and the lentil industry is a now major part of Canadian and the US prairie agriculture with a third of global lentil production now originating in Saskatchewan and the American Midwest [17]. Lentils are typically rotated with wheat or canola (*Brassica napus* L.) in North America, and with rice or wheat under rain-fed conditions in Asia. Annual lentil production in developing countries is declining, mainly due to low yields obtained from marginal soils with relatively few inputs. In Bangladesh, for example, farmers are shifting from lentils to high-yielding cultivars of rice and wheat. The main drivers of this shift are poor soil conditions, lack of drought tolerance, poor disease resistance, and prohibitively long harvest times in triple rotation cropping systems. In contrast, superior yields and an excellent fit into existing crop rotations have increased Canadian and the US red and green lentil production during the last two decades.

Table 20.2 The chemical composition of lentils (average of green and red varieties) grown in North America [14, 20, 24, 48]

Major nutrient component	Concentration
Carbohydrates (63.1 %) [47]	
– Starch (%)	35–53
– Oligosaccharides (%)	5–9
– Cellulose and hemicellulose (%)	10
Protein (%) [20]	25–30
Fat (%)	<1
Ash (%)	3.1
Micronutrients [24]	
– Iron (mg/kg)	73–90
– Zinc (mg/kg)	44–54
– Selenium (μg/kg)	425–673
– Beta carotene (μg/100 g)	110–313
Phytic acid (mg/g) [3]	2.5–4.4

Lentils are important pulse crops in sustainable cropping systems. They provide significant benefits through the fixation of atmospheric nitrogen (N), which improves soil fertility. Generally, grain legumes fix up to 450 kg N per ha. On average, lentils fix N in amounts ranging from 5 to 191 kg N per ha [18], which is in general low compared to other grain legumes. Lentil is well adapted to semi-arid, temperate climatic conditions, requiring only 10–12 in. of rain and a soil pH of 7 for high grain yields. Lentils have indeterminate (branching) growth, and plant height can range from 20 to 75 cm. Lentil leaves produce tendrils and flowering begins at the 11th or 12th node stage. Lentil flowers are self-pollinated. Generally, seed pods are <2.5 cm long, containing one or two seeds. Lentils are classified by seed size: large (Chilean) or small seeded (Persian). Seed coats can be red, green, brown, gray, or black, and cotyledons can be red, green, or/and yellow. Lentil grain yields range from 500 to 2,800 kg per ha [19]. Average yields range from 650 kg per ha in India to 1,345 kg per ha in North America [15, 19]; however, yields approaching 2,800 kg per ha are possible for some cultivars with appropriate crop management.

Lentil production and consumption have been increasing [15]. This is likely due to the convenience and economy of its short cooking time. The nutritional composition of lentils has been reported (Table 20.2); however, composition can vary with genotype and growing location/country. Lentils and peas produced in North America are typically high in Se as well as two other essential micronutrients: iron (Fe) and zinc (Zn). For example, 50 g of lentils or peas can provide a minimum of 25–50 % of the recommended daily allowances (RDA) of these three nutrients. Further, because lentils also contain relatively low concentrations of phytic acid [20], which forms nonabsorbable complexes with divalent cations, it can be expected that the Fe and Zn in lentils should be relatively highly bioavailable. Lentils also have a favorable amino acid profile that complements those of cereal grains to produce a dietary protein mixture of high biologic value. For these reasons, lentils can be an important source of nutrition in grain-based diets. Specifically, we have undertaken to determine the potential of Se-biofortification of lentils to the end of developing lentil as a sustainable, food-based approach to preventing Se deficiency.

Selenium Species in Lentils: Implications for Bioavailability

Plants uptake Se from the soil primarily as selenate or selenite and translocate it to the chloroplast where it follows the sulfur assimilation pathway. Selenate is reduced to selenide, which reacts with serine to form SeCys and is further metabolized to other organic Se forms including selenomethionine (SeMet). Therefore, the major Se-species in lentils have been thought to be SeCys and SeMet, which is predominantly protein-bound [21, 22]. Using synchrotron X-ray absorption spectroscopy (XAS), we found that most (86–95 %) of the Se in Saskatchewan lentils was present in organic forms with the remainder as selenate [22]. Using high performance liquid chromatography-inductively coupled plasma-mass spectrometry (HPLC-ICP-MS), we found that most (69 %) of the organic component was SeMet, with small amounts of SeCys (7 %) and other selenooligopeptides such as γ-glutamylselenocysteine [14]. More than half of the SeCys occurred in the embryo axis [14].

SeMet as the dominant Se-species suggests that lentil-Se is likely to have good biological availability. Free SeMet is well utilized [8], being actively absorbed by the methionine transport system and then trans-selenated to SeCys, which is catabolized to selenide, the obligate form of Se incorporated into selenoproteins [23]. SeMet is also incorporated, as a methionine mimics, in general protein synthesis; this nonspecific incorporation into proteins means that ingestion of SeMet supports significant tissue levels of Se [8, 23]. Because the same phenomenon occurs in plants, SeMet in lentil proteins may determine its bioavailability. We found that Se from Canadian lentils (727 μg Se per kg) was effective in raising blood Se concentrations in healthy Sri Lankan children [24]; children fed with 50 g Se-rich red lentils per day had significantly higher blood Se concentrations 2 h after their meal (82 ppb) compared to children fed with local lentils (64 ppb). Thus, we believe that lentils containing nutritionally significant amounts of bioavailable Se can make important contributions to public health, particularly in South Asia. Such lentils can be provided by sourcing from Se-rich production areas, by selecting lentil cultivars that efficiently utilize soil Se, or by using Se-containing fertilizers.

Sourcing High-Se Lentils

Soils are highly variable with respect to the distribution of Se in forms that can be utilized by plants. Most soils contain between 1.0 and 1.5 μg Se per kg [25]; those with <0.6 μg/kg are considered deficient. The species of Se in soils depend on pH, aeration, organic matter content, texture, microbial activity, and the presence/absence of competitive ions (sulphate, phosphate) and organic compounds such as polysaccharides [26]. Selenate (VI) tends to be the major species in aerobic and neutral to alkaline soils, whereas selenide (-II) and elemental Se (0) dominate in anaerobic soils [27]. In acidic soils, Se is poorly available to plants, occurring mainly as insoluble selenides. In lateritic soils, it binds strongly to Fe to form insoluble and unavailable ferric hydroxide-selenite complexes. Selenate is water-mobile and can be leached from soils, as has occurred in New Zealand and Tasmania [28]. Consequently, some regions of the world have soils with low or unavailable Se, resulting in a food chain that is Se-deficient; other regions with higher amounts of plant-available Se support the production of foods with greater Se contents. Examples of the latter include the major lentil growing regions of Saskatchewan, Canada, which have soil Se concentrations of 37–301 μg/kg [14].

A survey of the Se content of lentils grown in six major regions shows considerable variation, with Turkey and Morocco producing very low-Se lentils (<30 μg/kg), Nepal and Australia producing moderate-Se lentils (140–180 μg/kg), and Saskatchewan and North Dakota producing high-Se lentils (<1,600 μg/kg) (Fig. 20.1). These differences reflect differences in soil Se content, with soils in parts of the Northern Great Plains of North America being rich in plant-available forms of Se.

Utilizing Se-Efficient Cultivars

Lentils grown in the Se-rich soils of Saskatchewan are naturally rich in Se (425–673 μg/kg), with some genotypes having 40–50 % more Se than others [14]. The extra-small genotype, CDC Robin, and two of the large green lentil genotypes, CDC Sedley and CDC Grandora, had the greatest Se concentrations at 612–672 μg/kg. A single 100 g serving of such lentils would provide as much as 77–122 % of an adult's RDA of Se (Fig. 20.2).

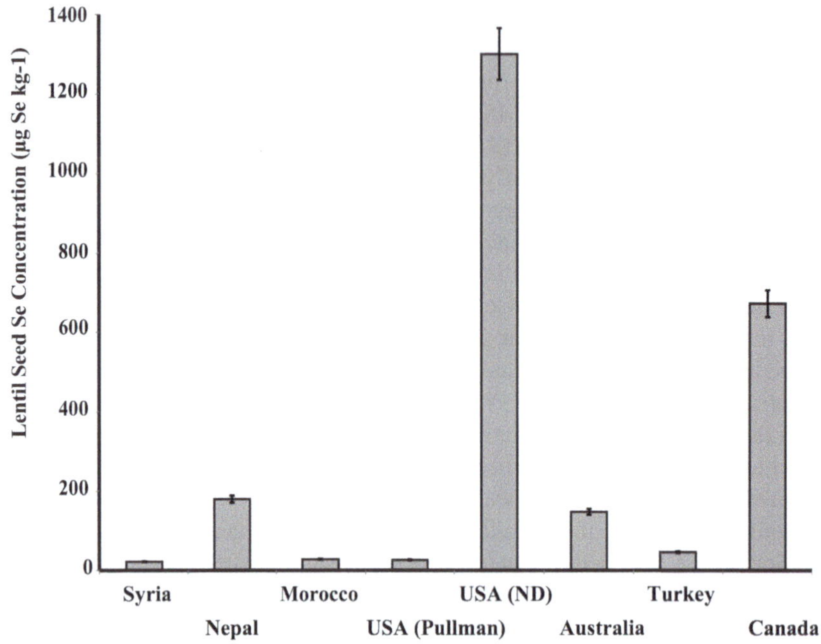

Fig. 20.1 Total Se concentration in lentils from different lentil growing countries (modified with new data from [24]). Number of samples from each region: Syria ($n=64$), Nepal ($n=255$), Morocco ($n=72$), the USA (Pullman, Washington, $n=216$), the USA (North Dakota, $n=150$), Australia ($n=57$), Turkey ($n=74$), Canada ($n=912$). Lentil seed selenium concentrations of major lentil producing and exporting countries

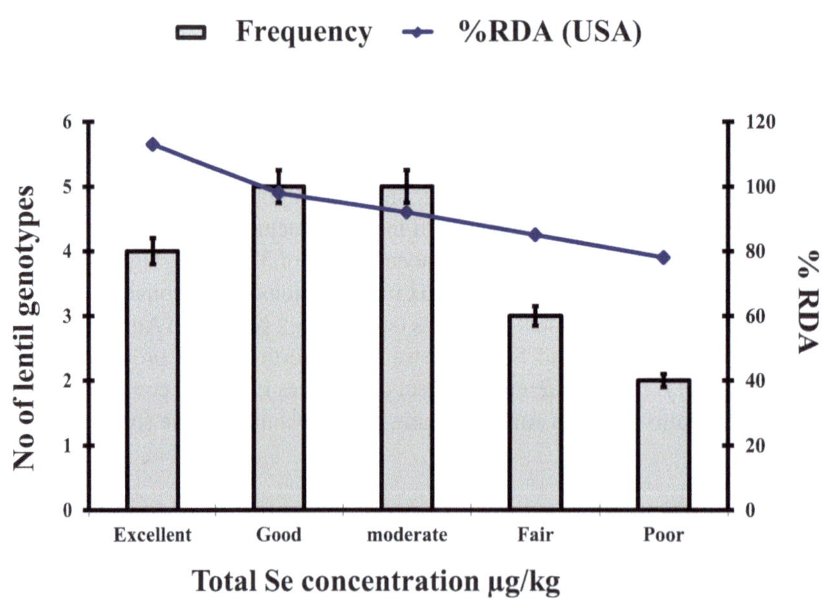

Fig. 20.2 Frequency distribution of Se uptake in lentils grown in Saskatchewan, Canada (data from Thavarajah et al. [14]). %RDA was calculated based on the mean Se concentration across eight location for 100 g of lentils. Variation in lentil genotypes in their ability to enrich seed selenium concentrations and %RDA of selenium from 100 g serving

Enhancing the efficiency of soil-Se uptake by lentils would be possible through selective breeding, using the approach termed "biofortification." The uptake of soils Se by the lentil plant is likely governed by several genes. The broad sense heritability of Se content in Canadian grown lentils was 40 %, with 4–5-fold differences in Se uptake among genotypes [14]. This suggests it may be worthwhile to screen available lentil germplasm for grain Se levels as a proxy for Se uptake capacity.

Selenium Fertilization

Selenium fertilization can increase crop Se contents. Allaway et al. [29] demonstrated that application of sodium selenate to Se-deficient Oregon, USA, soils increased the Se concentration of alfalfa (*Medicago sativa* L.) from 0.01–0.04 to 2.6–2.7 mg/kg. Since then, the efficacy of Se-fertilization has been well established as a means to prevent Se deficiencies in North America, Australia, Finland, and New Zealand [8, 30]. Se-containing fertilizers (16 mg/kg as sodium selenate) have been used in Finland since 1984 to elevate Se concentrations in their major food crops, and this practice resulted in increases in the daily Se intake of Finnish consumers from 39 to 110 μg of Se per day [31]. While either selenate or selenite can be used for Se-fertilization, selenate appears to be used by plants with greater efficacy. This has been shown for barley (*Hardeum vlugare* L.) [32, 33], red clover (*Trifolium pretense* L.) [34], perennial ryegrass (*Lolium perenne* L.) [35], and wheat (*Triticum aestivum* L.) [36]. Accordingly, we have found selenate more effective than selenite for the Se-fertilization of lentils, with application of aqueous solutions containing 2 ppm Se resulting in seed Se concentrations to 2.5–8.7 mg/kg [37] (Table 20.3). The mechanism of selenate uptake by plants was discussed above and plant roots are known to update selenate through the high affinity sulphate transporters [38, 39]. However, mechanism of selenite uptake is not well understood in plants and has yet to be studied in lentil. Arvy [40] suggests that selenite is taken up by plant roots through passive diffusion, yet a recent study indicates that uptake in wheat is an active process mediated through phosphate transporters. We have found that lentil genotypes differ in their responses to soil applications of Se. For example,

Table 20.3 Mean total Se concentration in seeds of selected lentil breeding lines grown under controlled conditions [37]

Lentil breeding line	Total Se concentration[a] (mg/kg)
PI320937	8.7 *a*
ILL 7537	8.1 *a*
CDC Robin	7.5 *ab*
LR 59-81	6.2 *bc*
PI572359	5.8 *c*
2670B	5.7 *c*
CDC Redberry	5.6 *cd*
964a-46	5.5 *cd*
S06-5P1-W08SI	5.4 *cd*
S06-1P1-W08SI	5.1 *cde*
ILL 7502	4.3 *de*
72815	3.7 *ef*
Ill 1704	2.8 *f*
Eston	2.5 *f*
Mean ± SE[b]	5.4 ± 0.1
Broad-sense heritability (%)[c]	88

These plants were treated with 2 ppm of selenate

[a]Means within a column followed by different letters are significantly different at $p < 0.05$

[b]SE, pooled standard error of the mean calculated from the mean square of ANOVA ($n = 84$)

[c]Broad-sense heritability is the proportion of genotypic to phenotypic variance

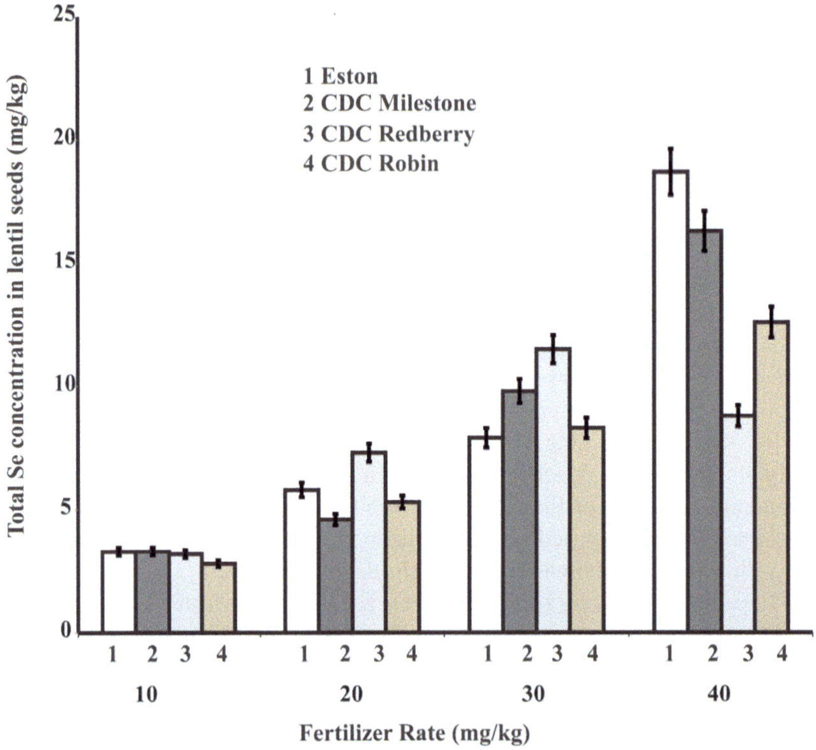

Fig. 20.3 Response of seed Se concentration to Se-fertilization for selected lentil genotypes grown under controlled conditions (Thavarajah et al., unpublished data). Changes of lentil seed selenium concentrations of different lentil genotypes to added selenium fertilizer rates

the small green lentil genotype Eston shows a significantly greater increase in Se uptake than other genotypes in high soil Se environments [37] (Fig. 20.3). Moreover, Se uptake in lentils is dose-dependent, with doses of 5–10 mg/kg increasing lentil Se concentrations 2–4-fold (Fig. 20.3).

Foliar application can be more effective than soil application of Se-fertilizer for increasing crop Se content [41]. Foliar application of Se has been demonstrated effective for the Se-enrichment of wheat [36], barley [41], rice [42], broccoli [43], and chicory [44]. Foliar application of Se has not been investigated for lentils, but there is no reason to expect it will be less effective than application of Se to the soil.

Selenium is not considered an element essential for higher plants. However, benefits have been reported for plants treated with Se [43, 45]. These include increased tuber yield in potato (*Solanum tuberosum* L.) and increased vegetative growth in rye grass (*Lolium perenne* L.) and lettuce (*Lactuca sativa* L.) exposed to UVB radiation [46, 47]. Lyons et al. [45] found a 43 % yield increase in mustard (*Brassica rapa* L.) in response to a low dose (22 μL of 0.001 M selenite) of Se to the soil, and noted that increased respiratory activity in leaves and flowers may have contributed to the greater seed production.

Conclusion

Lentil is an important food crop in many parts of the world. It also can contribute to the growing global demand for protein foods. Lentil is produced in and exported from regions relatively rich in the essential nutrient Se, which is limiting in several parts of the world. Lentil can also be enriched in Se through the use of Se-fertilizers. Moreover, this pulse crop shows genetic potential for biofortification in Se, which could further enrich Se in seeds produced in marginal soils. Current evidence suggests that lentils so enriched, when consumed in modest amounts (50–100 g/day), can provide daily Se needs. Thus, lentils may be a sustainable food-based approach to malnutrition, including the prevention of Se deficiency. Similar strategies are likely to be efficacious for other pulses.

Acknowledgements The authors thank members, collaborators, and funding agencies of the North Dakota State University Pulse Quality and Nutrition Program (2010–present), Fargo, ND, USA and the University of Saskatchewan Pulse Biofortification Team (2007–2010), Saskatoon, SK, Canada.

References

1. Berry MJ, Banu L, Chen Y, Mandel SJ, Kieffer JD, Harney JW, et al. Recognition of a UGA as a selenocysteine codon in Type 1 deiodinase requires sequences in the 3′ untranslated region. Nature (London). 1991;353:273–6.
2. Kryukov GV, Castellano S, Novoselov SV, Lobanov AV, Zehtab O, Guigo R, et al. Characterization of mammalian selenoproteomes. Science. 2003;300(5624):1439–43.
3. Brigelius-Flohé R. Glutathione peroxidases and redox-regulated transcription factors. Biol Chem. 2006;387:1329–35.
4. Tamura T, Stadman TC. A new selenoprotein from human lung adenocarcinoma cells: purification, properties, and thioredoxin reductase activity. Proc Natl Acad Sci U S A. 1996;93:1006–11.
5. Burk RF, Hill KE. Selenoprotein P-expression, functions and roles in mammals. Biochim Biophys Acta. 2009;1790:1441–7.
6. Vandeland SC, Beilstein MA, Yeh JY, Ream W, Whanger PD. Rat skeletal muscle selenoprotein W: cDNA clone and mRNA modulation by dietary selenium. Proc Natl Acad Sci U S A. 1995;92:8749–53.
7. Kim HY, Gladyshev VN. Mineral element composition of Finnish foods. Mol Biol Cell. 2004;15:1055–64.
8. Combs Jr GF. Selenium in global food systems. Br J Nutr. 2001;85(5):517–47.
9. Ellis DR, Salt DE. Plants, selenium and human health. Curr Opin Plant Biol. 2003;6(3):273–9.
10. Spallholz JE, Mallory BL, Rhaman MM. Environmental hypothesis: is poor dietary selenium intake an underlying factor for arsenicosis and cancer in Bangladesh and West Bengal, India? Sci Total Environ. 2004;323(1–3):21–32.
11. Combs Jr GF, Lu J. Selenium as a cancer preventive agent. In: Hatfield DL, Berry MJ, Gladyshev VN, editors. Selenium: its molecular biology and role in human health. 2nd ed. New York: Springer; 2001. p. 205–17.
12. Jackson MI, Combs Jr GF. Selenium and anticarcinogenesis: underlying mechanisms. Curr Opin Clin Nutr Metab Care. 2008;11:718–26.
13. Clark LC, Combs Jr GF, Turnbull BW, Slate EH, Chalker DK, Chow J, et al. Effects of selenium supplementation for cancer prevention in patients with carcinoma of the skin. A randomized controlled trial. Nutritional Prevention of Cancer Study Group. JAMA. 1996;276:1957–63.
14. Thavarajah D, Ruszkowski J, Vandenberg A. High potential for selenium biofortification of lentils (*Lens culinaris* L.). J Agric Food Chem. 2008;56(22):10747–53.
15. FAOSTAT Website. Available at http://faostat.fao.org/. Accessed 5 May 2010.
16. Vandenberg A. Expansion of lentil in Canada. In: Masood A, Kumar S, editors. Milestones in food legume research. Kanpur: IIPR; 2009. p. 58–72.
17. Northern Pulse Growers Association Website. Available at http://www.northernpulse.com/. Accessed 5 June 2011.
18. Unkovich MJ, Pate JS. An appraisal of recent field measurements of symbiotic N2 fixation by annual legumes. Field Crop Res. 2000;65:211–28.
19. Saskatchewan Pulse Growers Association Website. Available at http://www.saskpulse.com/. Accessed 5 June 2011.
20. Thavarajah P, Thavarajah D, Vandenberg A. Low phytic acid lentils (*Lens culinaris* L.): a potential solution for increased micronutrient bioavailability. J Agric Food Chem. 2009;57:9044–9.
21. Olson OE, Novacek EJ, Whitehead EI, Palmer IS. Investigations on selenium in wheat. Phytochemistry. 1970;9:1181–8.
22. Thavarajah D, Vandenberg A, George GN, Pickering IJ. Chemical form of selenium in naturally selenium-rich lentils (*Lens culinaris* L.) from Saskatchewan. J Agric Food Chem. 2007;55(18):7337–41.
23. Rayman MP. The argument for increasing selenium intake. Proc Nutr Soc. 2002;61:203–15.
24. Thavarajah D, Thavarajah P, Wejesuriya A, Rutzke M, Glahn R, Combs Jr GF, et al. The potential of lentil (*Lens culinaris* L.) as a whole food for increased selenium, iron, and zinc intake: preliminary results from a three year study. Euphytica. 2011;180:123–8.
25. Berrow ML, Ure AM. Geological materials and soils. In: Ihnat M, editor. Occurrence and distribution of selenium. Boca Raton, FL: CRC Press; 1989. p. 226–8.

26. Pezzarossa B, Petruzzelli G, Petacco F, Malorgio F, Ferri T. Chemosphere. Absorption of selenium by Lactuca sativa as affected by carboxymethylcellulose. Chemosphere. 2007;67:322–9.
27. Terry N, Zayed AM, De Souza MP, Tarun AS. Selenium in higher plants. Annu Rev Plant Physiol Plant Mol Biol. 2000;51:401–32.
28. Reilly C. Selenium: a new entrant into the functional food arena. Trends Food Sci Technol. 1998;9:114–8.
29. Allaway WH, Moore DP, Oldfield JE, Muth OH. Movement of physiological levels of selenium from soils through plants to animals. J Nutr. 1966;88:411–8.
30. Lee GP, Park KW. Quality improvement of 'Seoul' celery by selenium in the nutrient solution culture. Acta Hortic. 1999;483:185–92.
31. Wang WC, Naentoe V, Maekelae AL, Maekelae P. Effect of nationwide selenium supplementation in Finland on selenium status in children with juvenile rheumatoid arthritis. A ten-year follow-up study. Analyst. 1995;120:955–8.
32. Ylaranta T. Effect of applied selenite and selenate on the selenium content of barley (Hordeum vlugare). Ann Agric Fenn. 1983;22:164–74.
33. Gupta UC, Winter KA, Sunderson JB. Selenium content of barley as influenced by selenite and selenate enriched fertilizers. Commun Soil Sci Plant Anal. 1993;24:1165–70.
34. Flemming GA. Some factor affecting the uptake of selenium by plants. Iris J Agric Res. 1962;1:131–8.
35. Poggi V, Arcioni A, Filippini P, Pifferi PG. Foliar application of selenite and selenate to potato (Solanum tuberosum): effect of a ligand agent on selenium content of tubers. J Agric Food Chem. 2000;48:4749–51.
36. Lyons GH, Judson GJ, Ortiz-Monasterio I, Genc Y, Stangoulis JCR, Graham RD. Selenium in Australia: selenium status and biofortification of wheat for better health. J Trace Elem Med Biol. 2005;19:75–82.
37. Thavarajah D, Vandenberg A. Genetic improvement of bioavailable selenium content in lentil seeds. Final report, Agriculture Development Fund (project # 20070186), Saskatchewan Pulse Growers Association (project # BRE0802), 28 Feb 2011.
38. White PJ, Bowen HC, Parmaguru P, Fritz M, Spracklen WP, Spiby RE, et al. Interactions between selenium and sulphur nutrition in Arabidopsis thaliana. J Exp Bot. 2004;55:1927–37.
39. Li HF, McGrath SP, Zhao FJ. Selenium uptake, translocation and speciation in wheat supplied with selenate or selenite. New Phytol. 2008;178:92–102.
40. Arvy MP. Selenate and selenite uptake and translocation in bean plant (Phaseolus vulgaris). J Exp Bot. 1993;44:1083–7.
41. Gupta UC, MacLeod JA. Effect of various sources of selenium fertilization on the selenium concentration of feed crops. Can J Soil Sci. 1994;74:285–90.
42. Fang Y, Wang L, Xin Z, Zhao L, An X, Hu Q. Effect of foliar application of zinc, selenium and iron fertilizers on nutrients concentration and yield of rice grain in China. J Agric Food Chem. 2008;56:2079–84.
43. Finley JW. Selenium accumulation in plant foods. Nutr Rev. 2005;1:196–202.
44. Germ M, Stibilj V, Osvald J, Kreft I. Effect of selenium foliar application on chicory (Cichorium intybus L.). J Agric Food Chem. 2007;55:795–8.
45. Lyons GH, Gene Y, Soole K, Stangoulis JCR, Liu F, Graham RD. Selenium increases seed production in Brassica. Plant Soil. 2009;318:73–80.
46. Turakainen M, Hartikainen H, Seppanen MM. Effects of selenium treatments on potato (*Solanum tuberosum* L.) growth and concentration of soluble sugars and starch. J Agric Food Chem. 2004;52:5378–82.
47. Hartikainen H, Xue T. The promotive effect of selenium on plant growth as triggered by ultraviolet irradiation. J Environ Qual. 1999;28:1372–5.
48. Bhatty RS. Composition and quality of lentil (Lens culinaris Medik): a review. Can Inst Food Sci Technol. 1988;21(2):144–60.

Chapter 21
Tocotrienol Fortification in Eggs

Kiyotaka Nakagawa, Phumon Sookwong, and Teruo Miyazawa

Key Points

- Tocotrienol (T3) has a wide variety of health benefits.
- For example, T3 acts as an effective anti-angiogenic compound useful for preventing angiogenic-related disorders (i.e., diabetic retinopathy, rheumatoid arthritis, and cancers).
- Because the intake of T3 from dietary foods is low (few mg/day), it is highly encouraged to develop T3-fortified food for therapeutic purposes.
- It was found that commercial eggs contain a little amount of T3 (around 0.11 mg/egg), and that by adding extra T3 source (rice bran scum oil) into laying hen feeds, T3 is absorbed and accumulated in hen eggs.
- The maximum level of T3 was 0.56–0.62 mg/egg after 7 days of the experimental period.
- Eggs enriched with T3 would be produced and recommended as one of choices for T3 for its health benefits.

Keywords Tocotrienol • Eggs • Fortification • Health benefits • Vitamin E

Abbreviations

HPLC	High-performance liquid chromatography
PMC	2,2,5,7,8-Pentamethyl-6-hydroxychromane
RBO	Rice bran scum oil
T3	Tocotrienol
Toc	Tocopherol

K. Nakagawa, Ph.D. (✉) • T. Miyazawa, Ph.D.
Food and Biodynamic Chemistry Laboratory, Graduate School of Agricultural Science, Tohoku University, 1-1 Tsutsumidori-amamiyamachi, Aoba-Ku, Sendai 981-8555, Japan
e-mail: nkgw@biochem.tohoku.ac.jp; miyazawa@biochem.tohoku.ac.jp

P. Sookwong, Ph.D.
Department of Chemistry, Chiang Mai University, 239 Hauy Kaew Road, Suthep, Muang Chiang Mai 50-200, Thailand
e-mail: phumon@gmail.com

V.R. Preedy et al. (eds.), *Handbook of Food Fortification and Health: From Concepts to Public Health Applications Volume 1*, Nutrition and Health, DOI 10.1007/978-1-4614-7076-2_21,

Introduction

Structure and Distribution of Tocotrienol

In 1922, tocopherol (Toc) was discovered in green leafy vegetables as a micronutrient essential for reproduction [1]. More than 40 years later, tocotrienol (T3) was isolated from latex [2]. Structurally, these two vitamin E differ only in their side chains (Fig. 21.1). Toc has a saturated phytyl side chain, while T3 contains an unsaturated isoprenoid tail. To date, eight substances have been found in nature as vitamin E: α-, β-, γ-, and δ-Toc and α-, β-, γ-, and δ-T3. Vitamin E is synthesized in plastids of plants, and Toc is widely present in a variety of foods such as vegetable oils and nuts. However, T3-containing foods are limited. Rice bran, palm oil, and annatto seeds are rich in T3 [3].

Tocotrienol Has a Wide Variety of Health Benefits

Toc and T3 are classified on their ability (vitamin E activity) to prevent the resorption of rat fetuses. α-Toc displays the highest efficacy among the eight vitamin E, whereas α-T3 has about one-third of the activity of α-Toc. Regardless, all forms of vitamin E are able to induce antioxidative effect and to act as protective agents against lipid peroxidation in biological membranes. In some model membrane studies, T3 has been reported to be a more potent antioxidant than Toc [4]. Moreover, T3 has recently gained increasing interest due to its several health-promoting properties that differ somewhat from those of Toc.

For example, T3 protects neuronal cells against oxidative damage [5], and suppresses cancer [6]. We found that T3 acts as an effective anti-angiogenic compound [7, 8] useful for preventing angiogenic-related disorders (i.e., diabetic retinopathy, rheumatoid arthritis, and cancers) (Fig. 21.2). These unique effects of T3 could be partly explained by its abilities to induce cell cycle arrest [9], to activate p53 and caspase [10, 11], to suppress adhesion molecules [12], to inhibit nuclear factor-κB [13], and to down-regulate c-Myc and telomerase [14]. Besides these activities, T3 has also gained attention for its lipid-lowering properties, especially reduction of cholesterol. The cholesterol-lowering effects have been observed in cell cultures [15–17], animals [18–21], and human studies [22], and the mechanism may involve a repression of hepatic 3-hydroxy-3-methylglutaryl-coenzyme A reductase through a posttranscriptional process [15, 16]. These findings [4–22] suggest that T3 has a wide variety of health benefits.

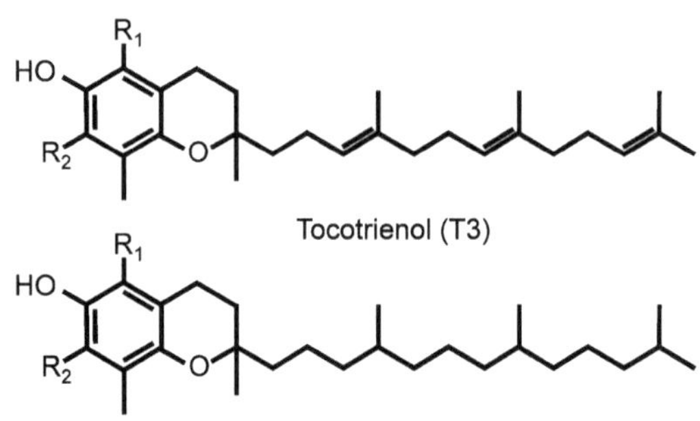

	α-	β-	γ-	δ-
R_1	CH_3	CH_3	H	H
R_2	CH_3	H	CH_3	H

Fig. 21.1 Chemical structures of tocotrienol (T3) and tocopherol (Toc). T3 consists of a chromanol ring and an unsaturated isoprenoid chain with three double bonds, while Toc possesses a chromanol ring and a fully saturated phytyl chain

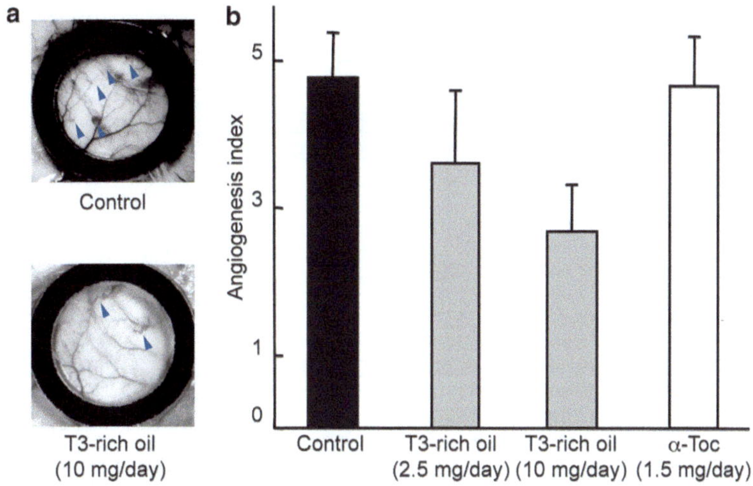

Fig. 21.2 Effects of T3-rich oil on tumor-cell-induced angiogenesis in human colon carcinoma-chamber-implanted mice. The figure shows angiogenesis index of tumor-cell-induced angiogenesis in human colon carcinoma-chamber-implanted mice fed with T3-rich oil (Tocomin 50; Koyo Mercantile, Tokyo, Japan) (2.5 and 10 mg) or α-Toc (1.5 mg), by gavage, once a day for 5 days. Control mice received only the vehicle (vitamin-E-stripped corn oil). Implanted chambers were removed and photographed (**a**), and the number of new blood vessels was counted and scored as the angiogenesis index (**b**). Values are presented as mean ± SD ($n = 10–12$)

Development of Tocotrienol-Fortified Eggs

As mentioned above, because T3 is limited only in some certain kinds of food sources (e.g., rice bran and palm oil), the intake of T3 from dietary foods is quite low (few mg/day) (Fig. 21.3) [23]. We are therefore interested in developing T3-fortified food for therapeutic purposes.

Recently, hen eggs have been received much attention, since eggs can be fortified with functional compounds by supplying the compounds into hen feeds. For example, Bourre and Galea reported that docosahexaenoic acid, folic acid, and Toc were able to concentrated up to 60 mg (threefold docosahexaenoic acid to normal egg), 0.1 μg (fourfold folic acid), and 4 mg (sixfold Toc)/egg, respectively [24]. These kinds of fortified eggs have been increasingly commercialized and consumed as ordinary foods or as foods for health purposes. Considering the results reported by Bourre and Galea [24], it may be possible that T3 can be accumulated and concentrated in hen eggs by adding T3 source into feed, because T3 has very similar structure to Toc (T3 has unsaturated isoprenoid chain, whereas Toc has saturated phytyl chain; Fig. 21.1).

In this chapter, we introduce our current research [25] on the T3 fortification in hen eggs by supplementing the feed with rice bran oil.

Tocotrienol Fortification in Eggs

Tocotrienol Concentrations in Commercial Eggs

To best of our knowledge, there is very few quantitative data concerning T3 concentrations in eggs. Therefore, we first measured T3 concentrations in commercial eggs by using high-performance liquid chromatography (HPLC) with fluorescence detection [3].

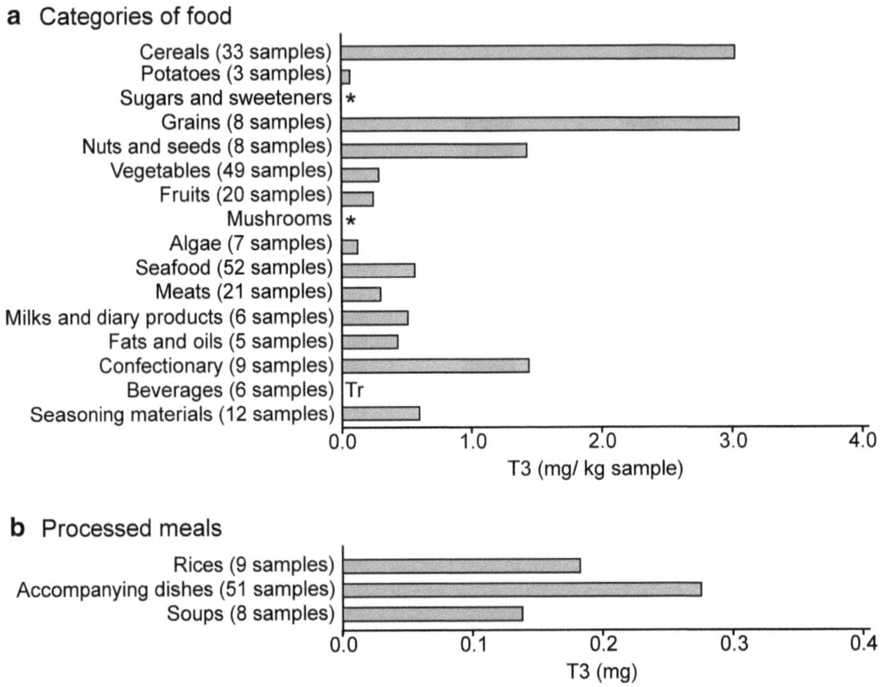

Fig. 21.3 Average T3 contents in foods by mean of food categories and processed meal items. The figure shows average T3 contents in foods by mean of categories of food as classified in the Japanese National Nutrition Survey (**a**) and by processed meal items (**b**). One meal consists of a dish of rice, a set of accompanying dishes (2–3 submenus), and a small bowl of soup. *Asterisks* denotes no quantitation determined in categories of sugars and sweeteners and of mushrooms because they have been reported to contain no Toc, implying a lack of T3. *Tr* trace

In brief, 11 kinds of hen eggs (four brown color eggs and seven white color eggs) were purchased from local market (Sendai, Japan). Egg yolk was separated from egg white, lyophilized, and ground into yolk powder. The yolk powder (0.25 g) was suspended in 0.5 mL of 1 % (w/v) NaCl aqueous solution. To the suspension, 9 mL of 3 % ethanolic pyrogallol, 1 mL of 50 μM ethanolic 2,2,5,7,8-pentamethyl-6-hydroxy-chromane (PMC, internal standard), and 0.5 mL of 60 % KOH aqueous solution were added and mixed. The mixture was incubated at 70 °C for 30 min. The saponified solution was cooled by ice, added with 22.5 mL of 0.9 % NaCl aqueous solution, and extracted with 15 mL of hexane:ethylacetate (9/1, v/v). After centrifugation at 1,000 × *g* for 5 min, the upper layer was collected. The extraction with hexane:ethylacetate (9/1, v/v) was then repeated. The upper layers were combined and dried. The residue was dissolved in hexane, and a portion of the extract was subjected to HPLC for vitamin E analysis.

The HPLC system consisted of a JASCO PU-980 pump (Japan Spectroscopic Co., Tokyo, Japan), a JASCO CO-860 column oven, and a Reodyne 7125 injector (Cotati, CA, USA). Inertsil SIL 100A-5 (4.6 × 250 mm; GL Science, Tokyo, Japan) was used as an HPLC column. A mixture of hexane/1, 4-dioxane/2-propanol (1,000:40:5, v/v/v) was used as mobile phase. The flow rate was adjusted to 1.0 mL/min, and the column temperature was maintained at 35 °C. T3 and Toc were detected by an RF-10AXL FLD detector (excitation 294 nm, emission 326 nm; Shimadzu, Kyoto, Japan). All peak areas were recorded using an SIC Chromatocorder 21J integrator (System Instruments, Tokyo, Japan). The concentrations of T3 and Toc in egg samples were calculated with calibration curves of standard T3 (Eisai, Tokyo, Japan) and Toc (Wako, Osaka, Japan), and then corrected using the peak area ratios of the vitamin E isoforms to PMC (internal standard). The determination was made 3 times in each sample.

T3 and Toc concentrations in 11 kinds of commercial eggs are shown in Table 21.1. White egg did not contain T3 or Toc (data not shown), but we detected vitamin E in egg yolk. The amounts of T3

Table 21.1 Tocotrienol (T3) and tocopherol (Toc) concentrations in 11 kinds of commercial eggs (mg/egg)

Egg sample	α-T3	α-T3	α-T3	α-T3	Total T3	Total Toc
a	n.d.	n.d.	0.06	0.01	0.07	17
b	0.16	n.d.	0.21	0.02	0.39	2.7
c	0.12	n.d.	0.11	n.d.	0.23	1.2
d	0.04	n.d.	0.01	n.d.	0.05	3.9
e	0.05	n.d.	0.04	n.d.	0.09	1.2
f	0.04	n.d.	n.d.	n.d.	0.04	0.77
g	0.04	n.d.	0.01	n.d.	0.05	1.1
h	0.02	n.d.	0.01	n.d.	0.03	7.9
i	0.06	n.d.	0.04	n.d.	0.10	9.4
j	0.04	n.d.	0.02	n.d.	0.06	2.7
k	0.05	n.d.	0.02	n.d.	0.07	1.6

The table shows T3 and Toc contents in commercial eggs (mg/egg). Egg yolk and egg white were lyophilized, ground into powder, and saponified with 60 % KOH solution. A portion of the extract was subjected to HPLC with fluorescence detection for vitamin E analysis
n.d. not detectable

were in range of 0.04–0.39 mg/egg, and α-T3 was found as the predominant form of T3. It is therefore likely that humans daily receive T3 from eggs, while eggs contain little amount of T3 (0.11 mg/egg as average). On the other hand, Toc in eggs varied from 0.77 to 17 mg/egg.

Tocotrienol Is Accumulated in Eggs by Supplementing Rice Bran Oil into Hen Feed

After confirming the presence of T3 in commercial eggs, we investigated whether T3 is accumulated and concentrated up in hen eggs by supplementing rice bran scum oil (RBO, Sanwa-Yushi Co. Ltd., Tendo, Japan) into hen feed. The RBO is composed of 1.3 % wt T3 (0.53 %, 0.75 %, and 0.05 % of α-, γ-, and δ-T3, respectively) as well as 1.7 % wt Toc (1.5 %, 0.04 %, 0.08 %, and 0.03 % of α-, β-, γ-, and δ-Toc, respectively).

Seventy two Julia hens were divided into three groups (24 hens/group, 4 hens/cage). Experimental diets (Toyohashi Feed Mills Co. Ltd., Shinshiro, Japan) contained essential nutrients (e.g., 17 % crude protein) and 4 % fat. The fats used were varied as: 0 % RBO group containing 4 % animal fat; 2 % RBO group containing 2 % animal fat and 2 % RBO; and 4 % RBO group containing 4 % RBO. T3 and Toc contents in experimental diets were as 18 mg T3/kg and 76 mg Toc/kg in 0 % RBO group, 170 mg T3/kg and 210 mg Toc/kg in 2 % RBO group, and 260 mg T3/kg and 300 mg Toc/kg in 4 % RBO group. The laying hens were given free access to feed and tap water, and eggs were collected at days 0, 7, 14, and 28. All egg samples were determined their contents of T3 and Toc in the same way for commercial eggs.

Eggs collected from each group on the days 0, 7, 14, and 28 had no significant differences in total weight (around 61 g), egg white weight (36 g), and yolk weight (17 g). Chromatograms of T3 and Toc of eggs collected on days 0 and 28 of 2 % RBO group are shown in Fig. 21.4a, and changes in T3 and Toc contents during the experiment period are expressed in Fig. 21.4b. Considering day-0 eggs (Fig. 21.4a), the predominant vitamin E were α-Toc and γ-Toc, whereas α-T3 and γ-T3 were found little compared with the Toc. The amounts of total T3 and total Toc in day-0 eggs were 0.08–0.09 mg T3/egg and 1.4–1.7 mg Toc/egg. In groups fed with RBO, the contents of both T3 and Toc were elevated up to reach the maximum levels on day-7 (2 % RBO group, 0.62 mg T3/egg, and 7.2 mg Toc/egg; 4 % RBO group, 0.56 mg T3/egg, and 7.6 mg Toc/egg). Then, T3 and Toc were gradually

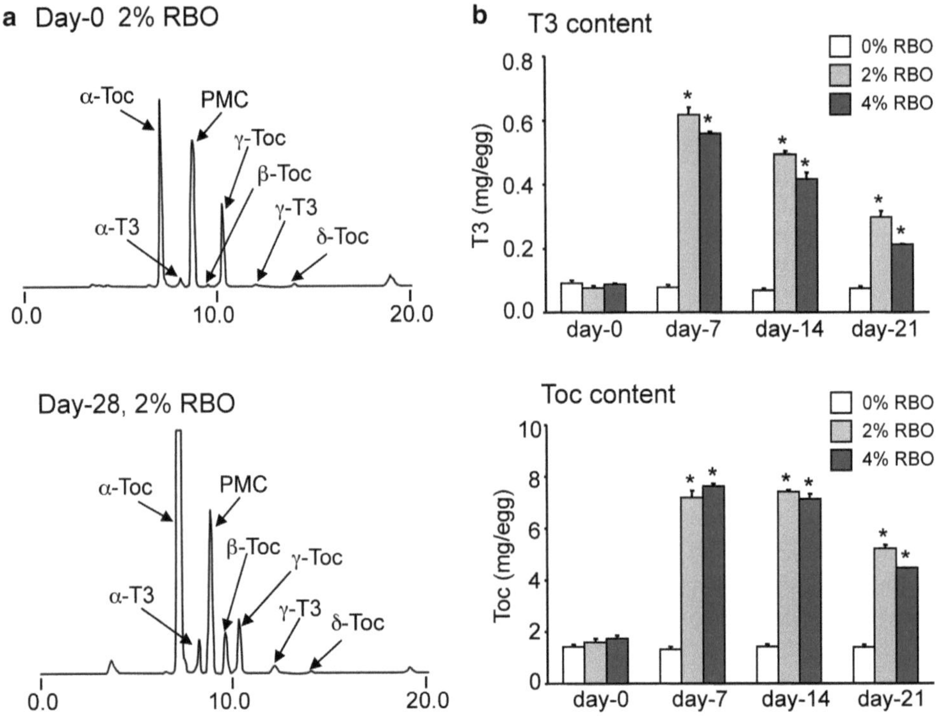

Fig. 21.4 Typical high-performance liquid chromatography (HPLC) chromatograms of T3 and Toc in eggs and time course changes of T3 and Toc concentrations in the experimental eggs. Typical HPLC chromatograms of T3 and Toc in eggs collected from day-0 to day-28 of 2 % rice bran scum oil (RBO) Group (**a**) and time course changes in T3 and Toc concentrations in eggs during the experiment (**b**). Laying hens were given free access to feed (0 % RBO, 2 % RBO, or 4 % RBO) and tap water, and eggs were collected at days 0, 7, 14, and 28. All egg samples were determined their contents of T3 and Toc by using HPLC. Values are mean ± SD ($n = 3$)

decreased on day-14 (2 % RBO group, 0.49 mg T3/egg, and 7.4 mg Toc/egg; 4 % RBO group, 0.41 mg T3/egg, and 7.1 mg Toc/egg) and day-28 (2 % RBO group, 0.30 mg T3/egg, and 5.2 mg Toc/egg; 4 % RBO group, 0.21 mg T3/egg, and 4.5 mg Toc/egg). These results clearly indicate that T3 as well as Toc can be accumulated to some extent in eggs by supplementing RBO into feed. Because RBO was rich in α-T3, γ-T3, and α-Toc, accumulations of these T3 and Toc isomers in eggs were met by RBO supplementation.

On the other hand, there are some reports about production of eggs enriched with Toc [26–29], but not T3. Toc accumulation in 2 % RBO group (7.2 mg Toc/egg) was lower or higher than previous studies supplementing the similar amount (200 mg/kg) of Toc or tocopheryl acetate [26, 27].

To More Improve Tocotrienol in Eggs

As shown in Fig. 21.4b, reduction of T3 and Toc in egg after they reached the maximum levels was observed. The reduction of T3 and Toc was by 52–62 % and 27–42 %, respectively. Some studies [26–28] reported such reduction of Toc (10–50 %), but others [29] showed no reduction. In our experiment, the reduction of T3 and Toc in eggs may be explained that they were used as antioxidants for protecting hens from unavoidable heat stress, because this study was conducted and finished in the middle summer.

On the other hand, for previous studies [29, 30], Toc accumulation in eggs seems to occur in a dose-dependent manner. However, in our experiment, no dose-dependent increase of both T3 and Toc was observed. This might be partly because the total amount of lipophilic compounds (22 mg/kg xanthophylls and 560 mg/kg vitamin E) in the feed of 4 % RBO group may be over-excessive. Therefore, no differences in Toc and T3 between 2 % RBO and 4 % RBO groups were observed.

For possibilities to more improve T3 in eggs, brown laying hens would be introduced instead of Julia hens (white laying hens), because brown laying hens have been reported to have better efficiency for vitamin E retention in eggs (2 or 3 times higher than the white ones) [31]. Although vitamin A is recommended for color enhancement in egg yolk and for natural antioxidant, vitamin A supplementation causes the competitive interaction in intestinal absorption between vitamin A and vitamin E [31]. Thus, by reducing the amount of vitamin A added into feed, T3 and Toc would be better absorbed and accumulated in eggs.

Fortification of Tocotrienol in Broiler Meat

Besides fortification of T3 in hen eggs, we did another fortification study of T3 in broiler meat. RBO was added into a basal experimental diet of broiler (Toyohashi Feed Mills Co. Ltd.). The feed of control group consisted of 5 % soybean (16.9 mg T3/kg feed and 77.2 mg Toc/kg feed), and the feed of 2 % RBO group was added with 3 % soybean oil and 2 % RBO (169.1 mg T3/kg and 215.8 mg Toc/kg). The Chunky broilers (6 birds/group) were given free accessed of feed and tap water for 14 days, and then meat samples (breast, thigh, and liver) were determined for their contents of T3 and Toc.

The contents of T3 and Toc in the breast, thigh, and liver samples of the broilers are reported in Table 21.2. To the 2 % RBO group, T3 contents were 3.0, 3.5, and 2.5 mg T3/kg of breast, thigh, and liver samples, respectively, whereas no T3 was detected in samples from the control group. The results indicate that T3 and Toc can be accumulated in broiler meat by adding RBO to broiler feeds. However, the accumulation of T3 in broiler meat was rather small comparing with T3 in eggs: the fortification of T3 in eggs was up to 0.62 mg T3/egg (equivalent to 10 mg/kg) but up to 3.68 mg/kg in broiler meat.

Table 21.2 The contents of T3 and Toc in broiler meat samples (mg/kg)

Sample	α-T3	β-T3	γ-T3	δ-T3	Total T3	Total Toc
Control—breast	n.d.	n.d.	n.d.	n.d.	n.d.	2.97
Control—thigh	n.d.	n.d.	n.d.	n.d.	n.d.	3.70
Control—liver	n.d.	n.d.	n.d.	n.d.	n.d.	10.51
2 % RBO—breast	2.7	n.d.	0.3	n.d.	2.95	14.05
2 % RBO—thigh	3.3	n.d.	0.2	n.d.	3.46	18.8
2 % RBO—liver	2.5	n.d.	n.d.	n.d.	3.68	102

The table shows contents of T3 and Toc in broiler meat samples (mg/kg). The meat samples were solidified with liquid nitrogen, ground into powder, and saponified. A portion of the extract was injected into HPLC with fluorescence detection for vitamin E analysis

n.d. not detectable

Conclusion

In summary, T3 has a wide variety of health benefits. We observed and found commercial eggs containing little amount of T3 (around 0.11 mg/egg). By adding extra T3 source (RBO) into laying hen feeds, T3 was absorbed and accumulated in hen eggs. In our study, the maximum level of T3 was 0.56–0.62 mg/egg after 7 days of the experiment. The accumulation of T3 in eggs would be improved by considering type of laying hen and proper amount of other lipophilic compounds that might be competitive in absorption of vitamin E. The accumulation of T3 was also found in broiler meat, but the fortification efficacy in meat appeared to be rather poor compared with fortification of T3 in eggs. Thus, the eggs enriched with T3 would be produced and recommended as one of the choices for T3 for its health benefits.

Acknowledgements A part of this study was supported by KAKENHI (S) (20228002, to T.M.) of JSPS, Japan. We thank Prof. Masaaki Toyomizu (Animal Nutrition, Graduate School of Agricultural Science, Tohoku University, Sendai 981-8555, Japan), Mr. Shin-ichi Nakajima (Technical Center, Toyohashi Feed Mills Co. Ltd., Shinshiro 444-1346, Japan), and Yoshikazu Amano (Sanwa-Yushi Co. Ltd., Tendo 994-0044, Japan) for excellent technical advices.

References

1. Evans HM, Bishop KS. On the existence of a hitherto unrecognized dietary factor essential for reproduction. Science. 1922;56:650–1.
2. Dunphy PJ, Whittle KJ, Pennock JF, Morton RA. Identification and estimation of tocotrienols in Hevea latex. Nature. 1965;207:521–2.
3. Sookwong P, Nakagawa K, Murata K, et al. Quantitation of tocotrienol and tocopherol in various rice brands. J Agric Food Chem. 2007;55:461–6.
4. Serbinova E, Kagan V, Han D, et al. Free radical recycling and intramembrane mobility in the antioxidant properties of α-tocopherol and α-tocotrienol. Free Radic Biol Med. 1991;10:263–75.
5. Khanna S, Roy S, Slivka A, et al. Neuroprotective properties of the natural vitamin E α-tocotrienol. Stroke. 2005;36:2258–64.
6. Hiura Y, Tachibana H, Arakawa R, et al. Specific accumulation of γ- and δ-tocotrienols in tumor and their antitumor effect in vivo. J Nutr Biochem. 2009;20:607–13.
7. Nakagawa K, Shibata A, Yamashita S, et al. In vivo angiogenesis is suppressed by unsaturated vitamin E, tocotrienol. J Nutr. 2007;137:1938–43.
8. Shibata A, Nakagawa K, Sookwong P, et al. Tumor anti-angiogenic effect and mechanism of action of δ-tocotrienol. Biochem Pharmacol. 2008;76:330–9.
9. Srivastava JK, Gupta S. Tocotrienol-rich fraction of palm oil induces cell cycle arrest and apoptosis selectively in human prostate cancer cells. Biochem Biophys Res Commun. 2006;346:447–53.
10. Agarwal MK, Agarwal ML, Athar M, et al. Tocotrienol-rich fraction of palm oil activates p53, modulates Bax/Bcl2 ratio and induces apoptosis independent of cell cycle association. Cell Cycle. 2004;3:205–11.
11. Shah S, Sylvester PW. Tocotrienol-induced caspase-8 activation is unrelated to death receptor apoptotic signaling in neoplastic mammary epithelial cells. Exp Biol Med. 2004;229:745–55.
12. Theriault A, Chao JT, Gapor A. Tocotrienol is the most effective vitamin E for reducing endothelial expression of adhesion molecules and adhesion to monocytes. Atherosclerosis. 2002;160:21–30.
13. Ahn KS, Sethi G, Krishnan K, et al. γ-Tocotrienol inhibits nuclear factor-κB signaling pathway through inhibition of receptor-interacting protein and TAK1 leading to suppression of antiapoptotic gene products and potentiation of apoptosis. J Biol Chem. 2007;282:809–20.
14. Eitsuka T, Nakagawa K, Miyazawa T. Down-regulation of telomerase activity in DLD-1 human colorectal adenocarcinoma cells by tocotrienol. Biochem Biophys Res Commun. 2006;348:170–5.
15. Pearce BC, Parker RA, Deason ME, et al. Hypocholesterolemic activity of synthetic and natural tocotrienols. J Med Chem. 1922;35:3595–606.
16. Parker RA, Pearce BC, Clark RW, et al. Tocotrienols regulate cholesterol production in mammalian cells by post-transcriptional suppression of 3-hydroxy-3-methylglutaryl-coenzyme A reductase. J Biol Chem. 1993; 268:11230–8.
17. Song BL, DeBose-Boyd RA. Insig-dependent ubiquitination and degradation of 3-hydroxy-3-methylglutaryl coenzyme a reductase stimulated by δ- and γ-tocotrienols. J Biol Chem. 2006;281:25054–61.

18. Watkins T, Lenz P, Gapor A, et al. γ-Tocotrienol as a hypocholesterolemic and antioxidant agent in rats fed atherogenic diets. Lipids. 1993;28:1113–8.
19. Khor H, Chieng D. Effect of dietary supplementation of tocotrienols and tocopherols on serum lipids in the hamster. Nutr Res. 1996;16:1393–401.
20. Black TM, Wang P, Maeda N, et al. Palm tocotrienols protect ApoE+/– mice from diet-induced atheroma formation. J Nutr. 2000;130:2420–6.
21. Qureshi AA, Salser WA, Parmar R, et al. Novel tocotrienols of rice bran inhibit atherosclerotic lesions in C57BL/6 ApoE-deficient mice. J Nutr. 2001;131:2606–18.
22. Qureshi AA, Qureshi N, Wright JJ, et al. Lowering of serum cholesterol in hypercholesterolemic humans by tocotrienols (palmvitee). Am J Clin Nutr. 1991;53:1021S–6.
23. Sookwong P, Nakagawa K, Yamaguchi Y, et al. Tocotrienol distribution in foods: estimation of daily tocotrienol intake of Japanese population. J Agric Food Chem. 2010;58:3350–5.
24. Bourre JM, Galea F. An important source of omega-3 fatty acids, vitamin D and E, carotenoids, iodine and selenium: a new natural multi-enriched egg. J Nutr Health Aging. 2005;10:371–6.
25. Sookwong P, Nakagawa K, Nakajima S, et al. Tocotrienol content in hen eggs: its fortification by supplementing the feed with rice bran scum oil. Biosci Biotechnol Biochem. 2008;72:3044–7.
26. Meluzzi A, Sirri F, Tallorico N, et al. Dietary vitamin E in production eggs enriched with n-3 fatty acids. In: Proceedings of the VIII European symposium on the quality of eggs and egg products. WPSA Italian Branch, Bologna; 1999. p. 153–9.
27. Surai PF, Ionov I, Buzhin A, et al. Vitamin E and egg quality. In: Proceedings of the VI European symposium on the quality of eggs and egg products. WPSA Italian Branch, Bologna; 1995. p. 387–94.
28. Galobart J, Barroeta AC, Cortinas L, et al. Accumulation of α-tocopherol in eggs enriched with ω3 and ω6 polyunsaturated fatty acids. Poult Sci. 2002;81:1873–6.
29. Chen JY, Latshaw JD, Lee HO, et al. α-Tocopherol content and oxidative stability of egg yolk as related to dietary α-tocopherol. J Food Sci. 1998;63:919–22.
30. Guang-Hai Q, Sim JS. Natural tocopherol enrichment and its effect in n-3 fatty acid modified chicken eggs. J Agric Food Chem. 1998;46:1920–6.
31. Grobas S, Mendez J, Bote CL, et al. Effect of vitamin E and A supplementation on egg yolk α-tocopherol concentration. Poult Sci. 2002;81:376–81.

Chapter 22
Vitamin A Fortification of Cooking Oils

Levente L. Diósady and M.G. Venkatesh-Mannar

Key Points

- Hundreds of millions of children in lower income countries are at increased risk of disease and early death due to vitamin A deficiency. It can cause eye disease, irreversible blindness, reduced resistance to infection, and an increased risk of morbidity and mortality.
- Fortification of food staples can have an impact on child health, both directly by increasing children's vitamin A intake and indirectly by raising levels obtained by children from breast milk.
- Vegetable oils are suitable vehicles for fortification with the fat-soluble vitamins A, D, and E, as the production and refining of the oils is a centralized process.
- Oil fortification consists of adding appropriate amounts of vitamin A concentrate to clarified, degassed oil. The final product concentration is governed by the expected per capita consumption of oil. Additional consideration should be given to such factors as loss of potency in cooking, reduced utilization with low-protein diets, and wastage.
- Potentially toxic levels are, for all practical purposes, too high to be of concern.
- Stability of vitamin A is key to the effectiveness of oil fortification. Vitamin A has to 'survive' the supply chain—from its own production, to processing, storage, retail, and ultimately household use through the course of the whole shelf life of the product.
- When fortified oil is packaged in light-protected, sealed containers that protect vitamin A and oil from light and air, losses of vitamin are negligible for up to a year.
- When vitamin A is used in oils that are subjected to severe heating, significant losses can occur, depending on temperature and time of heating.
- Usage of oil in the household is an important consideration in determining the choice of oil as a vehicle for vitamin A fortification.
- Oil fortification has gained considerable momentum in developing countries because of its reach into target groups, technical feasibility, and cost-effectiveness.

L.L. Diósady
Department of Chemical Engineering and Applied Chemistry, University of Toronto,
200 College Street, Toronto, ON, Canada M5S 3E5
e-mail: l.diosady@utoronto.ca

M.G. Venkatesh-Mannar, M.S. (✉)
Micronutrient Initiative, 180 Elgin Street, Suite 1000, Ottawa, ON, Canada K2P 2K3
e-mail: vmannar@micronutrient.org

V.R. Preedy et al. (eds.), *Handbook of Food Fortification and Health: From Concepts to Public Health Applications Volume 1*, Nutrition and Health, DOI 10.1007/978-1-4614-7076-2_22,

Keywords Vitamin A • Edible oils • Fortification • Carotenoids • Stability • Efficacy • Safety • Standards • Enforcement

Abbreviations

BHA	Butylated hydroxyanisole
BHT	Butylated hydroxytoluene
CSR	Corporate social responsibility
FAO	Food and Agriculture Organization
FSA	Food Standards Association
HPLC	High-performance liquid chromatography
IU	International unit
MI	Micronutrient Initiative
RAE	Retinol activity equivalents
RDI	Recommended dietary intakes
RE	Retinol equivalent
TBHQ	Tertiary-butylhydroquinone
VAD	Vitamin A deficiency
WFP	World Food Programme
WHO	World Health Organization

Introduction

Requirement for Vitamin A

Vitamin A is essential for normal tissue growth. Vitamin A functions in vision cell differentiation, embryonic development, spermatogenesis, the immune response, and epithelial cell integrity. Vitamin A deficiency (VAD), which mainly affects young children and pregnant women in lower income countries, can cause eye disease, irreversible blindness, reduced resistance to infection, and an increased risk of morbidity and mortality. VAD leads to a vicious cycle that increases susceptibility to infection such as diarrheal disease or measles, which in turn can cause loss of appetite, reduced absorption of vitamin A, and an increase in the body's excretion of vitamin A. While more severe VAD causes impaired vision and blindness, research indicates that even children with mild VAD and no clinical symptoms, if left unprotected, have a 24 % higher risk of death [1].

WHO's (World Health Organization) recommended dietary intakes (RDI) and basal requirements for vitamin A for different groups appear in Table 22.1. Basal requirements, which reflect the minimum needs of the body at rest, are substantially lower than the RDI.

Hundreds of millions of children are at increased risk of disease and early death due to VAD. It compromises the immune systems of approximately 33 % of the developing world's children under the age of 5 [2] and leads to the deaths of as many as one million children annually, making it a serious public health problem.

For this reason, and the difficulty in ensuring young children in resource-poor regions of the world consume sufficient amounts of vitamin A through their diet, WHO recommends that vitamin A supplementation be provided to infants and young children 6–59 months of age in areas where VAD is considered a public health problem. The suggested dose is 100,000 IU vitamin A on one occasion for infants 6–11 months of age and 200,000 IU vitamin A every 4–6 months for children 12–59 months of age.

Table 22.1 Vitamin A requirement and safe intake levels[a]

Life stage group	Estimated mean requirement (μg RE/day)	Safe intake levels (μg RE/day)
Infants		
0–6 mos	180	375
7–12 mos	190	400
Children		
1–3 y	200	400
4–6 y	200	450
7–9 y	250	500
Adolescents		
10–18 y	330–400	600
Men		
19–65 y	300	600
>65 y	300	600
Women		
19–65 y	270	500
>65 y	300	600
Pregnant women		
Pregnant	370	800
Lactating	450	850

[a]Data from WHO, FAO

Dietary Sources of Vitamin A

Animal sources of vitamin A are well absorbed and used efficiently by the body. Plant sources are not as well absorbed. In Western diets preformed vitamin A derived from animal sources, i.e. mother's milk, liver, egg yolk, butter, liver, cod-liver oil, and whole cow's milk, provides ~70 % daily intake [3]. However, in developing countries, where animal products are less available, carotenoids that the body converts to vitamin A provide as much as ~70 % of daily intake. Carotenoids are found in dark-green leafy and yellow- and orange-coloured vegetables and fruits. Many vegetable oils also contain carotenoid pigments.

Rationale for Vitamin A Fortification of Oil

Fortification of food staples, including those provided in food aid programmes, can impact child health—directly by increasing children's vitamin A intake and indirectly by raising levels obtained by children from breast milk. It may also reduce health problems associated with iron deficiency anaemia and improve the mother's overall health.

Oils and fats, along with carbohydrates and proteins, are major components of the human diet. Oils provide energy, fat-soluble vitamins (vitamins A, D, and E), and essential fatty acids that are required for proper growth and development. The production of vegetable oils (canola, corn, cottonseed, coconut, olive, palm, peanut, safflower, soybean, sunflower) is high throughout the world, and consumption is increasing (Table 22.2), especially among lower socioeconomic groups. Consumption of vegetable oils over animal fats is preferable because vegetable oils typically contain much less saturated fat, and they contain no cholesterol.

Table 22.2 Per capita vegetable oil consumption and percent daily energy intake from vegetable oils in selected countries[a]

Country	Consumption (g/day)	% Energy intake
Argentina	33	9
Brazil	27	9
Mexico	30	9
Costa Rica	35	11
Central Africa	12	5
Congo	34	12
Gambia	31	11
India	16	7
Indonesia	17	6
Philippines	12	4

[a]*Source*: FAO. Food Balance Sheets 1984–1986. Rome; 1991

The rationale for oil fortification is based on the following criteria, which are commonly applied to assess vehicles for fortification:

1. *Technical feasibility*. Vegetable oils are suitable vehicles for fortification with the fat-soluble vitamins A, D, and E, as the production and refining of oils is a centralized process. These vitamins form a true solution and are uniformly distributed in oil. The stability of vitamin A is greater in oils than in any other food, and oil facilitates the absorption of vitamin A by the body. Mixing is quite simple and can often be done with equipment readily available at mills, such as normal agitators and dosifiers. At low concentrations, vitamin A changes neither colour, taste, and shelf life nor other product parameters of oils, which are highly relevant for producers and consumers. Stabilized vitamin A forms remain active in the end product, even when used for frying.
2. *Human consumption levels*. Vegetable oils are consumed by almost everyone; thus, it is possible to improve people's access to fat-soluble vitamins through oil fortification. In many countries, oil consumption is uniform: 10–20 g/capita/day in African countries and up to 70–90 g/capita/day in Asia. The near-universal consumption of oils ensures a good coverage of populations, and the average consumption level allows moderate fortification levels for achieving public health impact. It is reasonable to assume that, ultimately, increased vitamin A intake from oils will result in a widely distributed, homogeneous improvement in the vitamin A status of affected populations.
3. *Domestic processing*. Oil fortification works best with domestic processors. As food producers, they are more open to consider improving the population's nutrition as part of their corporate social responsibility (CSR) than foreign manufacturers. Local enterprises are more likely to respond to the governments' demands for fortification and its quality control than foreign producers.
4. *Industry concentration*. Oil milling is usually capital-intensive and thereby concentrated, with only a few oil mills serving the majority of national demand. Small-scale community production is rare. Self-sufficient home growing and crushing of oil seeds, particularly in parts of Africa, constitutes only a small fraction of oil use.
5. *Low incremental cost*. Economically sustainable fortification calls for minimal increases of final retail prices of the fortified foods, so as to remain affordable and be the product of choice for the poor and undernourished with limited purchasing power. The cost increase of vitamin A-fortified oils amounts to only 0.1–0.3 % of the retail price or a fraction of a US$/kg. This allows producers to absorb the cost of fortification. This contrasts sharply with salt fortification, where the cost of iodization encourages the grey importation of unfortified products.
6. *Cost-effectiveness*. Oil fortification is very cost-effective. Since vitamin A can be added in concentrated and stable form, the cost of equipment is moderate [4]. Success requires widespread consumption of the fortified edible oil product, specific to each country. Where oil fortification is not yet possible or

established, the addition of vitamin A to existing flour fortification programmes can be technically feasible. Other vehicles are suitable for targeted fortification programmes but do not have equivalent nationwide reach (e.g. milk) or are technically and economically more challenging (e.g. rice).

Vitamin A Chemistry

Vitamin A (Retinol)

Vitamin A is a yellow, oil-soluble crystal that can be uniformly distributed in oil. The body easily absorbs added vitamin A in the presence of oil. Vitamin A is unstable when exposed to light (particularly UV), air, oxidizing agents, and heat. Heavy metals and acids, even in trace quantities, can accelerate decomposition.

Retinoids are insoluble in water but are soluble in alcohols, ether, chloroform, oils, and fats. β-carotene is less soluble than retinol but is still quite soluble in fats and oils. All vitamin A compounds and their precursors are sensitive to oxygen and light. Vitamin A is extremely sensitive to oxygen (undergoes oxidation), light (promotes *trans-cis* isomerization), heat (catalyzes isomerization), halogens (isomerization, particularly in the presence of light and high temperature), and is unstable in acidic environments (undergoes rearrangements of the double bonds and dehydrates).

Due to the wide range of compounds with vitamin A activity, a single unit called the retinol equivalent (RE) was established in 1967 by a Food and Agriculture Organization (FAO)/WHO Expert Group. The RE unit expresses and measures vitamin A activity relative to retinol where 1 μg of retinol = 1 RE. For example:

1 μg retinyl palmitate = 0.546 μg RE
1 μg retinyl acetate = 0.872 μg RE
1 μg β-carotene = 0.167 μg RE
1 μg other provitamin A carotenoids = 0.084 μg RE [2]

Vitamin A in dietary sources, preformed or provitamin A, can also be measured as μg/g or ppm and frequently as International Units (IUs). IUs measure biological activity. One IU is biologically equivalent to 0.3 μg of retinol or 0.3 μg of β-carotene in Canada. However, it is now recommended that weight or molar units replace the IU system to decrease confusion [2]. The Recommended Dietary Allowances (RDAs) for vitamin A are more recently listed as retinol activity equivalents (RAE) to account for the different activities of retinol and provitamin A carotenoids. Sometimes RDAs are also listed in IUs, because food and some supplement labels list vitamin A content in IUs (1 μg RAE = 3.3 IU).

Vitamin A Forms

Vitamin A is readily bioavailable, especially in the all-trans-retinol form. All-trans vitamin A palmitate is the most biologically active form of the vitamin A esters, which means it is the most absorbed, transported, and utilized physiologically by the body. Retinol, its metabolites, and synthetic analogues that have a similar structure and biological activity are referred to as retinoids. Dietary precursors of retinol, often referred to as provitamin A, include a number of pigments called carotenoids due to their typical orange colour. The most active among these is β-carotene, which can readily react to form two retinol molecules.

Table 22.3 Vitamin A and β-carotene content of typical oils

Oil	Vitamin A (μg/g)	β-carotene (μg/g)
Butter[a]	5.5–12	6–20
Tallow[b]	22	22
Margarine[b]	55	–
Coconut[b]		Trace
Palm[b]	–	5,650
Soy[b]	350	
Rapeseed[b]		330
Cottonseed[b]	–	300
Sunflower[b]	–	2.6
Corn oil[b]	–	14
Cod-liver oil[b]	3,000	

[a]Data from Swern D, ed. *Bailey's Industrial Oil and Fat Products*. 4th ed. New York: John Wiley and Sons New York; 1979
[b]Data from Souci SW, Fachmann W, Kraut H. *Food Composition and Nutrition Tables 1981/82*. International Publishers Service Inc; 1987

Vitamin A esters are significantly more stable than alcohols as the free hydroxyl group of their alcohol forms is highly sensitive to oxidation. To increase stability and solubility, it is common practice to utilize esters of vitamin A. Typically, retinol palmitate is used in lipid systems and retinol acetate in aqueous or alcohol systems.

Retinyl acetate and palmitate are the most common market forms of vitamin A used for oil fortification. Palmitate is slightly more stable and is slightly more soluble in oil. After storing the premix for 24 months at 20 °C, Roche Food Applications Laboratory reported 95.7 % retention of palmitate vs. 93.6 % retention of the acetate form [5]. Gopal et al. [6] reported higher recovery of palmitate under a range of temperatures in tests at Roche [7] in India. After 25 min at 180 °C, Gopal et al. found 56 % of the acetate was retained compared to 80 % of the palmitate. As expected in aqueous solution at 45 °C, tests at Unilever [8] indicated palmitate is more stable in coloured bottles.

DSM (formerly Hoffman LaRoche) and BASF are the dominant suppliers of retinol esters worldwide.

Vitamin A and Carotenoids in Edible Oils and Oil Products

When fats are extracted from plants, they typically contain several minor components including plant sterols, some of which have beneficial health effects, and pigments, including carotenes and chlorophyll. Oils from plant sources do not contain any vitamin A, but the carotenoid pigments have vitamin A activity (see Table 22.3).

Technology

Vegetable Oil Processing Technology

Plants store energy as starches (complex carbohydrates) and as triglycerides. Triglycerides are esters of fatty acids with glycerol. Fatty acids are usually linear hydrocarbon chains with a carboxylic end, with chain length varying from 2 to 26.

Vegetable oils also contain minor components that are typically removed by the refining process. The refining process typically consists of degumming, which removes phosphatides or lecithins. While these may have positive nutraceutical value, they smoke when heated and are undesirable in cooking oil.

The free fatty acids and other hydrolysis products are removed. In the conventional process, the oil is treated with alkali to neutralize the free fatty acids, forming soaps. In physical refining, they are removed by vacuum steam refining.

Pigments (including carotenoids and chlorophyll) and sterols, which also have positive nutraceutical functions, are conventionally removed by adsorption in a process termed 'bleaching'.

Finally the oil is deodorized, using high-temperature vacuum steam distillation. This removes all volatiles, including much of the tocopherols. Tocopherols are natural antioxidants with vitamin E activity.

Modern processes try to retain tocopherols, as well as trapping them for re-addition to oil or manufactured foods as stabilizers.

Oil Fortification Technology

Fortification of vegetable oils and their derivatives (margarine, mayonnaise, etc.) with fat-soluble vitamins is technologically feasible. Oil fortification consists of adding appropriate amounts of vitamin A concentrate to clarified, degassed oil at 45–50 °C. The solubility of commercially available vitamin A formulations in vegetable oils is excellent. The most common commercial vitamin A formulation contains 1,000,000 IU vitamin A palmitate (300,000 μg/g) in a liquid form, stabilized with vitamin E (α-tocopherol) or a butylated hydroxyanisole (BHA)/butylated hydroxytoluene (BHT) mixture.

To ensure that the vitamins are uniformly distributed, mixing takes place in vertical tanks that contain turbines or propeller agitators. Edible antioxidants (BHA and/or BHT) or natural antioxidants (e.g. α-tocopherol or ascorbyl palmitate) may be added to protect both the vitamin A and the oil; the stability of vitamin A in the oil depends greatly on the stability of the oil itself. Vitamin A oxidizes faster and loses its activity in the presence of oxidized oils. To maintain vitamin A activity, fortified oil needs to be packaged in light-protected, sealed containers. Replacing the container headspace with inert gas will help retain the stability of both the oil and vitamin A prior to the container being opened. However, this is impractical in developing countries, so the micronutrient losses are compensated for by overage.

The production and fortification of margarine-like semisolid products are carried out either in a batch or continuous process. The vitamin blend is premeasured according to the batch size of the margarine tanks and mixed with warm oil, in a ratio of 1:5, until a uniform solution is obtained. This premix is then incorporated into the margarine before the emulsifying process. This emulsion is chilled to partially crystallize the fat and packaged in continuously operating equipment. Usually the vitamin concentrate is supplied in containers, which hold the specified amount of vitamin to be added per batch of oil. This avoids weighing errors by plant staff.

Inclusion of vitamin A in vegetable oil does not require large investments in new technology. In continuous refining (see Fig. 22.1), investment is limited to piping, a small tank for pre-blending, a dosing pump, flow metres, and maybe an electronic control system, as illustrated below.

For batch production, a suitable tank should be equipped with an agitator and baffles in order to ensure an effective homogenization of the blend, as indicated in Fig. 22.2. Since vitamin A is readily soluble in edible oils, any degree of agitation of the oil that is being fortified is adequate to effect uniform distribution. Some agitation time must be allowed, depending on agitation intensity. In practically all cases, a 30-min agitation time is adequate. Intense agitation, which risks incorporation of air, must be avoided to prevent vitamin A oxidation.

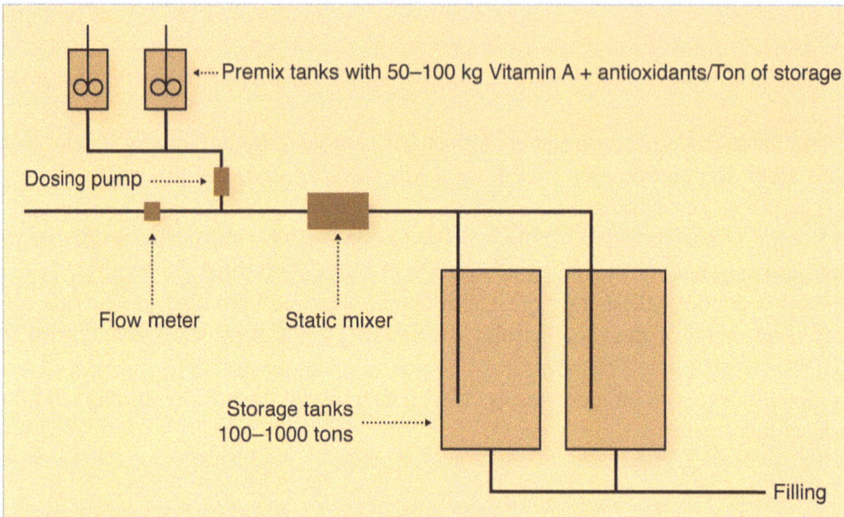

Fig. 22.1 Oil fortification in a continuous refining system (based on BASF illustration)

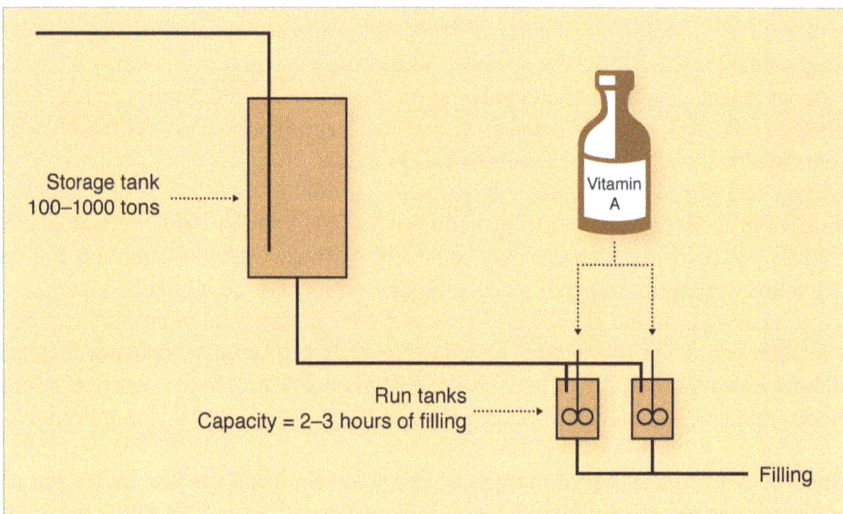

Fig. 22.2 Vitamin A fortification in a batch oil refining system (based on BASF illustration). *Source*: Figures 22.1 and 22.2 are original illustrations based on personal communication with BASF

To avoid air contact, the fortified oil must be packaged immediately after fortification, rather than stored in open tanks for any length of time. If short-term storage in an open tank is unavoidable, the agitator should be shut off.

Guidance on Oil Fortification Levels

The final product concentration is governed by the expected per capita consumption of oil. Additional consideration should be given to such factors as loss of potency in cooking, reduced utilization with low protein diets, and wastage. Potentially toxic levels are, for all practical purposes, too high to be of concern.

Daily intake of fat varies significantly between countries and within economic groups. Fortification levels must be targeted to provide 33–100 % of the daily requirement, based on the average daily fat intake, which can vary from 12 to 28 g/day. This translates to 20–100 RE/g oil.

The following equation has been proposed to set fortification levels in fortified foods to address the effects of RDI coverage, average daily intake of the fortified product, and retention of vitamin A after cooking:

$$\frac{\text{RD} \times \text{RDI coverage}}{\text{FF Level}} = \text{Retention} \times \text{Average daily intake}$$

RDI is the Recommended Daily Intake for an average population, in line with local laws or regulations.

RDI coverage is the target fortification level, expressed as % of RDI, and assumes that the rest of vitamin A is obtained from other food sources.

Retention is the fraction of vitamin A remaining after production, storage, and cooking: 60 % is widely assumed.

Average daily intake refers to the daily consumption of the vehicle and is calculated from either food consumption surveys or the average yearly consumption in a country calculated as intake per capita per day.

Here is a sample calculation for oil fortification in a region where per capita oil consumption is 30 g/day:

$$\text{Fortification Level} = \frac{2{,}000\,\text{IU} \times 33\%}{60\% \times 30\,\text{g}} = 37\,\text{IU}/\text{g}\ (37\,\text{IU}/\text{g is rounded off to } 40\,\text{IU}/\text{g})$$

Measuring the amount of micronutrients to add, and the process of their addition to oil or margarine, requires careful attention to ensure the final fortified product is both homogeneous and standardized.

Costs

The cost of fortification includes capital costs, such as blending equipment (tanks, agitators), and operating costs including those for the premix, personnel, monitoring, and evaluation. If margarine is fortified to provide 30,000 IU of vitamin A/kg, the cost of the fortificant would be in the order of US$0.0017/kg. These estimates do not take into account the ongoing cost of quality control nor the cost of new equipment and training of staff, which are one-time costs and are likely to be small.

Quality Control

The means for cost-effective quality control have been developed for testing of vitamin A levels in edible oils. Quantitatively, vitamin A is best analyzed in vegetable oil by high-performance liquid chromatography (HPLC). Semi-quantitative field test kits are available, which are based on colour indication. Screening of samples requires low skilled but trained personnel, and equipment should be routinely calibrated by HPLC.

For example, BioAnalyt, Germany, developed a handheld device costing ~10 % of an HPLC, with similar accuracy and sensitivity. This equipment can be operated by anyone after a few hours of training.

Stability of Vitamin A Activity

Stability of Vitamin A Forms

Stability of vitamin A is key to the effectiveness of oil fortification. Vitamin A has to survive the supply chain—from its own production to processing, storage, retail, and ultimately household use through the course of the whole shelf life of the product (often up to 24 months). Degradation of vitamin A cannot easily be countered by overages in dosage, as the variation in degradation is often unpredictable.

The quality of vitamin A used for fortification has the greatest impact on stability. Tests have shown variation in heat stability and potency in excess of 20 %. While vitamin A is sensitive to light, oxygen, moisture, and to some extent heat, in sealed containers vitamin A is stable, as it is well protected from moisture and oxygen.

Stability of vitamin A decreases significantly under direct UV light exposure, whereas indirect light, such as normal daylight hardly affects stability. In practice, direct light exposure of oils, even in transparent containers, is minimal. Producers supply oil bottles in light-proof cartons, and consumers rarely expose bottles to direct sunlight in order to avoid rancidity.

Effect of Antioxidants on Vitamin A in Oil

Fats are oxidized by a free-radical-initiated chain reaction. Under normal conditions, the oils oxidize to form aldehydes, which have the characteristic rancid flavour.

Free-radical oxidation is catalyzed by metal ions. The rate of oxidation depends on the availability of free radicals through the initiation step of hydroperoxide formation as well as on the presence of species that terminate the free-radical chain reaction. Thus, metal chelators that remove metal ions from the system and free-radical scavengers such as phenolic compounds can dramatically retard the rate of fat oxidation.

Since vitamin A oxidizes by the same mechanism as the fat, vitamin A dissolved in oil will be greatly affected by the availability of free radicals and antioxidants in the system. Peroxide value is a measure of the oxidative stability of oil and is a critical parameter in ensuring stable fortified oil. Vitamin A competes for free radicals with the oil and acts as an antioxidant. Accordingly, free-radical scavengers, such as phenolic antioxidants, will protect both the oil and the added vitamin A from oxidative degradation.

Tocopherols are good antioxidants for oils and vitamin A. When they supplement the naturally occurring tocopherol in crude vegetable oils or replace them after their reduction during refining, tocopherols are much more expensive than phenolic antioxidants. The most widely used synthetic antioxidants are BHA, BHT, and tertiary-butyl hydroquinone (TBHQ). BHA and BHT are allowed in food at levels up to 200 ppm in fats and oils. While TBHQ is more effective, its use is restricted in some jurisdictions. Natural, organic antioxidants such as rosemary extract contain mixtures of similar phenolic compounds. All these compounds can be used in conjunction with metal chelating agents such as phosphates or citric acid. As the phenolic antioxidants are volatile at high temperatures, they are less effective then tocopherols in protecting vitamin A at high frying temperatures.

Stability of Vitamin A During Storage in Sealed Containers

In sealed and opaque containers that protect vitamin A and oil from light and air, losses of vitamin are negligible for up to a year [9]. Studies by Favaro et al. [10] reported high retention after 9 months of storage in sealed containers at 23 °C but considerable losses at 18 months. Bauerenfeid et al. [11]

reported 91 % vitamin A retention after 6 months. Hoffman LaRoche [12] reported that 90–95 % of vitamin A was retained in soybean oil after 6 months' storage at 20–25 °C—superior to retention in margarine over the same time period (85–90 %). Studies of vitamin A retention during shipment (average 2–4 months) have shown values of 87–98 % [13].

Stability of Vitamin A During Storage in Open Containers

Bagriansky and Ranum [9] also reported on two studies that considered the stability of fortified oil in open cans. Studies by Favaro et al. [10] have shown no difference in stability between sealed cans and open cans for the first 6 months, even in the presence of light. However, after 3 additional months, only 48 % of original vitamin A level was retained in the opened cans exposed to light vs. 76 % in opened cans kept in the dark. Atwood et al. [13] reported an average of 70–88 % of the original vitamin A remaining after 30 days in open pails exposed to light, air, and temperatures of up to 35 °C.

Stability of Vitamin A During Food Preparation

Mag and Diosady reviewed oil fortification technology for the Micronutrient Initiative [14]. They reported that when vitamin A is used in foods that are subjected to severe heating, significant losses can occur, depending on temperature and time of heating. This is important in countries in which the practice of sautéing foods is widespread. Usual sautéing conditions involve heating the food with the oil to 150–160 °C for 5–10 min.

Synthetic antioxidants were found to have little effect. The lack of protection from these compounds is well known, i.e. they are volatile at high temperatures. Tocopherols, however, have been shown to persist under sautéing conditions (Food Standards Association [FSA]) and can therefore be expected to confer a measure of stability under these conditions. However, no direct evidence of this is available. Commercial vitamin A palmitate is available with alpha-tocopherol (vitamin E) added and may need to be considered for oil fortification in some markets.

Bagriansky and Ranum [9] reviewed the literature in more detail. The literature confirmed a wide variation in vitamin A stability during cooking, depending on time and temperature. The studies reviewed indicate that the deterioration of vitamin A in cooking oil is related primarily to the treatment temperature. They grouped studies by temperature.

1. *Boiling, simmering, and stewing*: *100–120 °C*
   At these temperatures, vitamin A is quite stable even when heated over an extended period of time. Studies by Favaro et al. [10], Atwood et al. [12], Bauerenfeind et al. [11], and Gopal and Ketyum [6] have reported vitamin A retention in the range of 88–100 % when oil was added to rice, pulses, onions, potatoes, or beans and cooked for 15–90 min. Only one study by Bauerenfeind et al. [11], where the oil was cooked with cornmeal for 30 min, reported lower retention rates of 66–75 %.
2. *Low-temperature frying*: *130–170 °C*
   When oil is subjected to light frying or deep-frying, vitamin A is lost at increasing rates. Favaro et al. [10] reported recovery of 83 % and 81 % of vitamin A after deep-frying four servings of potatoes at 130–170 °C. After the third and fourth fryings, 71 % and 52 % of the vitamin were retained. Sagredos [8] of Unilever Laboratories found that heating margarine to 150 °C suffered 41 % vitamin A loss, increasing to 41–55 % and 67–73 % after 10, 20, 30, and 45 min, respectively. Roche [12], on the other hand, reported retention of 90–95 % in frying oil held at 160 °C for 20 min.
3. *High-temperature frying*: *180–200 °C*
   Wok or deep-frying oils result in significant vitamin A losses. The loss depends on the number of times the same oil is used for frying foods. Studies by Favaro [10] showed that after the initial frying,

about 65 % of the original vitamin A remained. After 4 repeated fryings, less than 40 % of the original levels of vitamin A was retained. After 12 consecutive fryings, most of the vitamin A was lost. The manner in which oil is used at the household is therefore an important consideration in determining whether oil is a good vehicle for vitamin A.

Efficacy and Safety

Biological Efficacy of Fortified Oil

Vitamin A is readily absorbed in the presence of oils and fats. After the introduction of vitamin A-fortified margarine in Denmark at the end of 1917, the number of cases of xerophthalmia reported at a Copenhagen Hospital fell by more than 90 %. By 1918 the condition had disappeared [15]. Studies before and after the fortification of margarine in Newfoundland in 1944 report that the percent of subjects with serum vitamin A below 20 μg/dL declined from 48 to 2 % over 4 years [16]. More recently, a shelf-stable margarine in the Philippines was fortified with vitamin A. After the margarine was consumed for 6 months, the baseline prevalence of children with serum retinol levels below 20 μg/dL fell from 25.6 to 10.1 % [17].

The biological value of vitamin A-fortified oil has been reported in two studies. Dutra de Oliveira et al. demonstrated that soybean oil with vitamin A in the form of retinyl palmitate is well absorbed in humans given fortified oil along with a rice-based diet [18]. Significant increases in plasma retinol were reported. Differences in plasma retinol for subjects receiving uncooked vs. cooked soybean oil were not statistically significant. Favaro et al. [10] report increased weight gain, plasma retinol, and liver stores in rats consuming diets prepared with fortified soybean oil. However, the improvement in plasma retinol and liver stores for rats consuming diets of food cooked at 170 °C was 55 % less than those given diets cooked at 100 °C.

Safety and Toxicity Considerations

Vitamin A is toxic in excessive amounts. Toxicity symptoms are a function of amount and length of time of excessive intake.

Toxic symptoms have been reported from continued daily doses of 12,000–15,000 REs (40,000–50,000 IUs) with adults and 7,500 REs with children. These are more than 10 times the recommended dosages. The only potential toxicity hazard is overdose of highly concentrated pharmaceutical preparations of vitamin A.

The provitamins (carotenes) are not toxic. A fortification programme gains some additional safety from toxicity if a part of the vitamin A activity is supplied via β-carotene.

Edible oil fortification is generally considered safe. No incidents of intoxication have been reported. Even though vitamin A in pure form can be toxic in high dosage, in oil it is practically impossible for the consumer to exceed safety limits. For toxic effects, adults would need to consume more than a litre of edible oil daily.

Accidental major over-fortification has not been observed so far. Even though homogeneity in mixing the oil and vitamin A could be a technical challenge for some producers, the variation in vitamin A content in over-fortified batches remains far below safety levels. However, under-fortification—through technical challenges, unstable quality of vitamin A, or in a deliberate effort to cut costs—is observable in the absence of effective regulatory control systems.

Enabling Measures

Standards and Regulation

To ensure that a fortification programme is successful, an interdisciplinary task force with experts from all relevant sectors should be established. It should include oil processors, industry and trade organizations, nutrition institutes, universities, ministries of health, regulatory institutions, consumer associations, and donors. A fortification plan should specify the type of micronutrients and levels to be added, based on the consumption patterns of oil by all socioeconomic and age groups. It must also define precautions and food safety conditions to be observed during production, transportation, storage, and sale of the products.

Monitoring and Enforcement

Sustainability and reach of oil fortification into low-income, undernourished target groups depends on a proper legislative framework, as is the case in other forms of fortification, e.g. flour fortification. The majority of oils in developing countries—often up to 80 %—are sold in bulk at informal markets. These unbranded oils are taken from refillable barrels or buckets and packaged in small plastic bags in varying sizes. It is often not possible to trace unbranded oils back to their producers. Incentives for fortification, e.g. differentiation of brands, do not apply in these transparent and highly price-competitive market segments. Voluntary, industry-led oil fortification programmes comprising only branded and packed oils thereby stop short of reaching the main target groups served by unbranded bulk oils.

An enabling normative framework for fortification is necessary to ensure the sustainable reach of the programme into low-income target groups and at the same time provide industry with a level playing field favourable to uniform fortification of all products in the market. Governments increasingly prefer this option—exercised through technical norms in conjunction with labelling or even through food legislation. While technical norms are easier to issue, food laws requiring parliamentary approval are more permanent solutions, albeit much more time-consuming. Several countries such as Nigeria, Philippines, Mozambique, and Bolivia have chosen to mandate oil fortification with vitamin A.

Much of the reach of fortification depends on a proper monitoring and reporting system underpinning these hardware components. Little more than some personnel, technical training, and small budgets are needed to apply the screening tool, backed up by a quantitative testing method. However, many countries with mandatory oil fortification have still not yet defined such roles, responsibilities, and reporting lines nor have they dedicated the needed budgets.

Current Experiences in Fortification of Vegetable Oil

Developed Markets

The experiences in Denmark and Newfoundland were described in section ‘Biological Efficacy of Fortified Oil’.

Today in North America and Europe, margarine fortification with vitamin A (and D) is mandated, in most cases to levels that make it an equivalent source of vitamin A to butter, which it replaces in the diet. In Canada, the fortification provides ~10 % of the RDI per 10 g serving of margarine, i.e. 10 RE/g. Other countries fortifying margarine with vitamins A and D are presented in Table 22.4.

Table 22.4 Current fortification programmes for vitamin A in fats and oil[a]

	Oil/fats	
Region/country	Type of programme	Vitamin A in fats/oil
EAWA		
Belgium	M	Margarine 22,500–27,000 IU/kg
Burkina Faso	V	Cooking oil
Cote d'Ivoire	V	Cooking oil
Denmark	NS	Margarine 25,200 IU/kg
Egypt	V	Cooking oil
Ghana	V	Cooking oil
Mali	V	Cooking oil
Netherlands	NS	Margarine >20,000 IU/kg
Niger	NS	
Nigeria	M	Margarine 24,000–30,000 IU/kg; edible oils 20,000 IU/kg
Portugal	M	Margarine 1,800 IU/kg
Senegal	V	Cooking oil
South Africa	V	Margarine 30,000 IU/kg
Sweden	NS	Margarine >30,000 IU/kg
Togo	NS	
Turkey	NS	Table margarine 20,000 IU/kg
Uganda	V	Vegetable oil
UK	M	Margarine 24,000–30,000 IU/kg
Zimbabwe	P	Margarine 27,000–33,000 IU/kg
Asia-Pacific		
Australia	M	Table margarine >28,300 IU/kg
India	M	Vanaspati 25,000; margarine >30,000 IU/kg
Indonesia	M	Margarine 25,000–35,000 IU/kg
Malaysia	M	Table margarine 25,000–35,000 IU/kg
New Zealand	NS	Table margarine >28,300 IU/kg
Pakistan	M	Vegetable ghee, cooking oil 33,000 IU/kg
Philippines	M	Margarine >33,000 IU/kg; cooking oil 40,000–70,000 IU/kg
Singapore	M	Margarine >28,300 IU/kg
Taiwan	M	Margarine >45,000 IU/kg
Latin/Central America		
Brazil	M	Margarine 15,000–50,000 IU/kg
Chile	M	Margarine 30,000 IU/kg
Colombia	M	Margarine 30,000 IU/kg
Ecuador	M	Margarine 20,000–30,000 IU/kg
El Salvador	M	Margarine 15,000 IU/kg
Guatemala	M	Margarine 15,000–50,000 IU/kg
Honduras	M	Margarine 35,000 IU/kg
Mexico	M	Table margarine 20,000 IU/kg
Panama	M	Margarine 20,000 IU/kg
Peru	M	Margarine 30,000 IU/kg
Venezuela	M	Margarine 16,500 IU/kg
NAFTA		
Canada	M	Margarine >33,000 IU/kg
USA	M	Margarine 33,000 IU/kg

V industry-led; *M* mandatory; *NS* not specified; *P* permitted

[a]*Sources*:

SAFO—Food Fortification Standards (Mandatory and Voluntary Staple Food Fortification)—www.food-fortification.com

Nutriview Special Issue 2003—Mandatory food enrichment

MI—www.micronutrient.org

GAIN—www.gainhealth.org

Sweden fortifies canola oil used in food aid programmes with 15 mg vitamin A/g oil. In its food aid programmes, Canada has adopted an even higher level of 22.5 mg vitamin A/g.

Developing Countries

Oil fortification has gained considerable momentum in developing countries because of its reach into target groups, technical feasibility, and cost-effectiveness. Oil fortification has become an industry trend since 2006, with many producers having demonstrated their capability of turning the marginal cost of fortification into a business case. Front runners used fortification as differentiation criteria (unique selling point) on the market and consequently invested in marketing the added value of vitamin A to the consumer. This included TV commercials, customer (retail) road shows, scientific marketing, employee communication, and public relations work. Leading oil companies demonstrated how oil fortification can constitute a business case, based on multiple corporate benefits arising from their responsible engagement in improved nutrition.

However, it is not the private sector alone with its corporate leaders who are fostering the spread of oil fortification in developing countries. Public-private partnerships have been proven to add significant value to establishing and sustaining fortification programmes. A range of public interest organizations such as MI, GAIN, UNICEF, World Food Programme (WFP), and the World Bank and bilateral agencies such as GIZ have been engaged in oil fortification. Assistance in the form of grants and technical assistance to industry and governments have been essential for the establishment of fortification programmes.

Coordinating stakeholders remains a challenge, as multiple ministries often have a role in nutrition, not to mention the UN, NGOs, and various industry associations and companies. It has been proven to be valuable to establish or strengthen national alliances, which are coordinated by a nongovernmental body with expertise in fortification and supported by all stakeholders, predominantly by the government. Producers of quality fortificants provide valuable technical service and capacity-building expertise to food producers, e.g. in issues related to processing and quality control techniques. Multi-stakeholder partnerships, globally and at country levels, support producers who engage in oil fortification.

Relief and Development Programmes/Food Aid

The WFP has regularly supplied edible oils for food aid and disaster response programmes. Its policy nowadays is to source oils that are fortified and, when available at competitive prices, locally or regionally produced. Such programmes not only address the nutrition demands of those in severe need but often constitute a first additional market for front-running companies fortifying their oils voluntarily.

Recommendations

Governments in countries where VAD persists as a public health problem should consider the option of fortifying edible oils with vitamin A. Before embarking on a fortification programme, governments should conduct a comprehensive techno-economic feasibility study to assess: the stability of the nutrient under prevailing storage, transportation, packing, and cooking conditions; the variations in per capita consumption of oils and fats; and the feasibility of determining a dosage level that would provide meaningful quantities of nutrient to those at the lower end of the consumption spectrum while not reaching unacceptable levels for those at the higher end.

Once feasibility has been established, programmes should be designed with supporting standards and enforcement procedures that will ensure compliance by all manufacturers. Periodic evaluations should also be conducted to assess the effectiveness of the intervention in improving and maintaining adequate vitamin A status in the most vulnerable sections of the population.

Conclusions

Fortification of edible oils with vitamin A can have an impact on child health, both directly by increasing children's vitamin A intake and indirectly by raising levels obtained by children from breast milk. Potentially toxic levels are, for all practical purposes, too high to be of concern. Stability of vitamin A is key to the effectiveness of oil fortification. Vitamin A has to survive the supply chain—from its own production, to processing, storage, retail, and ultimately household use through the course of the whole shelf life of the product. Usage of oil in the household is an important consideration in determining the choice of oil as a vehicle for vitamin A fortification.

Oil fortification is very cost-effective. Since vitamin A can be added in concentrated and stable form, the cost of equipment is moderate. Success requires the widespread consumption of the fortified edible oil product, specific to each country.

References

1. Imdad A, et al. Vitamin A supplementation for preventing morbidity and mortality in children from 6 months to 5 years of age. Cochrane Database Syst Rev. 2010;(12):CD008524.
2. WHO. Global prevalence of vitamin A deficiency in populations at risk 1995–2005. WHO global database on vitamin A deficiency. Geneva: World Health Organization; 2009.
3. Tang G. Bioconversion of dietary provitamin A carotenoids to vitamin A in humans. Am J Clin Nutr. 2010; 91(5):1468S–73.
4. Anon. Enriching lives of the urban poor through food fortification. JFPR 9065: Asian Development Bank/Ministry of Health Indonesia; 2009.
5. Nagy K. Fortification of edible fats and oils with vitamin A and D. Nutley, NJ: Hoffman LaRoche; 1995.
6. Gopal SH, Ketyum FK. Vitamin A and D in ghee and vanaspati. J Sci Ind Res. 1956;15c(2):48–51.
7. Anon. Stability of vitamin A esters in partially skimmed milk and skim milk. Hoffman LaRoche.
8. Sagredos AN. Adding vitamins to fats. Unilever; 1988.
9. Bagriansky J, Ranum P. Vitamin A fortification of P.L. 480 vegetable oil. Washington, DC: Sustain; 1998.
10. Favaro RMD et al. Studies on fortification of refined soybean oil with all-trans-retinyl palmitate in Brazil: stability during cooking and storage. J Food Compost Anal. 1991;4(3).
11. Bauernfeind JC et al. Synthetic vitamin A and food fortification. Food Eng 81;1953.
12. Anon. Fortification and coloring of edible fats and oils. Hoffman LaRoche; 1995.
13. Atwood SJ et al. Stability of vitamin A in fortified vegetable oil and corn soy blend used in child feeding programs in India. J Food Compost Anal. 1995;8(1).
14. Mag T, Diosady LL. Vitamin A deficiency: a fortification strategy for deficient areas of the world. Unpublished report prepared for the Micronutrient Initiative; 1995.
15. Block CE. Effects of deficiency in vitamins in infancy. Am J Dis Child. 1931;42:271.
16. Aykroyd WR et al. Medical resurvey of nutrition in Newfoundland 1948. Toronto, ON: Murray Printing Company; 1949. p. 11–2.
17. Solon FS et al. Evaluation of the effect of vitamin A-fortified margarine on the vitamin A status of preschool Filipino children. Eur J Clin Nutr. 1996;50(11):720–3.
18. de Oliveira JED et al. Effect of heat treatment during cooking on the biological value of vitamin A fortified soybean oil in humans. Int J Food Sci Nutr. 1994;45:203–7.

Part IV
Biofortification: Biological Modes of Enhancing Nutrient Intake

Chapter 23
Iron and Zinc Enhancement in Rice Endosperm by Targeted and Synergistic Action of Genes

Navreet K. Bhullar, Kulaporn Boonyaves, Meng Wang, and Christof Sautter

Key Points

- Iron deficiency anemia and zinc deficiency are among the most recognized forms of micronutrient malnutrition.
- Monotonous diets based on staple cereals are in fact a poor source of iron and zinc.
- Biofortification of cereal grains, such as rice, has therefore emerged as a promising strategy.
- Traditional breeding alone is not a valid option for rice biofortification in many circumstances, owing to low genetic variability of micronutrients in the rice germplasm.
- Gene technology offers perspectives for efficiently improving iron and zinc content in rice grain.
- The biotechnology strategies used to date in order to improve rice for iron and zinc content and the genes controlling iron and zinc homeostasis are reviewed.

Keywords Biofortification • Rice • Iron • Zinc • Rice endosperm

Abbreviations

CGIAR	Consultative Group on International Agricultural Research
$FeSO_4$	Ferrous sulfate
Fe	Iron
Zn	Zinc
Mn	Manganese
Co	Cobalt
Cd	Cadmium
Ni	Nickel

N.K. Bhullar, Ph.D. (✉) • K. Boonyaves, M.Sc. • M. Wang, M.Sc. • C. Sautter, Ph.D.
Department of Biology, Institute of Agricultural Sciences, Swiss Federal Institute of Technology (ETH), Universitatsstrasse 2, 8092 Zurich, Switzerland
e-mail: bhullarn@ethz.ch; kboonyav@ethz.ch; yywang@ilsichina.org; csautter@ethz.ch

V.R. Preedy et al. (eds.), *Handbook of Food Fortification and Health: From Concepts to Public Health Applications Volume 1*, Nutrition and Health, DOI 10.1007/978-1-4614-7076-2_23,

Introduction

Iron deficiency anemia and zinc deficiency are among the most recognized forms of micronutrient malnutrition in humans. Various food fortification approaches have been suggested, but not many proved useful mainly due to socioeconomic or biological reasons. Monotonous diets based on staple cereals are frequently associated with human micronutrient malnutrition. Cereal grains constituting the most important basis of human food are in fact a poor source of iron and zinc. Biofortification of cereal grains, such as rice, has therefore emerged as a promising strategy. However, the variability for most micronutrients is very low in the rice germplasm and this does not leave traditional breeding alone to be a valid option for rice biofortification in many circumstances. Complementing the breeding efforts, gene technology offers perspectives for efficiently improving iron and zinc content in rice grain to dietary significant levels for human nutrition. In this chapter, the biotechnology strategies used to date in order to improve rice for iron and zinc content and the genes controlling iron and zinc homeostasis are reviewed.

Iron and Zinc Malnutrition in Humans

Deficiencies of various minerals and vitamins together are often addressed as "hidden hunger," which is one of the most serious challenges to global human health today. Iron deficiency anemia and zinc deficiency fall among the most recognized forms of micronutrient malnutrition, together with vitamin A deficiency and iodine deficiency [1]. Deficiencies from other nutrients including folate, calcium, proteins, and vitamins are also significant.

Serious consequences including mental retardation, decreased immune function, and increased mortality of mother and child at childbirth can result from iron deficiency [1, 2]. Approximately, two billion people in both developed and developing countries are known to be affected by iron deficiency anemia [1]. Human adults are recommended with daily iron intake between 8 mg/day (male) and 18 mg/day (female), with recommendations for 30 mg/day intake to pregnant women [3]. Similarly, zinc acts as a cofactor for more than 300 enzymes in humans, which are involved in synthesis and degradation of carbohydrates, lipids, proteins, and nucleic acids, and therefore, its deficiency proves crucial for human wellbeing. It is estimated that 49 % of world's population is at a risk of marginal to severe zinc deficiency, and various symptoms of zinc deficiency include growth retardation, delayed bone maturation, skin lesions, diarrhea, and weaker immune system [4]. The daily recommended zinc intake for human adults ranges between 7 and 10 mg/day [3], depending upon age and gender. The aforementioned health issues are not only limited to iron and zinc deficiencies, but other micronutrients play a vital role in normal body functioning, and lack of these components can therefore lead to severe consequences. However, in this chapter we will restrict our discussion to iron and zinc deficiencies and improvement of rice grain for the same.

More balanced diets would be required to fight micronutrient malnutrition, but unfortunately a large number of people in the world do not have the privilege of diversifying their diets to allow this balance. A number of food fortifying approaches have been suggested. However, not many of these proved useful mainly due to socioeconomic or biological reasons [5, 6]. Iron is one of the most difficult minerals for food fortification, because iron compounds that are most soluble and have high bioavailability, such as $FeSO_4$, are unpalatable and often provoke unacceptable color, while the less soluble compounds, such as elemental iron, are poorly absorbed [7].

Human nutritional deficiencies appear to be associated to monotonous diets based on staple crops, including cereals and little or no meat. Cereal grains constituting the most important basis of human food are in fact a poor source of iron and zinc. Most of the cereals are not only low in total concentrations of these elements but in addition contain antinutrient substances, such as phytic acid and phenolics, reducing their bioavailability. For example, rice that serves more than half of world's population as a staple is currently not an ideal source of essential nutrients. Starch contributes as a main component in rice grains (almost 90 %) with a little fraction of storage proteins [8]. Rice is already low in nutrient content, and furthermore these nutrients are present mainly in the outer layers of the grain (including husk, aleurone, and embryo) and thus get removed during grain polishing. As a consequence, polished rice grains contain very small amounts of micronutrients, for example, 2 μg iron per gram endosperm, no β-carotene, no vitamin D. Considering the facts above and severity of widespread micronutrient malnutrition, biofortification of cereal grains, such as rice, has emerged as a promising strategy.

Exploration of Genetic Diversity and Breeding for High Iron and High Zinc Content in the Rice Endosperm

Nutritional improvement of crops has lately become an important focus of crop breeding and there were initiatives and programs specifically launched to promote research in this direction. In 1992, CGIAR launched an initiative to increase the mineral content in staple crops [9, 10], which is further being complemented by the HarvestPlus Challenge Program launched in 2004 that supports biofortification of staple food crops, including rice, maize, wheat, cassava, pearl millet, beans, and sweet potato, primarily for increased iron, zinc, and vitamin A (http://www.harvestplus.org/). More recently, HarvestZinc Fertilizer Project was started in 2008 aimed at assessing the potential of Zn fertilizers in order to increase Zn content in cereal grains, mainly wheat and rice (www.harvestzinc.org).

In the past decades, genetic variability for iron and zinc content has been explored in different crops, to identify donor genotypes for high grain micronutrient content. Almost fourfold differences in grain iron content were identified in a study that screened 939 rice genotypes, with Fe content ranging between 7.5 and 24.4 mg/kg and zinc content between 15.9 and 58.4 mg/kg in the brown rice [11]. Despite these potential examples from diversity screens, iron biofortification of rice based on conventional breeding has met with only marginal success. The polished rice grains from most of the cultivated mega-rice varieties contain around 2 μg/g of iron. The iron levels achieved to date are still too low to address the required target levels set by HarvestPlus (around 14 μg/g) indicating that iron biofortification in rice remains a challenge. Other related concerns like processing (grain polishing in rice) and the bioavailability make the target levels further difficult to achieve.

Breeding of crop plants with promoter substances (e.g., ascorbate and cysteine) enhancing bioavailability of micronutrients or reduction of antinutrients (phytic acid) in the seeds has been another research direction. Mutants were developed for different staple crops, including rice, wheat, and maize [12, 13], with reduced phytic acid content in their seeds. The role of agronomic practices on biofortification is also being evaluated, where zinc biofortification met with relatively more success in wheat [14, 15], and is now being further explored in case of rice (HarvestZinc Program). Soil Zn status is described as a prominent determinant of grain Zn concentrations by some [16], where a range of 8–47 mg/kg grain Zn concentration was obtained for a single genotype grown over soils with different zinc status. Wissuwa and colleagues [16] further reported that fertilizer applications do not necessarily compensate for the low soil Zn availability, while intra-genotype differences in grain Zn concentrations are maintained over different soil types. Biofortification by fertilizer application appears rather difficult or even impossible for complex compounds such as vitamins; therefore, cultivars developed for high nutrient content have the potential to perform better, also on nutrient poor soils.

Since the variability for most micronutrients is very low in the rice germplasm, this does not leave traditional breeding alone to be a valid option for rice biofortification in many circumstances. Complementing the breeding efforts, gene technology offers perspectives for efficiently improving iron and zinc content of rice grain to dietary significant levels for human nutrition (reviewed below).

Iron and Zinc Enhancement in Rice Through Biotechnology

In the last some years, different strategies have been used to enhance iron (and zinc) in the rice grain, particularly in the endosperm. These strategies targeted on improving iron uptake and transport within the plant, storage in the grain, or increased bioavailability (Fig. 23.1). For storage of iron in the rice grains, overexpression of iron storage protein, ferritin, has been evaluated in different studies. Ferritin acts as an iron buffer inside the cell that can store up to 4,500 Fe molecules in a soluble, nontoxic and bioavailable form [17]. One of the first reports of iron biofortification through biotechnology included overexpression of soybean ferritin in the rice endosperm [18], driven under the control of rice seed storage protein glutelin promoter (GluB-1). The transgenic seeds exhibited up to threefold increase in the iron content as compared to the non-transformed ones. Since ferritin was expressed in transgenic seeds but not leaves, and iron content was increased in the endosperm as compared to that in the embryo, this confirmed that the iron increases were specific to endosperm [18]. Overexpression of *Phaseolus vulgaris* ferritin in rice under the control of glutelin promoter led to a twofold increase in iron content in the transformed rice seeds [19]. It is noteworthy that although glutelin promoter (GluB-1) is a good candidate for endosperm-specific expression of ferritin, it might not be the ideal choice. Studies suggested that glutelin promoter is most intensively expressed in the sub-aleurone and peripheral layers of the seed tissue as compared to rather central endosperm expression driven by globulin promoter, [18, 20] and therefore, the expression of ferritin under the control of glutelin promoter might lead to losses of iron stored in ferritin upon prolonged polishing of rice grain. Vasconcelos et al. [21] also observed accompanied increases in zinc content of the transgenic rice seeds, in addition to the increased iron content upon overexpression of soybean ferritin under control of glutelin promoter.

Considering that level of ferritin expression could be a bottleneck in further increasing the endosperm iron content, Qu et al. [22] produced double-ferritin lines by transforming rice with ferritin expressed under two different seed storage gene promoters: glutelin (GluB-1) and globulin (Glb-1) promoters. Although ferritin was expressed 13-fold higher in double-ferritin lines as compared to the single-ferritin lines, there were no significant differences in iron content of rice grains of single- and double-ferritin lines [22]. This implies that iron accumulation in the endosperm is also limited from uptake and transport of iron.

Improving bioavailability of iron and zinc has been targeted through overexpression of proteins promoting iron and zinc absorption in humans or by elimination of antinutrients, like phytic acid.

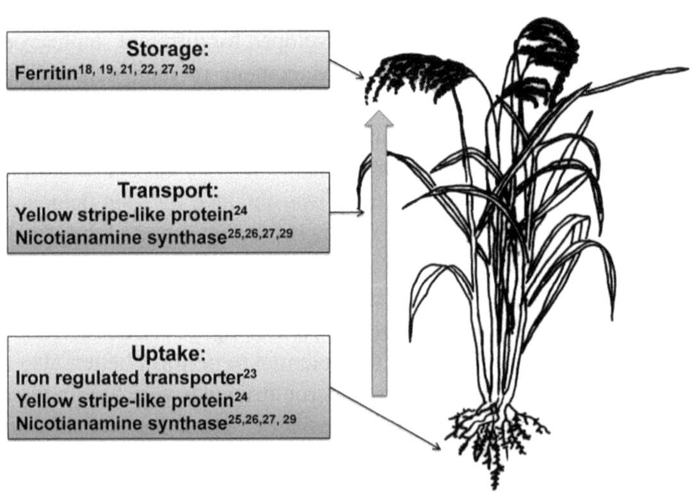

Fig. 23.1 Scheme of coordinated metal uptake, translocation within the plant, and storage in the grains. Legend: The enzymes and transporters used in the transgenic approaches to date to enhance iron or zinc uptake, transport, and storage are presented

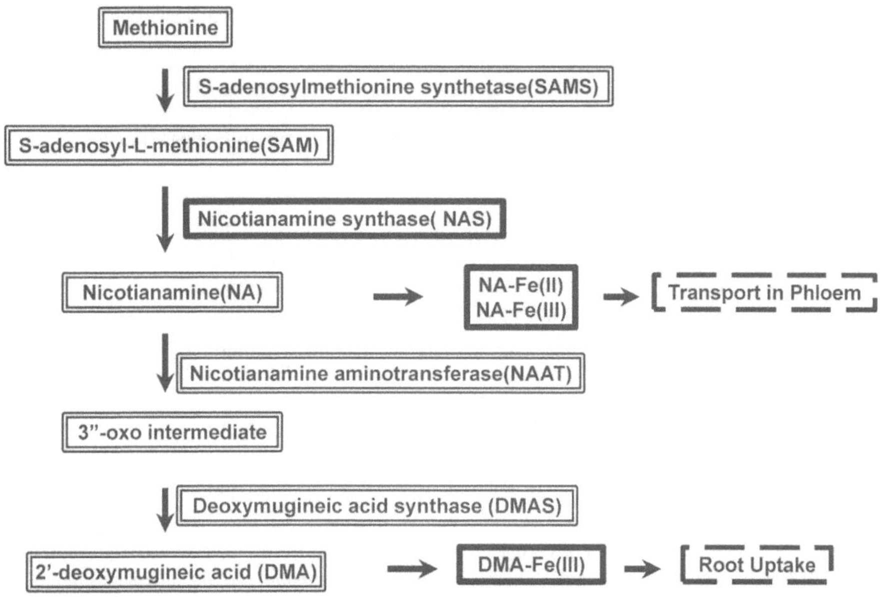

Fig. 23.2 Summary of phytosiderophore synthesis from methionine, with special emphasis on nicotianamine synthase (NAS). NAS is involved in production of nicotianamine, a metal ion transporter in the phloem and of 2′-deoxymugineic acid, phytosiderophore that facilitates transport of Fe(III) to the plant

Lucca et al. [19] produced rice plants that either overexpressed cysteine-rich metallothionein-like protein or phytase genes, respectively. They observed about sevenfold increase in cysteine content of the soluble seed protein, but bioefficacy of this strategy remains to be tested. Although phytase from *Aspergillus fumigatus* is recognized as a thermotolerant enzyme, Lucca et al. [19] reported low activity of the *in planta*-produced protein in the transgenic rice seeds upon cooking. For optimal expression in cereal grains, often requiring cooking, more heat stable phytase sources would need to be evaluated.

In the last decade, our knowledge increased considerably on the genes involved in iron and zinc uptake and transport within the plants. With the goal to improve grain iron content, researchers have transformed rice with key genes involved in iron uptake and translocation. Role of transporters, like *IRT1* (iron-regulated transporter 1), has been studied, and overexpression of the *OsIRT1* in rice plants increased iron and zinc concentrations in shoots, roots, and mature seeds and lead to increased iron deficiency tolerance at the seedling stage in the transformed plants [23]. More recently, Ishimaru et al. [24] expressed *OsYSL2*, a metal-nicotianamine transporter, under the control of sucrose transporter promoter and observed a 4.4-fold increase in Fe concentration in the polished rice grains as compared with the wild type. Additional experiments in this study also supported that *OsYSL2* is important for Fe translocation within the plants, especially shoots and endosperm.

Nicotianamine synthase (*NAS*), one of the key genes from phytosiderophore biosynthetic pathway, has been focused to a relatively greater extent (Fig. 23.2). The expression of barley nicotianamine synthase gene (*HvNAS*) under the control of CaMV35S and rice Actin1 promoters, led to an increased iron content of about 2.3-fold and 1.6-fold, respectively, in the polished T_2 seeds as compared to the non-transformed rice [25]. Zinc content in these lines increased by 1.5-fold (CaMV35S-*HvNAS*) and 1.3-fold (Actin1-*HvNAS*) [25]. Overexpression of *HvNAS* gene in these plants led to increased synthesis of nicotianamine (NA), a metal chelator known to play a role in long distance transport of iron and zinc, as well as to increased production of phytosiderophores, that facilitate iron uptake from soil for strategy II plants (for genes involved in Fe and Zn uptake, see section "Molecular Mechanisms

Table 23.1 Iron and zinc enhancement of rice through biotechnology approaches. The increases in grain iron and zinc content achieved to date and the strategies used for the same are presented

Promoter/gene used[†]	Increase in grain iron content of the transgenic rice as compared to the wild type	Increase in grain zinc content of the transgenic rice as compared to the wild type	Reference
GluB-1/SoyferH-1	Threefold	Not reported	[18]
GluB1/Pvferritin	Up to twofold	Not reported	[19]
GluB-1/SoyferH-1	Up to 3.7-fold	Up to 1.6-fold	[21]
GluB-1/SoyferH-1+ Glb-1/SoyferH-1	Up to twofold	Not reported	[22]
CaMV35S/HvNAS1	2.3-fold	1.5-fold	[25]
OsActin1/HvNAS1	1.6-fold	1.3-fold	[25]
OsNAS3 with downstream 35S enhancer element	2.9-fold	2.2-fold	[26]
Glb-1/Pvferritin+ CaMV35S/AtNAS1	6.3-fold	1.5-fold	[27]
OsSUT1/OsYSL2	Up to 4.4-fold	Not reported	[24]
CaMV35S/OsNAS	Up to 4.2-fold	Up to 2.2-fold	[29]

[†] *GluB-1,* rice seed storage protein glutelin promoter; *SoyferH-1*, soybean ferritin gene; *Pvferritin, Phaseolus vulgaris* ferritin gene; *Glb-1*, rice seed storage globulin promoter; *HvNAS1*, *Hordeum vulgare* nicotianamine synthase gene; *OsActin1*, *Oryza sativa* actin promoter; *OsNAS*, *Oryza sativa* nicotianamine synthase gene; *AtNAS1*, *Arabidopsis thaliana* nicotianamine synthase gene; *OsYSL2*, *Oryza sativa* yellow stripe-like 2 transporter; *OsSUT1*, *Oryza sativa* sucrose transporter 1 promoter; *CaMV35S*, cauliflower mosaic virus 35S promoter

Relating to Iron and Zinc Uptake and Translocation Within the Plant"). The efficacy of NAS genes in increased iron uptake was also supported by increased iron and zinc concentrations in the grains of an activation-tagged mutant rice lines in which *OsNAS3* was overexpressed [26]. Mature seeds of these rice lines showed increased iron, zinc, and copper content by 2.9-fold, 2.2-fold, and 1.7-fold, respectively, as compared to that of wild type [26].

A strategy combining genes for iron uptake and storage reported by Wirth et al. [27], where *Arabidopsis thaliana NAS1* (*AtNAS1*) and *P. vulgaris* ferritin (*Pvferritin*) exhibited a synergistic effect, has met with more than sixfold increases in the grain iron levels as compared to that of wild-type controls. *AtNAS1* was expressed constitutively in these plants, while *Pvferritin* and *phytase* genes were expressed in the endosperm. Zinc content of these lines was 1.3-fold higher than that of the control plants. Most of these iron and zinc rich transgenic lines were reported to have normal morphology [27, 28], and increased iron accumulation in the endosperm was found not to perturb iron homeostasis in the leaves. More recently, a four- and twofold increase in iron and zinc content, respectively, has been reported by Johnson et al. [29] in rice lines overexpressing *OsNAS2*, with two of these lines containing final concentration of 14 and 19 μg/g iron in the polished rice grains. The iron concentrations ranging between 14 and 19 μg/g appear promising, it should be noted however that iron content in these lines was fourfold higher as compared to the wild-type japonica rice cultivar used for transformation.

In view that most of the indica rice varieties, where the technology would need to be ultimately transferred, possess around 2 μg iron/g of endosperm, a four- to sixfold increase would still not be sufficient to reach the dietary significant levels. The biofortification strategies still need further optimization, and testing of different promoter and transporter combinations might prove useful in raising the endosperm iron content further. The information on metal uptake systems in rice and on the key genes playing roles in different tissues and developmental stages in this regard will contribute to further refine future biotechnology efforts. Table 23.1 summarizes important biotechnology strategies used for iron and zinc enhancement in the rice grain.

Further, following a successful proof-of-concept in the laboratory, the genetically engineered plants require evaluation of their performance in the field, and ultimately release for agronomic production and human consumption. The regulatory processes required prior to evaluation and release of transgenic plants can often be lengthy, and therefore might slow down their development and utilization. In many countries, including the United States, genetically modified plants are grown to a significant proportion [30], while most of the European countries have rather low or no acceptance towards the same. While the legal regulations associated with field research (and release) of genetically modified plants are strict in order to ensure biosafety, the long procedures could delay the reach of potentially beneficial product to the needy consumer. "Golden rice," improved for provitamin A in the grains, is an example that has faced such delay since its first report in 2000 [31]. Although golden rice has been demonstrated to be an effective source of vitamin A [32] and there are studies suggesting its potential to significantly reduce the burden of vitamin A deficiency [33], it is not yet available to affected rice consumers. It is only recent that golden rice is being incorporated into breeding programs in countries, like Philippines, India, Indonesia, and Vietnam, and it is expected that it might reach farmers in the Philippines soon. It is therefore necessary to raise public awareness about potential benefits and risks of the technology, so that a rational opinion can guide the deregulation process [34].

Molecular Mechanisms Relating to Iron and Zinc Uptake and Translocation Within the Plant

Biofortification relies considerably on the information of genes related to metal acquisition in plants (reviewed in section "Iron and Zinc Enhancement in Rice Through Biotechnology"). Research in this context continues to contribute candidate genes, whose individual and combinatorial expression could potentially be evaluated with respect to enhancing iron and zinc concentrations in the rice grains. The genes/mechanisms involved in iron and zinc uptake and translocation are summarized in this section (Table 23.2).

Metal Uptake Strategies in Plants

Iron uptake in plants can be broadly classified into reduction (strategy I) or chelation (strategy II) strategies, for non-grasses and grasses, respectively. The reduction strategy includes induction of three responses at the plasma membrane of root cells. Acidification marks the first step, during which protons are released to increase the solubility of iron via H^+-ATPases. The *AHA2*, belonging to *AHA* (*Arabidopsis* H^+-ATPase) gene family, was reported to mediate this function in *Arabidopsis* [35]. Fe(III) is reduced to Fe(II) by action of ferric chelate reductases, and in *Arabidopsis*, FRO2 (a membrane-bound ferric reductase oxidase), one of the eight members of the *FRO* protein family, serves this function [36]. Fe(II) is then moved across the plasma membrane and into the cells by an iron-regulated transporter (*IRT1*), a member of the zinc-regulated transporter (ZRT), IRT-like proteins (ZIP) divalent metal transporter family [37]. Although the essential role of *IRT1* is in iron uptake, metal uptake experiments and yeast growth assays have shown that *IRT1* is a broad range divalent metal ion transporter that is also capable of transporting Zn, Mn, Co, and Cd [38].

The strategy II, mainly used by grasses, involves four main steps, involving biosynthesis of mugineic acid family phytosiderophores, release of phytosiderophores (PS) to the rhizosphere, iron solubilization, and Fe(III)-PS transport to the plant [39]. The biosynthetic pathway of mugineic acid family phytosiderophores has been well studied now. S-adenosylmethionine synthetase (SAMS), nicotianamine synthase (NAS), nicotianamine aminotransferase (NAAT), and deoxymugineic acid synthase

Table 23.2 Genes involved in iron and zinc homeostasis in rice

Process involved	Gene	Role	Expression pattern	Reference
Metal uptake strategies in plants				
Reduction strategy (strategy 1)	*OsIRT1*, *OsIRT2* (*O. sativa* iron-regulated transporters)	Fe(II) transporter	Specifically upregulated in roots of iron-deficient plants	[48]
Chelation strategy (strategy 2)	*OsNAS1*, *OsNAS2*, *OsNAS3* (*O. sativa* nicotianamine synthase genes)	Phytosiderophores synthesis	Under iron deficiency, *OsNAS1*, *OsNAS2* transcripts are strongly induced in roots and leaves, while *OsNAS3* is induced in roots but suppressed in leaves. *OsNAS3* is upregulated in both roots and shoots under zinc deficiency	[40, 41]
	OsNAAT1 (*O. sativa* nicotianamine aminotransferase)	Phytosiderophores synthesis	Strongly induced in roots as well as in shoots under iron deficiency	[40]
	OsDMAS1 (*O. sativa* deoxymugineic acid synthase)	Phytosiderophores synthesis	Upregulated in roots and shoots under iron deficiency	[40]
	OsYSL15 (*O. sativa* yellow stripe-like gene)	Uptake of Fe(III)-phytosiderophore complexes	Strongly expressed in rice root epidermal cells under iron deficiency	[46]
	OsZIP1, *OsZIP3*,*OsZIP4*, *OsZIP5* (*O. sativa* zinc-regulated transporter, iron-regulated transporter-like protein (*ZIP*) family)	Zinc transporters	Highly expressed in roots and shoots under Zn deficiency conditions	[42, 51]
Inter- and intracellular metal transport	*OsFRDL1* (*O. sativa* Ferric reductase defective 3-like gene)	Iron-citrate translocation from rice roots to shoots	Localized at the root pericycle cells	[54]
	OsYSL2 (*O. sativa* yellow stripe-like gene)	Metal-NA transporters, involved in phloem transport of iron and its translocation to the grain	Phloem-specific expression	[58]
	OsMIR (*O. sativa* mitochondrial iron-regulated gene)	Mitochondrial iron homeostasis regulation	Iron-deficiency-inducible gene expression in roots as well as shoots	[66]
Transcription factors involved in metal homeostasis	*OsIDEF1*, *OsIDEF2*	Transcription factors directly interacting with iron-deficiency-responsive element 1 and 2, respectively	Regulate the genes involved in iron homeostasis	[68, 70]
	OsIRO2	Iron-deficiency-inducible basic helix-loop-helix transcription factor	Strongly expressed in roots and shoots upon iron deficiency	[71]

The table summarizes the function and expression pattern of the rice genes involved in iron and zinc acquisition and translocation within the plant

(DMAS) are the key genes involved in synthesis of phytosiderophores from methionine [40]. Under iron deficiency, *OsNAS1* and *OsNAS2* transcripts are strongly induced in roots and leaves of rice plants, while *OsNAS3* is induced in roots but is suppressed in leaves [41]. *OsNAS3* is reported to be upregulated in the Zn deficiency situation in both roots and shoots [42]. Among the six *OsNAAT* genes identified in rice, only *OsNAAT1* gene is reported to be strongly induced by iron deficiency, in roots as well as in shoots [43]. The rice *OsDMAS1* gene shows similar expression pattern under iron deficiency conditions, being strongly upregulated in the roots as well as in shoots [44].

The resulting Fe(III)-PS complexes are transported into root cells via transporters belonging to the yellow stripe (YS) family of proteins. The maize *ZmYS1* was identified to be a proton-coupled symporter for various phytosiderophore-bound metals, including, Zn(II), Cu(II), Ni(II), as well as for Fe(II)-NA, Fe(III)-NA, and Ni(II)-NA. However, unlike *ZmYS1*, the barley *HvYS1* is a specific transporter for Fe(III)-PS but not Fe–nicotianamine (NA) [45]. Eighteen *YSL* genes have been identified in rice, and among these *OsYSL15* is suggested to have potential role in uptake of Fe(III)-PS complexes since it is strongly expressed in the rice root epidermal cells under iron deficiency conditions [46].

In contrast to other grasses, rice also possesses an efficient Fe(II) uptake system. Cheng et al. [47] showed that rice plants carrying a mutation in the *NAAT* gene and thus not able to synthesize PS did not show any growth defects if external Fe(II) was supplied but showed strong growth defects if iron was supplied as Fe(III). *OsIRT1* and *OsIRT2*, the rice homologs of iron-regulated transporter *IRT1*, are specifically upregulated in roots of iron-deficient plants [48]. However, rice apparently cannot accomplish ferric reduction as strategy I plants do.

The molecular mechanisms for Zn uptake are not that well understood as compared to iron. Roots of graminaceous plants were considered to primarily take up non-chelated Zn(II) ions; however, phytosiderophores have been suggested to have a role in Zn uptake and transport [49]. The uptake and homeostasis of zinc and iron are closely linked as mediated by members of the zinc- and iron-regulated transporter protein (ZIP) family. Wirth et al. [27] observed that zinc content in the rice leaves decreases upon increased external iron supply to the rice plants, further supporting the idea that iron and zinc might compete for their transport within the plants. Among the Zn transporters, *ZIP1* and *ZIP3* are expressed in roots in response to zinc deficiency, suggesting their function in zinc transport from the soil into the plant. *ZIP4* is suggested to have a role in intracellular zinc transport or transport between plant tissues, as indicated by its induced expression in both shoots and roots of zinc-deficient plants [50]. Among the rice ZIP genes, *OsZIP1*, *OsZIP3*, *OsZIP4*, and *OsZIP5* are induced under Zn-deficient conditions and therefore documented as Zn transporters [42, 51].

Inter- and Intracellular Metal Transport in Plants

Recent studies have provided more information of genes involved in inter- and intracellular metal transport. After Fe and Zn are loaded into the xylem, chelators are needed for further transportation within the plant. Citrate is considered to be one of the main chelators in xylem for long distance transport [52]. *FRD3* (Ferric reductase defective 3), a member of the multidrug and toxin efflux (MATE) family, effluxes citrate into the *Arabidopsis* root vasculature and is important for iron transport to the shoot [53]. In rice, an *FRD3*-like gene, *OsFRDL1*, localized at the root pericycle cells, is involved in iron-citrate translocation from rice roots to shoots [54]. Besides, in Arabidopsis, two transporters (*IREG1/FPN1* and *IREG2/FPN2*) from the ferroportin (FPN) family have been identified. The *IREG1/FPN1* functions in vascular loading while *IREG2/FPN2* plays a role in buffering metal influx [55]. Zinc translocation in the xylem mainly relies on *HMA2* (heavy metal ATPase 2) and *HMA4* (heavy metal ATPase 4) transporters, which are expressed in the vascular tissues of roots, stems, and leaves [56].

Nicotianamine (NA), also a precursor of phytosiderophores, serves as another important chelator capable of binding to different metals such as Fe(II), Fe(III), Zn, Cu, and Ni [52], and thus plays an essential role in phloem loading and unloading of iron. Genes belonging to yellow stripe-like (YSL) family are also involved in transport of metal–NA complexes [57]. Among the rice YSL genes, *OsYSL2* is one of the rice metal-NA transporters, involved in phloem transport of iron including its translocation to the grain [58].

Relatively little is yet known about intracellular metal transport, involving vacuoles, chloroplasts, and mitochondria. The vacuoles serve as essential cell compartments for metal storage and the *VIT1* (Vacuolar iron transporter 1) present in the vacuolar membrane mediates iron sequestration into vacuoles [59]. During the seed germination, the natural resistance-associated macrophage protein (NRAMP) family of transporters is suggested to be crucial for iron mobilization for export from vacuoles [60]. The *AtNRAMP3* and *AtNRAMP4* are induced under Fe deficiency and mobilize vacuolar Fe stores in *Arabidopsis* during early development [61]. Zn homeostasis in *Arabidopsis* is influenced by the expression of vacuolar membrane localized *AtMTP1* (metal tolerance protein1) and *AtMTP3* (metal tolerance protein3), belonging to the CDF (cation diffusion facilitator) proteins family [62, 63].

Duy et al. [64] demonstrated *PIC1* (Permease in Chloroplasts1) to be involved in chloroplast Fe transportation. Besides, *FRO7* which also localizes in the chloroplast is essential for chloroplast iron acquisition [65]. A rice-specific, iron deficiency-induced, mitochondrial iron-regulated gene (*MIR*) has also been identified [66]. The *mir* plants enhanced the Fe-deficiency-inducible gene expression in roots as well as in shoots even when rice grows under Fe-sufficient conditions [66].

The Cis-Acting Elements and Transcription Factors Involved in Metal Homeostasis

From barely, two cis-acting elements, IDE1 (iron-deficiency-responsive element 1) and IDE2 (iron-deficiency-responsive element 2), were identified in the promoter of IDS2 (iron-deficiency-specific clone no. 2) [67] and were found to confer root-specific and iron-deficiency-inducible expression. The IDE1 homologous sequences have also been found in Fe-deficiency-inducible promoters in rice, barley, and tobacco, suggesting that these *cis*-acting elements are conserved among different species [40]. Transcription factors, IDEF1 and IDEF2 specifically interacting with *IDE1* and *IDE2*, respectively, were identified in rice [68, 69]. Recently, IDEF1 is suggested to be capable of binding directly to the divalent metal ions, including iron and zinc, and thus playing a crucial role in sensing cellular metal status [70]. Another transcription factor *OsIRO2* has been characterized, which is strongly expressed in roots and shoots of rice plants upon iron deficiency and is not induced by deficiencies in other metals, including zinc, manganese, and copper [71].

Together, iron and zinc homeostasis in plants is controlled by complex interplay of several genes in different plant tissues and cell types and at different developmental stages. The information reviewed above and research that is further continued in this regard allows better understanding of the metal uptake and transport within plants and thereby designing of targeted biofortification approaches.

Conclusions

It is evident from different biofortification examples, including those of vitamin A (Golden rice), high-folate rice and high iron, that right combination of target genes is critical for successful improvement of micronutrient composition in rice grains. Increased knowledge on genes involved in iron and zinc uptake from soil and translocation within the plant is continuously contributing to a better design of biofortification strategies targeting these nutrients. Further information on inter- and intracellular metal transport will allow to specifically target the nutrients to particular tissues, for example, grains.

For iron and zinc biofortification, further efforts should include transferring the strategy to widely grown indica rice varieties, and future research should also focus on combining different traits into single rice lines. All this has to be achieved without altering the agronomic performance and cooking qualities of modified rice. This requires field and feeding experiments, and therefore, public awareness and understanding about these scientific advancements is necessary. The regulatory processes also need adaptation in view of practical application and utility of crop biofortification achievements. If successful, rice biofortication has the potential to make substantial contributions by improving health and wellbeing of the undernourished populations around the globe.

Acknowledgements We thank ETH Zurich and Swiss State Secretariat for Education and Research for funding our research.

References

1. World Health Organization (WHO). Micronutrient deficiencies: iron deficiency anemia. http://www.who.int/nutrition/topics/ida/en/index.html. Assessed June 27, 2011.
2. Puig S, Andrés-Colás N, García-Molina A, Peñarrubia L. Copper and iron homeostasis in *Arabidopsis*: responses to metal deficiencies, interactions and biotechnological applications. Plant Cell Environ. 2007;30(3):271–90.
3. Institute of Medicine (IOM), Food and Nutrition information centre, USDA. http://www.iom.edu/Activities/Nutrition/SummaryDRIs/~/media/Files/Activity%20Files/Nutrition/DRIs/New%20Material/5DRI%20Values%20SummaryTables%2014.pdf. Assessed July 17, 2011.
4. Tauris B, Borg S, Gregersen PL, Holm PB. A roadmap for zinc trafficking in the developing barley grain based on laser capture microdissection and gene expression profiling. J Exp Bot. 2009;60(4):1333–47.
5. Frossard E, Bucher M, Mächler F, Mozafar A, Hurrell R. Potential for increasing the content and bioavailability of Fe, Zn and Ca in plants for human nutrition. J Sci Food Agric. 2000;80(7):861–79.
6. Mayer JE, Pfeiffer WH, Beyer P. Biofortified crops to alleviate micronutrient malnutrition. Curr Opin Plant Biol. 2008;11(2):166–70.
7. Hurrell R, Egli I. Iron bioavailability and dietary reference values. Am J Clin Nutr. 2010;91(5):1461S–7.
8. Kennedy G, Burlingame B, Nguyen VN. Nutritional contribution of rice and impact of biotechnology and biodiversity in rice-consuming countries. In: Proceedings of the 20th Session of the International Rice Commission; July 23-26; 2002; Bangkok; Thailand. http://www.fao.org/docrep/006/y4751e/y4751e05.htm#bm05. Assessed September 29, 2011.
9. Gregorio GB, Senadhira D, Htut H, Graham RD. Breeding for trace mineral density in rice. Food Nutr Bull. 2000;21:382–6.
10. Welch RM, Graham RD. Breeding for micronutrients in staple food crops from a human nutrition perspective. J Exp Bot. 2004;55(396):353–64.
11. Graham R, Senadhira D, Beebe S, Iglesias C, Monasterio I. Breeding for micronutrient density in edible portions of staple food crops: conventional approaches. Field Crop Res. 1999;60(1–2):57–80.
12. Guttieri M, Bowen D, Dorsch JA, Raboy V, Souza E. Identification and characterization of a low phytic acid wheat. Crop Sci. 2004;44(2):418–24.
13. Raboy V. Progress in breeding low phytate crops. J Nutr. 2002;132(3):503S–5.
14. Cakmak I. Enrichment of cereal grains with zinc: agronomic or genetic biofortification? Plant Soil. 2008; 302(1–2):1–17.
15. Cakmak I, Pfeiffer WH, McClafferty B. Biofortification of durum wheat with zinc and iron. Cereal Chem. 2010; 87(1):10–20.
16. Wissuwa M, Ismail AM, Graham RD. Rice grain zinc concentrations as affected by genotype, native soil-zinc availability, and zinc fertilization. Plant Soil. 2008;306(1–2):37–48.
17. Jin F, Frohman C, Thannhauser TW, Welch RM, Glahn RP. Effects of ascorbic acid, phytic acid and tannic acid on iron bioavailability from reconstituted ferritin measured by an in vitro digestion-Caco-2 cell model. Br J Nutr. 2009;101:972–81.

18. Goto F, Yoshihara T, Shigemoto N, Toki S, Takaiwa F. Iron fortification of rice seed by the soybean ferritin gene. Nat Biotechnol. 1999;17:282–6.
19. Lucca P, Hurrell R, Potrykus I. Genetic engineering approaches to improve the bioavailability and the level of iron in rice grains. Theor Appl Genet. 2001;102(2–3):392–7.
20. Furtado A, Henry RJ, Takaiwa F. Comparison of promoters in transgenic rice. Plant Biotechnol J. 2008; 6(7):679–93.
21. Vasconcelos M, Datta K, Oliva N, et al. Enhanced iron and zinc accumulation in transgenic rice with the *ferritin* gene. Plant Sci. 2003;164(3):371–8.
22. Qu LQ, Yoshihara T, Ooyama A, Goto F, Takaiwa F. Iron accumulation does not parallel the high expression level of ferritin in transgenic rice seeds. Planta. 2005;222(2):225–33.
23. Lee S, An G. Over-expression of *OsIRT1* leads to increased iron and zinc accumulations in rice. Plant Cell Environ. 2009;32(4):408–16.
24. Ishimaru Y, Masuda H, Bashir K, et al. Rice metal-nicotianamine transporter, OsYSL2, is required for the long-distance transport of iron and manganese. Plant J. 2010;62(3):379–90.
25. Masuda H, Usuda K, Kobayashi T, et al. Overexpression of the barley nicotianamine synthase gene *HvNAS1* increases iron and zinc concentrations in rice grains. Rice. 2009;2(4):155–66.
26. Lee S, Jeon US, Lee SJ, et al. Iron fortification of rice seeds through activation of the *nicotianamine synthase* gene. Proc Natl Acad Sci U S A. 2009;106(51):22014–9.
27. Wirth J, Poletti S, Aeschlimann B, et al. Rice endosperm iron biofortification by targeted and synergistic action of nicotianamine synthase and ferritin. Plant Biotechnol J. 2009;7(7):631–44.
28. Masuda H, Suzuki M, Morikawa KC, et al. Increase in iron and zinc concentrations in rice grains via the introduction of barley genes involved in phytosiderophore synthesis. Rice. 2008;1(1):100–8.
29. Johnson AAT, Kyriacou B, Callahan DL, et al. Constitutive overexpression of the *OsNAS* Gene family reveals single-gene strategies for effective iron- and zinc-biofortification of rice endosperm. PLoS One. 2011;6(9):e24476. doi:10.1371/journal.pone. 0024476.
30. ISAAA, Global Status of Commercialized Biotech/GM Crops: 2010. http://www.isaaa.org/resources/publications/briefs/42/executivesummary/default.asp. Assessed September 28, 2011.
31. Ye X, Al-Babili S, Klöti A, et al. Engineering the provitamin A (β-Carotene) biosynthetic pathway into (carotenoid-free) rice endosperm. Science. 2000;287(5451):303–5.
32. Tang G, Qin J, Dolnikowski GG, Russell RM, Grusak MA. Golden Rice is an effective source of vitamin A. Am J Clin Nutr. 2009;89(6):1776–83.
33. Stein AJ, Sachdev HPS, Qaim M. Genetic engineering for the poor: golden rice and public health in India. World Dev. 2008;3(1):144–58.
34. Potrykus I. Regulation must be revolutionized. Nature. 2010;466(7306):561.
35. Santi S, Schmidt W. Dissecting iron deficiency-induced proton extrusion in Arabidopsis roots. New Phytol. 2009;183(4):1072–84.
36. Robinson NJ, Procter CM, Connolly EL, Guerinot ML. A ferric-chelate reductase for iron uptake from soils. Nature. 1999;397(6721):694–7.
37. Connolly EL, Fett JP, Guerinot ML. Expression of the IRT1 metal transporter is controlled by metals at the levels of transcript and protein accumulation. Plant Cell. 2002;14(6):1347–57.
38. Korshunova YO, Eide D, Clark WG, Guerinot ML, Pakrasi HB. The IRT1 protein from Arabidopsis thaliana is a metal transporter with a broad substrate range. Plant Mol Biol. 1999;40(1):37–44.
39. Palmer CM, Guerinot ML. Facing the challenges of Cu, Fe and Zn homeostasis in plants. Nat Chem Biol. 2009;5(5):333–40.
40. Kobayashi T, Nakanishi H, Nishizawa NK. Recent insights into iron homeostasis and their application in graminaceous crops. Proc Jpn Acad Ser B Phys Biol Sci. 2010;86(9):900–13.
41. Inoue H, Higuchi K, Takahashi M, Nakanishi H, Mori S, Nishizawa NK. Three rice nicotianamine synthase genes, *OsNAS1*, *OsNAS2*, and *OsNAS3* are expressed in cells involved in long-distance transport of iron and are differentially regulated by iron. Plant J. 2003;36(3):366–81.
42. Ishimaru Y, Bashir K, Nishizawa NK. Zn uptake and translocation in rice plants. Rice. 2011;4(1):21–7.
43. Inoue H, Takahashi M, Kobayashi T, et al. Identification and localisation of the rice nicotianamine aminotransferase gene *OsNAAT1* expression suggests the site of phytosiderophore synthesis in rice. Plant Mol Biol. 2008; 66(1–2):193–203.
44. Bashir K, Inoue H, Nagasaka S, et al. Cloning and characterization of deoxymugineic acid synthase genes from graminaceous plants. J Biol Chem. 2006;281(43):32395–402.
45. Murata Y, Ma JF, Yamaji N, Ueno D, Nomoto K, Iwashita T. A specific transporter for iron(III)-phytosiderophore in barley roots. Plant J. 2006;46(4):563–72.
46. Inoue H, Kobayashi T, Nozoye T, et al. Rice OsYSL15 is an iron-regulated iron(III)-deoxymugineic acid transporter expressed in the roots and is essential for iron uptake in early growth of the seedlings. J Biol Chem. 2009;284(6):3470–9.

47. Cheng L, Wang F, Shou H, et al. Mutation in nicotianamine aminotransferase stimulated the fe(II) acquisition system and led to iron accumulation in rice. J Plant Physiol. 2007;145(4):1647–57.
48. Ishimaru Y, Suzuki M, Tsukamoto T, et al. Rice plants take up iron as an Fe^{3+}-phytosiderophore and as Fe^{2+}. Plant J. 2006;45(3):335–46.
49. Schaaf G, Ludewig U, Erenoglu BE, Mori S, Kitahara T, von Wirén N. ZmYS1 functions as a proton-coupled symporter for phytosiderophore- and nicotianamine-chelated metals. J Biol Chem. 2004;279(10):9091–6.
50. Grotz N, Fox T, Connolly E, Park W, Guerinot ML, Eide D. Identification of a family of zinc transporter genes from Arabidopsis that respond to zinc deficiency. Proc Natl Acad Sci USA. 1998;95(12):7220–4.
51. Lee S, Jeong HJ, Kim SA, Lee J, Guerinot ML, An G. OsZIP5 is a plasma membrane zinc transporter in rice. Plant Mol Biol. 2010;73(4–5):507–17.
52. Jeong J, Guerinot ML. Homing in on iron homeostasis in plants. Trends Plant Sci. 2009;14(5):280–5.
53. Durrett TP, Gassmann W, Rogers EE. The FRD3-mediated efflux of citrate into the root vasculature is necessary for efficient iron translocation. Plant Physiol. 2007;144(1):197–205.
54. Yokosho K, Yamaji N, Ueno D, Mitani N, Ma JF. OsFRDL1 is a citrate transporter required for efficient translocation of iron in rice. Plant Physiol. 2009;149(1):297–305.
55. Morrissey J, Baxter IR, Lee J, et al. The ferroportin metal efflux proteins function in iron and cobalt homeostasis in *Arabidopsis*. Plant Cell. 2009;21(10):3326–38.
56. Hussain D, Haydon MJ, Wang Y, et al. P-type ATPase heavy metal transporters with roles in essential zinc homeostasis in Arabidopsis. Plant Cell. 2004;16(5):1327–39.
57. Curie C, Cassin G, Couch D, et al. Metal movement within the plant: contribution of nicotianamine and yellow stripe 1-like transporters. Ann Bot. 2009;103(1):1–11.
58. Koike S, Inoue H, Mizuno D, et al. OsYSL2 is a rice metal-nicotianamine transporter that is regulated by iron and expressed in the phloem. Plant J. 2004;39(3):415–24.
59. Kim SA, Punshon T, Lanzirotti A, et al. Localization of iron in *Arabidopsis* seed requires the vacuolar membrane transporter VIT1. Science. 2006;314(5803):1295–8.
60. Conte SS, Walker EL. Transporters contributing to iron trafficking in plants. Mol Plant. 2011;4(3):464–76.
61. Lanquar V, Lelièvre F, Bolte S, et al. Mobilization of vacuolar iron by AtNRAMP3 and AtNRAMP4 is essential for seed germination on low iron. EMBO J. 2005;24(23):4041–51.
62. Kobae Y, Uemura T, Sato MH, et al. Zinc Transporter of *Arabidopsis thaliana* AtMTP1 is localized to vacuolar membranes and implicated in zinc homeostasis. Plant Cell Physiol. 2004;45(12):1749–58.
63. Arrivault S, Senger T, Krämer U. The Arabidopsis metal tolerance protein AtMTP3 maintains metal homeostasis by mediating Zn exclusion from the shoot under Fe deficiency and Zn oversupply. Plant J. 2006;46(5):861–79.
64. Duy D, Wanner G, Meda AR, von Wirén N, Soll J, Philippar K. PIC1, an ancient permease in *Arabidopsis* chloroplasts, mediates iron transport. Plant Cell. 2007;19(3):986–1006.
65. Jeong J, Cohu C, Kerkeb L, Pilon M, Connolly EL, Guerinot ML. Chloroplast Fe(III) chelate reductase activity is essential for seedling viability under iron limiting conditions. Proc Natl Acad Sci USA. 2008;105(30):10619–24.
66. Ishimaru Y, Bashir K, Fujimoto M, et al. Rice-specific mitochondrial iron-regulated gene (*MIR*) plays an important role in iron homeostasis. Mol Plant. 2009;2(5):1059–66.
67. Kobayashi T, Nakayama Y, Itai RN, et al. Identification of novel cis-acting elements, IDE1 and IDE2, of the barley *IDS2* gene promoter conferring iron-deficiency-inducible, root specific expression in heterogeneous tobacco plants. Plant J. 2003;36(6):780–93.
68. Kobayashi T, Ogo Y, Itai RN, et al. The transcription factor IDEF1 regulates the response to and tolerance of iron deficiency in plants. Proc Natl Acad Sci USA. 2007;104(48):19150–5.
69. Ogo Y, Kobayashi T, Itai RN, et al. A novel NAC transcription factor IDEF2 that recognizes the iron deficiency-responsive element 2 regulates the genes involved in iron homeostasis in plants. J Biol Chem. 2008; 283(19):13407–17.
70. Kobayashi T, Itai RN, Aung MS, Senoura T, Nakanishi H, Nishizawa NK. Rice transcription factor IDEF1 directly binds to iron and other divalent metals for sensing cellular iron status. Plant J. 2012;69(1):81–91. doi:10.1111/j.1365-313X.2011.04772.x.
71. Ogo Y, Itai RN, Nakanishi H, et al. Isolation and characterization of IRO2, a novel iron-regulated bHLH transcription factor in graminaceous plants. J Exp Bot. 2006;57(11):2867–78.

Chapter 24
Novel Fortification Strategies for Staple Gluten-Free Products

Jelena Jastrebova and Margaretha Jägerstad

Key Points

- The majority of gluten-free (GF) staple products available on the market today do not meet the nutritional requirements and need to be fortified.
- Traditional fortification with single vitamins and minerals improves the nutritional value of GF foods but cannot provide products that are fully comparable with whole-grain wheat products.
- Natural fortification by using nutritious ingredients and/or by improving nutritional value through bioprocessing is the best way to develop nutrient-rich GF products.

Keywords Gluten-free diet • Coeliac disease • Gluten intolerance • Vitamins • Antioxidants • Minerals • Dietary fibre • Natural fortification

Abbreviations

CD	Coeliac disease
FAO	Food and Agriculture Organization of the United Nations
GF	Gluten-free
RDI	Recommended daily intake
WG	Whole-grain
WHO	World Health Organization

Introduction

Gluten is the major storage protein in cereals such as wheat, rye and barley, or their crossbreds. In the wheat flour the gluten proteins contribute 80–85 % of the total protein content. These proteins contain peptides with high glutamine/proline content which are resistant to digestion by human proteases and may trigger damage to the small intestines. Gluten intolerance is a lifelong intolerance to gluten

J. Jastrebova, Ph.D. (✉) • M. Jägerstad, Ph.D.
Department of Food Science, Swedish University of Agricultural Sciences, Uppsala BioCenter, Almas Allé 5, P.O. Box 7051, Uppsala SE 750 07, Sweden
e-mail: jelena.jastrebova@gmail.com; margaretha.jagerstad@slu.se

V.R. Preedy et al. (eds.), *Handbook of Food Fortification and Health: From Concepts to Public Health Applications Volume 1*, Nutrition and Health, DOI 10.1007/978-1-4614-7076-2_24,

proteins [1]. A couple of decades ago, gluten intolerance was considered an uncommon disorder in the world, with prevalence rates of 1 in 1,000 or lower [2]. However, the development of novel sensitive and specific screening methods for gluten intolerance improved considerably diagnosis rates and resulted in an epidemiologic shift. Recent population studies have reported a much higher prevalence of gluten intolerance and it is now estimated to be 1:100–1:200 [1, 3].

Micronutrient Deficiencies and Health Risks Associated with Gluten Intolerance

The most common and severe form of gluten intolerance is coeliac disease (CD), characterised by immune-mediated damage of the small intestinal mucosa [3]. The "classic" symptoms of CD are diarrhoea and weight loss, but the range of symptoms is very broad and the severity of symptoms varies widely between patients [4]. In the Western world gluten intolerance is the most common cause of malabsorption of several important nutrients including folate, vitamins B6 and B12, calcium, iron, copper, zinc, selenium, and fat-soluble vitamins (Table 24.1) [3–5]. Several epidemiological studies have shown CD to be a risk factor for cancer, anemia, osteoporosis, thyroid disease, type 1 diabetes, female infertility, and dermatitis herpetiformis [4]. The prevalence of neurological and psychiatric disorders is also considerably increased in coeliac patients [1, 4] (Table 24.1 [5–13]).

Untreated CD is associated with 2–4-fold increased risk of death [2, 14]. The only effective treatment for gluten intolerance and related diseases is a lifelong withdrawal of gluten from the diet. Several studies have shown that a strict gluten-free (GF) diet results in clinical and mucosal recovery and improves considerably the health-related quality of life of coeliac patients [15]. However, to follow a GF diet is difficult. The availability of GF foods varies greatly in different countries and noncompliance with the diet is not uncommon, with rates between 17 and 44 % in those diagnosed as adolescents and more than 50 % of patients diagnosed as adults [4, 16]. Such behaviour may cause partial damage of the intestinal mucosa resulting in continued malabsorption also after CD diagnosis and prescription of a GF diet, which in turn may result in increased vitamin and mineral needs in noncompliant coeliac patients. Even compliant patients may need extra vitamins to improve their health status. As shown by Hallert et al. [17], B-vitamin supplementation in coeliac patients on strict GF diet resulted in normalised plasma total homocysteine levels and provided significant improvement in general well-being.

As seen from Table 24.1, many coeliac patients have reduced intake of minerals calcium, magnesium, iron, zinc, manganese, copper, selenium, and water-soluble vitamins B6 and folate as well as fat-soluble vitamins A and D. Even intake of fibres is considerably below recommended daily intake (RDI) according to most studies [18]. Bread is one of important sources of several nutrients including vitamins B1, B2, niacin, B6, and folate and minerals magnesium, iron, and zinc, whereas dairy and meat products are important sources of vitamin B12 and fat-soluble vitamins. However, the nutritional value of many GF breads available on the market is lower compared with their gluten-containing counterparts [18–20], which makes it difficult to meet RDI levels for B-vitamins, magnesium, iron, zinc, and fibres when following a GF diet.

Nutritional Requirements on Gluten-Free Foods and Needs for Fortification

The definition of GF food varies in different countries. In the United States a GF diet is based on rice and maize that are naturally GF [19, 20], whereas in Scandinavia and the UK a GF diet may include wheat starch that has been rendered GF [21]. According to the latest EU regulations the content of gluten should not exceed 20 mg/kg in GF foods and 100 mg/kg in foods specially processed to reduce gluten content from wheat [21].

Table 24.1 Micronutrients of special importance for coeliac patients

Nutrients	Deficiency symptoms and clinical prevalence in coeliac patients, (%)	% of patients on GF diet *not* meeting RDI	Major dietary sources of each nutrient
Calcium (Ca)	Impaired bone health, 30–50 [6]	46–82 [7, 8] 11 [9]	Dairy products
Magnesium (Mg)	Bone disease, 30–50 [6], cardiovascular dysfunction	69 [7] ~50 [10] 54 [9]	Dairy products, vegetables, bread
Iron (Fe)	Anemia, 49 [4], 46 [6], S-ferritin<cut-off 0–38 [11]	20–90 [7] 65 [12] 33 [9]	Meat, bread, vegetables
Zinc (Zn)	Impaired wound-healing, dermatitis, growth and sexual development retardation	40–45 [7] 18 [9]	Meat, dairy products, bread
Manganese (Mn)	Unclear	24–52 [7]	
Copper (Cu)	Hematologic and neurologic abnormalities [13]	33 [9]	
Selenium (Se)	Impaired antioxidant status, increased risk for cancer and vascular diseases	89–94 [7] ~50 [10]	Foods of animal origin
Retinol (vitamin A)	Night blindness, skin lesions	48 [9]	Foods of animal origin, vegetables, oils
Cholcalciferol (vitamin D)	Bone disease, 30–50 [6]	100 [8] 80 (in patients >65 years) [9] ~50 [10]	Foods of animal origin
Tocopherol (vitamin E)	Impaired antioxidant status	No data	Vegetable oils, germs, cereals
Vitamin K	Impaired blood coagulation, 10 [4]	No data	Green leafy vegetables
Thiamine (vitamin B1)	Nerve disease, beriberi	Average intakes meet RDI [12]	Meat, bread, dairy products
Riboflavin (vitamin B2)	Skin changes		Dairy products, meat, bread
Niacin	Skin disease, pellagra		Meat, bread, dairy products
Pyridoxin (vitamin B6)	Low B6, elevated homocysteine in blood, 20–37 [6]	0 [5]	Meat, vegetables, fruits, bread
	Low B6, 37 [5]	11 [9]	
Folate[a]	Low folate and elevated homocysteine in blood, 20–37 [6]	80–90 [7]	Vegetables, fruits, dairy products, bread
	Low erythrocyte folate, 3–34 [11]	65 [8, 9]	
	Low plasma-folate, 20 [5]	100 [5]	
	Increased risk for neural tube defects		
Cobalamin (B12)	Pernicious anemia, 8–41 [4]	10 [8]	Foods of animal origin
	Low serum vitamin B12, 0–27 [11]	4 [9]	
		0 [5]	

[a]RDI for folate in UK for adults is 200 μg. WHO recommends 400 μg folate/day

Codex Standard for GF foods requires that the GF products substituting important basic foods should supply approximately the same amount of vitamins and minerals as the original foods they replace (see Guidance on the levels to be added). However, many GF foods are still based on nutrient-poor starches and refined flours of rice, maize, potato, and wheat rendered GF and do not meet the nutritional requirements. According to our survey of 262 staple GF foods (breads, flour mixes, and pasta products) produced in Europe by some leading manufactures, starch is the main ingredient of 79 % GF soft breads and 83 % GF bread flour mixes (Table 24.2), which result in poor nutritional

Table 24.2 Comparison of 262 staple GF foods produced in Europe[a] in relation to their main ingredients and enrichment with vitamins and minerals

Product	Total number	Number[b] of products enriched with vitamins and minerals	Number[b] of products based on		
			Starch	Refined flour	Whole-grain flour
Flour mixes for bread	42	12 (29 %)	35 (83 %)	7 (17 %)	0
Soft breads	109	12 (11 %)	86 (79 %)	6 (5.5 %)	17 (15.5 %)
Crispbreads	20	2 (10 %)	4 (20 %)	11 (55 %)	5 (25 %)
Pasta products	91	0	32 (35 %)	51 (56 %)	8 (9 %)
All products	262	26 (10 %)	157 (60 %)	75 (29 %)	30 (11 %)

[a]GF staple foods from 11 manufactures of GF foods in Europe (BiAglut, DreiPauly, DS, Finax, Glutafin, Glutano, Hammermühle, Juvela, Minderleinsmühle, Orgran, Schär, Semper) are surveyed
[b]Numbers in brackets are expressed as percent of total number of corresponding products

quality of these products if fortification is not used. The content of B-vitamins and some minerals is commonly much lower in these foods compared with cereal products based on whole-grain (WG) wheat and rye or cereal products based on fortified refined flours. According to the comprehensive survey of GF products in the United States made by Thompson [19, 20] the great part of these products has content of thiamine, riboflavin, niacin, folate, and iron, which is only 66–80 % of content in their gluten-containing counterparts. Low folate content was also reported for some GF products in Sweden [22]. The content of dietary fibres in GF products is only 30–50 % of fibre content in corresponding gluten-containing products [20]. The reduced nutritional value of many GF foods may lead to low micronutrient intake (Table 24.1) and poor vitamin and mineral status in coeliac patients [5]. Even antioxidant status is much lower in celiac patients [23, 24], which may be partially caused by low content of antioxidants in GF foods based on starches and refined flours [25]. Therefore, the development of more nutrient-rich GF products is of great importance.

Despite the necessity of improving the nutritional value of GF foods there is no mandatory fortification of GF products in Western countries. GF foods available on the market vary greatly in content of proteins, fibres, vitamins, and minerals. For one decade ago the majority of these products were not fortified [19, 20] and the situation is similar even today. Fortified GF products represent only 10 % of GF staple foods in Europe (Table 24.2). Among starch-based GF soft breads produced in Europe only 5 % breads are fortified with five B-vitamins (B1, B2, niacin, B6, and folic acid) and iron and 9 % breads are fortified with folic acid and calcium, whereas 56 % of starch-based GF soft breads have low nutritional value (Table 24.3).

The use of starches as main ingredient in many GF foods makes it difficult to successfully implement common fortification with single micronutrients. Such fortification cannot provide nutritional value fully comparable with that of gluten-containing products, because starches lack or have low levels of many essential micronutrients and phytochemicals. As seen from Fig. 24.1a, b, maize starch contains no B-vitamins and the mineral content of maize starch is only 2–13 % of that of WG wheat. Other starches (potato, rice, and wheat starches) are similar to maize starch regarding low nutritional value (data not shown). This clearly demonstrates unsuitability of using starches as main ingredients in GF foods. Even refined flours of maize and rice are much lower in most micronutrients compared with corresponding WG products or WG wheat. The content of calcium, iron, magnesium, zinc, and copper is 3–17 times lower in refined flours of rice and maize compared to WG wheat and up to 5 times lower compared to corresponding WG flours (Fig. 24.1a). Refined flour of rice is also low in vitamins B1, B2, and folate, whereas refined maize flour is low in vitamins B1, B2, and B6 (Fig. 24.1b). Moreover, the absence of bran/germ fractions in refined flours results in much lower levels of dietary fibres and antioxidants compared to WG flours because bran/germ fraction has high content of fibres and contributes to a greater part of antioxidant capacity in WG flour [26, 27] (Fig. 24.1 [28]).

Table 24.3 Survey of 86 starch-based soft GF breads produced in Europe[a]

Ingredients improving nutritional value	Enrichment with vitamins and minerals	Number of breads (%)	Nutritional value
No	No	11.7	Low (56 % of breads)
Fibres[b]	No	7.0	
Fibres + proteins[c]	No	37.2	
Fibres +/or proteins	B-vitamins, iron	3.5	Improved (44 % of breads)
Proteins + seeds	B-vitamins, iron	1.2	
Whole grains[d]	No	2.3	
Fibres + proteins + whole grains	No	9.3	
Fibres + proteins + whole grains	Folic acid, calcium	7.0	
Fibres + proteins + seeds[e]		8.1	
Fibres + proteins + whole grains + seeds	No	10.5	
Fibres + proteins + whole grains + seeds	Folic acid, calcium	2.3	

[a]Breads from 11 manufactures of GF foods in Europe (BiAglut, DreiPauly, DS, Finax, Glutafin, Glutano, Hammermühle, Juvela, Minderleinsmühle, Orgran, Schär, Semper) are surveyed
[b]Fibres—psyllium, sugar beet fibre or apple fibres or their mixtures
[c]Proteins—soy protein isolate/soy flour, lupin proteins/flour, egg proteins, milk proteins, or their mixtures
[d]Whole grains—WG flours of maize, rice, buckwheat, millet, amaranth, teff, quinoa, sorghum, or their mixtures
[e]Seeds—seeds of sunflower, sesame, flax, or their mixtures

WG Flours and Nutrient-Rich Seeds as Valuable Natural Fortificants for GF Foods

Recently, a positive trend towards more nutritious GF foods is seen in many countries. More and more producers develop novel GF foods with higher nutritional value by using WG flours of rice, maize, buckwheat, millet, amaranth, teff, quinoa, and sorghum. In Europe, WG flours are used as the main ingredient in 15.5 % of soft breads, 25 % of crispbreads and 9 % of pasta products (Table 24.2). The use of WG flours as well as other nutrient-rich ingredients such as seeds (sesame, sunflower, and flax seeds) and flours of soy, lupine, chick-pea, and chestnut become more and more common when developing new GF breads (Table 24.3) and pasta products. This is also a common practice in production of GF cereals. A great part of breakfast cereals are based on whole grains and contain different nutrient-rich ingredients such as seeds and fruits (data not shown).

As seen from Fig. 24.1a, oat, buckwheat, millet, amaranth, quinoa, sorghum, and teff have mineral content, which is comparable or higher than that of WG wheat. The content of B-vitamins varies greatly between different cereals and pseudocereals (Fig. 24.1b). Compared to WG wheat, amaranth and quinoa are considerably higher in vitamins B2, B6, and folic acid, but lower in niacin, whereas oat is higher in B1, but lower in other B-vitamins. Buckwheat, millet, and teff are comparable with WG wheat or better regarding B-vitamin content. Several investigations have also shown that these alternative cereals/pseudocereals have beneficial composition regarding proteins, amino acids, and dietary fibres [29–32]. They have also high antioxidant capacity, especially buckwheat, sorghum, and quinoa [31, pp. 149–175, 33]. The substitution of starches and refined flours of rice, maize, and potato by WG flours of these cereals/pseudocereals can therefore multiply the nutritional value of GF foods by several times.

As shown in Table 24.4, the majority of WG-based GF products have WG (brown) rice as the main ingredient. This provides considerably higher nutritional value compared with starch-based GF foods. WG rice has high content of vitamins B1, B6, and niacin as well as minerals magnesium and zinc (Fig. 24.1a, b). The levels of vitamin B2 and minerals iron and copper are around 50 % of corresponding values for WG wheat and antioxidant activity is comparable with that for WG wheat [34].

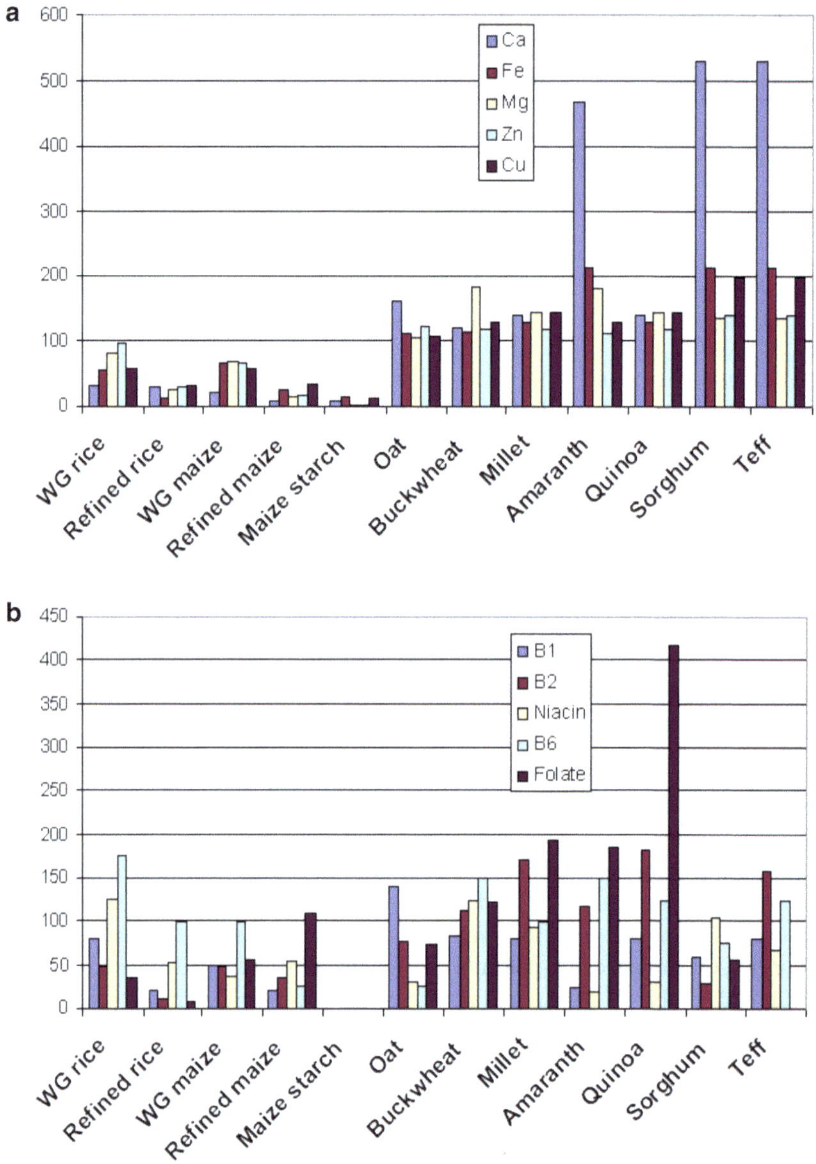

Fig. 24.1 Mineral (**a**) and vitamin (**b**) content in whole-grain (WG) and refined flours of rice and maize, maize starch, partially debranned oat flour and whole grains or WG flours of buckwheat, millet, amaranth, quinoa, sorghum, and teff related to their content in WG wheat flour which is taken as 100 %. Data are taken from USDA National Nutrient Database [28]

However, the levels of folate and calcium are 3 times lower in WG rice compared with WG wheat (Fig. 24.1a, b). Therefore the addition of other WG flours with higher nutrient content may be of great interest. For example, the addition of quinoa, amaranth, or millet can provide higher folate content, whereas higher calcium content can be obtained by the addition of amaranth, sorghum, or teff. As seen from Table 24.4, several breads available on the market contain mixtures of WG flours, which provide high nutritional value that is fully comparable with WG-based gluten-containing breads.

Only one WG bread product is based on oat as main ingredient (Table 24.4) despite good nutritional value of oat (Fig. 24.1a, b). The use of oats in GF diet is still controversial due to frequent contamination of commercial oats by wheat and barley. In Canada, for example, 88 % of oat samples from retail stores

Table 24.4 Some examples of whole-grain-based GF foods produced in Europe[a]

Product name	Main WG ingredient	Other WG ingredients	Producer
Soft breads			
Sliced bread with teff	Whole rice (40 %)	Teff (13 %), millet, buckwheat	Drei Pauly
Sliced bread with buckwheat and linseed	Whole rice	Millet (8 %), buckwheat bran (6 %)	Drei Pauly
Wholemeal sliced bread with teff	Whole rice (38 %)	Millet, teff (6 %), buckwheat	Drei Pauly
wholemeal sliced bread	Whole rice (39 %)	Whole maize 8 %, millet 8 %	Drei Pauly
Sliced bread with teff and seeds	Whole rice (37 %)	Teff (6 %), buckwheat, millet	Drei Pauly
Bread, 3-kernels	Whole rice (39 %)	Millet (8 %), whole maize (8 %)	Glutano
Bio-Amaranth Schnittbrot	Buckwheat	Amaranth 19 %	Hammermühle
Bio-Buchweizen Schnittbrot	Buckwheat (40 %)	–	Hammermühle
Bio-Hirsebrot Schnittbrot	Buckwheat (28 %)	Millet (18 %)	Hammermühle
Körnerbrot geschnitten	Whole rice	Buckwheat	Hammermühle
Vitalbrot mit Sonnenblumenkernen geschnitten	Whole rice	Millet, buckwheat	Hammermühle
Vollkornbrot haltbar	Whole rice	–	Hammermühle
Steinofenbrötchen frisch	Whole rice	–	Minderleinsmühle
Hausbrot in Scheiben	Whole rice	–	Minderleinsmühle
Sonnenblumenbrot in Scheiben	Whole rice	–	Minderleinsmühle
Vollkornbrot, ballaststoffreich	Whole rice	–	Minderleinsmühle
Solena whole-grain bread	Whole rice (34 %)	Millet (8 %), buckwheat (7 %)	Schär
Crispbreads			
Bio-Reiswaffeln	Whole rice (70 %)	–	Hammermühle
Essential Fibre Crispibread	Brown rice	Sorghum	Orgran
Multigrain Crispibread with Quinoa	Brown rice	Sorghum, quinoa (10 %)	Orgran
Crispbread with buckwheat	Buckwheat (68 %)	–	Orgran
Havreknäcke	Oat	Teff	Semper
Pasta products			
Gourmet Rice Pasta spirals	Brown rice	–	Orgran
Buckwheat Pasta spirals	Buckwheat (80 %)	–	Orgran
Vegetable Rice Pasta (penne)	Brown rice (99 %)	–	Orgran
Vegetable Rice Pasta (spirals)	Brown rice (99 %)	–	Orgran
Rice and Millet Pasta	Brown rice (94.5 %)	Millet (5.5 %)	Orgran
Essential Fibre Pasta (lasagnette)	Brown rice	–	Orgran
Essential Fibre Pasta (penne)	Brown rice	–	Orgran
Essential Fibre Pasta (spirals)	Brown rice	–	Orgran

[a]Breads and pasta products from 11 manufactures of GF foods in Europe (BiAglut, DreiPauly, DS, Finax, Glutafin, Glutano, Hammermühle, Juvela, Minderleinsmühle, Orgran, Schär, Semper) are surveyed

were found to contain gluten at levels higher than allowed level for GF foods (20 mg/kg) according to the study of Koerner et al. [35]. However, the use of pure oats in GF diet can significantly increase intakes of nutrients, e.g. iron, zinc, thiamine, and dietary fibres and make the GF diet more diverse and balanced [36, 37]. On the other hand, the bioavailability of iron may decrease due to higher content of phytate in oat; yet this seems not to have influenced the iron status of coeliac patients [36]. Pure oats are well tolerated by majority of coeliac patients, but around 5 % of coeliac patients can develop oat intolerance [38], therefore the introduction of oats in GF diet should be done with caution.

Buckwheat and millet are the most common minor ingredients in GF bread and pasta products. According to our survey of 109 soft GF breads produced in Europe, 22 % of breads contain buckwheat and 21 % contain millet. Buckwheat can also be used as main ingredient in WG GF products (Table 24.4). Compared to WG wheat, buckwheat has higher content of most micronutrients (Fig. 24.1a, b), similar protein and fibre content and high antioxidant capacity [39]. According to the findings of Krupa-Kozak et al. [40], the addition of buckwheat to GF flour mixtures provides breads with much higher protein and mineral content. Increasing concentration of buckwheat flour (10–40 %) affected proportionally the enrichment in proteins (up to fivefold) and minerals, e.g. Zn (twofold), Cu (fivefold), and Mn (tenfold) compared to control bread.

Millet is also a good source of micronutrients (Fig. 24.1a, b) and antioxidants [39] and has been used as a staple food by millions of people in Asia and Africa for thousands of years. Several other GF cereals and pseudocereals such as sorghum, teff, quinoa, and amaranth are also used as minor ingredients in GF breads, which helps to improve the nutritional value of breads [41]. However, only few GF products containing these nutritious cereals and pseudocereals are today available on the market (see, for example, Table 24.4).

Another way to improve the nutritional value of GF foods is to add highly nutritious ingredients such as soy, lupin, chick-pea, or chestnut flours or different seeds such as flax, sunflower, sesame, or pumpkin seeds. As seen from Fig. 24.2, the content of several micronutrients in these ingredients is 2–10 times higher compared with WG wheat. This means that the addition of small amounts, e.g. 5–10 %, may result in considerable improvements of nutritional value of GF products. For example, chick-pea, lupin, or soy flours can be used to fortify GF flours with folate; the addition of just 5 % of chick-pea flour can provide the same amount of folate as 50 % of WG wheat flour. Pumpkin, sesame, and sunflower seeds can be used to fortify GF breads with zinc and magnesium, whereas soy flour, and pumpkin seeds may be useful as natural iron and copper fortificants.

As shown in Table 24.5, WG flours of GF cereals and pseudocereals as well as nutritious seeds may be used as valuable natural fortificants to increase content of micronutrients and antioxidants in GF foods. Because these cereals/pseudocereals have different nutritional profiles, it is beneficial to combine several of these ingredients to achieve high nutritional value (Fig. 24.2 [28]).

The Use of Genetic Diversity and Engineering for Improving the Nutritional Quality of GF Foods

The content of micronutrients, minerals, and phytochemicals may vary widely between different cultivars or varieties. For example, variety has great effect on the content of several nutrients in millet [42]. The concentration of calcium is 40-fold higher in Finger millet than in Proso millet, whereas Japanese Barnyard millet has sixfold higher content of iron compared with Proso or Pearl millet. This gives the opportunity to enhance the nutritional value of GF foods by choosing the right variety. Another promising example is the large biodiversity of different yeast strains used in bread making. As shown by Hjortmo et al. [43], it is possible to increase up to fivefold the levels of folate in bread by using a high folate producing yeast strain instead of commercial baker's yeast.

Biofortification is another efficient way to enhance the content and bioavailability of micronutrients and beneficial phytochemicals in food crops through genetic engineering. Novel varieties of staple cereals with enhanced micronutrient content have been developed recently, e.g. rice biofortified with folate, rice biofortified with iron and zinc, multivitamin maize biofortified with ascorbic acid, β-carotene, and folate (see previous chapters). These novel varieties of GF cereals can be used in the future to enhance the nutritional value of GF products.

Natural Fortification Through Bioprocessing: Enhancing Vitamin Content in GF Products and Improving the Bioavailability of Minerals

Typical examples of bioprocessing are germination/malting/sprouting of seeds/kernels and fermentation by adding yeasts and/or bacteria. In contrast to traditional fortification, a natural way to increase vitamin levels is *germination* (*or malting/sprouting*) of plant seeds, which has been applied for decades.

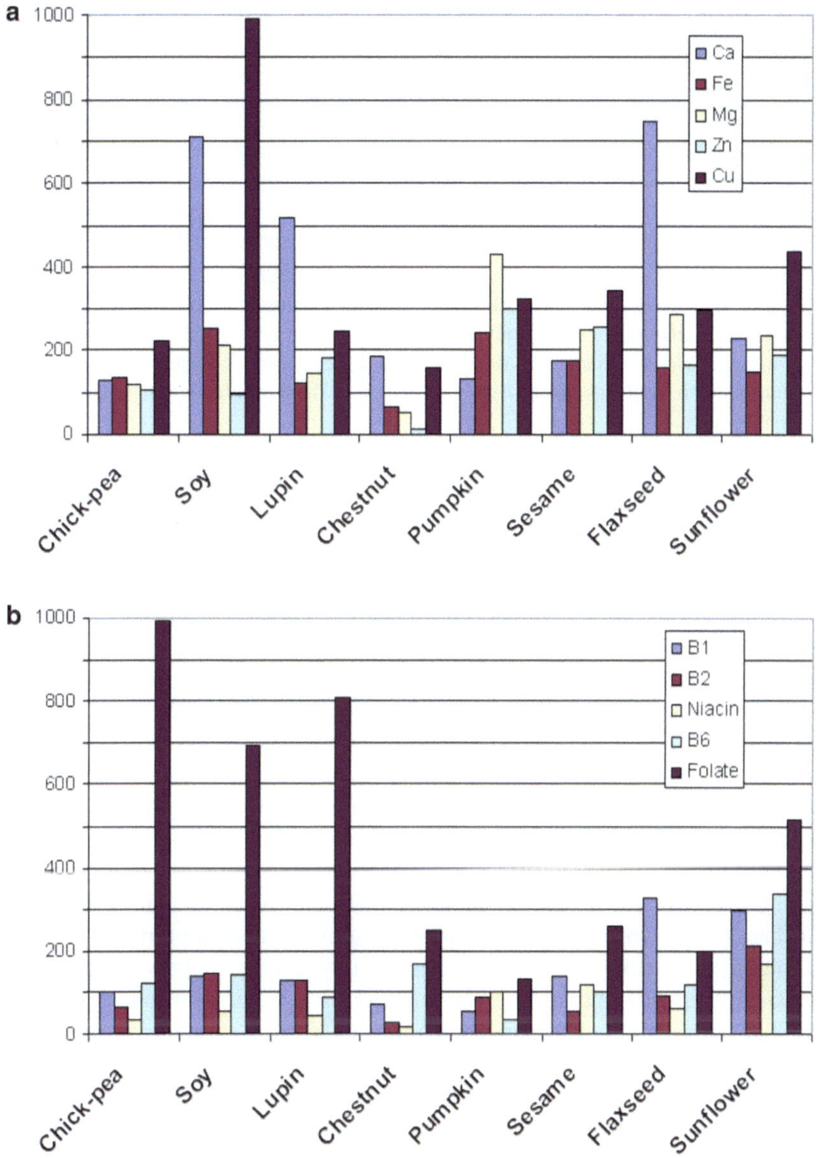

Fig. 24.2 Mineral (**a**) and vitamin (**b**) content in chick-pea and soy flours, seeds of lupin, chestnut (dried, peeled), and flax and seed kernels of pumpkin, sesame, and sunflower related to their content in WG wheat flour which is taken as 100 %. Data are taken from USDA National Nutrient Database [28]

By this way, levels of vitamins such as thiamine, riboflavin, folate, biotin, pantothenic acid, and tocopherols can be increased 2–4 times than those in ungerminated seeds [44–46]. Germination also increases endogenous phytase activity in cereals, legumes, and oil seeds through activation of intrinsic phytase [47] leading to reduction of total phytates, that compromise mineral and trace element absorption in humans.

Germination/malting might interfere negatively with baking performance due to increase of enzymatic activities such as protease and amylase leading to degradation of proteins and starch to provide the developing plant with nutrients. Hefni and Witthoft [48] could, however, replace about 50 % of the white wheat flour with germinated wheat flour, which together with added yeast doubled the folate

Table 24.5 The use of natural fortificants to enhance the nutritional value and health-promoting properties of GF products

	Natural fortificant[a]	
Nutrient	WG or bran	Seeds
Ca	Teff, amaranth, oat, quinoa, buckwheat	Flaxseed, soy, lupin, sunflower, chestnuts
Mg	Buckwheat, amaranth, quinoa, teff, oat	pumpkin, flaxseed, sesame, sunflower, soy
Fe	Teff, amaranth, quinoa, buckwheat	Soy, pumpkin, sesame, flaxseed, chick-pea
Zn	Teff, oat, quinoa, buckwheat, millet	Pumpkin, sesame, sunflower, lupin, flaxseed
Cu	Teff, quinoa, millet, amaranth, buckwheat	Soy, sunflower, pumpkin, sesame, flaxseed
B1	Oat	Flaxseed, sunflower, sesame, pumpkin
B2	Quinoa, millet, teff, amaranth, buckwheat	Sunflower, sesame, lupin
Niacin	Whole rice (brown), buckwheat, millet, sorghum	Sunflower, sesame, pumpkin
B6	Whole rice (brown), amaranth, buckwheat, quinoa	Sunflower, chestnuts, sesame, chick-pea, flaxseed
Folate	Quinoa, millet, amaranth, buckwheat	Chick-pea, lupin, soy, sunflower seed, sesame
Antioxidants	All WG and bran products	All seeds

[a]Placed in descending order regarding the content of nutrient

content in the bread. Their results demonstrate the possibility of using germinated seeds to increase the vitamin content in breads. Likewise, the antioxidative capacity and total phenolic content increased approximately twofold in sprouted pseudocereals (amaranth, buckwheat, quinoa) [41]. However, when making bread from 100 % buckwheat mixed with sprouted buckwheat, the antioxidative capacity decreased during baking. Still, though, this bread had significantly higher antioxidant capacity and total phenolic content than control breads made from either wheat or GF rice flour and potato starch [41].

Fermentation by yeast and or lactic acid bacteria is another well-known application of bioprocessing used in bread making. Bakery yeast is a rich source of zinc and B-vitamins, especially folate. Dry bakery yeast contains 4–24-fold higher concentrations of B-vitamins compared with WG wheat flour; for folate even 50-fold higher amounts [28]. Approximately 1 % of dry matter of bread constitutes bakery yeast, hence providing around half or more of the total folate in bread [49].

Bread making by yeast also hydrolyse phytates, especially when combined with sourdough fermentation, i.e. bacterial enzymes. The phytate concentration can under optimal conditions be reduced to near-zero values [50]. Such substantial decrease of phytates can improve mineral availability in humans. Sourdough is traditionally made by mixing flour and water allowing it to ferment. Bakeries typically have their own sourdoughs which are maintained by back-slopping procedure. The microorganism (lactic acid bacteria and yeast) originate mainly from the flour but also from the microflora, associated with bakery yeast often added to the sourdough. In addition to improved technological properties, fermentation creates a typical flavour and increases the shelf-life, mainly due to lactic acid production by lactic acid bacteria. Nutritional value is improved by better bioavailability of minerals due to destruction of phytates [31, p. 271].

The exploitation of sourdough in GF systems is still in its infancy, only few GF breads available on the market are made by using sourdough. The literature data available strongly indicate that sourdough may undoubtedly be considered as a technological tool for improving the texture and flavour characteristics of GF products.

Positive Effects of Nutrient-Rich and Healthy Ingredients on Sensory and Technological Properties of GF Products

The absence of gluten in GF flours makes them unsuitable for production of dough with good viscoelastic and extensible properties. Gluten proteins from wheat play a vital role in bread making because they form a continuous viscoelastic network in the fermenting dough, which is necessary to

Table 24.6 Positive effects of some natural fortificants on quality and sensory characteristics of GF breads

Fortificant and its labeled maximal content in commercial soft GF breads (%)	Literature data	
	Quality and sensory characteristics of breads compared to GF controls	Amount added (%)
Buckwheat (40)	Increasingly improved sensory quality	10–40 [52]
	Improved shape and volume	10–40 [40]
	Improved loaf volume, softer crumb, good sensory properties	25 (in batter) [53]
Amaranth (19)	Improved loaf volume	Used as main ingredient [54]
	Comparable bread quality	Less than 20 [55]
	Improved loaf volume, decreased hardness	10 [56]
	Softer crumb, good sensory properties	25 (in batter) [53]
Millet (18)	Improved loaf volume, better resistance to staling	15–70 [31, p. 131, 139]
Quinoa (10)	Improved loaf volume, softer crumb, good sensory properties	25 (in batter) [53]
Chestnut (4.5)	Bread quality comparable with wheat control	46.5 [57]
Lupin flour (4)	Good bread texture and pleasant taste	No data [58]
Pea isolate	Comparable bread quality	Less than 3 [55]
Soy proteins	Improved bread texture	7.5 [59]
Milk protein isolate/sodium caseinate	Improved shape and volume, softer crust and crumb texture	3–9 [51]
Calcium caseinate, calcium citrate	Better bread quality, softer and more elastic	0.7–2 [60]
Psyllium fibres	Better rheological properties of dough, comparable bread quality	2 [55]
Inulin	Increased loaf volume, reduced rate of crumb hardening, good flavour	5 [31, 61]

produce bread of high quality [51]. These properties are completely unique to wheat gluten proteins and cannot be replicated by GF cereals such as rice and maize. A lot of research was therefore carried out to find functional ingredients which could be used instead of gluten to improve the viscoelastic properties of GF dough [51]. A greater part of this research was performed, however, with starch-based GF flour mixes that lack most micronutrients. The result was development of GF breads with good baking and sensory properties but low nutritional value.

Nutritious pseudocereals such as amaranth, buckwheat, and quinoa have higher protein content than rice and maize and can be successfully used to improve baking properties of GF flours. As shown in Table 24.6, the addition of amaranth, buckwheat, and quinoa to bread flour mixes can considerably improve loaf volume, provide softer crumb as well as better sensory properties. Even other highly nutritious ingredients such as protein-rich soybeans, lupin beans, chick-pea, chestnut, or milk protein isolate can have positive effects on bread quality. Adding dietary fibres such as inulin or psyllium can also be useful from the technological point of view because they improve rheological properties of dough (Table 24.6 [31, 40, 52–61]).

Guidance on Levels to Be Added

Designing GF products generally means replacing of gluten-containing cereals by GF counterparts, which might include natural ingredients, e.g. nutrient-rich GF cereals/pseudocereals or nutritious seeds. These ingredients do not need to be restricted for healthy or nutritional reasons. Instead, technological aspects may limit their use, e.g. baking properties, sensory characteristics, impact on colour and shelf-life of products.

Traditional fortification with micronutrients, e.g. minerals and vitamins follow legislations outlined by international expert committees associated with World Health Organization (WHO) and

Food and Agriculture Organization of the United Nations (FAO). In 2008, *The Codex standard for foods for special dietary use for persons intolerant to gluten* was adopted [21].

Except for stating maximum levels of gluten allowed in products labelled as "gluten-free", the Commission made the following statement concerning essential composition and quality factors: "products covered by this standard substituting important basic foods, should supply approximately the same amounts of vitamins and minerals as the original foods they replace".

For more specific information on permitted vitamins and minerals that could be added to GF products, the legislation given for fortification of normal foods can be followed. Authorities on national levels give guidelines in this respect, usually by following recommendations originally set by Codex Alimentarius standards. Note that there might be upper limits for certain nutrients, for example some fat-soluble vitamins, folate, and iron to minimise health hazards.

Recommendations

- Starches as main ingredients in GF staple foods should be avoided.
- GF staple foods based mainly on refined flours should be fortified by adding B-vitamins (thiamine, riboflavin, niacin, B6, and folic acid) and iron (in accordance with legislation in each country) or by adding nutritious ingredients such as WG flours and seeds.
- WG flours of GF cereals/pseudocereals and their mixtures are recommended as main ingredients in GF products.
- The use of highly nutritious ingredients such as soy, lupin, chestnut, and chick-pea flours or seeds (sunflower, flax, sesame, or pumpkin) as minor ingredients in GF products is recommended.
- Bioprocessing such as germination or fermentation with yeast and/or sourdough can also be used to further improve the nutritional value of GF products.

Conclusions

A great part of GF staple products available on the market today are based on starches and do not meet the nutritional requirements. They have lower nutritional value compared with gluten-containing products and need to be fortified. The traditional fortification of starch-based GF products with single vitamins and minerals cannot, however, provide products that are fully comparable with WG wheat products. These fortified GF products still lack many micronutrients, antioxidants, and other health-promoting compounds. The best way to develop nutritious healthy GF products with high content of proteins, fibres, micronutrients, and antioxidants is natural fortification by using nutritious ingredients such as WG flours of GF cereals/pseudocereals, protein-rich flours of soy, lupin, chick-pea, chestnut, and different seeds as well as bioprocessing such as germination or fermentation with yeast and/or sourdough.

References

1. Rewers M. Epidemiology of celiac disease: what are the prevalence, incidence, and progression of celiac disease? Gastroenterology. 2005;128:S47–51.
2. Peters U, Askling J, Gridley G, et al. Causes of death in patients with celiac disease in a population-based Swedish cohort. Arch Intern Med. 2003;163:1566–72.
3. Mendoza N, McGough N. Coeliac disease: an overview. Nutr Food Sci. 2005;35:156–62.

4. Garcia-Manzanares A, Lucendo AJ. Nutritional and dietary aspects of celiac disease. Nutr Clin Pract. 2011;26:163–73.
5. Hallert C, Grant C, Grehn S, et al. Evidence of poor vitamin status in coeliac patients on a gluten-free diet for 10 years. Aliment Pharmacol Ther. 2002;16:1333–9.
6. Haines ML, Anderson RP, Gibson PR. Systematic review: the evidence base for long-term management of coeliac disease. Aliment Pharmacol Ther. 2008;28:1042–66.
7. Wild D, Robins GG, Burley VJ, et al. Evidence of high sugar intake, and low fibre and mineral intake, in the gluten-free diet. Aliment Pharmacol Ther. 2010;32:573–81.
8. Kinsey L, Burden ST, Bannerman E. A dietary survey to determine if patients with coeliac disease are meeting current healthy eating guidelines and how their diet compares to that of the British general population. Eur J Clin Nutr. 2008;62:1333–42.
9. McFarlane XA, Marsham J, Reeves D, et al. Subclinical nutritional deficiency in treated celiac-disease and nutritional content of the gluten-free diet. J Hum Nutr Diet. 1995;8:231–7.
10. Ohlund K, Olsson C, Hernell O, et al. Dietary shortcomings in children on a gluten-free diet. J Hum Nutr Diet. 2010;23:294–300.
11. Kemppainen T, Uusitupa M, Janatuinen E, et al. Intakes of nutrients and nutritional-status in celiac patients. Scand J Gastroenterol. 1995;30:575–9.
12. Hopman EGD, le Cessie S, von Blomberg BME, et al. Nutritional management of the gluten-free diet in young people with celiac disease in the Netherlands. J Pediatr Gastroenterol Nutr. 2006;43:102–8.
13. Halfdanarson TR, Kumar N, Hogan WJ, et al. Copper deficiency in celiac disease. J Clin Gastroenterol. 2009;43:162–4.
14. Rubio-Tapia A, Kyle RA, Kaplan EL, et al. Increased prevalence and mortality in undiagnosed celiac disease. Gastroenterology. 2009;137:88–93.
15. Johnston SD, Rodgers C, Watson RGP. Quality of life in screen-detected and typical coeliac disease and the effect of excluding dietary gluten. Eur J Gastroenterol Hepatol. 2004;16:1281–6.
16. Pietzak MM, Fasano A. Celiac disease: a new paradigm of an immune-mediated disorder due to dietary gluten. In: Preedy VR, Watson RR, editors. Reviews in food and nutrition toxicity, vol. 3. Boca Raton, FL: CRC Press; 2005. p. 243–65.
17. Hallert C, Svensson M, Tholstrup J, et al. Clinical trial: B vitamins improve health in patients with coeliac disease living on a gluten-free diet. Aliment Pharmacol Ther. 2009;29:811–6.
18. Hager AS, Axel C, Arendt EK. Status of carbohydrates and dietary fiber in gluten-free diets. Cereal Foods World. 2011;56:109–14.
19. Thompson T. Thiamin, riboflavin, and niacin contents of the gluten-free diet: is there cause for concern? J Am Diet Assoc. 1999;99:858–62.
20. Thompson T. Folate, iron, and dietary fiber contents of the gluten-free diet. J Am Diet Assoc. 2000;100:1389–96.
21. The Codex Standard for Special Dietary Use for Persons Intolerant to Gluten. 2008. http://www.codexalimentarius.net/download/standards/291/cxs_118e.pdf. Accessed Sept 2011.
22. Yazynina E, Johansson M, Jagerstad M, et al. Low folate content in gluten-free cereal products and their main ingredients. Food Chem. 2008;111:236–42.
23. Odetti P, Valentini S, Aragno I, et al. Oxidative stress in subjects affected by celiac disease. Free Radic Res. 1998;29:17–24.
24. Stojiljkovic V, Todorovic A, Pejic S, et al. Antioxidant status and lipid peroxidation in small intestinal mucosa of children with celiac disease. Clin Biochem. 2009;42:1431–7.
25. Zhokhov SS, Broberg A, Kenne L, et al. Content of antioxidant hydroquinones substituted by beta-1,6-linked oligosaccharides in wheat milled fractions, flours and breads. Food Chem. 2010;121:645–52.
26. Adom KK, Sorrells ME, Liu RH. Phytochemicals and antioxidant activity of milled fractions of different wheat varieties. J Agric Food Chem. 2005;53:2297–306.
27. Kong S, Lee J. Antioxidants in milling fractions of black rice cultivars. Food Chem. 2010;120:278–81.
28. US Department of Agriculture, Agricultural Research Service. USDA national nutrient database for standard reference. http://www.nal.usda.gov/fnic/foodcomp/search/. Accessed Sept 2011.
29. Gabrovska D, Fiedlerova V, Holasova M, et al. The nutritional evaluation of underutilized cereals and buckwheat. Food Nutr Bull. 2002;23:246–9.
30. Krkoskova B, Mrazova Z. Prophylactic components of buckwheat. Food Res Int. 2005;38:561–8.
31. Arendt EK, Dal Bello F. Gluten-free cereal products and beverages. In: Taylor SL, editor. Food science and technology international series. 1st ed. Burlington, MA: Academic; 2008. p. 1–445.
32. Belton PS, Taylor JRN. Pseudocereals and less common cereals. 2nd ed. Berlin: Springer; 2011. p. 1–287.
33. Brindzova L, Zalibera M, Simon P, et al. Screening of cereal varieties for antioxidant and radical scavenging properties applying various spectroscopic and thermoanalytical methods. Int J Food Sci Technol. 2009;44:784–91.
34. Adom KK, Liu RH. Antioxidant activity of grains. J Agric Food Chem. 2002;50:6182–7.
35. Koerner TB, Cleroux C, Poirier C, et al. Gluten contamination in the Canadian commercial oat supply. Food Addit Contam Part A Chem Anal Control Expo Risk Assess. 2011;28:705–10.

36. Storsrud S, Hulthen LR, Lenner RA. Beneficial effects of oats in the gluten-free diet of adults with special reference to nutrient status, symptoms and subjective experiences. Br J Nutr. 2003;90:101–7.
37. Kemppainen TA, Heikkinen MT, Ristikankare MK, et al. Nutrient intakes during diets including unkilned and large amounts of oats in celiac disease. Eur J Clin Nutr. 2010;64:62–7.
38. Lundin KEA, Nilsen EM, Scott HG, et al. Oats induced villous atrophy in coeliac disease. Gut. 2003;52:1649–52.
39. Hall C. Sources of natural antioxidants: oilseeds, nuts, cereals, legumes, animal products and microbiological sources. In: Pokorny J, Yanishlieva N, Gordon M, editors. Antioxidants in food: practical applications. Cambridge: Woodhead Publishing; 2001. p. 159–209.
40. Krupa-Kozak U, Wronkowska M, Soral-Smietana M. Effect of buckwheat flour on microelements and proteins contents in gluten-free bread. Czech J Food Sci. 2011;29:103–8.
41. Alvarez-Jubete L, Arendt EK, Gallagher E. Nutritive value of pseudocereals and their increasing use as functional gluten-free ingredients. Trends Food Sci Technol. 2010;21:106–13.
42. Leder I. Sorghum and millets. In: Füyleky G, editor. Cultivated plants, primarily as food sources, in Encyclopedia of Life Support Systems (EOLSS), developed under the auspices of the UNESCO. Oxford, UK: Eolss Publishers; 2004. p. 1–18. http://www.eolss.net/. Accessed Sept 2011.
43. Hjortmo S, Patring J, Jastrebova J, et al. Biofortification of folates in white wheat bread by selection of yeast strain and process. Int J Food Microbiol. 2008;127:32–6.
44. Plaza L, de Ancos B, Cano MP. Nutritional and health-related compounds in sprouts and seeds of soybean (Glycine max), wheat (Triticum aestiivum L.) and alfalfa (Medicago sativa) treated by a new drying method. Eur Food Res Technol. 2003;216:138–44.
45. Koehler P, Hartmann G, Wieser H, et al. Changes of folates, dietary fiber, and proteins in wheat as affected by germination. J Agric Food Chem. 2007;55:4678–83.
46. Ochanda SO, Akoth OC, Mwasaru MA, et al. Effects of malting and fermentation treatments on group B-vitamins of red sorghum, white sorghum and pearl millets in Kenya. J Appl Biosci. 2010;34:2128–34.
47. Egli I, Davidsson L, Juillerat MA, et al. The influence of soaking and germination on the phytase activity and phytic acid content of grains and seeds potentially useful for complementary feeding. J Food Sci. 2002;67:3484–8.
48. Hefni M, Witthoft CM. Increasing the folate content in Egyptian baladi bread using germinated wheat flour. LWT-Food Sci Technol. 2011;44:706–12.
49. Patring J, Wandel M, Jagerstad M, et al. Folate content of Norwegian and Swedish flours and bread analysed by use of liquid chromatography-mass spectrometry. J Food Compost Anal. 2009;22:649–56.
50. Fretzdorff B, Brummer JM. Reduction of phytic acid during breadmaking of whole-meal breads. Cereal Chem. 1992;69:266–70.
51. Gallagher E, Gormley TR, Arendt EK. Recent advances in the formulation of gluten-free cereal-based products. Trends Food Sci Technol. 2004;15:143–52.
52. Wronkowska M, Zielinska D, Szawara-Nowak D, et al. Antioxidative and reducing capacity, macroelements content and sensorial properties of buckwheat-enhanced gluten-free bread. Int J Food Sci Technol. 2010;45:1993–2000.
53. Alvarez-Jubete L, Auty M, Arendt EK, et al. Baking properties and microstructure of pseudocereal flours in gluten-free bread formulations. Eur Food Res Technol. 2010;230:437–45.
54. Calderon de la Barca AM, Elvira Rojas-Martinez M, Rosa Islas-Rubio A, et al. Gluten-free breads and cookies of raw and popped amaranth flours with attractive technological and nutritional qualities. Plant Foods Hum Nutr. 2010;65:241–6.
55. Mariotti M, Lucisano M, Pagani MA, et al. The role of corn starch, amaranth flour, pea isolate, and psyllium flour on the rheological properties and the ultrastructure of gluten-free doughs. Food Res Int. 2009;42:963–75.
56. Marciniak-Lukasiak K, Skrzypacz M. Gluten-free bread concentrate with addition of amaranthus flour. Zywnosc Nauka Technologia Jakosc. 2008;15:131–40.
57. Demirkesen I, Sumnu G, Sahin S, et al. Optimisation of formulations and infrared-microwave combination baking conditions of chestnut-rice breads. Int J Food Sci Technol. 2011;46:1809–15.
58. Vavreinova S, Ouhrabkova J, Paulickova I, et al. Gluten-free mixtures and their utilization in the special diet products. In: Proceedings of third international congress 'Flour-Bread 05' and fifth Croatian congress of cereal technologists, Opatija, 26–29 Oct 2005; 2006. p. 201–7.
59. Sanchez HD, Osella CA, de la Torre MA. Use of response surface methodology to optimize gluten-free bread fortified with soy flour and dry milk. Food Sci Technol Int. 2004;10:5–9.
60. Krupa-Kozak U, Troszynska A, Baczek N, et al. Effect of organic calcium supplements on the technological characteristic and sensory properties of gluten-free bread. Eur Food Res Technol. 2011;232:497–508.
61. Korus J, Grzelak K, Achremowicz K, et al. Influence of prebiotic additions on the quality of gluten-free bread and on the content of inulin and fructooligosaccharides. Food Sci Technol Int. 2006;12:489–95.

Chapter 25
Biofortified Rice to Fight Folate Deficiency

Dieter Blancquaert, Oscar Navarrete, Sergei Storozhenko, Hans De Steur, Jeroen Van Daele, Wei Dong, Cailin Lei, Chunyi Zhang, Christophe Stove, Xavier Gellynck, Jacques Viaene, Willy Lambert, and Dominique Van Der Straeten

Key Points

- Folates (vitamin B9) are essential for human health.
- Combating folate deficiency, a widespread phenomenon, is a major challenge in the twenty-first century.
- A thorough understanding of folate functions and its metabolism both in humans and in plants is indispensable for successfully reaching this goal.
- Folic acid supplementation and food fortification have been widely implemented so far, but recently some concern has been raised about their possible negative impact on human health.
- Folate biofortification of crops, and rice in particular, through metabolic engineering is a valuable alternative and/or complement in fighting folate deficiency, especially among poor and rural populations.

Keywords Folic acid • Folate • Fortification • Biofortification • Metabolic engineering • Neural tube defects • Rice

Abbreviations

10-FDF	10-FormylTHF deformylase
10-FS	10-FormylTHF synthase

D. Blancquaert • O. Navarrete, Ph.D. • S. Storozhenko, Ph.D. • D. Van Der Straeten, Ph.D. (✉)
Department of Physiology, Ghent University, K.L. Ledeganckstraat 35, Ghent 9000, Belgium
e-mail: dieter.blancquaert@ugent.be; Oscar.navarrete@ugent.be; Serguei.storojenko@ugent.be; dominique.vanderstraeten@ugent.be

H. De Steur, Ph.D. • X. Gellynck, Ph.D. • J. Viaene, Ph.D.
Department of Agricultural Economics, Ghent University, K.L. Ledeganckstraat 35, Ghent 9000, Belgium
e-mail: Hans.Desteur@ugent.be; Xavier.Gellynck@ugent.be; Jacques.Viaene@ugent.be

J. Van Daele • C. Stove, Ph.D. • W. Lambert, Ph.D.
Department of Bioanalysis, Ghent University, K.L. Ledeganckstraat 35, Ghent 9000, Belgium
e-mail: Jeroen.Vandaele@ugent.be; Christophe.Stove@ugent.be; Willy.Lambert@ugent.be

W. Dong, Ph.D. • C. Lei, Ph.D. • C. Zhang, Ph.D.
Chinese Academy of Agricultural Sciences, Beijing 100081, China
e-mail: sdu_dw@163.com; leicl@mail.caas.net.cn; Chunyi.Zhang@caas.net.cn

V.R. Preedy et al. (eds.), *Handbook of Food Fortification and Health: From Concepts to Public Health Applications Volume 1*, Nutrition and Health, DOI 10.1007/978-1-4614-7076-2_25,

ADC	Aminodeoxychorismate
ADCL	Aminodeoxychorismate lyase
ADCS	Aminodeoxychorismate synthase
C1	Carbon-one
DALY	Disability-adjusted life years
DHC	5,10-Methylene THF dehydrogenase/5,10-methenylTHF cyclohydrolase
DHF	Dihydrofolate
DHFR	Dihydrofolate reductase
DHFS	Dihydrofolate synthetase
DHNA	Dihydroneopterin aldolase
DHP	Dihydropteroate
DHPS	Dihydropteroate synthase
dTMP	Deoxythymidine monophosphate
dUTP	Deoxyuridine triphosphate
FA	Folic acid
FPGS	Folylpolyglutamate synthase
FW	Fresh weight
GDC	Glycine decarboxylation complex
Glb-1	Globulin-1
GluB1	Glutelin B1
GMO	Genetically modified organism
GRAS	Generally regarded as safe
GTP	Guanosine triphosphate
GTPCHI	Guanosine triphosphate cyclohydrolase 1
HMDHP	Hydroxymethyldihydropterin
HPPK	Dihydropterin pyrophosphokinase
MS	Methionine synthase
MTases	Methyltransferases
MTHFR	5,10-MethyleneTHF reductase
NTD	Neural tube defect
p-ABA	*Para*-aminobenzoate
RDI	Recommended/reference daily intake
SAH	*S*-adenosylhomocysteine
SAM	*S*-adenosylmethionine
SHMT	Serine hydroxymethyltransferase
THF	Tetrahydrofolate

Introduction

Folates are water-soluble tripartite B-vitamins (B9), which are important cofactors in C1 metabolism, where they act as one-carbon donors and acceptors [1–4]. They play an important role in DNA biosynthesis, methylation, histidine catabolism, and serine and glycine interconversion. Folates are also necessary in the biosynthesis of vitamin B5 (pantothenate). In plants, they are indispensable in photorespiration and, indirectly, through *S*-adenosylmethionine (SAM), in lignin, betaine, alkaloid, chlorophyll, and tocopherol biosynthesis [4, 5].

Only plants and micro-organisms are capable of synthesizing folates de novo. Therefore, humans rely entirely on their diet as the sole source of vitamin B9. Green leafy vegetables, certain fruits (such as oranges and strawberries), liver, eggs, and yeast are quite rich in folates, as well as beers, yoghurt, and other fermented products (although alcohol counteracts the intestinal folate uptake). It is worth mentioning that genetically modified micro-organisms can be used to biofortify fermented products [6]. Staple crops, such as rice and other cereals, potatoes, and bananas are very poor folate sources [7]. Hence, folate deficiency is an important problem in developing as well as in certain regions of developed countries [8]. It can cause a whole range of diseases and disorders, such as neural tube defects (NTDs, e.g., spina bifida and anencephaly) and megaloblastic anemia. An association between low folate status and neurodegenerative disorders, such as Alzheimer disease [9], stroke [10], and several cancers (e.g., leukemia, colorectal, breast, pancreatic, cervical, and bronchial cancer) [11] and a higher risk of cardiovascular diseases [12] have been reported. In this chapter, we focus on folate metabolism in plants, and on approaches for biofortification of staple crops through metabolic engineering. The different attempts made and suggested to fight folate deficiency are discussed, as well as recent progress made in biofortifying folates in food crops, in particular rice, and its importance, applicability, and acceptance to fight folate deficiency worldwide.

Chemical Properties of Folates and Folate Functions

Folates consist of a pteridine moiety, a *para*-aminobenzoate (*p*-ABA) ring and a tail of one or more γ-linked L-glutamates (Fig. 25.1). They comprise a family of related molecules, which can differ in their oxidation state, the attached one-carbon (C1) unit and the length of the glutamate tail. The different C1 units occur as methyl, methenyl, methylene, formyl, and formimino groups, each having specific functions in C1 metabolism. These C1 units can be attached to the pteridine ring (N5 position) and/or to *p*-ABA (N10 position). The most reduced folate form is tetrahydrofolate (THF), which can be further oxidized to folic acid (FA). The latter is commercially produced and considered to be nonexisting in

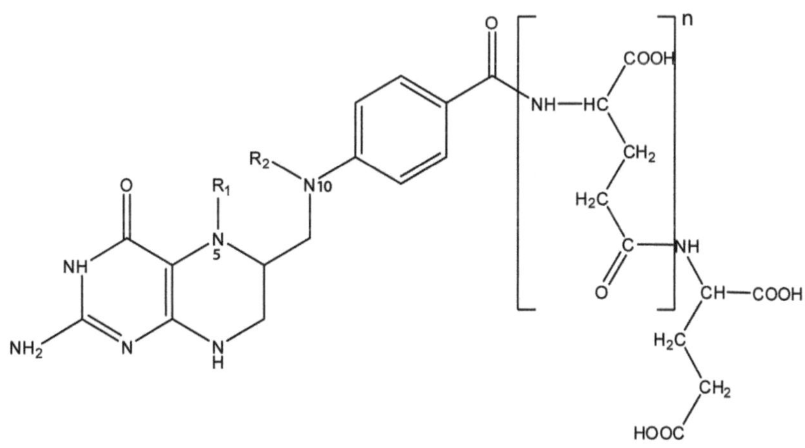

R_1	R_2	C1- unit
H	H	THF
CH_3	H	5 - methyl
CHO	H	5 - formyl
CH=NH	H	5 - formimino
H	CHO	10 - formyl
- CH_2 -		5,10 - methylene
= CH -		5,10 - methenyl

Fig. 25.1 The chemical structures of folates. The C1-unit is attached to the main structure at the pteridine ring (R1) and/or *p*-ABA (R2). Folates can differ in their oxidation state, the attached C1-unit, and the length of the glutamate tail

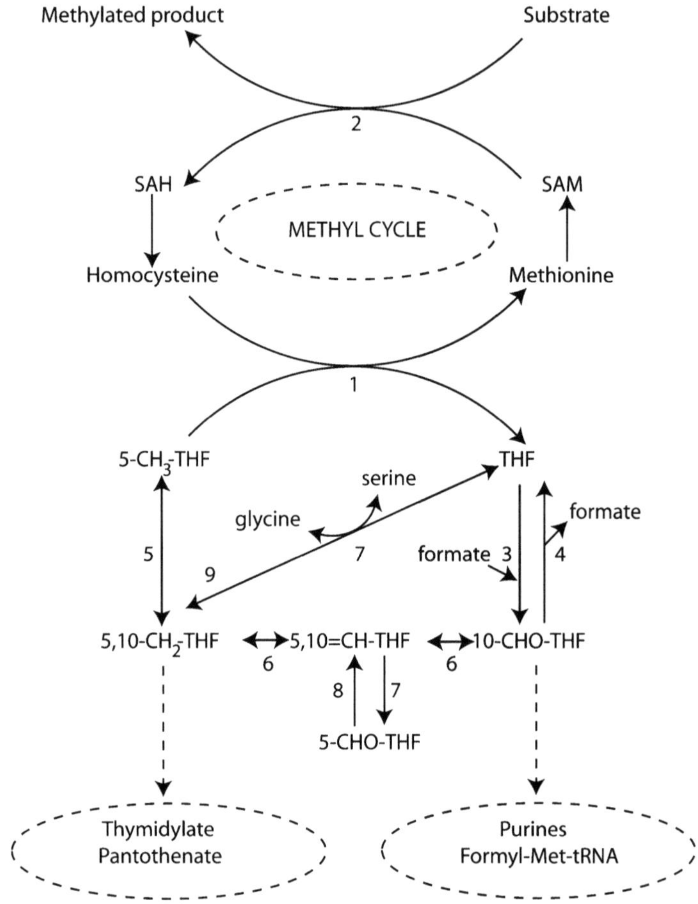

Fig. 25.2 Schematic overview of folate metabolism and functions (in *dashed ovals*) in C1-metabolism. Folate forms: 5-CH_3-THF, 5-methylTHF; 5,10-CH_2-THF, 5,10-methyleneTHF; 5,10=CH-THF, 5,10-methenylTHF; 10-CHO-THF, 10-formylTHF; 5-CHO-THF, 5-formylTHF. Enzymes: 1, methionine synthase (MS); 2, methyltransferases (MTases); 3, 10-formylTHF synthase (10-FS); 4, 10-formylTHF deformylase (10-FDF); 5, 5,10-methyleneTHF reductase (MTHFR); 6, 5,10-methyleneTHF dehydrogenase/5,10-methenylTHF cyclohydrolase (DHC); 7, serine hydroxymethyl transferase (SHMT); 8, 5-formylTHF cycloligase (5-FCL); 9, glycine decarboxylation complex (GDC)

nature. When taken up by the body, FA is reduced to dihydrofolate (DHF) and subsequently to THF in the gut mucosa, rendering it biologically active. It will then be further converted to 5-methylTHF [1]. The glutamate tail can reach a length up to 14 glutamate moieties [2] and plays an important role in cellular and subcellular folate retention. Moreover, the length of the glutamate tail correlates with the binding with folate-dependent enzymes (with the exception of folate transporters) and hence enzyme activity [4]. Upon consumption, folate polyglutamates are converted to monoglutamates in the intestinal brush border, from where they are transported to the rest of the body. Upon arrival in the different tissues, they are reconverted to polyglutamylated folates.

Folates are important cofactors in different aspects of C1 metabolism, such as the methyl cycle and the biosynthesis of DNA and pantothenate (Fig. 25.2). 5-MethylTHF donates its methyl group to homocysteine, which leads to the formation of methionine. This reaction is mediated by the cobalamin (vitamin B12)-dependent enzyme methionine synthase. Methionine is further converted to SAM, which will be used in the methylation of an onset of substrates, such as lipids, DNA, hormones, and proteins. 10-FormylTHF is of great importance in the biosynthesis of purines and formyl-methionine-tRNA, whereas 5,10-methyleneTHF is necessary in the formation of thymidine (TMP) from uracil (UMP), a reaction catalyzed by thymidylate synthase, and the biosynthesis of pantothenate. 5,10-MethyleneTHF acts together with THF as a cofactor in the interconversion of glycine and serine, reactions mediated by serine hydroxymethyltransferase (SHMT) and the glycine decarboxylation complex (GDC). Upon histidine catabolization, 5-formiminoTHF is formed, which is further converted to 5,10-methenylTHF. These two reactions, which are not proven to exist in plants, are mediated by the bifunctional enzyme formiminotransferase cyclodeaminase. So far, the function of

5-formylTHF in C1 metabolism is unknown. Since this is one of the folates with the highest stability, it is thought to be an important folate storage form [2]. Depending on the demands, interconversions between different folate species can occur, providing high plasticity to the folate pool.

Folate Biosynthesis

Only bacteria, fungi, and plants are capable of synthesizing folates. In plants, the biosynthesis is characterized by a compartmentalization in three subcellular locations: the cytosol, the plastids, and the mitochondria (Fig. 25.3). A total of seven reactions are required to obtain THF, similar to those in micro-organisms.

Pteridine is synthesized in the cytosol from guanosine triphosphate (GTP). Four subsequent reactions are necessary to form hydroxymethyldihydropterin (HMDHP). The first step is mediated by guanosine triphosphate cyclohydrolase 1 (GTPCHI), an enzyme which forms dihydroneopterin triphosphate [13, 14]. The plant enzyme is considered to be directly feedback inhibited [15], while the mammalian counterpart requires feedback regulatory proteins for feedback regulation [16]. The following two reactions are required to remove the triphosphate group. First, a nudix aldolase ensures the cleavage of the pyrophosphate group. Second, the remaining phosphate group is removed by a nonspecific phosphatase with dihydroneopterin as the product of this reaction. The latter is converted to HMDHP by dihydroneopterin aldolase (DHNA).

The second building block, *p*-ABA, is produced in the plastids from chorismate in two reactions. Aminodeoxychorismate (ADC) is formed as an intermediate by aminodeoxychorismate synthase (ADCS). With the exception of prokaryotic ADCS, this enzyme is inhibited by methotrexate, which makes it a suitable candidate for anti-folate drugs [17]. Aminodeoxychorismate lyase (ADCL) uses ADC as a substrate to form *p*-ABA. In plants, most of the free *p*-ABA is enzymatically converted to its β-D-glucopyranosylester [18]. This reaction is reversible. Since 88 % of the esterified *p*-ABA is located in the vacuoles, it is considered to be an important *p*-ABA storage form [18, 19].

The actual folate formation occurs in the mitochondria. HMDHP and *p*-ABA are condensed with the formation of dihydropteroate (DHP) by a bifunctional enzyme. First, HMDHP is activated by addition of a pyrophosphate group, a reaction which is catalyzed by dihydropterin pyrophosphokinase

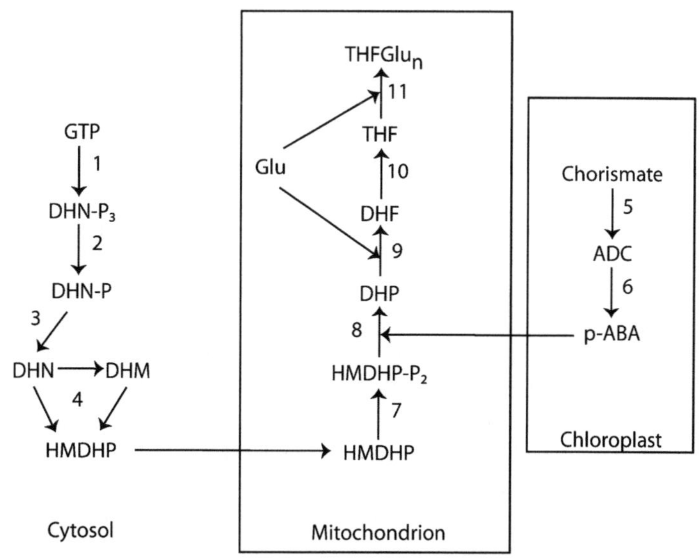

Fig. 25.3 Schematic representation of folate biosynthesis and its compartmentalization. *p*-ABA is synthesized in the plastids, pteridine in the cytosol, and both are condensed to form THF in the mitochondria. Enzymes: *1* GTPCHI; *2* dihydroneopterin triphosphate pyrophosphatase; *3* nonspecific phosphatase; *4* DHNA; *5* ADCS; *6* ADCL; *7* HPPK; *8* DHPS; *9* DHFS; *10* DHFR; *11* FPGS

(HPPK). The condensation itself is mediated by dihydropteroate synthase (DHPS). This reaction is feedback inhibited by its product and the monoglutamate forms of DHP and THF, thus considered to be a regulatory point of plant folate biosynthesis [20]. Interestingly, a cytosolic isoform of HPPK/DHPS was found in Arabidopsis, which could play a role in stress response [21]. Next, a first glutamate unit is attached to DHP, producing DHF. This mitochondrial reaction is catalyzed by dihydrofolate synthetase (DHFS). A reduction of DHF is mediated by dihydrofolate reductase (DHFR) to form THF monoglutamate. Polyglutamylation takes place in the cytosol, mitochondria, and plastids by the action of different isoforms of folylpolyglutamate synthase (FPGS).

Folate Deficiency

Folate deficiency can cause an onset of numerous health problems. Megaloblastic anemia results from aberrant maturation of the bone marrow and impaired development of erythrocytes, in which folates are very important. NTDs comprise a whole range of congenital malformations, resulting from incomplete neurulation. The best known examples are encephalocele (1.20/10,000 births), spina bifida (5.01/10,000 births), and anencephaly (3.83/10,000 births) (figure pertain to Europe) [8]. Encephalocele is a condition in which the failure of the neural tube to close completely results in protrusions of the brain and/or its covering membranes through openings in the skull. Spina bifida occurs when the neural tube fails to close completely and the overlying vertebral arches fail to develop. Anencephaly is a disorder in which the brain represents an exposed mass of undifferentiated tissue. In most of the cases, anencephalic embryos will be liveborn, but die soon after birth. Several studies, conducted in the developed world, reported on a higher prevalence of NTD's among light-skinned populations, most likely because people with a deeply melanized skin profit a higher protection against folate photolysis, caused by UV radiation [22]. Indeed, this hypothesis was supported by a study, in which the mothers of NTD babies appeared to be exposed to UV light in tanning salons during the first weeks of their pregnancy [23]. A causal relationship between NTD occurrence and folate deficiency has been established and several studies showed a great reduction of NTD frequency upon FA supplementation and fortification [24]. Similar to the role of folates in embryonic development, their importance in spermatogenesis has been shown, suggesting the use of anti-folate drugs as contraceptives [22]. Other conditions have been proven to occur more often with low folate status. The underlying mechanisms of these conditions are still unclear, but in general they can be divided in three groups by cause: homocysteinemia, hypomethylation, and a shortage of deoxythymidine monophosphate (dTMP). Homocysteine is converted to methionine in the methyl cycle, in which folates play an important role as cofactors. Inadequate folate intake can thus cause high levels of homocysteine, a condition which is called homocysteinemia. This is known to be correlated with higher risk to stroke [10], coronary, and cardiovascular diseases [12]. A combination of folate deficiency and high homocysteine levels can cause susceptibility to β-amyloid toxicity in hippocampal neurons, which possibly acts as a trigger for Alzheimer disease [25]. It can also induce Alzheimer disease pathogenesis by being a risk factor for cerebrovascular disease [26]. Concurrent with these high homocysteine levels, methionine concentrations, and SAM levels are considerably low, resulting in a lower capacity of the organism to methylate DNA and other substrates. This hypomethylation can change the expression of certain oncogenes and thus result in a whole range of cancers [11]. Since folates are necessary in the biosynthesis of dTMP, folate deficiency triggers the incorporation of deoxyuridine triphosphate (dUTP) during DNA duplication. Transient nicks in DNA strands made in order to repair the uracil mis-incorporation might lead to point mutations, chromosomal damage, and breakage [27]. Although a causal relationship remains to be proven, it has been suggested that an adequate intake of folate can prevent these diseases and disorders [28].

The recommended daily intake (RDI) of folates is 400 μg for adults and 600 μg for pregnant women. Since most of the diets provide approximately 200 μg/day [1], folate deficiency is a global

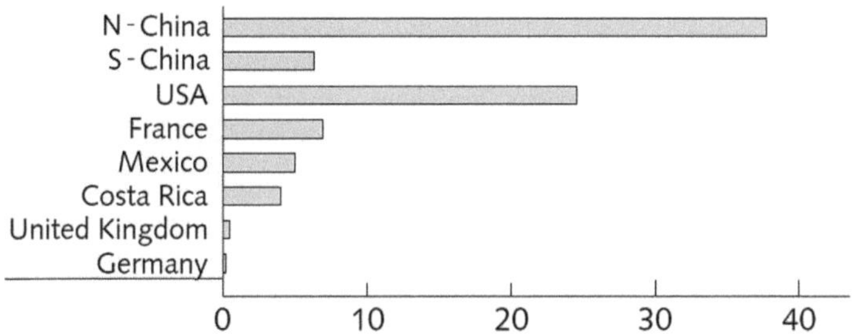

Fig. 25.4 Folate deficiency is a global problem, affecting both developing and developed countries. Percentage of adults with folate deficiency in eight countries (*X*-axis). For Costa Rica and United States, values before the fortification program are shown. Calculations for China are based on previous reports [59, 60]

problem (Fig. 25.4). It manifests in the Western world, where related congenital disorders show an increased region-specific prevalence [8, 29]. The consequences of low folate intake in the developing world have been studied in detail in Asian countries such as China, Japan, and India. In Shanxi, a province in Northern China, NTD incidence is 10 times higher than in the Western world (up to 199.38 in 10,000 live births), with anencephaly occurring most (41.4 %), followed by spina bifida (19.5 %) [30, 31]. Similar results have been reported in the Balrumpur district in India (NTD prevalence rate of 65.7–82.1/10,000 live births) [32]. In Japan, between 1994 and 2003, the occurrence of NTDs ranged from 3.58 to 5.12/10,000 births [33].

There are several ways to fight folate deficiency. Dietary diversification, enriching a diet with folate rich food sources, requires educational efforts and changes in dietary habits. However, due to the accessibility and affordability of folate rich products, this strategy is less successful in practice [34].

Intake of folic acid supplements before and during pregnancy to prevent NTDs can be useful, but shows limited and often temporary success in practice. The neural tube is formed after 21–27 days upon fertilization. Ideally, women should take folic acid pills on a regular basis from the peri-conceptional phase until 3 months of pregnancy. However, women's pregnancy awareness often occurs far beyond neural tube formation. Moreover, studies showed that approximately half of the pregnancies in the United States are unplanned [4], making folic acid supplementation alone insufficient to prevent NTDs on a broader scale. In addition, FA supplementation targets a specific population group and is often unavailable in rural areas of developing countries.

Fortification of food with folic acid is a widely used strategy to fight folate deficiency. Since 1998, fortification of cereal-based food such as pasta, breakfast cereals, cornmeal, and flour is mandatory in the United States and Canada [35]. Later, this policy was adopted by other countries worldwide. Predictions showed that globally approximately 250,000 children could be saved with fortification [36]. Indeed, NTD prevalence rates dropped significantly with 20–53 % for spina bifida and 38 % for anencephaly [37, 38]. In Chile, NTD occurrence decreased with 43 % since the start of the fortification program [38]. The goal was to reach a daily intake of 100 μg of folic acid. Analysis of the effects of the FA fortification program in Canada revealed that folate levels in the circulatory system of test persons raised continuously and did not stabilize, even after 6 years of FA fortification [39]. Moreover, blood homocysteine levels dropped shortly after the start of the fortification program, albeit a temporary effect [39].

Nevertheless, the opinion on whether FA fortification should be mandatory or not differs greatly among scientists and policy makers. Although beneficial effects on NTD prevalence rates have been convincingly proven, its influence on other diseases and disorders is highly debated. For instance, possible associations between high folic acid intake and an increased risk on colorectal and prostate cancer have been suggested [40]. In this respect, the timing of folic acid supplementation is extremely important to ensure a protective effect against cancer. On the other hand, a worrisome increase in prescribed dosage of the anti-folate drug methotrexate to fight rheumatoid arthritis, cancer, and psoriasis, has been reported, indicating a reduction of effectiveness of anti-folate medication upon folic acid food fortification [41]. Moreover, folic acid fortification has apparently no effect on ischemic heart disease incidence [42]. In seniors, high serum folate levels in combination with low vitamin B12 status were associated with cognitive impairment and anemia [43]. Very high folic acid intake (>1 mg/day) may even camouflage the diagnosis of vitamin B12 deficiency [44]. Upon intake of folic acid in a single dose of more than 300 μg, the excess cannot be converted to the biologically active 5-methylTHF and will appear unaltered in the body [1]. The effects of this phenomenon are not completely elucidated, but it was suggested to promote tumor growth and mask pernicious anemia, when combined with vitamin B12 deficiency [1]. From a practical point of view, specialized infrastructure and control mechanisms are necessary to successfully apply folic acid fortification. Therefore, fighting folate deficiency by folic acid supplementation and food fortification can be quite easily implemented in developed countries, but is less suitable for developing countries.

Increasing the natural folate content in staple crops using biotechnology or conventional plant breeding can offer an alternative, or at least a complement to the abovementioned strategies. Moreover, since folic acid and natural folates influence folate metabolism differently [45], the adverse effects of folic acid intake possibly do not occur with folate biofortified food. Indeed, a study of 25,000 postmenopausal women clearly showed a higher risk of breast cancer (32 % increase) upon high doses of folic acid supplementation, an effect not observed with natural folates from food [46].

Folate Biofortification

Folate biofortification can theoretically be achieved in two ways: by traditional plant breeding and by metabolic engineering. Classical breeding has been used over a thousand of years by farmers, horticulturists, and scientists. It involves interbreeding to produce new cultivars with desirable characteristics. Since crossing is only possible between closely related species natural variation can be quite limited for some traits, such as vitamin levels. This is the main disadvantage of the method, besides being very time consuming. Nowadays, traditional breeding can be simplified and accelerated through the mapping of quantitative trait loci (QTL), in combination with a molecular marker-assisted selection. However, QTLs have not been used in enhancing crop folate levels so far. In order to create a basis for breeding wheat with an enhanced folate content, natural variation of total folate content was investigated in 130 winter and 20 spring genotypes of bread wheat [47]. A twofold variation was observed in both wheat types, with folate content in winter wheat ranging from 36.4 to 77.4 μg/100 g dry weight and in spring genotypes from 32.3 to 74.1 μg/100 g dry weight. A twofold difference was also observed in 12 greenhouse-grown rice varieties, with the highest levels found in the Blue belle variety (having a folate content of 68 μg/100 g fresh weight, FW) and the lowest in Rok 5 (32 μg/100 g FW) [4]. These data suggest that folate biofortification through classical breeding is not sufficient, at least in wheat and rice, to meet the recommended daily dose.

Folate biofortification through metabolic engineering appeared a feasible solution to enhance natural folate levels in crops. In this approach folate biosynthesis enzymes were overexpressed to create an efficient flux towards folate accumulation. Initially, it was suggested that GTPCHI, the first enzyme in the pteridine branch of folate biosynthesis, was a rate-limiting step, thus overexpression was expected to result in higher folate levels. GTPCHI overexpressor lines were created in Arabidopsis [48], tomato [49], lettuce [50], and white corn [51]. To avoid a possible feedback inhibition, the bacterial FolE gene from Escherichia coli was overexpressed in Arabidopsis. Although pteridine levels in transgenic lines were 750–1,250-fold higher than in control lines (mainly attributed by neopterin, which was enhanced 1,100-fold), folate levels raised only two- to fourfold, with a maximum of 3.4 nmol/g fresh weight. Tomato has also been subjected to folate biofortification attempts because of its global importance as a staple crop and its low folate content. Overexpression of a synthetic gene, based on mammalian GTPCHI, under the control of the fruit-specific E8 promotor resulted in a 3–140-fold increase of pteridines, mainly neopterin, monapterin, hydroxymethylpterin (an oxidation product of the folate biosynthesis intermediate HMDHP) and pteridine glycosides, the latter not previously reported to occur in plants. Folate levels increased moderately, with a twofold difference compared to empty-vector controls, with a maximum of 4 nmol/g FW. This equals approximately 180 μg/100 g, which is supposed to meet child folate requirements, but only half of the RDI of adults. The main folate forms present in transgenic as well as in control lines were 5-methylTHF and 5,10-methenylTHF. Interestingly, the highest folate content was observed in transgenic lines with moderate pteridine levels. Moreover, fruit that was allowed to ripen on the plant contained much more folate than those ripened after harvesting, most likely owing to folate degradation in the latter. More recently, a codon-optimized gchI gene, based on the native chicken (Gallus gallus) GTPCHI gene, was overexpressed in lettuce. Folate content in the transgenic lines was 2.1–8.5 times higher than in control lines, with a maximum folate concentration of 188.5 μg/100 g FW. Since a single serving contains approximately 56 g of lettuce, this would account for 26 % of the RDI. Although data on pteridine content were not reported, it can be predicted that a massive accumulation of pteridines occurs in this transgenic lettuce. Finally, a transgenic multivitamin white corn was created with enhanced levels of β-carotene, ascorbate, and folate. Overexpression of *Escherichia coli* FolE gene under the control of the endosperm specific barley D-hordein promotor doubled folate levels up to 1.94 μg/g dry weight [51].

In GTPCHI overexpressing tomato fruits, a depletion of the *p*-ABA pool was observed, with 90–97 % being used for folate synthesis [49]. Together, these findings showed that the *p*-ABA branch of the folate biosynthesis pathway represents a second limiting step towards high folate accumulation in staple crops. Indeed, when *p*-ABA was exogenously supplied to ripening tomatoes, harvested at breaker stage, total folate levels were 2.5–10-fold enhanced [49]. Consequently, a second round of engineering involved the overexpression of both ADCS, the first enzyme in the *p*-ABA branch of folate biosynthesis, and GTPCHI. Transgenic tomato lines were created overexpressing Arabidopsis cDNA encoding ADCS, under the control of the fruit-specific E8 promotor [52]. These tomatoes showed no significant enhancement in folate content, but a 19-fold raise of *p*-ABA levels (56 nmol/g fresh weight) compared to the empty-vector controls. Interestingly, approximately 85 % of the accumulating *p*-ABA was conjugated as a glucose ester. Upon crossing these lines with the previously obtained GTPCHI overexpressor tomato lines, a folate content up to 840 μg/100 g fresh weight was obtained, which is approximately 25-fold higher than in control fruit and sufficient to meet adult folate requirements in less than one standard serving. 5-MethylTHF was the predominant folate form. Interestingly, *p*-ABA and pteridine levels were still high in these folate enhanced lines, suggesting another flux constraint in folate biosynthesis in tomato fruit. Since DHF, DHP, and HMDHP pyrophosphate did not accumulate, HPPK is most likely the bottleneck in folate overproduction in tomato. Other possible explanations are an insufficient transport of pteridines into the mitochondria and the fast oxidation of pteridines, making them incapable to enter the folate biosynthesis pathway. Most of the folates accumulating in these tomatoes were monoglutamylated, whereas the majority of folates in the control fruit were polyglutamylated. In parallel with the biofortified tomato lines, a successful folate enhancement in rice seeds was reported [53]. Rice is one of the most important staple crops, being the main source of carbohydrates for half of the world population. Rice, and cereals in general, are poor in vitamins and micronutrients. Moreover, upon milling, the hull, bran, and germ are removed, improving rice storage. However, most of the vitamins and nutrients are present in the bran (pericarp and aleurone layer), thus milling lowers the nutritional value of the seeds. Therefore, the aim was to accumulate folates in the remaining rice endosperm. This was assured by the use of endosperm specific promoters. Rice was transformed with three different constructs: Arabidopsis cDNA encoding GTPCHI under the control of the globulin-1 (Glb-1) promoter (G lines), ADCS driven by the glutelin B1 (GluB1) promoter (A lines), and a single T-DNA locus containing both genes (GA lines). Although no difference in folate content was observed in G-lines, pteridines highly accumulated (up to 25-fold higher than in wild type and empty-vector controls), neopterin being the main contributor to the pteridine pool (approximately 70 %). Rice A-lines showed 49-fold higher *p*-ABA levels than the control lines. Interestingly, total folate levels in these lines were 6 times lower than in wild type seeds, suggesting a possible inhibitory effect of *p*-ABA and its intermediates on folate biosynthesis. Since this phenomenon was not observed in the folate biofortified tomatoes, different folate biosynthesis regulatory mechanisms may occur in these two species. The GA transgenic rice lines showed no phenotypic difference with wild type and empty-vector control plants, while displaying a massive folate enhancement up to 1,723 μg/100 g of polished raw seeds, which is 100 times higher than the wild type and empty-vector control. The main folate form found in GA lines is 5-methylTHF, which accounts for 89 % of the folate pool. A 100 g of GA rice contained up to 4 times the adult RDI. Taken into account that 45 % of folates are lost during 30 min of cooking and an estimated bioavailability of approximately 50 % [53], a single standard serving is still sufficient to meet the adult daily requirements and almost that of pregnant women. Regardless the high folate levels, considerable amounts of *p*-ABA were present in GA rice. However, the *p*-ABA concentrations were twice as low as in the A-lines and 4.5–10 times lower than in folate engineered tomato. Theoretically, this should not pose a concern for human health, since *p*-ABA is listed as a GRAS (generally regarded as safe) compound with a daily intake limit of 30 mg, while a single serving of the best performing GA line only corresponds to a *p*-ABA intake of 0.17 mg. Moreover, some vegetables, such as Brussels sprouts, naturally contain high *p*-ABA concentrations. Pteridine levels were fourfold higher in folate biofortified rice as compared to wild type and empty-vector controls. However, they were still much lower than in G-lines and in engineered tomato. In conclusion, possible health issues, caused by the presence of folate biosynthesis intermediates upon consumption of GA rice, are assumed to be extremely low. Since *p*-ABA and pteridine levels in GA rice are considerably lower than in biofortified tomato, the flux towards folate in transgenic rice is presumably stronger than in engineered tomato. Moreover, since a plant GTPCHI was successfully applied in these transgenic rice lines, the use of a mammalian or bacterial GTPCHI gene to prevent inhibitory feedback control in plants is questionable. Altogether, the folate content in folate biofortified rice is the highest reported in plants.

Implementation of Folate Biofortified Rice

One of the biggest advantages using biofortification of crops to fight folate deficiency is that there are no recurrent costs; seeds can be harvested and resown each growth season and there is no need for a specialized infrastructure. Moreover, consumers do not have to change their dietary habits. Therefore, this strategy can reach poor and rural populations who would gain most profit upon consumption of folate biofortified crops. Cultivation of different rice varieties can differ regionally and it is known that farmers stay quite loyal to the locally grown varieties. Therefore, it is important to introduce the beneficial traits of the folate biofortified prototypes into these local rice varieties, in order to gain both farmer's and consumer's acceptance. The engineered rice line with the highest folate content, originally created in Oryza sativa ssp. japonica cv. Nippon Bare, was crossed with four other commonly consumed japonica varieties: Jijing 88, Kong Yu 131, Liaojing 9, and Xu Dao 38 (Fig. 25.5). Folate content in the F2 of each crossed variety was measured and ranged between approximately 200 and 500 μg/100 g of unpolished rice seeds. These levels are lower than in the original GA Nippon Bare lines, most likely because of folate degradation between harvest and analysis. Nevertheless, these data prove that folate biofortification of local rice was successful and can be implemented to fight folate deficiency worldwide, even in developed countries, where they can be used as a complementary strategy next to food fortification and folic acid supplementation.

Studies on the possible impact of folate biofortified rice on global folate deficiency are limited, but quite promising. Since prevalence data of other diseases and disorders linked to inadequate folate consumption are scarce, and scientists and policy makers mainly focus on alleviation of NTDs, the latter was used as a proxy to measure the benefits of folate engineered rice. The theoretically

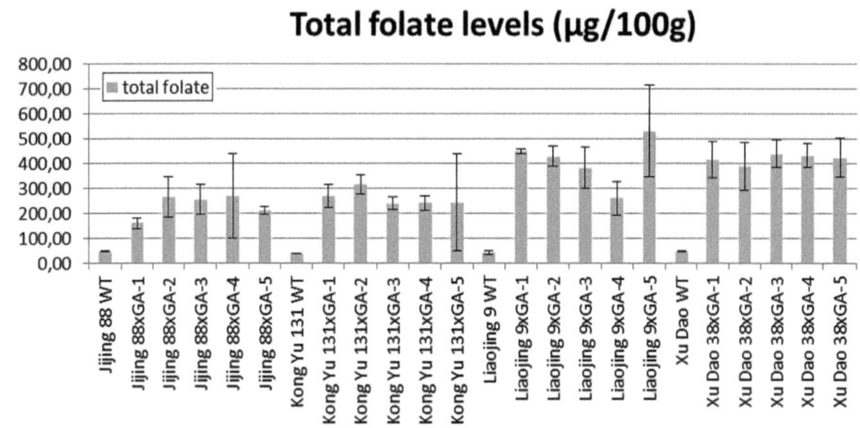

Fig. 25.5 Four local rice japonica varieties were crossed with folate biofortified rice (GA-line). Seed folate content (in µg/100 g FW) of five individual F2 plants, originating from the same cross, of each variety was measured and compared to wild type (WT) levels. Error bars indicate standard deviations ($n = 2$)

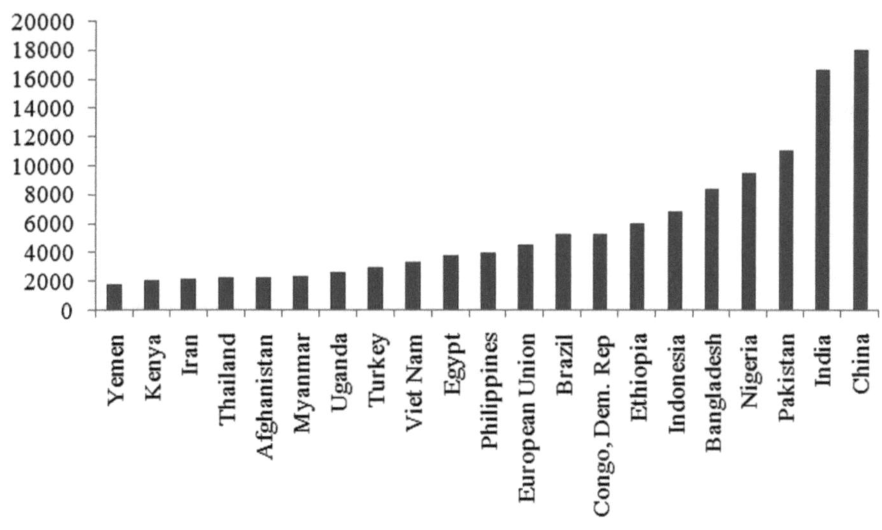

Fig. 25.6 The top 20 countries with the highest annual neural tube defect (NTD) prevalence [32, 61, 62]. On the *Y*-axis, the annual estimated number of NTDs is shown. Asian countries are the most affected, with China and India on top

calculated impact of this introduction[1] is expressed in terms of DALYs (disability-adjusted life years). This equals the sum of the "years lived with disability" and "years of life lost". Globally, folate deficiency accounts for 2.3 million DALYs lost per year [54] (Fig. 25.6). A recent study on six regions in China showed that the current burden (expressed as annual DALYs lost) in northern China is significantly higher than in southern China [55]. Nine hundred and forty-four face-to-face interviews with rice consumers in the Shanxi province were taken and revealed that 62.2 % of the persons questioned were willing to accept folate engineered rice and 34 % even wants to pay more for it [56]. The acceptance rate for female rice consumers is 55.4 %. Altogether, this means that introduction of folate biofortified rice could save between 3,443 and 3,705 births (on a total of 394,674 births [57]) from a NTD, which accounts for a theoretical reduction of 44–47 % of the latter.

[1] For more information on the implementation of folate biofortified rice, we refer to the contribution of De Steur et al. in this handbook.

Guidance on Safe Levels

Although an increasing number of studies report on possible negative effects of FA overconsumption, advised upper thresholds of natural folate intake are still lacking. Folate instability, losses during processing and bioavailability at least quarters the amount of folate taken up by the body. Therefore, the highest folate levels obtained in biofortified rice should not be the subject of concern. Nevertheless, if future data contradict this hypothesis, engineered rice lines with intermediate folate levels can be adopted.

Recommendations

Over the past 15 years the importance of folate deficiency on global public health was realized, documented, and mapped. Different folic acid food fortification policies have been implemented in the Western world, with promising results. Nevertheless, a great deal of concern rises upon the possible adverse effects of folic acid fortification. Therefore, it is extremely important to investigate the beneficial as well as the negative effects of FA fortification on human health. Biofortification is most likely the best intervention to combat folate deficiency in poor and rural regions of the world. However, policy changes, proper education, and an affordable implementation are necessary to successfully reach this goal. Even though possible negative impacts of folate biofortified food consumption on human health are considered to be much less than FA supplementation and food fortification, profound research in this matter is of utmost importance. Since many food crops are poor in vitamins and nutrients, it is desirable to create "nutritionally complete crops." The transgenic multivitamin corn [51] is a first prototype, but there is still a long way to go. Nevertheless, a multi-biofortification approach would be a highly cost-effective intervention [58] to expel global nutrient deficiency.

Conclusions

The second generation of genetically modified organisms (GMOs) is ready to reach consumers all over the world and to improve their nutrition. In particular, folate biofortified rice can save and ameliorate a huge number of lives, especially in the poorest regions in the world.

Acknowledgement Ghent University and the Fund for Scientific Research-Flanders are gratefully acknowledged for financial support to DVDS, WL, and JV (Bijzonder Onderzoeksfonds-GOA-1251204, GOA 2009-004, and G.0126.09). DB is a researcher of the Fund for Scientific Research-Flanders.

References

1. Scott J, Rébeillé F, Fletcher J. Folic acid and folate: the feasibility for nutritional enhancement in plant foods. J Sci Food Agric. 2000;80:795–824.
2. Rébeillé F, Ravanel S, Jabrin S, et al. Folates in plants: biosynthesis, distribution and enhancement. Physiol Plant. 2006;126:330–42.
3. Bekaert S, Storozhenko S, Mehrsahi P, et al. Folate biofortification in food plants. Trends Plant Sci. 2008;13:28–34.
4. Blancquaert D, Storozhenko S, Loizeau K, et al. Folates and folic acid: from fundamental research toward sustainable health. Crit Rev Plant Sci. 2010;29:14–35.

5. Mène-Saffrané L, DellaPenna D. Biosynthesis, regulation and functions of tocochromanols in plants. Plant Physiol Biochem. 2010;48:301–9.
6. Rossi M, Amaretti A, Raimondi S. Folate production by probiotic bacteria. Nutrients. 2011;3:118–34.
7. USDA National Nutrient Database for Standard References. http://www.nal.usda.gov/fnic/foodcomp/search/. Accessed 3 Oct 2011.
8. European Surveillance of Congenital Anomalies. http://www.eurocat-network.eu/. Accessed 16 Nov 2011.
9. Seshadri S, Beiser A, Selhub J, et al. Plasma homocysteine as a risk factor for dementia and Alzheimer's disease. N Engl J Med. 2002;346:476–83.
10. Wald NJ, Watt HC, Law MR, et al. Homocysteine and ischaemic heart disease: results of a prospective study with implications on prevention. Arch Intern Med. 1998;158:862–7.
11. Choi SW, Friso S. Interactions between folate and aging for carcinogenesis. Clin Chem Lab Med. 2005;43:1151–7.
12. Stanger O. The potential role of homocysteine in percutaneous coronary interventions (PCI): review of current evidence and plausibility of action. Cell Mol Biol. 2004;50:953–88.
13. Fan CL, Brown GM. Partial purification and properties of guanosine triphosphate cyclohydrolase from Drosophila melanogaster. Biochem Genet. 1976;14:259–70.
14. Basset G, Quinlivan EP, Ziemak MJ, et al. Folate synthesis in plants: the first step of the pterin branch is mediated by a unique bimodular GTP cyclohydrolase I. Proc Natl Acad Sci U S A. 2002;99:12489–94.
15. Sohta Y, Ohta T, Masada M. Purification and some properties of GTP cyclohydrolase I from spinach leaves. Biosci Biotechnol Biochem. 1997;61:1081–5.
16. Yoneyama T, Hatakeyama K. Decameric GTP cyclohydrolase I forms complexes with two pentameric GTPCH feedback regulatory proteins in the presence of phenylalanine or of a combination of BH 4 and GTP. J Biol Chem. 1998;273:20102–8.
17. Sahr T, Ravanel S, Basset G, et al. Folate synthesis in plants: purification, kinetic properties, and inhibition of aminodeoxychorismate synthase. Biochem J. 2006;396:157–62.
18. Quinlivan EP, Roje S, Basset G, et al. The folate precursor p-aminobenzoate is reversibly converted to its glucose ester in the plant cytosol. J Biol Chem. 2003;278:20731–7.
19. Eudes A, Bozzo GG, Waller JC, et al. Metabolism of the folate precursor p-aminobenzoate in plants. Glucose ester formation and vacuolar storage. J Biol Chem. 2008;283:15451–9.
20. Mouillon JM, Ravanel S, Douce R, et al. Folate synthesis in higher plant mitochondria: coupling between the dihydropterin pyrophosphokinase and the dihydropteroate synthase activities. Biochem J. 2002;363:313–9.
21. Navarrete O, Van Daele J, Stove C, et al. A folate independent role for cytosolic HPPK/DHPS upon stress in Arabidopsis thaliana. Phytochemistry. 2012;73(1):23–33. doi:10.1016/j.phytochem.2011.09.008.
22. Jablowski NG, Chaplin G. The evolution of skin coloration. J Hum Evol. 2000;39:57–106.
23. Lapunzina P. Ultraviolet light-related neural tube defects? Am J Med Genet. 1996;67:106.
24. Lumley J, Watson L, Watson M, et al. Periconceptional supplementation with folate and/or multivitamins for preventing neural tube defects. Cochrane Database Syst Rev. 2001;(3):CD001056.
25. Kruman II, Kumaravel TS, Lohani A, et al. Folic acid deficiency and homocysteine impair DNA repair in hippocampal neurons and sensitize them to amyloid toxicity in experimental models of Alzheimer's disease. J Neurosci. 2002;22:1752–62.
26. Seshadri S, Wolf PA. Homocysteine and the brain: vascular risk factor or neurotoxin? Lancet Neurol. 2003;2:11.
27. Blount BC, Mack MM, Wehr CM, et al. Folate deficiency causes uracil misincorporation into human DNA and chromosome breakage: implications for cancer and neuronal damage. Proc Natl Acad Sci U S A. 1997; 94:3290–5.
28. Berry RJ, Li Z. Folic acid alone prevents neural tube defects: evidence from the China study [letter]. Epidemiology. 2002;13:114–6.
29. EUROCAT Database. http://www.bio-medical.co.uk/eurocatlive. Accessed 6 Oct 2011.
30. Li ZW, Ren AG, Zhang L, et al. Extremely high prevalence of neural tube defects in a 4-county area in Shanxi Province, China. Birth Defects Res A Clin Mol Teratol. 2006;76:237–40.
31. Gu X, Lin L, Zheng X, et al. High prevalence of NTDs in Shanxi Province: a combined epidemiological approach. Birth Defects Res A Clin Mol Teratol. 2007;79:702–7.
32. Cherian A, Seena S, Bullock RK, et al. Incidence of neural tube defects in the least-developed area of India: a population-based study. Lancet. 2005;366:930–1.
33. Matsuzaki M, Haruna M, Ota E, et al. Dietary folate intake, use of folate supplements, lifestyle factors, and serum folate levels among pregnant women in Tokyo, Japan. J Obstet Gynaecol Res. 2008;34:971–9.
34. CDC. CDC grand rounds: additional opportunities to prevent neural tube defects with folic acid fortification. MMWR Morb Mortal Wkly Rep. 2010;59:980–4.
35. Food and Drug Administration. Food standards: amendments of standards of identity for enriched grain products to require addition of folic acid. Final Rule 21 CFR Parts 136, 137, 139. Fed Regist. 1996;61:8781–807.
36. Bell KN, Oakley GP. Tracing the prevention of folic acid-preventable spina bifida and anencephaly. Birth Defects Res A Clin Mol Teratol. 2006;76A:654–7.

37. De Wals P, Tairou F, Van Allen MI, et al. Reduction in neural-tube defects after folic acid fortification in Canada. N Engl J Med. 2007;357:135–42.
38. Wald NJ, Oakley GP. Should folic acid fortification be mandatory? Yes. Br Med J. 2007;334:1252.
39. Garcia AA, Day AG, Zanibbi K, et al. Longterm effects of folic acid fortification and B-vitamin supplementation on total folate, homocysteine, methylmalonic acid and cobalamin in older adults. Can J Public Health. 2008;99:428–33.
40. Cole BF, Baron JA, Sandler RS, et al. Folic acid for the prevention of colorectal adenomas. A randomized clinical trial. JAMA. 2007;297:2351–9.
41. Arabelovic A, Sam G, Dallal GE, et al. Preliminary evidence shows that folic acid fortification of the food supply is associated with higher methotrexate dosing in patients with rheumatoid arthritis. J Am Coll Nutr. 2007;26:453–5.
42. Wald DS, Wald NJ, Morris JK, et al. Folic acid, homocysteine, and cardiovascular disease: judging causality in the face of inconclusive trial evidence. Br Med J. 2006;333:1114–7.
43. Morris MS, Jacques PF, Rosenberg IH, et al. Folate and vitamin B-12 status in relation to anemia, macrocytosis, and cognitive impairment in older Americans in the age of folic acid fortification. Am J Clin Nutr. 2007;85:193–200.
44. Mills JL, Von Kohorn I, Conley MR, et al. Low vitamin B-12 concentrations in patients without anemia: the effect of folic acid of grain. Am J Clin Nutr. 2003;77:1474–7.
45. Ross J, Green J, Baugh CM, et al. Studies on the polyglutamate specificity of methylenetetrahydrofolate dehydrogenase from pig liver. Biochemistry. 1984;23:1796–801.
46. Stolzenberg-Solomon RZ, Chang SC, Leitzmann MF, et al. Folate intake, alcohol use, and postmenopausal breast cancer risk in the prostate, lung, colorectal, and ovarian cancer screening trial. Am J Clin Nutr. 2006; 83:895–904.
47. Piironen V, Edelmann M, Kariluoto S, et al. Folate in wheat genotypes in the HEALTHGRAIN diversity screen. J Agric Food Chem. 2008;56:9726–31.
48. Hossain T, Rosenberg I, Selhub J, et al. Enhancement of folate in plants through metabolic engineering. Proc Natl Acad Sci U S A. 2004;101:5158–63.
49. Diaz de la Garza R, Quinlivan EP, Klaus SM, et al. Folate biofortification in tomatoes by engineering the pteridines branch of folate synthesis. Proc Natl Acad Sci U S A. 2004;101:13720–5.
50. Nunes ACS, Kalkmann DC, Aragão FJL. Folate biofortification of lettuce by expression of a codon optimized chicken GTP cyclohydrolase I gene. Transgenic Res. 2009;18:661–7.
51. Naqvi S, Zhu C, Farre G, et al. Transgenic multivitamin corn through biofortification of endosperm with three vitamins representing three distinct metabolic pathways. Proc Natl Acad Sci U S A. 2009;106:7762–7.
52. Diaz de la Garza RI, Gregory III JF, Hanson AD. Folate biofortification of tomato fruit. Proc Natl Acad Sci U S A. 2007;104:4218–22.
53. Storozhenko S, De Brouwer V, Volckaert M, et al. Folate fortification of rice by metabolic engineering. Nat Biotechnol. 2007;25:1277–9.
54. Blencowe H, Cousens S, Modell B, et al. Folic acid to reduce neonatal mortality from neural tube disorders. Int J Epidemiol. 2010;39:110–21.
55. De Steur H, Gellynck X, Storozhenko S, et al. Health impact in China of folate-biofortified rice. Nat Biotechnol. 2010;28:554–6.
56. De Steur H, Gellynck X, Storozhenko S, et al. Willingness-to-accept and purchase genetically modified rice with high folate content in Shanxi Province, China. Appetite. 2010;54:118–25.
57. Shanxi Province Statistical Bureau. Shanxi statistical yearbook 2007. Beijing: Shanxi Statistics Press; 2007.
58. De Steur H, Gellynck X, Van Der Straeten D, et al. Potential impact and cost-effectiveness of multi-biofortified rice in China. N Biotechnol. 2012;29(3):432–42.
59. Mclean E, Benoist B, Allen L. Review of the magnitude of folate and vitamin B12 deficiencies worldwide. Food Nutr Bull. 2008;29:S38–51.
60. Hao L, Ma J, Stampfer M, et al. Geographical, seasonal and gender differences in folate status among Chinese adults. J Nutr. 2003;133:3630–5.
61. UNICEF. Vitamin and mineral deficiency: a global damage assessment report. New York: UNICEF; 2004.
62. Busby A. Preventing neural tube defects in Europe: population based study. Br Med J. 2005;330:574–5.

Chapter 26
Transgenic Multivitamin Biofortified Corn: Science, Regulation, and Politics

Gemma Farré, Shaista Naqvi, Uxue Zorrilla-López, Georgina Sanahuja, Judit Berman, Gerhard Sandmann, Gaspar Ros, Rubén López-Nicolás, Richard M. Twyman, Paul Christou, Teresa Capell, and Changfu Zhu

Key Points

- Combinatorial nuclear transformation was developed as a technique to dissect and modulate the carotenoid biosynthesis pathway in corn.
- The same strategy was then used to generate corn plants simultaneously engineered to produce higher levels of provitamin A, vitamin B9, and vitamin C (β-carotene, folate, and ascorbate).
- The best-performing lines contained 169-fold more β-carotene, 6.1-fold more ascorbate, and double the amount of folate as found in wild-type endosperm of the same variety.

G. Farré, Ph.D. • U. Zorrilla-López • G. Sanahuja • J. Berman • T. Capell, Ph.D. • C. Zhu, Ph.D.
Department of Plant Production and Forestry Science, ETSEA, University of Lleida-Agrotecnio Center, Av. Alcalde Rovira Roure, 191, 25198 Lleida, Spain
e-mail: g.farre@pvcf.udl.cat; uzorrilla@pvcf.udl.cat; georgina.sanahuja@pvcf.udl.cat; jberman@hbj.udl.cat; teresa.capell@pvcf.udl.cat; Zhu@pvcf.udl.cat

S. Naqvi, Ph.D.
MRC Protein Phosphorylation Unit, College of Life Sciences, Sir James Black Complex, University of Dundee, Dundee, UK

Department of Plant Production and Forestry Science, ETSEA, University of Lleida- Agrotecnio Center, Av. Alcalde Rovira Roure, 191, 25198, Lleida, Spain
e-mail: s.naqvi@dundee.ac.uk

G. Sandmann, Ph.D.
Bisynthesis Group, Molecular Biosciences, Johann Wolfgang Goethe Universität, 60054 Frankfurt, Germany
e-mail: sandmann@bio.uni-frankfurt.de

G. Ros, Ph.D. • R. López-Nicolás, Ph.D.
Department of Food Science and Nutrition, Faculty of Veterinary Sciences, Regional Campus of International Excellence "Campus Mare Nostrum", University of Murcia, Spain
e-mail: gros@um.es; rubenln@um.es

R.M. Twyman, Ph.D.
TRM Ltd., P.O. Box 93, York, YO43 3WE, UK
e-mail: richard@writescience.com

P. Christou, Ph.D. (✉)
Department of Plant Production and Forestry Science, ETSEA, University of Lleida-Agrotecnio Center, Av. Alcalde Rovira Roure, 191, 25198 Lleida, Spain

Institució Catalana de Recerca I Estudis Avançats, 08010 Barcelona, Spain
e-mail: christou@pvcf.udl.es

V.R. Preedy et al. (eds.), *Handbook of Food Fortification and Health: From Concepts to Public Health Applications Volume 1*, Nutrition and Health, DOI 10.1007/978-1-4614-7076-2_26,

- Genetic engineering provides a rapid way to generate nutritionally enhanced traits in local breeding varieties and this has a great potential to improve human health in developing countries.
- However, several nontechnical constraints need to be addressed for the benefits of nutritionally enhanced crops such as multivitamin corn to reach poor people in the developing world.
- The use of genetically engineered plants could not only help to prevent micronutrient deficiency, it could also reduce the need for vitamin supplements and therefore avoid many cases of hypervitaminosis.

Keywords Plant biotechnology • Genetic engineering • Transgenic crop • Vitamin • Reference daily intake • Subsistence agriculture • Developing country • Vitamin deficiency • Multivitamin corn • Hypervitaminosis

Abbreviations

Adcs	Aminodeoxychorismate synthase
CRTB	Bacterial phytoene synthase
CRTI	Bacterial phytoene desaturase/isomerase
CRTY	Bacterial lycopene cyclase
Dhar	Dehydroascorbate reductase
DHPS	7,8-Dihydropteroate synthase
EU	European Union
folE	*E. coli* GTP cyclohydrolase
FPGS	Folypolyglutamate synthetase
GalLDH	L-Galactono-1,4-lactone dehydrogenase
gch1	GTP cyclohydrolase 1
GGP	GDP-L-galactose phosphorylase
GGPP	Geranylgeranyl diphosphate
Glbch	*Gentiana lutea* β-carotene hydroxylase
Gllycb	*Gentiana lutea* lycopene β-cyclase
GLOase	L-Gulono1,4-lactone oxidase
GME	GDP-D-mannose-3′,5′-epimerase
HGA	Homogentisic acid
HMDHP	Hydroxymethyldihydropterin
HPP	ρ-Hydroxyphenylpyruvic acid
HPPD	ρ-Hydroxyphenylpyruvic acid dioxygenase
HPPK	6-Hydroxymethyl-7,8-dihydropterin pyrophosphokinase
HPT1	Homogentisate phytyltransferase
MDHA	Monodehydroascorbate
MPBQ	2-Methyl-6-phytylbenzoquino
MPBQ MT	MPBQ methyltransferase
Or	Orange
PABA	*p*-Aminobenzoate
PacrtI	*Pantoea ananatis* phytoene desaturase
ParacrtW	*Paracoccus* β-carotene ketolase
PSY1	Phytoene synthase
RAE	Retinol activity equivalent
RDI	Reference daily intake
RNAi	RNA interference

TC	Tocopherol cyclase
TyrA	Prephenate dehydrogenase
Zmpsy1	*Zea mays* phytoene synthase 1
γ-TMT	γ-Tocopherol methyltransferase

Introduction

Micronutrient deficiency is a major global challenge because at any one time up to 50 % of the world's population may suffer from diseases caused by a chronic insufficient supply of vitamins and minerals, and this largely reflects the lack of access to a diverse diet [1]. In developed countries, micronutrient deficiency is addressed by encouraging the consumption of fresh fruits and vegetables, along with supplementation and fortification programs to enhance the nutritional value of staple foods [2]. In contrast, the populations of developing countries typically subsist on a monotonous diet of milled cereal grains such as rice or corn, which are poor sources of vitamins and minerals. Strategies that have been proposed to overcome micronutrient deficiencies in developing countries include supplementation, fortification, and the implementation of conventional breeding and genetic engineering programs to generate nutrient-rich varieties of staple crops. Unfortunately, the first two strategies have been largely unsuccessful because of the insufficient funding, poor governance, and dysfunctional distribution network in developing country settings [3]. Biofortification programs based on conventional breeding have enjoyed only marginal success because of the limited available genetic diversity and the time required to develop crops with enhanced nutritional properties as well as desirable agronomic characteristics. It is also impossible to conceive of a conventional breeding strategy that would ever produce "nutritionally complete" cereals [2]. More promising results have been obtained by engineering the metabolic pathways leading to provitamin A, vitamin B9, and vitamin C (β-carotene, folate, and ascorbate) in the same transgenic corn line multivitamin corn [4]. Genetic engineering therefore has immense potential to improve the nutritional properties of staple crops and contribute to better health, although a number of technical, economical, regulatory, and sociopolitical constraints remain to be addressed.

Biofortification by Genetic Engineering

Vitamin A (Retinol)

Humans can store retinol obtained as retinyl esters from meat and dairy products but can also synthesize the reduced form (retinal) directly from β-carotene, one of more than 700 fat-soluble pigments known as carotenoids that accumulate in the flowers, fruits, and storage organs of plants and confer red, orange, and yellow coloring [5]. Cereal grains do not accumulate β-carotene, so vitamin A deficiency is therefore prevalent in developing country populations that subsist on cereal-based diets. Several strategies have been used alone and in combination to increase the levels of β-carotene in cereals, such as increasing flux through the carotenogenic pathway by making more precursors available, modifying the activity of carotenogenic enzymes, blocking pathway branch points, and creating sinks to store β-carotene and relieve feedback inhibition.

The first committed step in carotenoid biosynthesis is the conversion of geranylgeranyl diphosphate (GGPP) into phytoene by phytoene synthase (PSY), and this is recognized as a major pathway bottleneck. Therefore, increasing the activity of this enzyme by expressing a plant PSY transgene or the bacterial equivalent CRTB has increased total carotenoid levels in tomato, canola, and corn by up to 50-fold, predominantly in the form of α- and β-carotene [6–8]. Phytoene is desaturated and isomerized in several steps to form lycopene, but one bacterial enzyme (CRTI) can accomplish all these reactions. Lycopene is then cyclized at each end by lycopene β-cyclase (LYCB, bacterial equivalent

CRTY) to form β-carotene or at one end by lycopene ε-cyclase (LYCE) and at the other by LYCB to form α-carotene. Several attempts have been made to increase the β-carotene content of plants by overexpressing LYCB or suppressing the activity of LYCE, thus shifting flux into the β-branch. For example, in canola lines expressing CRTB, CRTI, and CRTY, there was not only a higher total carotenoid content than wild-type seeds (1,229 μg/g fresh weight), but the β- to α-carotene ratio increased from 2:1 to 3:1 showing that the additional LYCB activity skewed the competition for the common precursor lycopene and increased flux specifically towards β-carotene [9].

Some cereal grains do not produce carotenoids at all and it is therefore necessary to introduce new functionality. One of the most interesting examples is rice endosperm, where the expression of PSY leads to the accumulation of phytoene but no other carotenoids, thus the entire carotenoid pathway has to be imported to produce "Golden Rice" containing β-carotene [10]. Similar methodology can be used to extend partial pathways and generate additional carotenoid products in plants, e.g., ketocarotenoids such as adonixanthin, echinenone, and astaxanthin were obtained in transgenic corn by expressing corn PSY1, *Paracoccus* CRTW and CRTI, and *Gentiana lutea* LYCB and BCH [8].

Blocking the α-carotene branch to prevent competition for the common precursor lycopene can also direct flux towards β-carotene synthesis. This was achieved by using RNA interference (RNAi) to block LYCE expression in canola, increasing total carotenoids 42.5-fold to 227 μg/g fresh weight and increasing β-carotene levels 185.2-fold to 90.76 μg/g fresh weight [11].

Carotenoids such as β-carotene accumulate in specialized lipoprotein-sequestering structures within chromoplasts, so a final strategy to enhance carotenoid accumulation in plants is to modify the storage capacity by increasing the number of storage compartments or encouraging chromoplast differentiation. For example, a spontaneous mutation in the cauliflower *Orange* (*Or*) gene generates deep orange cauliflower heads associated with the hyperaccumulation of carotenoids in chromoplasts [12, 13], and when this dominant allele was cloned and expressed in potato tubers, a tenfold increase of β-carotene levels was achieved and the tubers became golden in color [14].

Vitamin C (Ascorbate)

Ascorbate is a potent antioxidant and an essential cofactor for many different human enzymes. Plants can produce ascorbate through several different pathways, although the predominant route involves the enzyme L-gulono1,4-lactone oxidase (GLOase), which is the rate-limiting step [15]. Oxidized ascorbate can also be recycled through the activity of specific reductases. Therefore, strategies to increase the levels of ascorbate in plants include the overexpression of enzymes in the biosynthesis pathway such as GLOase, the overexpression of reductases that recycle ascorbate and the suppression of ascorbate oxidase, which converts ascorbate into the unstable derivative monodehydroascorbate (MDHA) [16].

Because of its rate-limiting status, GLOase is the key target enzyme for metabolic engineering, and as an example the overexpression of rat GLOase in lettuce resulted in double the normal ascorbate levels [17]. The main enzyme responsible for recycling ascorbate in plants is dehydroascorbate reductase (DHAR), and a six-fold increase in ascorbate levels was achieved by expressing the rice *dhar* gene in corn under the control of an endosperm-specific promoter [4]. Two DHAR isoforms are present in potato leaves, one expressed constitutively and located in the cytosol, and the other expressed specifically in green tissue and targeted to the plastids. Transgenic potatoes expressing cytosolic *dhar* accumulated higher ascorbate levels in green tissues and tubers, but those expressing plastidic *dhar* accumulated higher levels of ascorbate only in the leaves [18].

Vitamin B_9 (Folate)

Folate is required in humans for the synthesis of tetrahydrofolate, an important intermediate in nucleic acid biosynthesis and many other core metabolic reactions. Deficiency in adults causes cardiovascular

Table 26.1 Recommended daily allowance and tolerable upper intake level of vitamins A, C, and E and folic acid [36, 37, 47, 48]

	RDA (recommended daily allowance; mg/day)	TUL (tolerable upper intake level; mg/day)
Vitamin A[a]	0.7–0.9	3
Vitamin C	75–90	2,000
Vitamin E[b]	15	1,000
Folate[c]	0.4	1

[a]As retinol activity equivalent (RAE). 1 RAE = 12 μg of dietary β-carotene = 24 μg of the three other dietary provitamin-A carotenoids (α-carotene, γ-carotene, and β-cryptoxanthin)

[b]As α-tocopherol. α-Tocopherol includes *RRR*-α-tocopherol, the only form of α-tocopherol that occurs naturally in foods, and the 2*R*-stereoisomeric forms of α-tocopherol (*RRR*-, *RSR*-, *RRS*-, and *RSS*-α-tocopherol) that occur in fortified foods and supplements. It does not include the 2*S*-stereoisomeric forms of α-tocopherol (*SRR*-, *SSR*-, *SRS*-, and *SSS*-α-tocopherol), also found in fortified foods and supplements

[c]Also known as folic acid, folacin, and pteroylpolyglutamates. As dietary folate equivalents (DFE). 1 DFE = 1 μg food folate = 0.6 μg of folic acid from fortified food or as a supplement consumed with food = 0.5 μg of a supplement taken on an empty stomach

disease [19], but the impact in pregnant women is much more severe, leading to the neural tube defect spina bifida in the fetus [20]. Cereal-based diets are not sufficient to achieve the reference daily intake (RDI) of folate (Table 26.1), and whereas fortification programs have been successful in the developed world, these are difficult to implement sustainably in developing countries [21].

The biofortification of staple crops by genetic engineering offers a sustainable solution, but these strategies must take into account that folate is a tripartite molecule formed by three separate metabolic pathways (pteridine, *p*-aminobenzoate [PABA], and glutamate) in different compartments (Fig. 26.1). The modulation of individual branches does increase the total folate content, but only to the extent that bottlenecks are revealed in the other branches. For example, GTP cyclohydrolase 1 (GCH1) is the first enzyme of the pterin branch, and its expression in tomato resulted in a 2-fold increase of folate levels but the PABA pool was depleted [22]. By combining GCH1 with the PABA branch enzyme aminodeoxychorismate synthase (ADCS) in transgenic rice plants, it was possible to increase folate levels 100-fold in the grain [23].

As well as the rate-limiting enzymes in the separate branches converging on folate, further targets include enzymes such as 6-hydroxymethyl-7,8-dihydropterin pyrophosphokinase (HPPK), 7,8-dihydropteroate synthase (DHPS), and folypolyglutamate synthetase (FPGS) which catalyze folate transformation steps and, in the case of FPGS, the sequential addition of glutamate residues to form the polyglutamate tetrahydrofolates that are the major forms of folate in plants (Fig. 26.1). The polyglutamate tail provides greater affinity for folate-dependent enzymes and helps retain folates within cells and subcellular compartments [24].

Vitamin E (Tocochromanols)

Vitamin E is the collective name for a group of eight molecules known as tocochromanols, comprising a common head decorated with various combinations of methyl groups to yield α, β, γ, and δ derivatives, plus an aliphatic tail derived from phytyldiphosphate (PDP), which forms the tocopherols, or GGPP, which forms the tocotrienols. The most potent form of vitamin E is α-tocopherol, so strategies to enhance vitamin E levels in plants focus on increasing total tocochromanol levels and/or increasing the proportion represented by α-tocopherol.

Tocochromanols are synthesized on the inner chloroplast membrane from precursors derived from the shikimate and methylerythritol phosphate (MEP) pathways. The shikimate pathway contributes the head-group precursor homogentisic acid (HGA), which requires the enzymes TyrA and ρ-hydroxyphenylpyruvic acid dioxygenase (HPPD), whereas the MEP pathway gives rise to the side-chain precursors PDP and GGPP. The first committed step in the reaction is the cytosolic conversion of

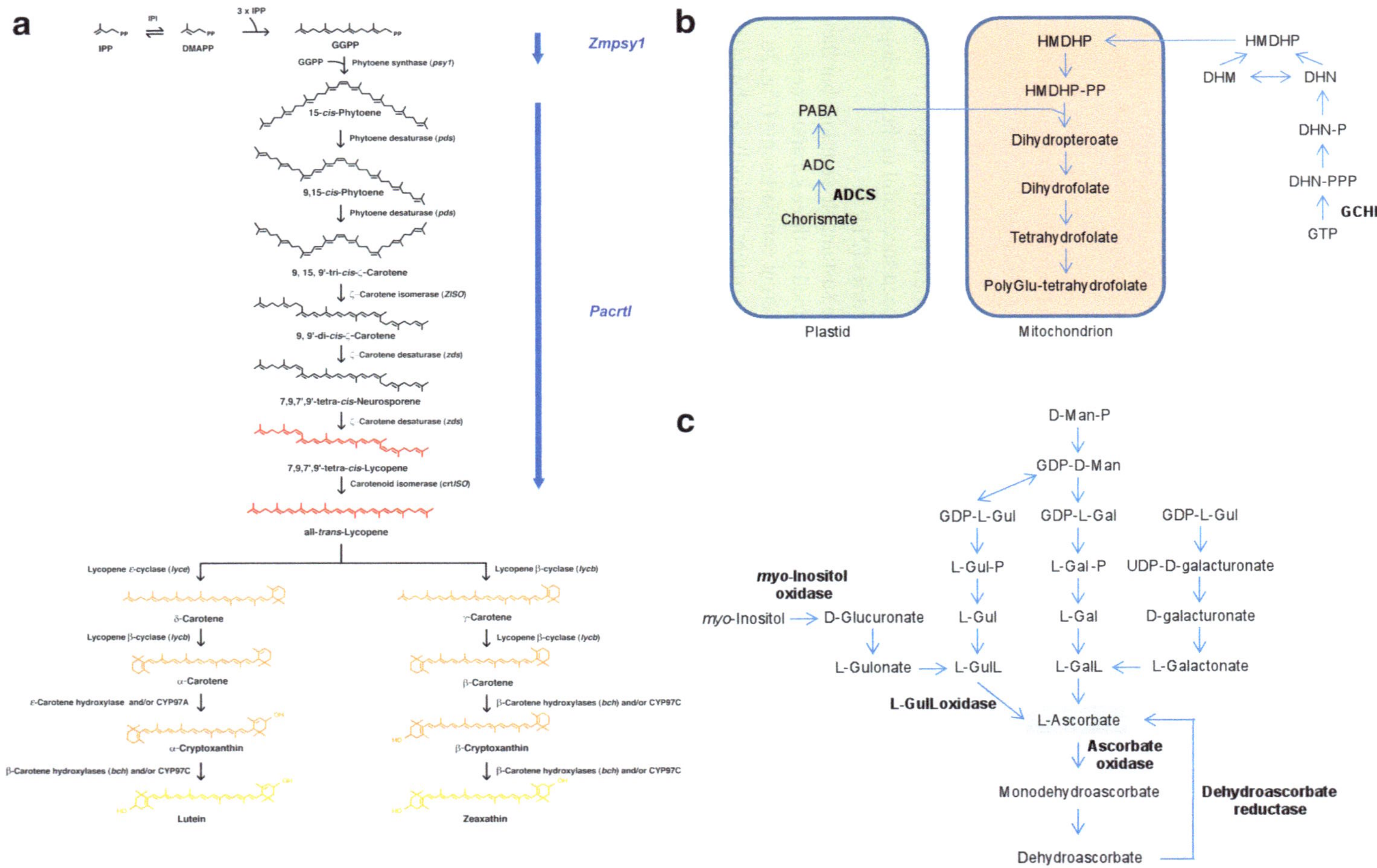

Fig. 26.1 Metabolic pathways engineered in multivitamin corn. (**a**) Enzymatic steps and metabolic products in the β-carotene biosynthesis pathway that are missing in cereal grains. (**b**) The plant folate biosynthesis pathway. *ADC* aminodeoxychorismate; *GCHI* GTP cyclohydrolase I; *ADCS* ADC synthase; *DHN* dihydroneopterin; *-P*/*-PP*/*-PPP* mono/di/triphosphate; *DHM* dihydromonapterin; *HMDHP* hydroxymethyldihydropterin. (**c**) The network of proposed biosynthetic pathways for ascorbate in plants. L-*Gal* L-galactose; L-*GalL* L-galactono-1,4-lactone; *GDP* guanosine diphosphate; L-*Gul* L-gulose; L-*GulL* L-gulono-1,4-lactone; D-*Man* D-mannose; *UDP* uridine diphosphate [4]

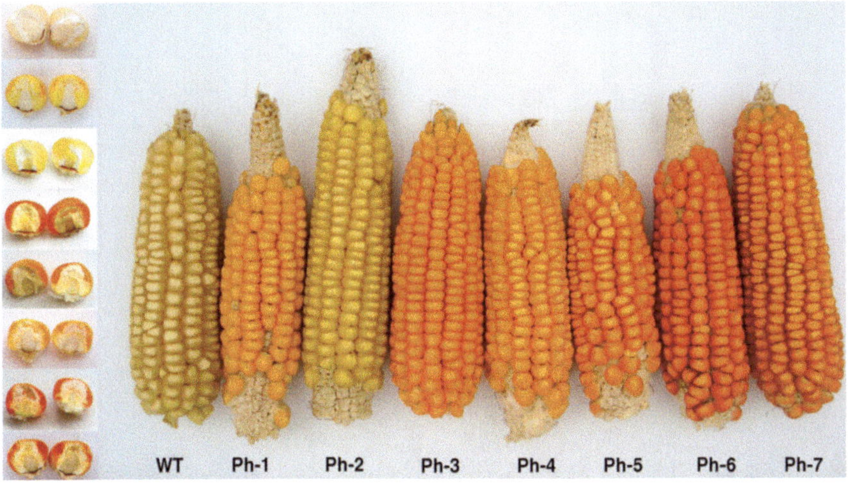

Fig. 26.2 Seven different phenotypes based on endosperm color were obtained by combinatorial nuclear transformation. Five carotenogenic genes (*Zea mays* phytoene synthase 1 (*Zmpsy1*), *Pantoea ananatis* phytoene desaturase (*PacrtI*), *Gentiana lutea* lycopene β-cyclase (*Gllycb*), *Gentiana lutea* β-carotene hydroxylase (*Glbch*), and *Paracoccus* β-carotene ketolase (*ParacrtW*)) were cotransformed in M37W

ρ-hydroxyphenylpyruvic acid (HPP) to HGA by HPPD. HGA is then prenylated with either PDP or GGDP to produce intermediates that can be methylated in different ways and converted by tocopherol cyclase (TC) into the δ- and γ-tocopherols and tocotrienols. These are further methylated by γ-tocopherol methyltransferase (γ-TMT) to yield α- and β-tocopherols and tocotrienols.

The simplest strategy to boost overall tocochromanol levels in plants is therefore to express the early enzymes TyrA, HPPD, and homogentisate phytyltransferase (HPT1), which produce the key pathway intermediates. The expression of all three of these genes in canola seeds increased the total vitamin E levels by 3.7-fold [25]. Boosting the flux in the latter part of the pathway can also increase vitamin E levels, albeit to a lesser extent. For example, the overexpression of TC resulted in a 20–50 % increase in total vitamin E levels in canola seeds [26]. By focusing on the tocopherol branch of the pathway, it has been possible to skew the ratio from γ-tocopherol to α-tocopherol, e.g., through the expression of Arabidopsis γ-TMT in soybean with or without the coexpression of MPBQ methyltransferase (MPBQ MT) [27].

Combinatorial Transformation as a Conduit to Multivitamin Engineering

Combinatorial nuclear transformation [8] was developed as a technique to dissect and modify the carotenoid biosynthesis pathway in corn and was initially applied to the transformation of the South African elite white corn inbred M37W with multiple carotenogenic genes. This corn variety lacks the variety carotenoids in the endosperm because the enzyme phytoene synthase (PSY1) is not expressed, and the variety also has low levels of other nutrients including ascorbate and folate.

In the original report [8], seven different phenotypes were obtained by combinatorial transformation with five carotenogenic genes, i.e., corn phytoene synthase 1 (*Zmpsy1*), *Pantoea ananatis* phytoene desaturase (*PacrtI*), *Gentiana lutea* lycopene β-cyclase (*Gllycb*), *Gentiana lutea* β-carotene hydroxylase (*Glbch*), and *Paracoccus* β-carotene ketolase (*ParacrtW*). The diverse phenotypes, which were easily scored on the basis of endosperm color (Fig. 26.2), represented a library of random transformants with a wide range of metabolic profiles. The population was therefore screened for metabolic variants reflecting the expression of the different combinations of transgenes, allowing the detailed analysis of the carotenoid biosynthesis pathway and the functions of the corresponding

a

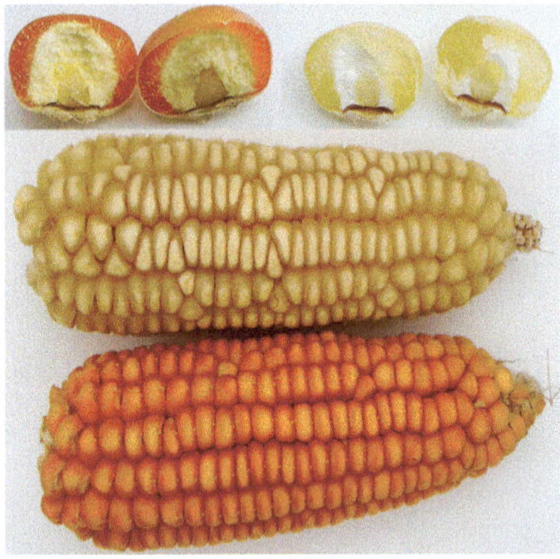

b

	Lyc	γ-Car	α-Car	β-Car	α-Cryptox	β-Cryptox	Lut	Zeax	CAR	Asc	Fol
M37W	0	0.09±0.02	0.12±0.05	0.35±0.06	ND	ND	0.57 ± 0.18	0.32 ± 0.05	1.45 ± 0.21	17.53 ± 2.90	0.93 ± 0.32
L-1	22.78±2.56	4.79±1.08	7.26±0.87	59.32±3.65	13.42±2.0	5.28±0.84	14.68 ± 2.16	35.76 ± 4.35	163.29 ± 8.61	106.94 ± 7.56	1.94 ± 0.17
Conventionally bred corn (Harjes et al 2008)	ND	ND	ND	1.65	ND	ND	11.36	8.187	23.06	-	-
Golden Rice 2 (Paine et al 2005)	ND	ND	ND	31	ND	ND	ND	ND	37	-	-

Fig. 26.3 (**a**) Accumulation of carotenes in the endosperm of transgenic multivitamin corn line. Phenotype of the transgenic endosperm compared with that of the wild-type M37W endosperm. (**b**) Comparison of the levels of carotenoids and other vitamins in wild-type M37W corn and transgenic line L-1 presented as μg/g DW + standard deviation (n = 3–5 mature T3 seeds). Also compared are a corn line bred conventionally [51] and genetically engineered Golden Rice 2, expressing *Zmpsy1* and *PacrtI* [52]. *WT* wild-type M37W; *L-1* transgenic line L-1; *Lyc* lycopene; *γ-Car* γ-carotene; *α-Car* α-carotene; *β-Car* β-carotene; *α-Cryptox* α-cryptoxanthin; *β-Cryptox* β-cryptoxanthin; *Lut* lutein and lutein epoxide; *Zeax* zeaxanthin; *CAR* total carotenoids; *Asc* ascorbate; *Fol* folate; *ND* not determined [4]

enzymes. Novel discoveries included the complementation of rate-limiting steps in the pathway and the competition between β-carotene hydroxylase and bacterial β-carotene ketolase for substrates in four sequential steps of the extended pathway [8]. The transgenic plants contained high levels of β-carotene, lycopene, zeaxanthin, lutein, and also commercially relevant ketocarotenoids that are not normally synthesized in plants such as astaxanthin and adonixanthin [8].

The Development and Characterization of Multivitamin Corn

The combinatorial transformation technique discussed above (Fig. 26.2) used to engineer multivitamin corn, a staple cereal crop that simultaneously accumulated higher levels of b-carotene, ascorbate, and folate in the endosperm [4]. These three vitamins are known to enhance human health and help to prevent a range of chronic diseases [28–35]. The M37W corn inbred was transformed with four transgenes affecting three metabolic pathways: the corn *psy1* and *P. ananatis crt*I genes for carotenoid synthesis, the rice *dhar* gene for ascorbate recycling, and the *E. coli* GTP cyclohydrolase (*folE*) for folate synthesis (Fig. 26.3). The best-performing transgenic line (Fig. 26.3) contained 59.32 μg/g dry weight β-carotene (169-fold increase), 106.94 μg/g dry weight ascorbate (6.1-fold increase), and 1.94 μg/g dry weight folate (twofold increase) [4].

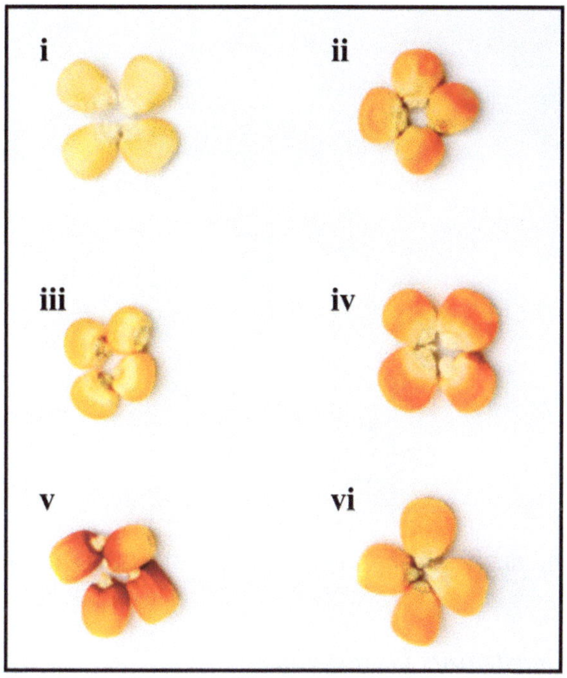

Fig. 26.4 Color phenotypes show carotenoid accumulation in endosperm38: (i) M37W; (ii) Ph-4 expressing *zmpsy1*, *PacrtI*, and *Gllycb*; (iii) EP42; (iv) Ph-4 x EP42 expressing *zmpsy1*, *PacrtI*, and *Gllycb*; (v) A632; (vi) Ph-4A x 632 expressing *zmpsy1*, *PacrtI*, and *Gllycb*

The food matrix plays an important role in determining the bioavailability of β-carotene, and 6 mg of β-carotene in a typical plant-based diet is equivalent to 1 mg of pure β-carotene dissolved in oil or 0.5 mg of retinol (the form of vitamin A stored in the human body before conversion to the active form, retinal) [36]. Therefore, we calculated that 182 g of the multivitamin corn would be sufficient to achieve the dietary reference intake (DRI) for adults, which is 900 retinol activity equivalents (RAEs), i.e., 900 mg of retinol, 1.8 mg of pure β-carotene, or 10.8 mg of β-carotene in food [36] (Table 26.1). Similarly, the DRI for ascorbate is 90 mg [36], which means 849 g of the multivitamin corn would be required, and the DRI for folate is 0.4 mg [37], which means 206 g of the multivitamin corn would be required (Table 26.1). In conclusion, 200 g of multivitamin corn provides the complete adult DRI for vitamin A and folate and nearly 25 % of the adult DRI for ascorbate [4].

Subsequent Development of Multivitamin Corn

We have crossed the multivitamin corn line with other, well-characterized corn lines to look at the impact of hybridization on the carotenoid pathway. For example, we have introgressed the transgenic mini-pathway into two yellow-endosperm varieties [38], one accumulating lutein (the end product of the α-carotene pathway) and the other accumulating zeaxanthin (Fig. 26.4). Lutein and zeaxanthin both confer yellow pigmentation to the endosperm, but they are two different carotenoids that accumulate according to the balance of LYCB and LYCE activity at the branch point (Figs. 26.1a). When multivitamin corn was crossed with the high-zeaxanthin variety, the bias towards the β-branch was exacerbated and the hybrids contained unprecedented levels of zeaxanthin (56 μg/g dry weight) [38]. In the future, it may be possible to increase overall β-carotene levels further by introducing the cauliflower *Or* gene that induces the creation of a carotenoid sink or by using RNAi to block LYCE activity and the activity of enzymes that further metabolize β-carotene [12, 39, 40]. Other potential future activities include crossing the multivitamin corn plants with other transgenic lines expressing additional genes involved in ascorbate synthesis (e.g., *gme*, *ggp*, and *galldh*), additional genes involved in folate synthesis (e.g., *adcs*), and also genes involved in the synthesis of further vitamins, such as vitamin E.

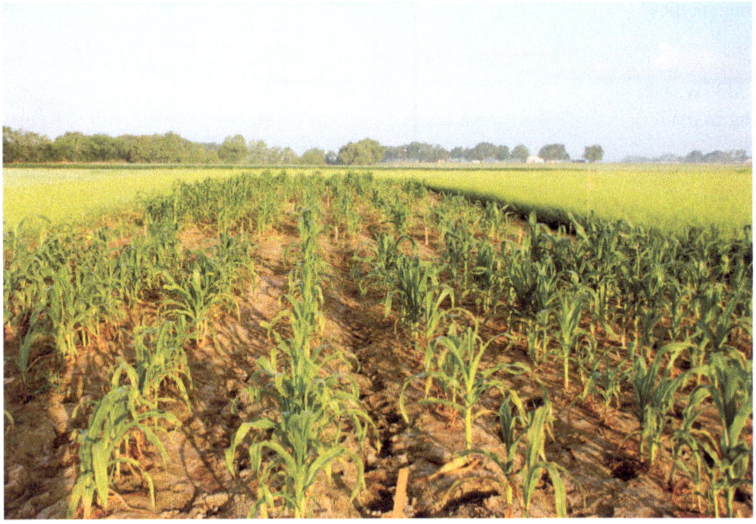

Fig. 26.5 Field trail conducted by Dr. Steve Linscombe, Rice Research Station, Crowley, LA (USA)

Constraints to Adoption

Although the technical limitations of genetically engineered crops are being addressed successfully, there are still a number of regulatory and sociopolitical constraints that prevent their adoption. Genetically engineered crops have been grown on a commercial basis for more than 15 years, and the number of countries adopting the technology continues to grow, as does the land area given over for their cultivation. There are still many countries that remain firmly attached to conventional agriculture, but most of these countries nevertheless import genetically engineered foods and other commodities from abroad or approve the marketing of food products containing genetically engineered ingredients [41]. However, the impact of scientific progress is being neutralized by politicians focusing on immediate popular support who are unwilling to take politically controversial decisions that would in the short to medium term save millions of lives and in the long term would make a significant impact on the health, well-being, and economic prosperity of the world's poorest people [42, 43].

The development and adoption of biotechnology is also hampered by discordant international regulations relating to research, biosafety, and the trade and use of genetically engineered crops and their products, particularly disagreements between the EU and the USA [43, 44]. Regulators must therefore focus on science-based estimates about the magnitude of any potential risks posed by genetically engineered crops, without political interference, and the media should be required to report on these matters responsibly, accurately, and without deliberately exaggerating the risks associated with new technologies [21, 43, 45]. At the same time, the public should be educated on the realistic nature of risk and the balance between risk and benefits that is daily used in all areas of life. Scientists should get involved in this process and aim to increase the public awareness and understanding of science through means other than newspapers [21].

Recommendations

Many people take dietary supplements to augment the nutrition obtained from food, so RDI tables now include a new value, the "tolerable upper intake level," which is the largest daily intake unlikely to cause harm. The concept of a tolerable upper level for vitamins is pertinent only for supplementary vitamins because it is difficult to ingest toxic levels of vitamins with a natural diet, although excess levels of the fat-soluble vitamins can be achieved through the overconsumption of highly fortified processed food [46]. Vitamin A toxicity (nausea, irritability, vomiting, blurred vision, headaches, hair loss, abdominal pain, muscle weakness, drowsiness, and loss of concentration [47]) has been reported in individuals who take more than the recommended dose of vitamin supplements, particularly combined with rich diets containing adequate vitamin A (e.g., diets with a high content of liver, carrots, and spinach), and therefore exceed the tolerable upper intake level of 3 mg/day in adults and 0.6–0.9 mg/day in children (Table 26.1).

The tolerable upper intake level for vitamin E is 1 g/day and for vitamin C is 2 g/day (adult values) [36], although clinical trials have not revealed a consistent pattern of adverse effects and those observed may have reflected comorbidities [48]. The risk of toxicity from folic acid is low because the tolerable upper intake level is 1 mg/day for adults, which is difficult to achieve [37]. Supplemental folic acid should not exceed the tolerable upper intake level to prevent folic acid from masking the symptoms of vitamin B_{12} deficiency, and several reports suggest that excess folate may be carcinogenic [49, 50]. Up to 1.5 kg of multivitamin corn can be consumed per day without reaching the tolerable upper intake level for vitamin A, and nearly 20 kg would be required before there was any risk of vitamin C toxicity. More than 0.5 kg would need to be consumed before folic acid levels reached the tolerable upper intake level. Since these refer to dry weight values, the amount of cooked corn that would be required to reach anywhere near the tolerable upper intake level of the three vitamins would be vastly in excess of any standard consumption.

Conclusion

Genetic engineering is the most effective way to generate nutritionally enhanced traits in staple food crops, and this has a great potential to improve human health in developing countries. The use of genetically enhanced plants will not only help to prevent micronutrient deficiency; it could also reduce or even eliminate the need for alternative non-sustainable interventions such as supplementation and food fortification which are not practical in developing countries. However, several nontechnical barriers such as political expediency, interference from a number of environmental organization with vested interests against the technology, and an overburdening and nonscience-based regulatory system need to be addressed in order to allow these crops to benefit the people most in need of them, resource-poor farmers and their families in the developing world.

Acknowledgement Research at the Universitat de Lleida is supported by MICINN, Spain (BIO2011-23324; BIO02011-22525; BIO2012-35359; PIM2010PKB-00746); European Union Framework 7 Program-SmartCell Integrated Project 222716; European Union Framework 7 European Research Council IDEAS Advanced Grant (to PC) Program-BIOFORCE; RecerCaixa; COST Action FA0804: Molecular farming: plants as a production platform for high value proteins; Centre CONSOLIDER on Agrigenomics funded by MICINN, Spain.

References

1. Zhu C, Naqvi S, Gomez-Galera S, Pelacho AM, Capell T, Christou P. Transgenic strategies for the nutritional enhancement of plants. Trends Plant Sci. 2007;12:548–55.
2. Gomez-Galera S, Rojas E, Sudhakar D, Zhu C, Pelacho AM, Capell T, et al. Critical evaluation of strategies for mineral fortification of staple food crops. Transgenic Res. 2010;19:165–80.
3. Nantel G, Tontisirin K. Policy and sustainability issues. J Nutr. 2002;132:S839–44.
4. Naqvi S, Zhu C, Farré G, Ramessara K, Bassie L, Breitenbach J, et al. Transgenic multivitamin corn through biofortification of endosperm with three vitamins representing three distinct metabolic pathways. Proc Natl Acad Sci U S A. 2009;106:7762–7.

5. Farré G, Sanahuja G, Naqvi S, Bai C, Capell T, Zhu C, et al. Travel advice on the road to carotenoids in plants. Plant Sci. 2010;179:28–48.
6. Fraser PD, Enfissi EMA, Halket JM, Truesdale MR, Yu D, Gerrish C, et al. Manipulation of phytoene levels in tomato fruit: effects on isoprenoids, plastids and intermediary metabolism. Plant Cell. 2007;19:3194–211.
7. Shewmaker CK, Sheehyl JA, Daley M, Colburn S, Ke YD. Seed-specific overexpression of phytoene synthase: increase in carotenoids and other metabolic effects. Plant J. 1999;20:401–12.
8. Zhu C, Naqvi S, Breitenbach J, Sandmann G, Christou P, Capell T. Combinatorial genetic transformation generates a library of metabolic phenotypes for the carotenoid pathway in corn. Proc Natl Acad Sci U S A. 2008;105:18232–7.
9. Ravanello MP, Ke D, Alvarez J, Huang B, Shewmaker CK. Coordinate expression of multiple bacterial carotenoid genes in canola leading to altered carotenoid production. Metab Eng. 2003;5:255–63.
10. Burkhard PK, Beyer P, Wünn J, Klöti A, Armstrong GA, Schledz M, et al. Transgenic rice (*Oryza sativa*) endosperm expressing daffodil (*Narcissus pseudonarcissus*) phytoene synthase accumulates phytoene, a key intermediate of provitamin A biosynthesis. Plant J. 1997;11:1071–8.
11. Yu B, Lydiate DJ, Young LW, Schäfer UA, Hannoufa A. Enhancing the carotenoid content of *Brassica napus* seeds by downregulating lycopene epsilon cyclase. Transgenic Res. 2008;17:573–85.
12. Li L, Paolillo DJ, Parthasarathy MV, Dimuzio EM, Garvin DF. A novel gene mutation that confers abnormal patterns of beta-carotene accumulation in cauliflower (*Brassica oleracea* var. botrytis). Plant J. 2001;26:59–67.
13. Lu S, Van Eck J, Zhou X, Lopez AB, O'Halloran DM, Cosman KM, et al. The cauliflower *Or* gene encodes a DnaJ cysteine-rich domain-containing protein that mediates high levels of beta-carotene accumulation. Plant Cell. 2006;18:3594–605.
14. Lopez AB, Van Eck J, Conlin BJ, Paolillo DJ, O'Neill J, Li L. Effect of the cauliflower *Or* transgene on carotenoid accumulation and chromoplast formation in transgenic potato tubers. J Exp Bot. 2008;59:213–23.
15. Jain AK, Nessler CL. Metabolic engineering of an alternative pathway for ascorbic acid biosynthesis in plants. Mol Breed. 2000;6:73–8.
16. Ishikawa T, Dowdle J, Smirnoff N. Progress in manipulating ascorbic acid biosynthesis and accumulation in plants. Physiol Plant. 2006;126:343–55.
17. Hemavathi CP, Upadhyaya AN, Akula N, Young KE, Chun SC, Kim DH, et al. Enhanced ascorbic acid accumulation in transgenic potato confers tolerance to various abiotic stresses. Biotechnol Lett. 2010;32:321–30.
18. Qin A, Shi Q, Yu X. Ascorbic acid contents in transgenic potato plants overexpressing two dehydroascorbate reductase genes. Mol Biol Rep. 2010;38:1557–66.
19. Quinlivan EP, McPartlin J, McNulty H, Ward M, Strain JJ, Weir DG, et al. Importance of both folic acid and vitamin B12 in reduction of risk of vascular disease. Lancet. 2002;359:227–8.
20. Geisel J. Folic acid and neural tube defects in pregnancy—a review. J Perinat Neonatal Nurs. 2003;17:268–79.
21. Farré G, Twyman RM, Zhu C, Capell T, Christou P. Nutritionally enhanced crops and food security: scientific achievements versus political expediency. Curr Opin Biotechnol. 2011;22:245–51.
22. Díaz de la Garza RI, Quinlivan EP, Klaus SM, Basset GJ, Gregory JF, Hanson AD. Folate biofortification in tomatoes by engineering the pteridine branch of folate synthesis. Proc Natl Acad Sci U S A. 2004;101:13720–5.
23. Storozhenko S, De Brouwer V, Volckaert M, Navarrete O, Blancquaert D, Zhang GF, et al. Folate fortification of rice by metabolic engineering. Nat Biotechnol. 2007;25:1277–9.
24. McIntosh SR, Henry RJ. Genes of folate biosynthesis in wheat. J Cereal Sci. 2008;48:632–8.
25. Karunanandaa B, Qi Q, Haoa M, Baszis S, Jensen P, Wong Y, et al. Metabolically engineered oilseed crops with enhanced seed tocopherol. Metab Eng. 2005;7:384–400.
26. Kumar R, Raclaru M, Schusseler T, Gruber J, Sadre R, Lühs W, et al. Characterisation of plant tocopherol cyclases and their overexpression in transgenic *Brassica napus* seeds. FEBS Lett. 2005;579:1357–64.
27. van Eenennaam AL, Lincoln K, Durrett TP, Valentin HE, Shewmaker CK, Thorne GM, et al. Engineering vitamin E content: from Arabidopsis mutant to soy oil. Plant Cell. 2003;15:3007–19.
28. Fraser P, Bramley PM. The biosynthesis and nutritional uses of carotenoids. Prog Lipid Res. 2004;43:228–65.
29. Chatterjee IB, Majumder AK, Nandi BK, Subramanian N. Synthesis and some major functions of vitamin C in animals. Ann N Y Acad Sci. 1975;258:24–47.
30. Zhu C, Sanahuja G, Yuan D Farre G, Arjo G, Berman J, Zorrilla-Lopez U, et al. Biofortification of plants with altered antioxidant content and composition: genetic engineering strategies. Plant Biotechnol J 2013;11:129–41.
31. Ames BN. Cancer prevention and diet: help from single nucleotide polymorphisms. Proc Natl Acad Sci U S A. 1998;96:12216–8.
32. Green R, Miller JW. Folate deficiency beyond megaloblastic anemia: hyperhomocysteinemia and other manifestations of dysfunctional folate status. Semin Hematol. 1999;36:47–64.
33. Naqvi S, Farré G, Sanahuja G, Capell T, Zhu C, Christou P. When more is better: multigene engineering in plants. Trends in Plant Sci. 2010;15:48–56.
34. Stanger O. The potential role of homocysteine in percutaneous coronary interventions (PCI): review of current evidence and plausibility of action. Cell Mol Biol. 2004;50:953–88.

35. Choi SW, Friso S. Interactions between folate and aging for carcinogenesis. Clin Chem Lab Med. 2005;43:1151–7.
36. Institute of Medicine (IOM), Food and Nutrition Board. Dietary reference intakes for vitamin C, vitamin E, selenium, and carotenoids. A report of the panel on dietary antioxidants and related compounds, subcommittees on upper reference levels of nutrients and interpretation and uses of dietary reference intakes, and the standing committee on the scientific evaluation of dietary reference intakes. Washington, DC: National Academy Press; 2001.
37. Institute of Medicine (IOM). Dietary reference intakes for thiamin, riboflavin, niacin, vitamin B6, folate, vitamin B12, pantothenic acid, biotin, and choline. Washington, DC: National Academy Press; 1998.
38. Naqvi S, Zhu C, Farré G, Sandmann G, Capell T, Christou P. Synergistic metabolism in hybrid corn indicates bottlenecks in the carotenoid pathway and leads to the accumulation of extraordinary levels of the nutritionally important carotenoid zeaxanthin. Plant Biotechnol. 2011;9:384–93.
39. Bai C, Twyman RM, Farré G, Sanahuja G, Christou P, Capell T, et al. A golden era—pro-vitamin A enhancement in diverse crops. In Vitro Cell Dev Biol Plant. 2011;47:205–21.
40. Paolillo DJ, Garvin DF, Parthasarathy MV. The chromoplasts of Or mutants of cauliflower (*Brassica oleracea* L. var. botrytis). Protoplasma. 2004;224:245–53.
41. Yuan D, Bassie L, Sabalza M, Miralpeix B, Dashevskaya S, Farré G, et al. The potential impact of plant biotechnology on the millennium development goals. Plant Cell Rep. 2011;30:249–65.
42. Sabalza M, Miralpeix B, Twyman RM, Capell T, Christou P. EU legitimizes GM crop exclusion zones. Nat Biotechnol. 2011;29:315–7.
43. Farré G, Ramessar K, Twyman RM, Capell T, Christou P. The humanitarian impact of plant biotechnology: recent breakthroughs vs bottlenecks for adoption. Curr Opin Plant Biol. 2010;13:219–25.
44. Ramessar K, Capell T, Twyman RM, Christou P. Going to ridiculous lengths European coexistence regulations for GM crops. Nat Biotechnol. 2010;28:133–6.
45. Twyman RM, Ramessar K, Quemada H, Capell T, Christou P. Plant biotechnology: the importance of being accurate. Trends Biotechnol. 2009;27:609–12.
46. Sizer F, Sienkiewicz F, Whitney E. Nutrition: concepts and controversies. 11th ed. Belmont, CA: Thomson Wadsworth; 2008. p. 221–35.
47. Maqbool A, Stallings VA. Update on fat-soluble vitamins in cystic fibrosis. Curr Opin Pulm Med. 2008;14:74–581.
48. Hathcock JN, Azzi A, Blumberg J, Bray T, Dickinson A, Frei B, et al. Vitamins E and C are safe across a broad range of intakes. Am J Clin Nutr. 2005;81:736–45.
49. Baggott JE, Morgan SL, Ha T, Vaughn WH, Hine RJ. Inhibition of folate-dependent enzymes by non-steroidal anti-inflammatory drugs. Biochem J. 1992;282:197–202.
50. Baggott JE, Oster RA, Tamura T. Meta-analysis of cancer risk in folic acid supplementation trials. Colorectal Dis. 2011;13:132–7.
51. Harjes CE, Rocheford TR, Bai L, Brutnell TP, Kandianis CB, Sowinski SG, et al. Natural genetic variation in lycopene epsilon cyclase tapped for maize biofortification. Science. 2008;319:330–3.
52. Paine JA, Shipton CA, Chaggar S, Howells RM, Kennedy MJ, Vernon G, et al. Improving the nutritional value of Golden Rice through increased pro-vitamin A content. Nat Biotechnol. 2005;23:482–7.

Chapter 27
Selenium Biofortified Wheat

Michael Fenech, Jing Wu, Robin Graham, and Graham Lyons

Key Points

- Selenium is essential for the function of important selenoproteins which include glutathione peroxidases, thioredoxin reductases and deiodinases and selenoprotein P.
- Selenium deficiency in foods is not uncommon and is largely due to geological variations in selenium abundance in soil.
- Selenium deficiency can cause infertility, increased oxidative stress, immune and thyroid dysfunction, cardiomyopathy, cognitive impairment and increased risk for specific cancers such as prostate cancer.
- The selenium content of wheat can be increased by agronomic biofortification which involves fertilising the growing crop with an appropriate inorganic form of the micronutrient, which the plant converts to several organic Se forms, notably selenomethionine, which are more suitable for human consumption.
- A recent intervention study has shown that moderate consumption of selenium-biofortified wheat can substantially increase blood plasma selenium concentration in healthy older men.

Keywords Selenium • Selenomethionine • Biofortified • Biofortification • Wheat

Abbreviations

Se	Selenium
Se-met	Selenomethionine

M. Fenech, Ph.D. (✉)
CSIRO Food and Nutritional Sciences, Gate 13 Kintore Avenue, Adelaide BC, SA 5000, Australia
e-mail: Michael.fenech@csiro.au

J. Wu, Ph.D.
Population Research and Outcome Studies, The University of Adelaide, Adelaide, SA 5005, Australia
e-mail: jing.wu@adelaide.edu.au

R. Graham, Ph.D. • G. Lyons, Ph.D.
School of Agriculture, Food and Wine, The University of Adelaide,Waite Campus, Glen Osmond, Adelaide, SA 5005, Australia
e-mail: robin.graham@adelaide.edu.au; graham.lyons@adelaide.edu.au

V.R. Preedy et al. (eds.), *Handbook of Food Fortification and Health: From Concepts to Public Health Applications Volume 1*, Nutrition and Health, DOI 10.1007/978-1-4614-7076-2_27,

Introduction

Selenium (Se) is essential to human and animal health but can be toxic in excess. Hesketh [1] recently reviewed the importance of selenium in cellular metabolism via its essential role in the function of specific selenoproteins or enzymes. The best characterised selenoproteins are the glutathione peroxidases, the thioredoxin reductases and deiodinases and selenoprotein P. Recently Johnson et al. [2] explained in a detailed review the importance of geology in determining the extent to which Se is accessible in the soil to food sources of agronomic importance. For example, because of these geological differences, US wheat has 10 times more Se than UK wheat, attributed to the fact that soils from the wheat-growing belt of America are more enriched in Se to a similar order of magnitude. For the same reasons, Se deficiency is endemic in specific regions of China such as Keshan where Se-deficiency disease was first reported and associated with cardiomyopathy [3]. Effective biofortification of crops with Se-rich fertilisers can counter the deficiencies due to geological variation in abundance of this important element.

Biofortification of Grains with Selenium

In countries where wheat products are widely consumed, wheat is usually a major source of dietary Se. In Australia, for example, it is estimated that most people obtain around half their Se from wheat [4, 5]. The Se content of wheat can be increased by agronomic biofortification (Fig. 27.1). This involves fertilising the growing crop with an appropriate inorganic form of the micronutrient, which the plant converts to several organic Se forms, notably Se-methionine, which are more suitable for human consumption [5, 6]. The relative effectiveness of soil or foliar application of Se depends on Se form, soil characteristics, method of basal application and time of foliar application. Ylaranta [7] found basal and foliar selenate to be equally effective at the low (10 g/ha) rate, foliar better at 50 g/ha, and both equal at the high rate of 500 g/ha. In further trials, foliar selenate applied at the three- to

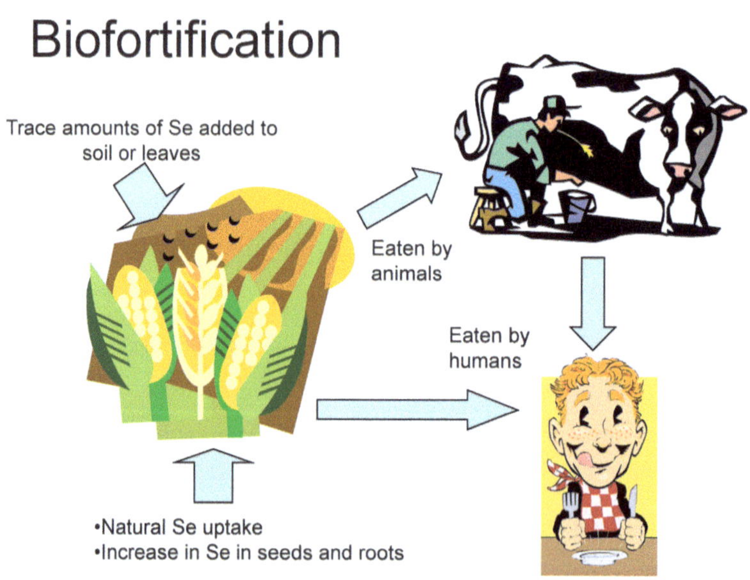

Fig. 27.1 Schematic diagram of selenium biofortification process. For more details refer to ref. [6]

four-leaf stage was found to be more effective than basal application on clay soil of pH 6.3; of similar effectiveness on high-humus, fine sandy soil of pH 4.6; and slightly less effective than basal fertiliser on a fine sandy soil of pH 5.0. Foliar selenate, at the level of 10 g/ha, using a wetting agent, raised the wheat-grain Se level from 16 to 168 μg/kg on the clay soil, while 9 g basally applied raised it to just 77 μg/kg. Overall, foliar application was the more effective method for wheat and barley, except where growth was poor due to low rainfall [8].

Health Effects of Deficiency and Excess of Selenium Intake

Moderate deficiency of selenium (Se) in humans is associated with various pathological conditions including infertility, increased oxidative stress, immune and thyroid dysfunction, cognitive impairment and increased risk for specific cancers such as prostate cancer [9–12]. Several essential structural proteins and enzymes in the body have improved function when seleno-amino acids such as selenomethionine (Se-met) and selenocysteine are incorporated into the protein instead of their sulphur-containing amino acid analogues [1, 13, 14]. There is emerging evidence that increased intake of organic Se may reduce the risk of certain degenerative diseases, but there is also concern that excessive Se intake may have unwanted toxic effects [15].

Se may also play an important role at the fundamental genome level through its role in selenoenzymes such as glutathione peroxidases involved in antioxidant response pathways that are required to prevent oxidation of DNA which is mutagenic and may reduce the regenerative potential of cells. Within the physiological concentration range of 3–430 μg Se/L, Se, as Se-met, had no impact on baseline or γ-ray-induced chromosome breakage or loss measured as micronuclei in human lymphocytes in vitro; however, spontaneous frequencies of nucleoplasmic bridges (biomarker of DNA misrepair or telomere dysfunction) and nuclear buds (biomarker of gene amplification) declined significantly as the dose increased, but higher concentrations of Se-met (>430 μg Se/L) caused strong inhibition of nuclear division and increased cytotoxicity [16]. Dietary selenium supplementation in dogs reduced DNA damage in prostate tissue as measured by the alkaline Comet assay but was not associated with glutathione peroxidase activity in plasma; however, excessive intake of Se appeared to increase DNA damage suggesting a U-shaped dose–response [17, 18]. In a study of men at high risk for prostate cancer, DNA strand breaks in lymphocytes measured by Comet assay were shown to be inversely associated with serum Se concentration for those with serum Se less than 98 μg/L but not for those with higher concentrations [19, 20]. Increased Se intake has been associated with decreased risk for cardiovascular disease (CVD), but it is unknown whether this is due to Se-mediated reduction in lipid peroxidation, inhibition of inflammation, or an improved lipid profile in the blood [21].

Until recently the effect of increased consumption of Se via Se-biofortified wheat on genome damage and immune function had not been tested previously. We aimed to investigate whether improving Se status, by increased dietary intake of Se-biofortified wheat, affects biomarkers of cancer risk, CVD risk, oxidative stress and immune function in healthy South Australian older men (aged 40–70 years) who had lower but not Se-deficient plasma concentration [22]. A 24-week placebo-controlled double-blind intervention was performed with increasing doses of Se intake every 8 weeks comparing the selenium bioavailability and bioefficacy effect of wheat that was biofortified with selenium (BIOFORT), wheat that was process fortified with selenomethionine (PROFORT) and wheat that was not fortified (CONTROL) (Fig. 27.2). Wheat was provided as 1, 2 and 3 puffed wheat biscuits, during weeks 1–8, 9–16 and 17–24, respectively. The Se content of the biscuits and the intake of Se in the three treatment groups are detailed in Tables 27.1 and 27.2. Blood was collected to measure a wide range of disease risk biomarkers. Consumption of Se-biofortified wheat was found to increase plasma Se concentration from a baseline level of 122–192 μg/L following intake of three biscuits per day,

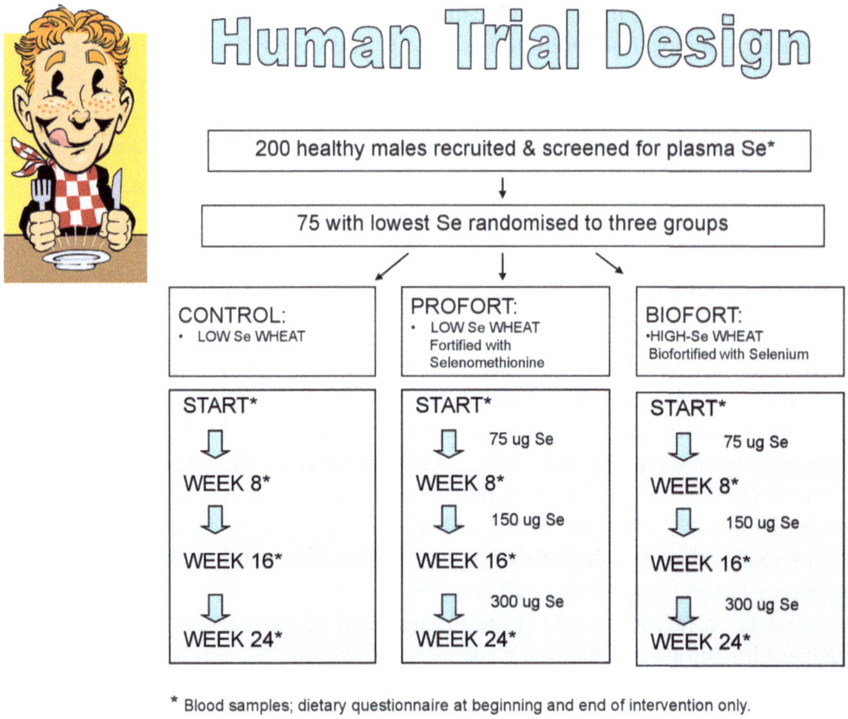

Fig. 27.2 Design of human trial investigating the bioavailability and bioefficacy of wheat biofortified with selenium (BIOFORT) in comparison to wheat that was process fortified by addition of selenomethionine (PROFORT) and wheat that was not fortified with selenium (CONTROL). For more details refer to ref. [22]

Table 27.1 Se concentration, weight and Se content of trial wheat biscuits

	Se conc. (mg/kg)	Weight (g)	Se content
	Mean (range)	Mean (range)	(μg/biscuit)
CONTROL	0.07 (0.06–0.08)	10.1 (10.1–10.4)	0.7
BIOFORT	9.0 (8.7–9.2)	9.6 (9.4–9.9)	86.0
PROFORT	9.8 (8.7–10.5)	10.7 (10.0–11.0)	105.0

Table 27.2 Estimated daily Se intakes from the intervention biscuits of trial participants at different time points during the intervention (μg/day)

	Weeks (biscuits/day)		
Dietary group	1–8 (1)	9–17 (2)	18–24 (3)
CONTROL	0.7	1.4	2.1
BIOFORT	86.0	172.0	258.0
PROFORT	105.0	210.0	315.0

which provided 267 μg Se (Fig. 27.3). Platelet glutathione peroxidase, chromosome aberrations and DNA damage in lymphocytes measured using the cytokinesis-block micronucleus cytome assay and with the Comet assay, plasma F2-isoprostanes, protein carbonyls, plasma C-reactive protein and leukocyte number were unaffected by the improved Se status. The results of this study also showed that there were no toxic side effects of increased intake of biofortified wheat even in a population that was already well nourished for selenium (>120 μg/L Se in plasma is considered to be optimal for disease prevention).

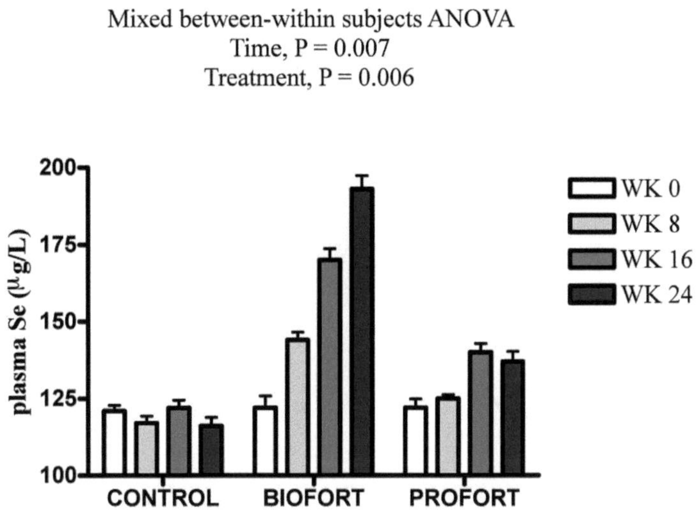

Fig. 27.3 Changes in plasma Se concentration during an intervention trial in healthy older men aged 40–70 years who were required to consume increasing amounts of whole grain wheat biscuits made with unfortified wheat (CONTROL), biofortified wheat (BIOFORT) and wheat that was process fortified with synthetic selenomethionine (PROFORT). Trial participants were required to consume one biscuit per day for the first 8 weeks, then two biscuits daily for the next 8 weeks, then three biscuits daily for the final 8 weeks. The intention of the study design was that each BIOFORT and PROFORT biscuit would deliver approximately 75 μg Se so that the daily amount of Se from the biscuits would increase progressively from 75 μg, to 150 μg, to 225 μg during each phase of the trial. The biscuits were developed by Laucke Flour Mills (Strathalbyn, South Australia) and were made by soaking whole grain wheat in water for 24 h, then heating to expand the grain, and compressing into a 'puffed wheat' biscuit. The actual Se content per biscuit (mean value (range) in micrograms) was 0.71 (0.64–0.75), 89.1 (86.4–94.5) and 101.9 (97.0–105.8) for CONTROL, BIOFORT and PROFORT biscuits, respectively. N=22, 19, 21 for CONTROL, BIOFORT and PROFORT groups, respectively. The statistical analysis was performed using delta value of result of each follow-up time point relative to baseline result, and the baseline value was included as covariate using mixed between within subjects ANOVA. Results were mean ± SEM (┬)

Kirby et al. [23] developed a species-unspecific isotope dilution and reverse phase ion pairing-inductively coupled plasma-mass spectrometry technique for the identification and quantification of Se species in biofortified grains (i.e. wheat and triticale), flour and wheat biscuits. This method was used to obtain information on Se species which is important for understanding of the bioavailability of Se in biofortified wheat biscuits and wheat biscuits that were process fortified with synthetic Se-met in the above clinical trial. The major Se species identified in biofortified (BIOFORT) and process-fortified (PROFORT) wheat biscuits were Se-met (76–85 %) and Se-met selenoxide (51–60 %), respectively (Fig. 27.4). Total plasma Se concentrations in the biofortified Se exposure group were found to increase steadily by 57 % throughout the 24-week trial period; in contrast, the trial group exposed to process-fortified Se biscuits only showed a modest 15 % increase in plasma Se by the end of the intervention (Fig. 27.3). The difference in total Se plasma concentrations following consumption of BIOFORT and PROFORT wheat may be due to the presence and bioavailability of different Se species in biofortified and process-fortified biscuits. Se speciation in fortified foods is recommended for a better understanding of their potential benefits for animals and humans. It is evident that BIOFORT wheat is a better source of bioavailable selenium and Se-met, the predominant organic form in wheat, appears to be less susceptible to oxidation during food processing than when it is added as a synthetic form to wheat.

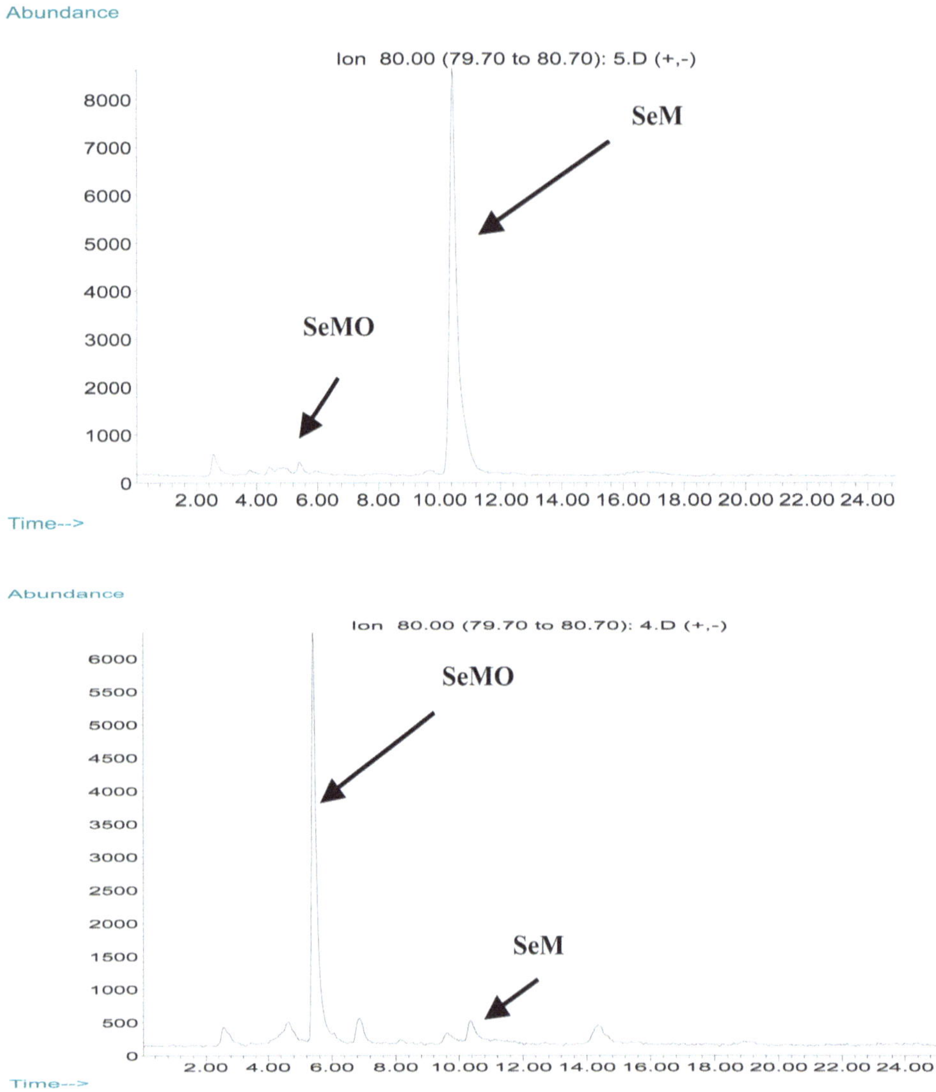

Fig. 27.4 Speciation of organic selenium forms in BIOFORT (*top panel*) and PROFORT biscuits (*bottom panel*) using ICPMS. *SeM* selenomethionine; *SeMO* methionine selenoxide (i.e. oxidised SeM)

Conclusion

In conclusion biofortified wheat is a suitable food for improving selenium status in humans. However, further research is needed to verify its bioefficacy in selenium-deficient populations.

Guidance on Safe Levels

Based on our intervention study, it appeared that daily consumption of up to 300 μg Se as organic selenium in Se-biofortified wheat is safe for human consumption over a 24-week period. Concentration of organic Se-met at or greater than 430 μg Se/L causes cytostatic and cytotoxic effects in human cells.

Recommendations

It is evident that wheat biofortified with Se is a safe and bioavailable source of organic Se and is recommendable for human consumption. Furthermore, biofortification appears to be preferable to process fortification with regard to prevention of Se-met oxidation during high temperature processing of wheat into puffed wheat biscuits. Se speciation in fortified foods is recommended for a better understanding of their potential benefits for animals and humans.

References

1. Hesketh J. Nutrigenomics and selenium: gene expression patterns, physiological targets, and genetics. Annu Rev Nutr. 2008;28:157–77.
2. Johnson CC, Fordyce FM, Rayman MP. Symposium on 'Geographical and geological influences on nutrition': factors controlling the distribution of selenium in the environment and their impact on health and nutrition. Proc Nutr Soc. 2010;69(1):119–32.
3. Hou J, Wang T, Liu M, Li S, Chen J, Liu C, et al. Suboptimal selenium supply-a continuing problem in Keshan disease areas in Heilongjiang province. Biol Trace Elem Res. 2011;143(3):1255–63.
4. Lyons G, Judson G, Stangoulis J, Palmer L, Jones J, Graham R. Trends in selenium status of South Australians. Med J Aust. 2004;180(8):383–6.
5. Lyons G, Ortiz-Monasterio I, Stangoulis J, Graham G. Selenium concentration in wheat grain: is there sufficient genotypic variation to use in breeding? Plant Soil. 2005;269:369–80.
6. Lyons G, Stangoulis J, Graham R. High-selenium wheat: biofortification for better health. Nutr Res Rev. 2003; 16:45–60.
7. Ylaranta T. Effect of applied selenite and selenate on the selenium content of barley (Hordeum vulgare). Ann Agric Fenniae. 1983;22:164–74.
8. Ylaranta T. Raising the selenium content of spring wheat and barley using selenite and selenate. Ann Agric Fenniae. 1984;23:75–84.
9. Rayman M. The importance of selenium to human health. Lancet. 2000;356:233–41.
10. Rayman MP. Selenium in cancer prevention: a review of the evidence and mechanism of action. Proc Nutr Soc. 2005;64(4):527–42.
11. Gromadzinska J, Reszka E, Bruzelius K, Wasowicz W, Akesson B. Selenium and cancer: biomarkers of selenium status and molecular action of selenium supplements. Eur J Nutr. 2008;47 Suppl 2:29–50.
12. Gronberg H. Prostate cancer epidemiology. Lancet. 2003;361(9360):859–64.
13. Gromer S, Eubel JK, Lee BL, Jacob J. Human selenoproteins at a glance. Cell Mol Life Sci. 2005;62(21): 2414–37.
14. Hatfield DL, Carlson BA, Xu XM, Mix H, Gladyshev VN. Selenocysteine incorporation machinery and the role of selenoproteins in development and health. Prog Nucleic Acid Res Mol Biol. 2006;81:97–142.
15. Zwolak I, Zaporowska H. Selenium interactions and toxicity: a review: selenium interactions and toxicity. Cell Biol Toxicol. 2012;28(1):31–46.
16. Wu J, Lyons GH, Graham RD, Fenech MF. The effect of selenium, as selenomethionine, on genome stability and cytotoxicity in human lymphocytes measured using the cytokinesis-block micronucleus cytome assay. Mutagenesis. 2009;24(3):225–32.
17. Waters D, Shen S, Cooley D, Bostwick D, Qian J, Combs Jr G, et al. Effects of dietary selenium supplementation on DNA damage and apoptosis in canine prostate. J Natl Cancer Inst. 2003;95(3):237–41.
18. Waters DJ, Shen S, Glickman LT, Cooley DM, Bostwick DG, Qian J, et al. Prostate cancer risk and DNA damage: translational significance of selenium supplementation in a canine model. Carcinogenesis. 2005;26(7): 1256–62.
19. Karunasinghe N, Han DY, Zhu S, Yu J, Lange K, Duan H, et al. Serum selenium and single-nucleotide polymorphisms in genes for selenoproteins: relationship to markers of oxidative stress in men from Auckland, New Zealand. Genes Nutr. 2012;7(2):179–920.
20. Karunasinghe N, Ryan J, Tuckey J, Masters J, Jamieson M, Clarke LC, et al. DNA stability and serum selenium levels in a high-risk group for prostate cancer. Cancer Epidemiol Biomarkers Prev. 2004;13(3):391–7.
21. Ravn-Haren G, Bugel S, Krath BN, Hoac T, Stagsted J, Jorgensen K, et al. A short-term intervention trial with selenate, selenium-enriched yeast and selenium-enriched milk: effects on oxidative defence regulation. Br J Nutr. 2008;99(4):883–92.

22. Wu J, Salisbury C, Graham R, Lyons G, Fenech M. Increased consumption of wheat biofortified with selenium does not modify biomarkers of cancer risk, oxidative stress, or immune function in healthy Australian males. Environ Mol Mutagen. 2009;50(6):489–501.
23. Kirby JK, Lyons GH, Karkkainen MP. Selenium speciation and bioavailability in biofortified products using species-unspecific isotope dilution and reverse phase ion pairing-inductively coupled plasma-mass spectrometry. J Agric Food Chem. 2008;56(5):1772–9.

Chapter 28
Market Potential of Folate Biofortified Rice in China

Hans De Steur, Xavier Gellynck, Dieter Blancquaert, Sergei Storozhenko, Ge Liqun, Willy Lambert, Dominique Van Der Straeten, and Jacques Viaene

Key Points

- Provision of a conceptual framework to investigate the market potential of folate biofortified rice (FBR).
- FBR would be a cost-effective health intervention to reduce folate deficiency in China.
- The key target groups of FBR are generally in favor of, and willing to pay more for FBR.
- Regulatory hurdles and weaknesses in the Chinese Intellectual Property Rights (IPRs) protection are key bottlenecks to speed up the commercialization of biofortified crops.
- Implementation issues refer to appropriate variety selection, genetically modified (GM) labeling and the need to address different stakeholders, such as farmers, governmental agencies, and seed producers.

Keywords Acceptance • Cost-effectiveness • China • Folate deficiency • Folate biofortified rice • GM rice • Policy • Willingness-to-pay

Abbreviations

CEA Cost-effectiveness analysis
DALY Disability-adjusted life year
FBR Folate biofortified rice
GM Genetically modified

H. De Steur, Ph.D. (✉) • X. Gellynck, Ph.D. • J. Viaene, Ph.D.
Department of Agricultural Economics, Ghent University, K.L. Ledeganckstraat 35, Ghent 9000, Belgium
e-mail: Hans.Desteur@ugent.be; Xavier.Gellynck@ugent.be; Jacques.Viaene@ugent.be

D. Blancquaert • S. Storozhenko, Ph.D. • D. Van Der Straeten, Ph.D.
Department of Physiology, Ghent University, K.L. Ledeganckstraat 35, Ghent 9000, Belgium
e-mail: Dieter.Blancquaert@UGent.be; serguei.storojenko@ugent.be; Dominique.VanDerStraeten@UGent.be

G. Liqun
Rural Economy Research Institute, Liaoning Academy of Agricultural Sciences,
Dongling District, 110161 Shenyang, Liaoning, People's Republic of China
e-mail: glqeml@yahoo.com.cn

W. Lambert, Ph.D.
Department of Bioanalysis, Ghent University, K.L. Ledeganckstraat 35, Ghent 9000, Belgium
e-mail: Willy.Lambert@ugent.be

V.R. Preedy et al. (eds.), *Handbook of Food Fortification and Health: From Concepts to Public Health Applications Volume 1*, Nutrition and Health, DOI 10.1007/978-1-4614-7076-2_28,

GR	Golden rice
IPR	Intellectual Property Rights
NTD	Neural-tube defect
WHO	World Health Organization
WTP	Willingness-to-pay

Introduction

Worldwide, micronutrient malnutrition or a chronic lack of essential vitamins and minerals affects over two billion people, particularly pregnant women and children in less developed regions [1]. Due to its far-reaching consequences for global health and development, international organizations have set specific nutritional goals in the 2015 UN millennium development goals. Today, despite the progress made towards eliminating the global burden of this "hidden hunger," these goals are far from being reached [2], necessitating an increase in efforts to support, develop, introduce, or improve micronutritional interventions.

In addition to the current policy tools to address micronutrient malnutrition, e.g., supplementation, fortification, and dietary diversification, biofortification has been explored and advocated as a novel, potential strategy, at both the policy and research level. By enriching the natural micronutrient content of staple crops, such as rice, wheat, or potatoes, biofortification aims to alleviate the burden of micronutrient deficiencies. In particular for the people who need it the most. In this respect, folate biofortified rice (FBR)[1] was recently developed through genetic engineering in order to tackle folate deficiency (<400 μg folate per day) [3]. As such, FBR is considered a genetically modified (GM) food product with health benefits. Due to the controversial nature of this micronutrient enriched staple crop, governments, decision-makers, and health planners are interested in the consumer reactions to this product as well as the benefits and costs of introducing it as an alternative health intervention. In order to justify the allocated resources of setting FBR as a priority to address folate deficiency, stakeholders should have access to information about the importance of this micronutrient deficiency on the one hand, and understand how FBR would contribute to reduce its burden on the other.

Because transgenic crops like FBR are still under development, little is known about the acceptance [4], purchase intentions [5], and public health impacts [6] of GM crops with health benefits, especially in high-risk regions. However, as the asynchronous approval of currently available GM foods demonstrates, consumer acceptance will also play an important factor in political support and farmer adoption. Not surprisingly, market failure of novel products or technologies is often caused by a lack of, or inadequate consumer market research [7].

This article anticipates these issues by providing a framework to investigate ex-ante the market potential of FBR, which is applied to its potential introduction in China and Shanxi Province, a poor, rural high-risk region in Northern China. Figure 28.1 presents the rationale behind the selection of China and Shanxi Province as the research location to evaluate the market potential of FBR. The research topic is a novel, controversial good, namely folate-enriched GM rice. The higher folate content is beneficial as it reduces the occurrence of several folate-related diseases, such as the risk to deliver a baby with a neural-tube defect (NTD) [9]. Due to its health benefits, FBR is oriented towards the consumer and, thus, categorized as a second-generation GM food product. By using the world's most consumed crop as the food vehicle for folate biofortification, the aim is to maximize the potential health impact of consuming FBR and, as a consequence, help to further alleviate the burden of micronutrient malnutrition.

Broadly three reasons can be cited for the selection of the research location. First, China is one of the key players in research, development, and production of GM crops, and rice in particular [10]. It is the sixth largest GM producer of the world [11] and will likely be the first to commercialize GM

[1] For more information on folate biofortification, we refer to the contribution of Blancquaert et al. in this handbook.

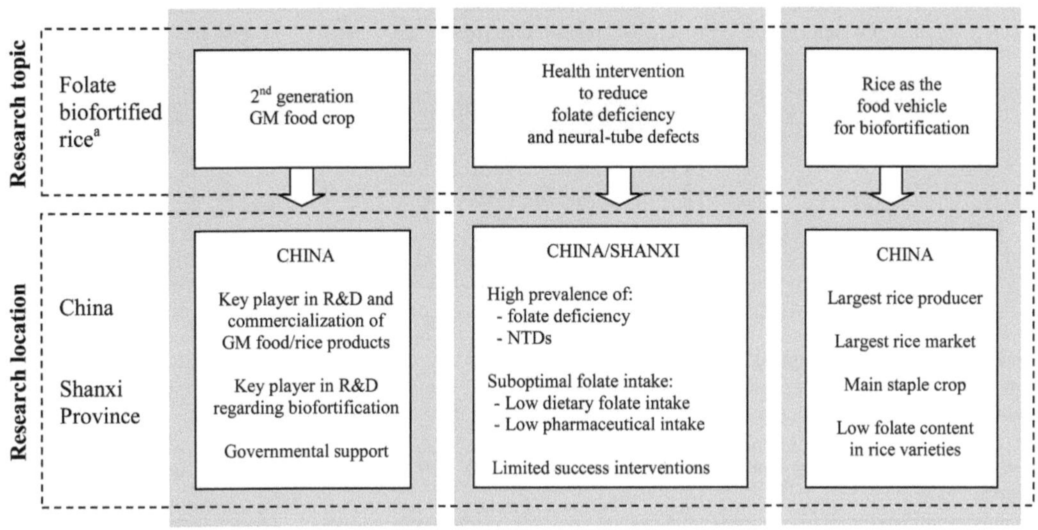

Fig. 28.1 Rationale behind the research location to investigate the market potential of FBR. The figure shows that China and Shanxi Province are relevant research locations to investigate the market potential of FBR as both a second-generation GM food product and a potential health strategy. *GM* genetically modified; *NTD* neural-tube defects. *Source*: Own compilation, based on Storozhenko et al. [3] and De Steur et al. [8]

rice [12]. Due to the governmental support towards biotechnology and reducing malnutrition, it is one of the main actors in conventional and transgenic biofortification research [13].

Second, China is characterized by a high prevalence of folate deficiency, with about 258 million people assumed to be folate-deficient [8], and a high prevalence rate of NTDs, i.e., the main adverse health outcome of maternal folate deficiency. The reason to improve folate consumption is even more relevant in Shanxi Province, where suboptimal folate intake levels occur in 43.8 % of all pregnant women [14], leading to one of the highest numbers of NTDs, i.e., up to 1 NTD per 50 births [15]. This is confirmed by the currently low use of folic acid supplements and the low dietary folate intake [16]. Moreover, past folic acid supplementation programs were not successful [17] and folic acid fortification is less feasible when aiming to tackle poor, developing regions, like Shanxi Province [18].

Third, biofortifying rice would be particularly relevant to China, as it is the world leader in rice production with the largest rice consumer market.

In the next section, the conceptual framework to determine the market potential of FBR in Shanxi Province and China is described. Hereby, four main lines of inquiry are proposed, namely acceptance, willingness-to-pay (WTP), disease burden, and cost-effectiveness analysis (CEA). For each of these research domains, findings will be presented based on previous research studies. Furthermore, specific attention will be drawn to policy issues to successfully commercialize FBR in China. A final section summarizes the main conclusions.

Conceptual Framework

Figure 28.2 presents the conceptual framework to analyze the market potential of FBR in China. In the center is the investigated research topic, i.e., FBR, a GM rice crop as a potential health intervention to tackle folate deficiency. Four different research domains are distinguished, namely consumer acceptance, WTP, disease burden, and cost-effectiveness. While the former two are examined at consumer level, the latter two refer to a policy-oriented ex-ante evaluation. Below, the main components of this framework and the rationale to investigate them will be briefly discussed in relation to the current research literature.

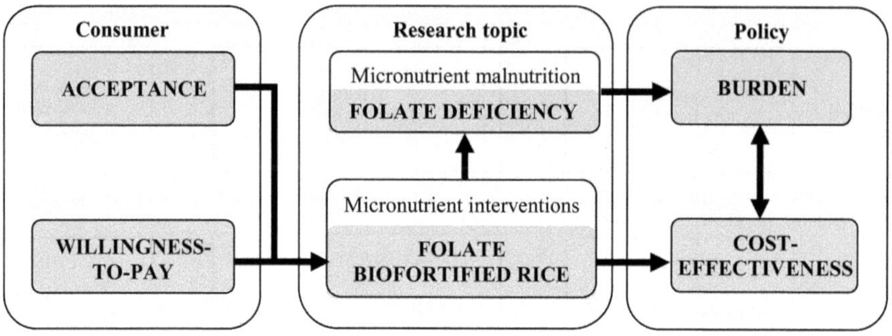

Fig. 28.2 Simplified conceptual framework to evaluate the market potential of folate biofortified rice. The figure demonstrates that the market potential of a biofortification strategy is measured on both the macro- (policy) and micro-level (consumer). *Source*: Own compilation, based on De Steur et al. [8, 19, 20]

Table 28.1 Overview of the main types of willingness-to-pay (WTP) values, based on the applied value elicitation method

WTP value	Value elicitation method	Specific types/examples
Stated WTP	Stated preference methods	
	Contingent valuation	Open-ended; closed-ended, e.g., dichotomous choice; payment card; bidding game
	Choice modeling	Conjoint analysis; contingent ranking
Revealed WTP	Revealed preference methods	
	Market data analysis	Panel data analysis, store scanner data analysis
	Travel cost	Recreational value of places of interest
	Hedonic pricing	House pricing
	Experimental auctions	Laboratory experiment; field experiment

Source: Own compilation, based on Bateman et al. [25] and Breidert et al. [26]
This table shows the different tools to measure the economic value of a good. Although experimental auctions are often categorized as revealed preference methods, they actually combine the strengths of both revealed and stated preference methods

Acceptance

The concept acceptance measures whether a consumer is favorable, indifferent or unfavorable to FBR. Due to its health benefits, this second-generation GM food product is expected to be more appreciated than its first-generation counterparts and may compensate for the negative perception that is associated with GM food technology [21]. To date, only two studies examined consumer acceptance of another biofortified food crop, i.e., conventionally bred provitamin A-enriched maize [22, 23]. Except for a qualitative study on golden rice (GR) which reported high farmer acceptance rates in the Philippines [24], consumer research on acceptance of transgenic biofortified crops is needed.

Willingness-to-Pay

Following acceptance, the next step to determine the market potential of novel goods, like FBR, is to analyze consumers' WTP. As the economic value of a good refers to the value consumers place on it, i.e., what this product is worth to consumers, WTP of a GM biofortified food product is understood as the highest amount a consumer is prepared to pay for it.

There are several approaches to define the concept of WTP which can be broadly categorized into stated or revealed values or preferences, i.e., economic values that are measured, respectively, directly or indirectly. Table 28.1 classifies the most commonly used WTP values, namely stated and revealed preferences. These concepts are defined by the technique that is applied to measure WTP, i.e., the value elicitation method. Although they should all obtain the same WTP value in theory, a discrepancy between different WTP values is often observed in practice [27]. According to Lusk et al. [21], the value elicitation method is a crucial factor that accounts for differences in WTP values between GM food studies. Here, we will present stated preferences for FBR in Shanxi Province, based on an open-ended contingent valuation approach, as described in De Steur et al. [19].

There is scientific evidence that the improved health benefits of GM food products lead to higher WTP values compared to GM food products that are not directly oriented towards the consumer [28]. Despite the large body of scientific studies on WTP and purchase intentions of GM food [21], biofortified crops with proven health benefits received little attention thus far [29]. Valuation studies focused solely on provitamin A-enriched products, such as maize in Kenya [30] or GR in Brazil [4], India [31], and the United States [5]. Together with the optimistic consumer reactions to GM rice in China [32], one could expect relatively large WTP valuations for FBR, especially in regions where the need is the highest.

Burden and Cost-Effectiveness

When evaluating the impact of health interventions that aim to tackle a specific disease in a society, like biofortification intends to do with micronutrient malnutrition, and to adequately inform decision-makers and health planners about the potential of such strategies, it is essential to analyze the current status of the targeted disease, i.e., the "burden of disease." According to the definition of the World Health Organization (WHO) [33], this concept is defined as the overall impact of the disease and its outcomes at the societal level. It represents the health gap between the health status and a hypothetical, ideal situation without diseases.

To evaluate the potential of health policy interventions, such as biofortification, one needs to determine the potential health benefits (effectiveness) and take into account the costs (cost-effectiveness). While a health impact analysis primarily quantifies the improved health outcomes, a full economic evaluation, such as CEA, compares the consequences (e.g., health benefits) and costs of an intervention in order to contribute to priority-setting and to facilitate decision-making about the resource allocation [34].

Table 28.2 presents an overview of the different approaches to describe the current burden of disease and to evaluate health interventions. This overview does not aim to offer an exhaustive overview, but focuses on the most commonly used approaches in economic health literature and health impact studies, and the underlying evaluation methods.

Regarding FBR, the disability-adjusted life year (DALY) approach and CEA were selected because of their historical use in World Bank [36] and WHO reports on developing countries [37] as well as in biofortification studies [38]. As previous cost-effectiveness studies solely refer to crops biofortified with one of the main micronutrients (zinc, iron, or vitamin A), there is a need to extend CEA to folate biofortification, especially in countries with a large prevalence of folate deficiency, such as China. Folate biofortification of the world's major staple crop is expected to have a large impact on folate-related health problems, especially in rice consuming countries. Building upon a health impact study on FBR [8] and intervention cost estimates (i.e., R&D costs, country-specific costs, social marketing costs, and maintenance breeding costs), the cost-effectiveness of FBR in China is explored.

Given the evidence on the cost-effectiveness of micronutrient interventions [39], including biofortification [38], FBR is expected to be a cost-effective strategy to reduce folate deficiency and its main health outcomes.

Table 28.2 Approaches to the estimation of disease burden, health impact assessment, and economic evaluation of interventions

Approach	Description	Unit	Examples
Burden of disease			
Health approach, e.g. DALY framework	Estimation of the burden of a disease through health outcome measures. The DALY framework, for example, calculates the number of DALYs lost	Natural units	DALYs lost; mortality; morbidity
Evaluation of interventions			
Health impact			
Health approach, e.g., DALY framework	The health impact is evaluated in terms of improved health outcomes. The DALY framework, for example, estimates the number of DALYs lost that can be averted through an intervention	Natural units	DALYs saved; deaths averted
Economic evaluation			
Cost-effectiveness analysis	All costs are related to a single health index, i.e., the outcome measure, and expressed as the additional cost spent per unit of health outcome	Natural and monetary units	US$ per DALY saved
Cost-benefit analysis	Both costs and benefits are converted into monetary units and outcomes are expressed as the value of the benefits per dollars expended; sometimes referred to as benefit-cost analysis	Monetary units	Benefit-cost (B/C); net benefit (B-C)

Source: Own compilation, based on Ngorsuraches [35] and Drummond et al. [34]
This table summarizes the main methods to conduct a health impact study, a cost-analysis or an economic evaluation study of a health intervention
DALY disability-adjusted life year

The Market Potential of FBR

Acceptance of FBR

In their consumer survey in the Chinese Shanxi Province, De Steur et al. [19] found a large acceptance rate of FBR (62.2 %). Only 11.2 % of the Shanxi rice consumers stated to be reluctant to this GM rice crop with health benefits, while 26.6 % is rather indifferent. Based on their dataset, Table 28.3 presents how the acceptance rate of FBR differs according to the target group of this intervention. Depending on the objective of the intervention, three main target groups can be distinguished. First, females are considered the key target group to reduce the number of NTDs, i.e., the most important outcome of folate deficiency. Although their acceptance rate is significantly lower than for males, the share of reluctant women is low. Second, low educated, poor consumers from rural areas are most vulnerable to become folate-deficient [40]. The results show that consumers with a low education and income level are significantly more indifferent to FBR, but their acceptance rate is still above 60 %. Moreover, nearly 68 % of the rural consumers accept FBR. Third, farmers are crucial stakeholders of FBR as their adoption will determine the coverage rate of this health intervention. Merely 7 % indicated to be reluctant to this GM rice crop, which further underpins its potential.

Willingness-to-Pay for FBR

This section presents the results based on a consumer study in Shanxi Province, where WTP for FBR was measured in 2008 [19]. The results are adapted from the open-ended contingent valuation

Table 28.3 Folate biofortified rice (FBR) acceptance in Shanxi Province, per target group and socio-demographic variable, significant differences by χ^2 test ($n=944$)

			FBR acceptance			χ^2	
Target group	Variable	Categories	Reluctance	Indifference	Acceptance	Value	p
Women	Gender	Female	12.3	32.3	55.4	22.09	0.00
		Male	10.0	20.1	69.9		
High-risk consumers	Education[a]	Low	10.3	28.9	60.8	7.84	0.02
		High	13.6	20.4	66.0		
	Income[b]	Low	11.2	27.1	61.8	2.07	0.36
		High	11.8	19.1	69.1		
	Residence	Rural	10.6	21.5	67.9	13.79	0.00
		Urban	11.8	31.4	56.8		
Farmers	Farmer status	Farmer	6.7	26.7	66.7	5.32	0.07
		Nonfarmer	12.4	26.4	61.1		

The results indicate that males, consumers with a high education and income level, people living in rural areas, and farmers are significantly more represented in the category of FBR acceptance
The applied methodology and the χ^2 values are based on the study of De Steur et al. [19]
[a]A high education level is defined as a college degree or higher
[b]A yearly income above ¥40,000 or US$6,288 is defined as a high income level

Table 28.4 WTP for FBR in Shanxi Province, mean value and standard deviation, in ¥, per target group and socio-demographic variable, and significant differences by one-way ANOVA ($n=801$)

					One-way ANOVA	
FBR target group	Variable	Categories	Mean WTP	Standard deviation	Value	p
Women	Gender	Female	2.49	2.63	22.77	0.00
		Male	1.79	1.18		
High-risk consumers	Education[a]	Low	2.00	1.76	10.99	0.01
		High	2.54	2.73		
	Income[b]	Low	2.08	2.03	12.84	0.00
		High	3.08	2.57		
	Residence	Rural	1.76	1.10	26.59	0.00
		Urban	2.51	2.65		
Farmers	Farmer status	Farmer	1.85	1.33	3.91	0.00
		Nonfarmer	2.23	2.22		

The results indicate that females, consumers with a high education and income level, people living in urban areas, and nonfarmers are willing to pay significantly more for FBR
The applied methodology and the one-way ANOVA values are based on the study of De Steur et al. [19]
[a]A high education level is defined as a college degree or higher
[b]A yearly income above ¥40,000 or US$6,288 is defined as a high income level

question "Considering that 1 kg of conventional rice costs ¥3 (in 2008), at what price would you think this GM rice product is expensive, but you would still purchase it?" and refer to indifferent and favorable consumers who are willing to purchase it. In general, these consumers stated to be willing to pay ¥2.15 (or US$0.34) more for 1 kg of FBR. The ones that are not willing to buy it (4.4 %) are excluded from the analysis. As this percentage is substantially low, this might reveal potential hypothetical bias. This occurs when people state higher values than they actually would pay, because of the hypothetical nature of the stated preference method [41].

Based on the socio-demographic profile of the consumers, Table 28.4 summarizes the WTP values of the different target groups of FBR. Although female are less favorable to FBR, those who are not reluctant are prepared to pay more than males. Consumers with a high risk stated lower values for

Table 28.5 Current burden of folate deficiency, potential health benefits, intervention costs, and cost-effectiveness of folate biofortified rice in China

Current burden of folate deficiency (in DALYs lost per year)	314,180[a]
Effectiveness (in DALYs saved per year)	
Low impact scenario	62,836[b,c]
High impact scenario	188,508[b,c]
Intervention costs (in million US$)	32.3[b]
Basic R&D (8 years)	5.7[b,d]
Country-specific (6 years)	9.5[b,e]
Social marketing (18 years)	15.0[b,f]
Maintenance breeding (18 years)	2.1[b]
Cost-effectiveness (in US$ per DALY saved)[g]	
Pessimistic scenario	64.2[b]
Optimistic scenario	21.4[b]

FBR could be a highly effective and cost-effective strategy to reduce the negative health impact of folate deficiency in China
DALY disability-adjusted life year
[a]De Steur et al. [8]
[b]De Steur et al. [20]
[c]The method to apply the DALY framework to investigate the health benefits of FBR is thoroughly described in De Steur et al. [8, 20]. Figures differ from the health impact study of FBR [8], due to the inclusion of more conservative coverage rates, i.e., 20 % and 60 % [20]
[d]The basic R&D cost is weighted by its share in the total rice production of other rice producing target countries (Bangladesh, India, and the Philippines), i.e., 48 % [42]
[e]Country-specific costs mainly consist of the regulatory costs, estimated at US$8 million [43]. Also adaptive breeding costs are included, i.e., US$1.5 million [44]
[f]Unlike the yellowish GR, the visual traits of folate-enriched rice are expected to be similar as regular rice. Therefore, the social marketing costs of the former, i.e., 30 million [45], are halved
[g]Based on a 30-year time horizon

FBR, which might be due to their low income level, rather than their attitude towards FBR. Regarding the farmer status, farmers are willing to pay less for FBR than nonfarmers. As they are significantly more favorable, these results could indicate a strategic bias, by which the values reflect a production strategy to buy low and sell high.

Cost-Effectiveness of FBR

The CEA of FBR in China builds upon two studies of De Steur et al., i.e., a health impact study of FBR [8] and a cost-effectiveness study on multibiofortification [20]. In the former study, the current burden of folate deficiency in China (and its provinces) is assessed in terms of the number of DALYs that are lost due to the occurrence of NTDs, caused by maternal folate deficiency, i.e., 314,180 DALYs (see Table 28.5).

Regarding the potential health benefits, lower, more conservative coverage rates were applied, as shown the multibiofortification study. This reduced the initial health impact of the pessimistic and optimistic scenario by 45.9 % and 26.8 %, respectively. Each year, between 62,836 and 188,508 DALYs could be saved through the introduction of FBR in China [20].

As FBR is still in a laboratory phase, the intervention cost figures are based on expert estimates. A 30-year time frame is applied (2002–2031), in line with health impact studies on other biofortified crops [6]. Broadly five categories are included, namely the basic R&D costs to develop FBR, country-specific costs, including the adaptive breeding costs and the costs to comply with regulatory requirements, social marketing costs to promote FBR, and maintenance breeding costs to maintain the purity of the FBR seeds. While the costs incurred by R&D and the in-country costs refer to the development process of

FBR, social marketing and maintenance breeding start when FBR is assumed to be launched, i.e., in 2014. Taken together, the total cost to introduce FBR in China is estimated at US$31.6 million [20].

In line with previous biofortification research [46], the cost-effectiveness of FBR in China is calculated by comparing the net present value of the potential health benefits and the costs incurred by introducing FBR. The discount rate is 3 %, which is widely recognized in cost-effectiveness analyses [37, 47]. De Steur et al. [20] showed that the introduction of FBR in China would save a DALY at cost between US$64.2 and US$21.4 in the low and high impact scenario, respectively (see Table 28.5). Given the World Bank cut-off level for cost-effective health interventions, i.e., US$86.04 in 2011 [36], biofortifying rice with folate can be assumed as a highly cost-effective intervention.

Policy Issues and Recommendations to Advance to a Successful Commercialization of FBR

Despite its key role in the development and commercial introduction of transgenic plant varieties, China has not yet commercialized a transgenic crop for consumption. This "commercialization slowdown" took place on a global scale [48], by which any optimistic expectation towards a fast, successful implementation of FBR based on the previous section should take into account the broad policy context. In this section, some key barriers and challenges to successfully introduce FBR in China are discussed.

Regulatory Issues

Apart from its financial implications, the regulation of GM food is often seen as the main reason for the 10-year delay in the commercialization of transgenic biofortified crops, such as GR [49]. In China, biosafety regulations on agricultural GM products are defined and implemented by the Chinese Ministry of Agriculture and its Office of Agricultural Genetic Engineering Biosafety Administration in particular [50]. The National Agricultural GMO Biosafety Committee is in charge of the risk assessment evaluation, while the Ministry of Health is involved to ensure the food safety of biotechnology products.

The Chinese regulatory process requires applicants to pay specific attention to biodiversity risks, such as cross-pollination and the preservation of locally grown crops [13]. Despite the fact that China has one of the most advanced biosafety regulatory and monitoring systems throughout Asia, there is still a need to improve efficiency and transparency of evaluation and approval procedures [51]. This could speed up and improve the adoption of GM technology.

Intellectual Property Rights

Although a lot of progress has been made to protect IPRs in China, its IPR framework is still criticized for a lack of coordination, monitoring, and enforcement [13]. Patent registration likely needs to be reformed and centralized in order to improve IPR-protection for biofortified crops [13].

When dealing with IPRs for FBR as a pro-poor, pro-rural health strategy, the introduction of humanitarian licenses in developing countries deserves attention. In the case of GR, this institutional arrangement allows poor farmers (i.e., earning less than US$10,000 per year) from developing countries to use it royalty-free and creates a free transfer of the rights to public research institutions in the targeted countries [52].

Table 28.6 The position of main stakeholders regarding biofortified crops in China

Stakeholder	Position towards GM food and transgenic biofortification
Government	
MOST (Ministry of Science and Technology)	Pro-GM; continues to invest in transgenic crop R&D
MoA (Ministry of Agriculture)	Initially in favor, but might be affected by the international political climate or public resistance
SEPA (State Environmental Protection Administration)	Most opposed Chinese Ministry; collaborates with Greenpeace
Foreign companies	Interested in entering the Chinese market, especially if the IPR framework is improved and China would further open their markets
Seed companies	Both government-owned and private seed companies are interested, if the demand is sufficient or when the distribution to the poor is organized by government
NGOs, e.g., Greenpeace, Utopia	Against GM adoption, could influence political actions and consumers
Farmers	Generally in favor (see Tables 28.3 and 28.4); could be attracted through incentives, e.g., improved agronomic traits, royalty-free production, or a price premium
Consumers	Generally in favor (see Tables 28.3 and 28.4)

This table shows that there is a potential to introduce biofortified crops in China, but incentives should be taken to attract farmers and seed companies

GM genetically modified; *IPR* Intellectual Property Right

Source: Pray and Huang [56], Campos-Bowers and Wittenmyer [13], and expert interviews with Chinese researchers and biotechnology industry representatives

Variety Selection

It is important that the selected FBR event will be tailored to local varieties in order to reach the poorest consumers in the rural regions. South-East Asia, and China in particular, is characterized by a heterogeneous, segmented market for rice varieties, grown by various substance farmers on numerous small-scale farms. One needs to take into account these market characteristics when aiming to address the various regions of China.

Stakeholder Approach

As the large-scale adoption of transgenic Bt-cotton in China demonstrated, a well-adapted and integrated strategy is a prerequisite for success [53]. With respect to biofortification, the involvement of stakeholders should go beyond the agricultural research community, as it is also a nutrition and health intervention. It should address the bottlenecks of nutrition programs, by ensuring accessibility and availability, adequately allocating resources, installing an efficient monitoring and supervising system, defining distribution strategies and a social marketing strategy, and integrating key stakeholders [18, 54, 55].

The most important stakeholders involved in the introduction of FBR, besides the consumers, are the farmers, the government and its relevant ministries, private companies, millers, and seed companies. Table 28.6 shows how the main stakeholders are expected to react towards FBR as a transgenic (biofortified) crop in China. Government agencies, except for SEPA, are generally supporters, while NGOs are the main opponents of transgenic (biofortified) crops in China. Foreign biotechnology companies, seed producers, and farmers are initially in favor, but could be further attracted by ensuring a sufficient coverage rate of FBR.

Farmers

When looking at farmers in particular, the aforementioned humanitarian license for poor, subsistence farmers, the provision of a governmental subsidized credit to purchase biofortified seeds (e.g., Bt cotton in South Africa [57]), crossing the folate trait into a variety that has a high yielding potential or is better resistant to diseases (e.g., GR in the Philippines [58]) or creating a mobilized political organization [56] could further help to deploy the adoption of this GM rice.

Seed Production and Distribution

Since 2000, private companies are allowed to enter the Chinese seed market and sell their seeds all over China, next to the initial state-owned seed producers [59]. This led to a complex situation of several large distribution and retail networks alongside thousands of small, local seed distributers. As a consequence, Chinese farmers are still facing difficulties to discover attractive rice varieties [60], which support the need for a successful distribution strategy for biofortified crops. One option could be to subsidize the production and/or consumption through public distribution systems in order to facilitate farmer adoption and consumption in poor areas [52].

Governmental Support and Political Climate

Although most governmental agencies support transgenic (biofortified) crops, political acceptance could be hampered by the political climate, both at national or international level. The insect-resistant Bt rice in China is an illustrative example on how transgenic biofortified foods may be struggling to pass the biosafety regulatory process and obtain political approval. Despite its biosafety approval in 2009, its commercialization is currently delayed due to the reactions from Greenpeace and Utopia [61]. Nevertheless, this GM rice variant is expected to be released within 10 years [61]. Once approved, some argue that it would be a catalyst for the release of future GM staple crops [62].

The impact of international events can be illustrated by the US Starlink™ Bt maize incident in 2000, after which China has put their GM crop releases temporary on-hold [48] (other cases in China are extensively described by Pray and Huang [56]). Trade issues such as potential trade bans are expected to have a marginal effect on GM rice in China, due to its low international rice exports [63]. However, there might be pressure from a rice exporting country to avoid cross-border contamination.

GM Labeling

Since 2001, China requires GM-labels for food products based on GM technology, as outlined by the Chinese State Council [13]. Their mandatory labeling policy is the first to apply a 0 % level of detection, i.e., a zero tolerance approach. A GM-label for FBR could be beneficial as it might increase consumer confidence through informed food choices, i.e., the “right-to-know” [64]. It also allows one to position a GM biofortified crop in a segmented market, especially when external rice attributes do not differ from regular rice. One of the downsides is the associated cost (market segregation, identity preservation), which is expected to increase the retail price by 10 % [64]. This is especially valid for China, as such costs are negatively associated with the targeted detection level [65].

Conclusions

This article summarizes the results of studies on the market potential of FBR in China based on four research lines: acceptance, WTP, disease burden, and cost-effectiveness. The findings support FBR as a cost-effective health intervention to reduce folate deficiency in China, and show that there is a potential market for FBR in high-risk regions like Shanxi province, where the main target groups (women, farmers, people at risk) generally accept FBR and are willing-to-pay for it. Despite the promising market potential, several policy issues, especially the regulatory hurdles and the incorporation of stakeholders, need to be adequately addressed before one could successfully implement this health intervention.

References

1. Micronutrient Initiative. Investing in the future, a united call to action on vitamin and mineral deficiencies, Global Report 2009. Ontario: Micronutrient Initiative; 2009.
2. United Nations. The millennium development goals report. New York: United Nations; 2010.
3. Storozhenko S, De Brouwer V, Volckaert M, et al. Folate fortification of rice by metabolic engineering. Nat Biotechnol. 2007;25:1277–9.
4. Gonzalez C, Johnson N, Qaim M. Consumer acceptance of second-generation GM foods: the case of biofortified cassava in the north-east of Brazil. J Agr Econ. 2009;60(3):604–24.
5. Lusk JL. Effects of cheap talk on consumer willingness-to-pay for golden rice. Am J Agr Econ. 2003;85:840–56.
6. Stein AJ. Micronutrient malnutrition and the impact of modern plant breeding on public health in India: how cost-effective is biofortification? Göttingen: Cuvillier; 2006.
7. Lusk JL, Norwood FB. Social desirability bias in willingness-to-pay for products with normative attributes. American Agricultural Economics Association Annual Meeting, Long Beach, CA; 2006.
8. De Steur H, Gellynck X, Storozhenko S, et al. The health benefits of folate biofortified rice in China. Nat Biotechnol. 2010;28:554–6.
9. Blancquaert D, Storozhenko S, Loizeau K, et al. Folates and folic acid: from fundamental research towards sustainable health. Crit Rev Plant Sci. 2010;29:14–35.
10. Wang Y, Johnston S. The status of GM rice R&D in China. Nat Biotechnol. 2007;25:717–8.
11. James C. Global status of commercialized Biotech/GM crops: 2009. ISAAA brief no. 41. Ithaca, NY: ISAAA; 2009.
12. Waltz E. China's GM, rice first. Nat Biotechnol. 2010;28:8.
13. Campos-Bowers M, Wittenmyer B. Biofortification in China: policy and practice. Health Res Policy Syst. 2007;5:1–7.
14. Ren A, Zhang L, Hao L, Li Z, Tian Y, Li Z. Comparison of blood folate levels among pregnant Chinese women in areas with high and low prevalence of neural tube defects. Public Health Nutr. 2007;10:762–8.
15. Gu X, Lin L, Zheng X, et al. High prevalence of NTDs in Shanxi Province: a combined epidemiological approach. Birth Defects Res A Clin Mol Teratol. 2007;79:702–7.
16. Zhang B, Zhang T, Lin L, et al. Correlation between birth defects and dietary nutrition status in a high incidence area of China. Biomed Environ Sci. 2008;21:37–44.
17. Li Z, Hao L. National neural tube defects prevention program in China. Food Nutr Bull. 2008;29:S196–204.
18. Alavi S, Bugusu B, Cramer G, et al. Rice fortification in developing countries: a critical review of the technical and economic feasibility. Washington, DC: Academy for Educational Development; 2008.
19. De Steur H, Gellynck X, Storozhenko S, et al. Willingness to accept and purchase genetically modified rice with high folate content in Shanxi Province, China. Appetite. 2010;54:118–25.
20. De Steur H, Gellynck X, Blancquaert D, Lambert W, Van Der Straeten D, Qaim M. Potential impact and cost-effectiveness of multi-biofortified rice in China. N Biotechnol. 2012;29(3):432–42.
21. Lusk JL, Jamal M, Kurlander L, Roucan M, Taulman L. A meta-analysis of genetically modified food valuation studies. J Agr Resour Econ. 2005;30:28–44.
22. De Groote H, Kimenju S. Comparing consumer preferences for color and nutritional quality in maize: application of a semi-double-bound logistic model on urban consumers in Kenya. Food Policy. 2008;33:362–70.
23. Stevens R, Winter-Nelson A. Consumer acceptance of provitamin A-biofortified maize in Maputo, Mozambique. Food Policy. 2008;33:341–51.
24. Chong M. Acceptance of golden rice in the Philippine 'rice bowl'. Nat Biotechnol. 2003;21:971–2.

25. Bateman IJ, Carson RT, Day B, et al. Economic valuation with stated preference techniques: a manual. Cheltenham: Edward Elgar Publishing; 2002.
26. Breidert C, Hahsler M, Reutterer R. A review of methods for measuring willingness-to-pay. Innov Market. 2006;4:8–32.
27. Balistreri E, McClelland G, Poe G, Schulze W. Can hypothetical questions reveal true values? A laboratory comparison of dichotomous choice and open-ended contingent values with auction values. Environ Resour Econ. 2001;18:275–92.
28. Rousu MC, Monchuk D, Shogren JF, Kosa K. Consumer willingness to pay for "second-generation" genetically engineered products and the role of marketing information. J Agr Appl Econ. 2005;37:647–57.
29. Chowdhury S, Meenakshi JV, Tomlins K, Owori C. Are consumers willing to pay more for biofortified foods? Evidence from a field experiment in Uganda. Washington, DC: International Food Policy Research Institute; 2009.
30. De Groote H, Kimenju S, Morawetz U. Estimating consumer willingness to pay for food quality with experimental auctions: the case of yellow versus fortified maize meal in Kenya. Agr Econ. 2011;42:1–16.
31. Deodhar S, Ganesh S, Chern W. Emerging markets for GM foods: a study of consumer's willingness to pay in India. Int J Biotechnol. 2008;10:570–87.
32. Li Q, Curtis K, McCluskey J, Wahl T. Consumer attitudes toward genetically modified foods in Beijing. China AgBioForum. 2002;5:145–52.
33. Lopez AD, Mathers CD, Ezzati M, Jamison DT, Murray CJL. Measuring the global burden of disease and risk factors, 1990–2001. New York: Oxford University Press; 2006.
34. Drummond MF, Sculpher MJ, Torrance GW, O'Brien B, Stoddart GL. Methods for the economic evaluation of health care programmes. 3rd ed. New York: Oxford University Press; 2005.
35. Ngorsuraches S. Defining types of economic evaluation. J Med Assoc Thai. 2008;91:21–7.
36. World Bank. World development report 1993. New York: Oxford University Press; 1993.
37. Evans DB, Tan-Torres Edejer T, Adam T, Lim SS. Methods to assess the costs and health effects of interventions for improving health in developing countries. Br Med J. 2005;331:1137–40.
38. Meenakshi JV, Johnson N, Manyong V, et al. How cost-effective is biofortification in combating micronutrient malnutrition? An ex-ante assessment. HarvestPlus working paper no. 2. Washington, DC: International Food Policy Research Institute; 2007.
39. Fiedler JL, Sanghvi TG, Saunders MK. A review of the micronutrient intervention cost literature: program design and policy lessons. Int J Health Plann Manage. 2008;23:373–97.
40. Li Z, Ren A, Zhang L, Guo Z, Li Z. A population-based case-control study of risk factors for neural tube defects in four high-prevalence areas of Shanxi Province, China. Paediatr Perinat Epidemiol. 2006;20:43–53.
41. List JA, Gallet CA. What experimental protocol influence disparities between actual and hypothetical stated values? Evidence from a meta-analysis. Environ Resour Econ. 2001;20:241–54.
42. FAOSTAT Database. Paddy rice production (000 t), by country and geographical region, 1961–2007. 2008. http://faostat.fao.org/faostat/.
43. Kalaitzandonakes N, Alston JM, Bradford KJ. Compliance costs for regulatory approval of new biotech crops. Nat Biotechnol. 2007;25:509–11.
44. Stein AJ, Meenakshi JV, Qaim M, Nestel P, Sachdev HPS, Bhutta ZA. Potential impacts of iron biofortification in India. Soc Sci Med. 2008;66:1797–808.
45. Stein AJ, Sachdev HPS, Qaim M. Potential impact and cost-effectiveness of golden rice. Nat Biotechnol. 2006;24:1200–1.
46. Stein AJ, Sachdev HPS, Qaim M. Genetic engineering for the poor: golden rice and public health in India. World Dev. 2008;36:144–58.
47. Zimmermann R, Qaim M. Potential health benefits of golden rice: a Philippine case study. Food Policy. 2004;29: 147–68.
48. Paarlberg R. The real threat to GM crops in poor countries: consumer and policy resistance to GM foods in rich countries. Food Policy. 2002;27:247–50.
49. Potrykus I. Regulation must be revolutionized. Nature. 2010;466:561.
50. Pray CE, Ramaswami B, Huang J, Hu R, Bengali P, Zhang H. Costs and enforcement of biosafety regulations in India and China. Int J Technol Global. 2006;2:137–57.
51. Huang J, Zhang DL, Yang J, Rozelle S, Kalaitzandonakes N. Will the biosafety protocol hinder or protect the developing world: learning from China's experience. Food Policy. 2008;33:1–12.
52. Dawe D, Unnevehr L. Crop case study: GMO golden rice in Asia with enhanced vitamin A benefits for consumers. AgBioForum. 2007;10:154–60.
53. Raney T. Economic impact of transgenic crops in developing countries. Curr Opin Biotechnol. 2006;17:174–8.
54. Brooks S. Rice biofortification: lessons for global science and development. London: Earthscan; 2010.
55. Faillace S, Ray J, Harvey P. Barriers and enablers in the start up and implementation of large scale micronutrient programs. Washington, DC: Academy for Educational Development; 2008.

56. Pray CE, Huang J. Biofortification for China: political responses to food fortification and GM technology, interest groups, and possible strategies. AgBioForum. 2007;10:161–9.
57. Gouse M, Pray CE, Kirsten J, Schimmelpfennig D. A GM subsistence crop in Africa: the case of Bt white maize in South Africa. Int J Biotechnol. 2005;7:84–94.
58. Barry G. Golden rice and progress towards GMO-deregulation. In: Bertebos Foundation, editor. Golden rice and other biofortified food crops for developing countries. challenges and potential, vol. 7. Slöige: KSLA; 2008. p. 75–80.
59. Huang J, Hu R, Rozelle S, Pray C. Development, policy and impacts of genetically modified crops in china: a comprehensive review of China's agricultural biotechnology sector. Working paper, presented at the 75th anniversary of the IAAE. Ithaca, NY: Cornell University; 2005.
60. Falck-Zepeda J. Evaluation of the project biosafety management of genetically modified crops—China. Final evaluation report. Washington, DC: IFPRI; 2010.
61. Stone R. Activists go on warpath against transgenic crops—and scientists. Science. 2011;331:1000–1.
62. James C. China approves biotech rice and maize in landmark decision. ISAAA crop biotech update. Manila: ISAAA; 2009.
63. Huang J, Hu R, Van Meijl H, Van Tongeren F. Biotechnology boosts to crop productivity in China: trade and welfare implications. In: Van Tongeren F, Huang J, editors. China's food economy in the early 21st century. Development of China's food economy and its impact on global trade and on the EU. Report 6.04.04 ed. The Hague: Agricultural Economics Research Institute (LEI); 2004. p. 217–38.
64. Tegene A, Huffman WE, Rousu MC, Shogren JF. The effects of information on consumer demand for biotech foods: evidence from experimental auctions. ERS/USDA research briefs technical bulletin no. 1903. Washington, DC: United States Department of Agriculture; 2003.
65. Qaim M. The economics of genetically modified crops. Ann Rev Resour Econ. 2009;1:665–93.

Chapter 29
Biofortified Crops with a Visible Trait: The Example of Orange-Fleshed Sweet Potato in Sub-Saharan Africa

Jan W. Low

Key Points

- Orange-fleshed sweet potato (OFSP) is the first biofortified vitamin A staple food to be developed and promoted in sub-Saharan Africa (SSA), where traditionally most varieties grown are white-fleshed (containing no beta-carotene).
- During the past decade research has demonstrated that OFSP is bioavailable, and lab studies have demonstrated efficacy and determined 13 units of beta-carotene:1 unit of retinol ratio.
- Research has also shown that when OFSP is introduced with an additional demand creation and nutrition education approach, significant increases in vitamin A consumption result, and in Central Mozambique, a 15 % decline in prevalence of vitamin A deficiency (VAD) was attributable to the intervention.
- The integrated agriculture-nutrition approach can be cost-effectively taken to scale.
- Because of sweet potato's image as a crop of the poor, policy makers in SSA often ignore its potential contribution to nutrition and health. Implementation of well-designed demand creation strategies can be very effective in changing the mind-set of policy makers.
- Unexpectedly, the visible orange flesh color trait turned out to be a positive marketing tool, not a negative constraint.
- Since the emergence of the food crisis in 2008, global policy makers have begun significantly reinvesting in agriculture.
- The benefits of linking nutrition and agriculture to address micronutrient malnutrition and overall food security are increasingly recognized, and OFSP is a tested intervention for effectively linking the two to address VAD in young children.
- Ten key critical steps should be considered when undertaking a new OFSP dissemination effort.

Keywords Orange-fleshed sweet potato • Vitamin A • Biofortification • Micronutrient malnutrition • Beta-carotene • Sub-Saharan Africa • Nutrition • Food security

J.W. Low, Ph.D. (✉)
International Potato Center, Box 25171, Nairobi 00603, Kenya
e-mail: j.low@cgiar.org

V.R. Preedy et al. (eds.), *Handbook of Food Fortification and Health: From Concepts to Public Health Applications Volume 1*, Nutrition and Health, DOI 10.1007/978-1-4614-7076-2_29,

Abbreviations

CBO	Community-based organization
CGIAR	Global agriculture research partnership for a food secure future
GDP	Gross domestic product
g	Grams
NGO	Nongovernmental organization
OFSP	Orange-fleshed sweet potato
RAE	Retinol activity equivalents (vitamin A unit of measure)
SPHI	Sweetpotato for Profit and Health Initiative
SSA	Sub-Saharan Africa
SUN	Scaling-up nutrition
VAD	Vitamin A deficiency
VITAA	Vitamin A for Africa

Introduction

The term biofortification refers to the intentional breeding of staple food crops rich in micronutrients. The extensive use of this term began around 2002, with the explicit aim of being a strategy specifically aimed to improve the health of poor people since over 60–70 % of their energy intake comes from staple food crops [1]. Biofortification is envisaged as being particularly suitable for reaching the rural poor, who typically have limited access to commercially fortified foods. Hence, it is seen as being complementary to industrial fortification. By integrating micronutrient breeding into traditional breeding regimes, the use of the approach can continue even if specific support for micronutrient interventions diminishes in the future [2].

To date, the biofortification effort has focused on the three most limiting micronutrients in the human diet: iron, zinc, and vitamin A. Incorporation of vitamin A is distinct from iron and zinc in that beta-carotene, the precursor to vitamin A in plants, turns the grain, root, or tuber to varying shades along the yellow-orange spectrum, with deep-orange varieties having the highest levels of beta-carotene. It was hypothesized that introducing varieties with such a visible trait would be more difficult than a micronutrient-enhanced variety without such a trait [1].

One of the primary determinants of micronutrient malnutrition is poor diet quality. Animal and fish sources are often highly bioavailable but very costly. Fruits, lentils, beans, and vegetables at times are expensive, difficult to grow in certain environments, or, if available, not regular parts of diet, particularly for poor rural children under 5 years of age. Critics of biofortification argue that efforts would be better spent on promoting diet diversification, greater use of fruits and vegetables [3], and agricultural commercialization as a source of improved incomes. Evidence, however, indicates that diet improvement as a consequence of gradual economic improvement is a slow process [4].

The policy reality is that interventions to combat micronutrient malnutrition in developing countries have until recently been dominated by supplementation efforts. Supplementing with vitamin A capsules targeted at risk children under 5 years of age requires a distribution system that can provide a capsule to a child every 6 months. Increasingly, there are greater efforts to artificially fortify key commodities such as sugar, cooking oil, and maize flour with vitamin A. The research community bemoans the lack of studies with convincing evidence that food-based approaches improve micronutrient status [5]. Advocates of food-based approaches recognize that initial setup and implementation takes longer but the potential for sustained impact on health may be greater. Due to their complexity and duration, obtaining funding to provide the evidence is particularly challenging, hence perpetuating the image that food-based approaches are less effective than supplementation. However, biofortification as a

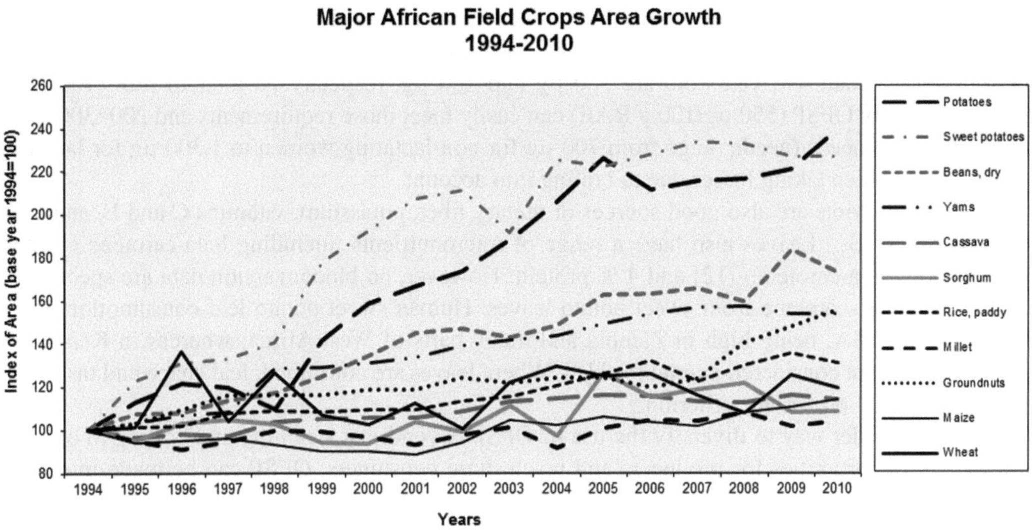

Fig. 29.1 Area expansion of major African food crops 1994–2010. *Source*: FAOSTAT (2011), except for Malawi (Ministry of Agriculture)

cost-effective approach has been increasingly recognized, for example, as one of the top approaches for addressing malnutrition cited by the Copenhagen Convention of 2008 [6].

It is within this context that the introduction and promotion of orange-fleshed sweet potato (OFSP) in sub-Saharan Africa (SSA) needs to be understood. Vitamin A deficiency (VAD) is widespread among young children in SSA, affecting at least 47.8 million children (2007) [7]; insufficient intake of vitamin A-rich foods is widely recognized as a major cause of VAD alongside high morbidity. In contrast to the Americas, most sweet potato varieties grown in SSA are white-fleshed (completely lacking in beta-carotene) or light-yellow-fleshed. Thus, the visible trait must be addressed as part of the introduction of OFSP to producers and consumers. Second, sweet potato is widely grown as a secondary staple throughout SSA, and in a few countries (Uganda, Rwanda, Burundi, and Malawi), it is a primary staple with over 80 kg per capita being consumed [8]. However, its image is that of the classic food security crop that is there when the maize fails and as a crop of the poor, mostly women, grown for subsistence, and not for sale. Hence, it often receives little attention from national research and development programs. In spite of that, the rate of sweet potato area expansion since 1994 has been impressive, reflecting its high energy output per unit area per unit time (see Fig. 29.1). Therefore, the introduction of OFSP offers the opportunity to work with a crop that already is grown by households most at risk of VAD yet faces the challenge of not being on many policy makers or donor priority lists, either in agriculture or nutrition.

Guidance on Levels to Be Consumed

Research has demonstrated that OFSP is such a rich source of bioavailable beta-carotene that impact on human health is possible in SSA, even when it is a secondary staple. It takes 13 units of beta-carotene from OFSP to convert into one unit of retinol (vitamin A) [9]. Loss of beta-carotene during preparation occurs, but typically only by 20–25 % when boiling [10], which is the most common form of root consumption in SSA.

There are wide range of OFSP varieties in use in SSA and the amount of beta-carotene found is highly correlated with the intensity of the orange color, ranging from 250 μg/100 g retinol activity equivalents (RAE) in pale orange varieties to over 1,300 μg/100 g RAE in dark orange varieties. Given that recommended daily vitamin A intakes [11] for infants 7–12 months of age are 500 μg and for children 1–3 and 4–8 years old are 300 μg and 400 μg, respectively, a small root (100 g) of medium intensity OFSP (550 μg/100 g RAE) can easily meet those requirements and 200–300 g can meet most adult needs (needs range from 700 μg for non-lactating women to 1,300 μg for lactating women), even when taking losses due to boiling into account.

Sweet potato roots are also good sources of dietary fiber, potassium, vitamins C and E, and all B vitamins except B_{12}. Leaves also have a range of micronutrients, including beta-carotene (cooked 500 μg/100 g beta-carotene) [12] and 4 % protein. However, no bioconversion data are specifically available for beta-carotene from sweet potato leaves. Human sweet potato leaf consumption varies enormously in SSA, being high in Zambia and many parts of West Africa; whereas in Kenya and Uganda, leaves are considered animal feed [8]. Where leaves are consumed, leaf shape and taste is an important varietal preference criterion.

Efforts are under way to diversify the use of OFSP beyond just steaming and boiling to open up new market opportunities for producers and reach more consumers. OFSP can be made into flour, preferably packed in paper not plastic to minimize beta-carotene degradation. Losses during storage of dried chips or flour under ambient conditions can be significant after 2 months [13]. Boiled and mashed sweet potato puree is being tried on a pilot scale in many countries as an ingredient in a wide range of bakery products (bread, biscuits, doughnuts, cakes) and juices. When processing, use of lower-intensity OFSP varieties (<500 μg/100 g RAE) should be avoided to ensure adequate beta-carotene content in the final product. For example, *golden bread* made by substituting 38 % of wheat flour with OFSP puree resulted in a deep yellow-colored product highly acceptable to Mozambican consumers that contained at least 135 RAE per 110 g bun [14]. A product can be considered a good source of vitamin A if it contains 10–19 % of the daily value per reference amount and an excellent source if it contains 20 % or more of the daily value per reference amount (United States Department of Agriculture standards). On this basis, a 110-g golden bread bun is an excellent source of vitamin A for children and nonpregnant women and a good source for all other adults.

Turning the Concept into Practice

During the past 15 years, considerable research undertaken in several SSA countries (especially Mozambique, Uganda, and Kenya) has built the evidence base demonstrating that OFSP can be successfully introduced and is an effective tool for combatting VAD among children under 5 years of age [15]. To turn such concepts into practice, several key questions had to be addressed: (1) Will the OFSP varieties be competitive with existing local varieties? (2) Are producers and consumers willing to accept a sweet potato variety with a distinct color difference? (3) How can we ensure that OFSP will be consumed by those target groups most at risk of VAD (young children and women of reproductive age)? (4) Will donors and governments support OFSP-based interventions?

In Kenya, sweet potato production is largely under the control of women, so initial work on OFSP began in the mid-1990s as part of a broader effort to develop and test women-based approaches for addressing micronutrient deficiencies. That work compared women's groups receiving agricultural extension advice and the new OFSP varieties to women's groups receiving the agricultural intervention *plus* nutrition education. The study found that the latter was essential for the frequency of vitamin A intake to increase among young children [16]. Several OFSP varieties used in the study (selected from introduced and local materials, but not bred) were found to be agronomically competitive with dominant local white- or yellow-fleshed varieties. Children were found to like OFSP varieties that were lower in dry matter content (more watery) than adults, who preferred higher dry matter content varieties similar to dominant existing varieties. Breeding programs began selecting for OFSP varieties with high dry matter content.

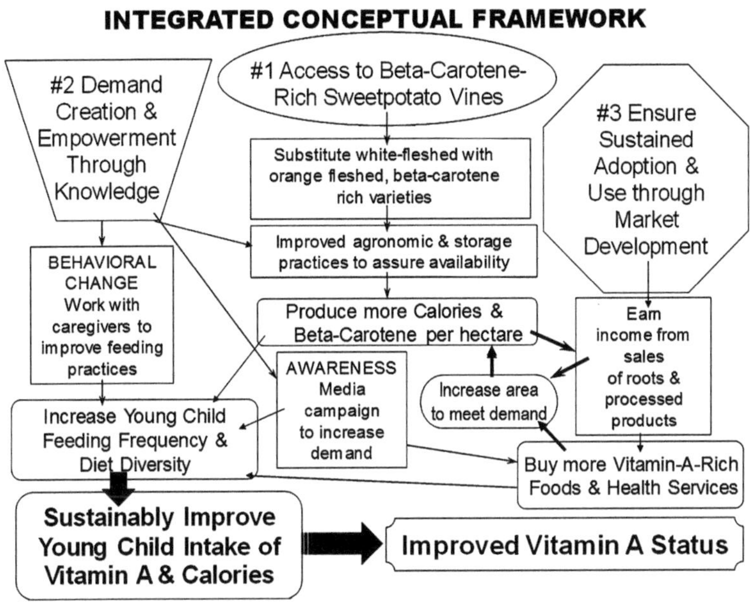

Fig. 29.2 Conceptual framework for the integrated approach

The next major research efforts did not occur in the early twenty-first century, reflecting the difficulty in raising funds for food-based approaches in the late 1990s. While the agricultural community had begun to recognize the potential contribution of OFSP, the nutrition community to a large extent was not yet convinced, often citing lack of convincing evidence. An interest group spearheaded by the International Potato Center, the Vitamin A for Africa (VITAA) Platform was created in 2001 to raise awareness and serve as a forum for exchange initially among five SSA countries. A 2001 ex-ante study drawing on available data detailing where sweet potato was produced and where VAD existed estimated that switching from white fleshed to OFSP could significantly contribute to reducing VAD in 50 million African children [17]. Around the same time, a major program looking at biofortification across several crops, HarvestPlus, received significant funding. OFSP emerged at the forefront of the biofortification concept effort because very high levels of beta-carotene already existed in the germplasm, and the breeding effort could focus on developing OFSP materials adapted to target areas in SSA and Asia. In other crops, the amount of the micronutrient within the crop had to first be increased to biologically significant levels.

An OFSP efficacy study conducted among school children (5–10 years old) in South Africa in 2002 measured vitamin A status using the modified-relative-dose response test [18]. The treatment group ($n=90$) consumed 125 g of boiled, mashed OFSP, while the control group ($n=90$) ate white-fleshed sweet potatoes for 53 school days. The treatment group showed significant improvement in vitamin A liver stores compared to the control group, with the proportion of children in the former group with normal vitamin A status increasing from 78 % to 87 % after the intervention. There was no significant change in vitamin A liver stores among the control group (86–82 %). This evidence was bolstered by a community-level intervention in a very resource-poor area of Mozambique, where VAD prevalence among the children at the beginning of the study was 71 % [19]. The intervention consisted of an integrated approach along three intersecting pathways (see Fig. 29.2):

1. Agriculture: *Introduction of a new source of vitamin A and energy, biofortified OFSP*. Intervention farmers organized in groups receive planting material of high-yielding OFSP varieties (see Fig. 29.3), combined with lessons on how to improve crop management and storage practices to maximize the availability of OFSP in the diet throughout the year.

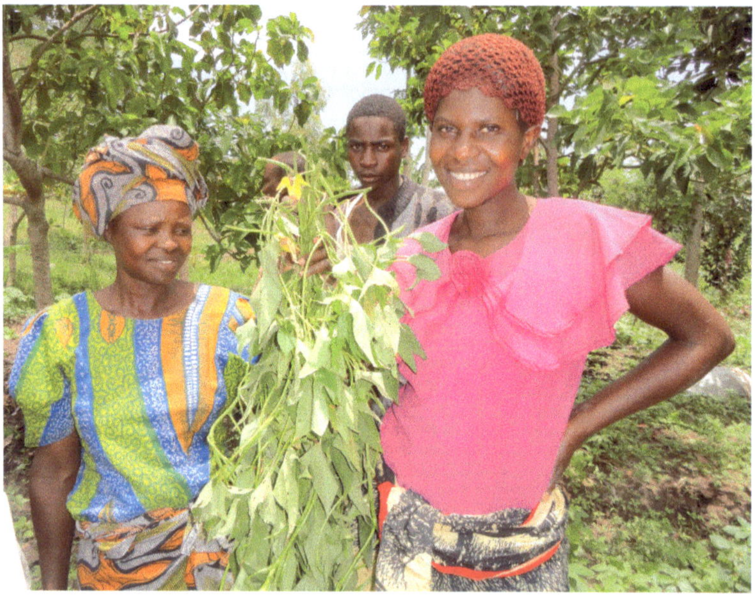

Fig. 29.3 Woman receiving quality sweet potato vines from trained multiplier in Tanzania (Credit: J. Low)

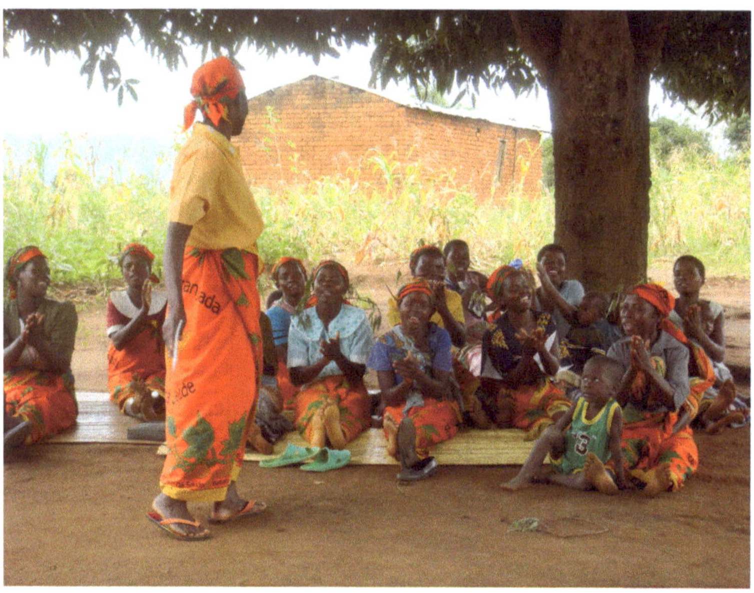

Fig. 29.4 Nutrition extensionists giving session with village promoters in Mozambique (Credit: J. Low)

2. Nutrition: *Demand creation and empowerment through knowledge*. At the village level, principal caregivers, both women and men, are encouraged and enabled to improve infant and young child feeding practices and hygiene practices and diversify the household diet. A nutrition extensionist conducts monthly group sessions for a year (see Fig. 29.4). Demand creation efforts focus on building awareness among the broader community to create (1) demand for the new OFSP cultivars and its derivatives, (2) demand for other vitamin A-rich foods, and (3) a supportive environment to accelerate behavior change at the household level. These included six provincial-wide radio programs, three community theater performances, painted stalls and signs in local markets, t-shirts,

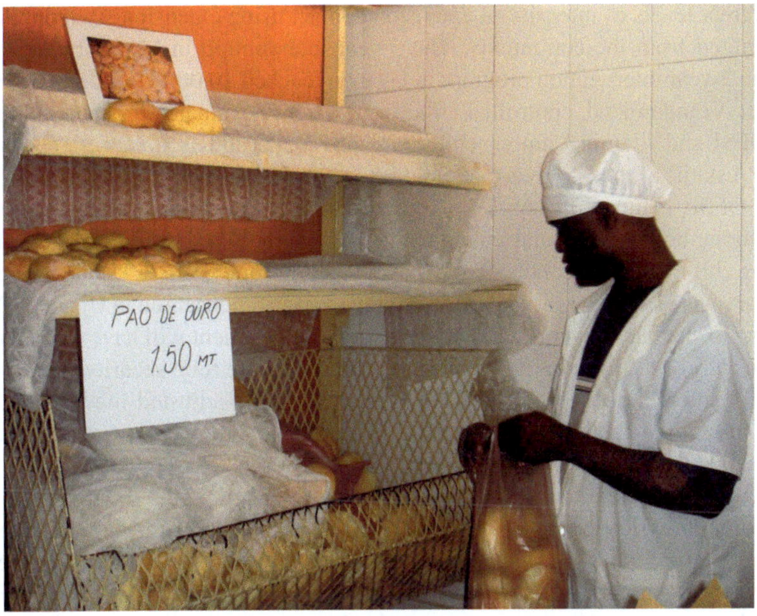

Fig. 29.5 Golden bread, made with OFSP, on sale in Mozambique (Credit: J. Low)

caps, and long cloths worn by women as skirts decorated with the slogan *O doce que dá saúde* (the sweet that gives health).

3. Marketing: *Market development for OFSP roots and processed products*. This component aims to link farmers to traders and to inform consumers about where they can purchase OFSP. Farmers with identified market outlets are more likely to expand area under production. Thus, generated demand combined with market development stimulates production, enhances producer income, and spreads the health benefits of OFSP to a wider population, all of which contribute to farmers' willingness to retain OFSP and expand production. Demand for OFSP is enhanced if profitable processed products using OFSP as a major ingredient are developed (see Fig. 29.5).

The intervention lasted 18 months in two of the poorest districts in rural Zambézia, Mozambique. World Vision, an international nongovernmental organization (NGO), posted a pair of extensionists at the community level: one for agriculture and marketing and the other for nutrition. Each pair served 14 farmer groups. In total there were 498 mother-child pairs captured in the study that were compared to 243 mother-child pairs from "control" areas where no intervention was made.

By the end of the study, 90 % of intervention households produced OFSP. Vitamin A intakes among intervention children ($n=498$) were much higher than those of control children ($n=243$) (median 426 μg vs. 56 μg RAE, $P<0.001$). OFSP contributed 35 % to the vitamin A intakes of all children in the intervention area and 90 % among those who had consumed it the previous day. Serum retinol data were obtained as a proxy for vitamin A status. Controlling for infection/inflammation and other cofounders, a 15 % decline in the prevalence of VAD was attributable to the integrated intervention [20]. OFSP was well accepted and liked by both adults and children. In fact, the color orange proved to be an effective tool for demand creation and marketing and became clearly associated with healthy foods.

Armed with this evidence, interest in OFSP interventions began to grow and the VITAA Platform expanded to 11 SSA countries. The next important step was to investigate whether such an OFSP-led food-based integrated approach could be taken to scale at reasonable cost. Drawing on a modified version of the three pathways outlined above, simultaneous studies conducted in Uganda and Mozambique tested two different levels of intensity of extension contact using extensionists supported by nonpaid promoters recruited from the community. The 3-year intervention in Mozambique reached 14,000 households; the 2-year intervention program in Uganda reached 10,000 Ugandan farmer group member households. A randomized, controlled effectiveness study evaluated the intervention's impact on the intake of OFSP and vitamin A among children 6–35 months and 3–5 years of age, and women, and on the vitamin A status of the 3–5-year-old children and women [21]. In Mozambique 77 % of households adopted OFSP, compared to 65 % in Uganda. In both countries, vitamin A intakes increased significantly among both women and young children, with OFSP contributing 78 % of total vitamin A intake among children 6–35 months of age in Mozambique and 53 % in Uganda. Average costs per target beneficiary were $86/household in Mozambique and $56/household in Uganda. OFSP vines are easy for farmers to share and over time; hence, the initial investment will have considerable spillover effects. In terms of just the vitamin A benefit (not considering the food security and other micronutrient benefits), the intervention costs $15–20 USD per disability-adjusted life years (DALYs) saved [22]. This amount falls within the "highly cost-effective" category of interventions as defined by the World Health Organization.

For governments, the experience indicates that "seeing is believing." Inviting local and national officials and community leaders to demonstration-based events and hearing farmer testimonies has been the most effective strategy for government buy-in and public sector resource investment. Good radio and television coverage of such events accelerates the buy-in process. For donors, a solid evidence base and country-specific government recognition of the crop's potential have been critical factors for generating further investments.

Building on growing donor support, the International Potato Center and over 30 partner organizations launched the 10-year Sweetpotato for Profit and Health Initiative (SPHI) in October 2009. The SPHI emerged from a 7-month consultative process to identify the constraints blocking the full exploitation of sweet potato and develop interventions in breeding, propagation, and dissemination of healthy planting material, crop management, human nutrition, and marketing. The Initiative's vision is to reposition sweet potatoes in African food economies, particularly in expanding urban markets, to reduce child malnutrition and improve smallholder incomes. It seeks to positively affect the lives of ten million African families by 2010 and is establishing support platforms in three subregions (East and Central Africa, Southern Africa, West Africa) to enable the creation of a vibrant community of practice. SPHI targets 17 countries and breeding or varietal selection activities are under way in 14 of those countries [23].

A major outcome of increased support is that sweet potato breeding work *in* Africa *for* Africa has been significantly strengthened, enabling the creation of better adapted disease and drought-tolerant varieties. Good varieties are the foundation of success, and approximately 70 % of breeding resources are focused on the development of the orange-fleshed types. Using a new breeding approach known as *accelerated breeding*, the time for new variety development has been lowered from 8 to 4 years. The first 15 OFSP drought-tolerant varieties developed using the accelerated approach in Mozambique (the support platform for Southern Africa) were released in February of 2011. Second-generation (bred in Africa) OFSP varieties that have started being released since 2005 are far superior to most first-generation OFSP varieties (often bred outside of Africa) in terms of agronomic performance and organoleptic characteristics desired by African consumers. In 2000, only two SSA countries (Uganda and South Africa) were breeding sweet potato; in 2012, 12 have sweet potato breeding programs and an additional 2 are selecting varieties based on seed generated from those programs.

In summary, it took 14 years to turn this concept into accepted practice. Returning to our key questions:

1. *Will the OFSP varieties be competitive with existing local varieties*? Yes, particularly if investments are made in breeding programs at the country level when beta-carotene-rich varieties are crossed with adapted local varieties with taste preferences desired by local producers and consumers.

2. *Are producers and consumers willing to accept a sweet potato variety with a distinct color difference?* Yes, the orange color is well liked and has proved to be a useful marketing tool for promoting adoption, knowledge about all types of vitamin A-rich foods, and appropriate young child feeding practices. In some SSA countries where there is significant fear of genetically modified products, clear messages must be communicated that the orange color is natural, drawn from the very diverse sweet potato germplasm available throughout the world.
3. *How can we ensure that OFSP will be consumed by those target groups most at risk of VAD?* Integrating nutrition education targeting caregivers with 5–7 group nutrition education sessions (emphasizing practical demonstrations) and larger educational efforts (using radio, meetings, community theater) at those who influence dietary practices (especially husbands, mother-in-laws, and community leaders) have proven to be effective in ensuring OFSP adoption and integration into the young child and general household diet.
4. *Will donors and governments support OFSP-based interventions?* Government officials are convinced when they visit pilot OFSP interventions and watch young children and families consume OFSP and describe how easy it is to produce and prepare. Governments are more willing to invest their own resources when sweet potato is viewed as an important food security crop in their country. Donors begin to significantly support OFSP interventions once sufficient scientific evidence on impact is available, there is some relevant buy-in by government officials for such investments within the specific country, and the investment is not at odds with their current development strategy.

Policy Environment

With the publication of findings and their presentation in recognized international nutrition conferences, support from the nutrition community for biofortification as an effective tool for combatting micronutrient deficiencies on an international level began to increase. In 2008, a recognized panel of experts in Copenhagen reviewing many different types of interventions to combat micronutrient malnutrition included biofortification as one with high potential for cost-effective impact. The year 2008 is most notable, however, for the steep risk in world food prices for basic grains such as wheat and rice that served as a wake-up call for the need to reinvest in agriculture to meet growing population demand. Sweet potato's traditional role as a rustic crop able to produce within SSA in a broad range of agroclimatic conditions and give much higher energy output per unit land per unit time than other grain crops has become increasingly acknowledged. Kenya, for instance, now has public sector programs promoting the utilization of the so-called *orphan* crops (those important for food security but have been underinvested in to date), including sweet potato in this category. Adequate resources remain a challenge. Although African leaders meeting in Maputo in 2003 committed to increasing investments into their agricultural sectors to 10 % of their gross domestic product (GDP), only a few (Malawi, Ghana, Zambia) had achieved that goal by 2009 [24].

Moreover, international organizations, developed countries, and donors increasingly began to recognize the potential synergies to be gained by better strengthening the links between agriculture and nutrition. For example, the United States Agency for International Development explicitly included nutrition as part of their *Feed the Future* global hunger and food security initiative launched in 2009. OFSP is posted as case study number 4 on their website. The nutrition community recognized that to address stubborn chronic malnutrition rates among young children would require community-level interventions, working on behavioral change as part of a comprehensive package of health, nutrition, and agricultural interventions. In September 2012, the scaling-up nutrition (SUN) movement was launched at the *1,000 Days: Change a Life, Change the Future* event cohosted by the United States and Ireland during the United Nations Summit on the Millennium Development Goals. To date 12 SSA countries have committed to the Initiative's strategic plan. In Malawi, OFSP is fully integrated as part of SUN activities and the potential exists to similarly integrate OFSP into other participant countries.

In SSA, sweet potato is one of the priority crops for the Alliance for a Green Revolution program and appears in subregional and country-level food security and nutrition strategies. At the country level, it takes a cadre of interested scientist and practitioners (OFSP advocates) to get OFSP and biofortification in general explicitly recognized and included in relevant strategies and implementation plans. Specific policy briefs, stakeholder workshops, and demand creation campaigns accelerate this process.

OFSP has an advantage in SSA in that, depending its role in the food economy, it can be promoted as food crop, a vegetable (part of home or school garden programs), a feed crop (especially for dairy cattle, dairy goats, and pigs), a food security crop, a famine relief food, a woman's crop, a snack food (chips, crisps, juice), or as a partial wheat flour substitute in bakery products. This means it has diverse entry points through relevant strategies and policies for the crop, livestock, health, education, social action, community development, and agro-processing sectors.

Recommendations

During the past decade, significant progress has been made in East, Central, and Southern Africa utilizing OFSP to change the image of sweet potato from being a crop of the poor to being a health food for all. Much remains to be done as only Mozambique and Uganda have significantly advanced programs, with many countries still at the early stages of OFSP development and promotion (see Table 29.1).

Experience to date has revealed ten critical steps to consider when designing an OFSP intervention:

1. *Understand how sweet potato fits into the current food system.* Collect information on:
   - How sweet potato fits into dominant farming systems
   - Its importance relative to other crops
   - The extent to which it is commercialized
   - Gender roles in sweet potato production, marketing, and decision making
   - Consumer and farmer perceptions about the crop (it may be viewed as inferior, debilitating to virility, unhealthy, etc.)
   - Its status in country-level food security and nutrition policies
2. *Find out if disease-free, adapted OFSP varieties already exist.*
   - Are officially released OFSP varieties available, or a breeding program developing new OFSP varieties in the country? How do the OFSP varieties compare to the most popular local sweet potato varieties in terms of yield and taste? To be competitive, OFSP varieties should perform at least as well as the dominant local varieties.
   - If there is no released, competitive OFSP variety, you will need to build in 18–24 months of time to introduce and select varieties to use before you can start a major dissemination effort. Material to test may be available from your national research center or can be requested through the International Potato Center from support platform countries (Uganda, Mozambique, and Ghana).
   - Even if there is a good released OFSP variety, if it has never been introduced in the area you plan to work in, investing in one season of on-farm trials is advisable at the beginning of the project.
   - Find out if the national program has disease-free foundation material. If it does not, you may need to build in a component to get the material "cleaned up" (which can take up to a year) while you use the best material available in the interim.

Table 29.1 Current status of SPHI target countries

	Average (2005–2007)							
Country	Sweet potato production ("000 metric tons)	% of total sweet potato grown in SSA	Estimated % children under 5 years with vitamin A deficiency (various years)	Desired number of direct beneficiaries by 2020	Has active breeding program	1st- or 2nd-generation OFSP varieties available	Experience with OFSP dissemination	Level of awareness among policy makers
Uganda	2,591	20.5	28	1,926,667	Yes	2nd	Large-scale	High
Nigeria	1,578	12.5	30	618,667	Yes	1st	Small-scale	Beginning
Malawi	1,146	9.1	59	1,592,270	Yes	2nd	Large-scale	Very high
Tanzania	960	7.3	24	1,515,000	Yes	2nd	Large-scale	Moderate
Madagascar	874	6.9	42	371,856	No	1st	Moderate	Low
Rwanda	872	6.9	6	1,241,633	Yes	1st	Moderate	Moderate
Burundi	838	6.6	28	625,000	No	1st	Small-scale	Low
Kenya	769	6.1	84	350,000	Yes	2nd	Moderate	Moderate
Angola	689	5.4	64	409,909	No	2nd	Moderate	Low
Ethiopia	409	3.2	46	347,592	Yes	1st	Large-scale	Moderate
Mozambique	388	3.1	69	970,000	Yes	2nd	Large-scale	Very high
DR Congo	228	1.7	61	182,596	No	1st	Small-scale	Low
Zambia	138	1.4	54	236,958	Yes	2nd	Moderate	Moderate
Ghana	91	0.7	76	456,750	Yes	2nd	Small-scale	Low
Burkina Faso	72	0.6	54	51,300	Yes	1st	Small-scale	Low
Benin	56	0.4	71	67,758	No	1st	Small-scale	Low
South Africa	46	0.4	17	15,438	Yes	2nd	Moderate	Moderate
Subregions (no. of countries)								
East and Central (7)	6,667	52		6,188,488	5			
Southern (6)	3,281	26		3,596,431	4			
West (4)	1,797	14		1,194,475	3			
All countries (17)	11,745	93		10,979,393	12			
	12,652	100.0						

Source of production data: FAOSTAT (2005–2007)
Source of vitamin A data: Micronutrient Initiative Call to Action Report (2009) (www.unitedcalltoaction.org/documents/Investing_in_the_future.pdf)

3. *Determine the extent of the VAD problem, how widespread knowledge of the role of vitamin A is, and whether combatting VAD and improving nutrition area priorities for the government.*

   - Obtain the most recent data, by district if possible, on VAD prevalence and rates of stunting (chronic malnutrition) among children less than 5 years old, the group most at risk of VAD. If you find that food-based approaches to combatting VAD are not part of existing nutrition or food security strategies, you will need to build in an advocacy component targeting key decision makers into your project.
   - If you find that knowledge of vitamin A and its importance is low at the community level, you will need to take this into account when designing the nutrition education campaign. It makes sense to prioritize districts for intervention that have high rates of VAD or chronic undernutrition and where sweet potato is already well known in the community.

4. *Decide what dissemination strategy makes sense for your environment.* Sweet potato is propagated by vines which perish in 2 days if not cared for properly. There are two major approaches for disseminating vines:

   - Mass multiplication and dissemination to a large number of households on a given day in a given location.
   - Establishing a cadre of trained quality vine multipliers at the community level from whom farmers pick up vines when they are ready to plant.

   The first method can reach larger numbers of households at lower per unit cost faster but, if not well organized, can lead to a high loss of material. The second method is preferred in drought-prone areas, where mechanisms are needed for sustaining access to quality planting material once the project is over. The cost per beneficiary will depend on factors such as population density, quality of infrastructure (roads, irrigation), and availability of good extension personnel.

5. *Understand existing vine conservation and exchange systems to decide on whether and how to subsidize vine dissemination.*

   - Find out how farmers are conserving their vines during the dry season and whether farmers who lack material purchase vines. If vines are sold, find out the price and typical volumes purchased.
   - Estimate the cost of producing vines. This helps determine how much it would cost the project to fully or partially subsidize vine dissemination.
   - To make an impact on production, a minimum of 200 vines (approximately 4 kg) should be provided to each household. Some type of subsidy is advisable the first year to stimulate interest.

6. *Decide whether to include a marketing component.* Experience has shown that it typically takes 4–5 years to build up successful marketing projects. If your time frame is short (2–3 years), consider focusing on production and consumption of OFSP by vulnerable groups. To engage in marketing, you first need to understand existing sweet potato value chains and then actively facilitate the formation of farmer marketing groups and the development of trader-producer linkages.
7. *Choose the major elements to include in your promotion campaign.* Develop a brand image and marketing campaign to promote and raise awareness of OFSP, taking advantage of the color orange. Choose a slogan (e.g., The Healthy Choice). It is best to use several promotional approaches to reinforce key messages—consider radio programs or jingles, billboards, community theater, songs, and promotional materials such as t-shirts and caps depending on your target audience and budget.

8. *Build on existing materials when developing nutrition and utilization messages.*

   - Develop nutritional messages that focus on how OFSP provides vitamin A and reduces deficiency among young children and pregnant and breastfeeding women. Do not have too many messages and keep them simple. Emphasize the importance of diet diversification.
   - Check with government and NGO nutritionists to learn what other nutrition training materials are available and can easily be adapted to meet your specific needs. Learn what approaches for changing behaviors have worked successfully at the community level.
   - Note that nutrition messaging should also target men and other influencers of dietary practice (community leaders, mother-in-laws) as they play important roles in deciding on child-feeding practices and use of health-care facilities.

9. *Find out who the other actors are in the nutrition and agriculture arena and decide whether you want to partner with them.* Potential partners include government agencies (ministries of agriculture, health, education, women's affairs, etc.); NGOs and community-based organizations (CBOs); research organizations, such as universities and CGIAR agricultural research centers; private sector partners; and community leaders. Building multi-sectoral programs often requires bringing different partners together. You should consider whether OFSP can be built into an existing agriculture or nutrition/health intervention or to approach it as a stand-alone project. Village promoters can be effectively used to expand the reach of extension personnel, but covering more than 30 persons per promoter is not recommended.
10. *Determine the essential package of agronomic messages.* Demonstrations, as opposed to lectures, are more effective for convincing farmers to change. Consider topics such as:

    - Characteristics of the new varieties and how to test new varieties
    - Planting one cutting per hole to efficiently use planting material
    - Spacing to obtained desired average root size
    - Identifying and removing plants with virus symptoms
    - Adopting cultural practices for weevil control
    - Harvesting carefully to increase postharvest shelf life
    - Conserving and multiplying vines
    - Storing fresh roots or dried chips

The Triple S Method is a new way to conserve roots as sources of future vines that makes sense when the dry season lasts more than 3 months.

The SPHI is building community of practice and encouraging members to share information on the Sweetpotato Knowledge Portal (www.sweetpotatoknowledge.org). It contains informational flyers that can be used by advocates to change policies and promote OFSP investment, research findings, and additional technical recommendations.

Conclusions

OFSP is the first biofortified crop that has begun to reach its intended target audience: women and children under 5 years of age at risk of VAD. The process of taking the idea that a biofortified crop could significantly contribute to combatting VAD in SSA from the conceptual stage to practice required building up an evidence base to convince the professional nutrition community and country-level policy makers of its potential. Based on the lessons learned from experiences in several SSA countries on how to best deliver OFSP for impact, the global policy environment is now poised to support innovative approaches such as biofortification that leverage agricultural investments to support positive nutrition outcomes.

References

1. Bouis H. A new tool for fighting micronutrient malnutrition. J Nutr. 2002;132:491S–4.
2. Bouis HE, Hotz C, McClafferty B, Meenakshi JV, Pfeiffer WH. Biofortification: a new tool to reduce micronutrient malnutrition. Food Nutr Bull. 2011;32(1 Suppl):S31–40.
3. Keatinge JDH, Waliyar F, Jamnadas RH, et al. Relearning old lessons for the future of food—by bread alone no longer: diversifying diets with fruit and vegetables. Crop Sci. 2010;50(March–April):S1–12.
4. Mebrahtu S, Pelletier D, Pinstrup-Andersen P. Agriculture and nutrition. In: Pinstrup-Andersen P, Pelletier D, Alderman H, editors. Child growth and nutrition in developing countries. Ithaca, NY: Cornell University Press; 1995. p. 220–42.
5. Masset E, Haddad L, Cornelius A, Isaza-Castro J. A systematic review of agricultural interventions that aim to improve nutritional status of children. London: EPPI-Centre, Social Science Research Unit, Institute of Education, University of London; 2011.
6. Horton S, Alderman H, Rivera J. Copenhagen consensus 2008: malnutrition and hunger, executive summary. Copenhagen: Copenhagen Consensus Center; 2008.
7. Standing Committee on Nutrition. 6th report on the world nutrition situation: progress in nutrition. Geneva: United Nations System; 2011.
8. Low JW, Lynam J, Lemaga B, et al. Sweetpotato in sub-Saharan Africa. In: Loebenstein G, Thottappilly G, editors. The sweetpotato. Heidelberg: Springer; 2009. p. 359–90.
9. Haskell MJ, Jamil KM, Hassan F, et al. Daily consumption of Indian spinach (Basella alba) or sweet potatoes has a positive effect on total body vitamin A stores in Bangladeshi men. Am J Clin Nutr. 2004;80:705–14.
10. Jaarsveld PV, Marais DW, Harmse E, Rodriguez-Amaya D. Retention of B-carotene in boiled, mashed orange-fleshed sweet potato. J Food Compos Anal. 2006;19:321–9.
11. Institute of Medicine. Dietary reference intakes for vitamin A, vitamin K, arsenic, boron, chromium, copper, iodine, iron, manganese, molybdenum, nickel, silicon, vanadium, and zinc. Washington, DC: National Academy Press; 2001.
12. U.S. Department of Agriculture (USDA) Agricultural Research Service. USDA national nutrient database for standard reference, release 16. Available from http://wwwnalusdagov/fnic/foodcomp; 2003. Cited 26 March 26, 2006.
13. Bechoff A. Investigating carotenoid loss after drying and storage of orange-fleshed sweet potato. Greenwich: University of Greenwich; 2010.
14. Low JW, van Jaarsveld P. The potential contribution of bread buns fortified with beta-carotene-rich sweetpotato in Central Mozambique. Food Nutr Bull. 2008;29(2):98–107.
15. Low JW, Kapinga R, Cole D, Loechl C, Lynam J, Andrade MI. Challenge theme paper 3: nutritional impact with orange-fleshed sweetpotato. In: Low J, editor. Unleashing the potential of sweetpotato in sub-Saharan Africa: current challenges and way forward. Lima: International Potato Center; 2009.
16. Hagenimana V, Oyunga MA, Low JW, Njoroge SM, Gichuki S, Kabira J. The effects of women farmer's adoption of orange-fleshed sweet potatoes: raising vitamin A intake in Kenya. Washington, DC: International Center for Research on Women, ICRW/OMNI Research Program, Research report no. 3; 1999.
17. Low JW, Walker T, Hijmans R. The potential impact of orange flesh sweetpotatoes on vitamin A intake in sub-Saharan Africa. Lima: The International Potato Center; 2001.
18. Jaarsveld PV, Faber M, Tanumihardjo SA, Nestel P, Lombard CJ, Benade AJ. Beta-carotene-rich orange-fleshed sweet potato improves the vitamin A status of primary school children assessed with the modified-relative-dose–response test. Am J Clin Nutr. 2005;81:1080–7.
19. Low JW, Arimond M, Osman N, Cunguara B, Zano F, Tschirley D. Ensuring supply and creating demand for a biofortified crop with a visible trait: lessons learned from the introduction of orange-fleshed sweet potato in drought-prone areas of Mozambique. Food Nutr Bull. 2007;28:S258–70.
20. Low JW, Arimond M, Osman N, Cunguara B, Zano F, Tschirley D. A food-based approach introducing orange-fleshed sweet potatoes increased vitamin A intake and serum retinol concentrations in young children in rural Mozambique. J Nutr. 2007;137:1320–7.
21. Hotz C, Loechl C, de Brauw A, et al. A large-scale intervention to introduce orange sweet potato in rural Mozambique increases vitamin A intakes among children and women. Br J Nutr. 2011;10:1–14.
22. HarvestPlus. Disseminating orange-fleshed sweet potato: findings from a HarvestPlus project in Mozambique and Uganda. Washington, DC: HarvestPlus; 2010.
23. Low JW. Unleashing the potential of sweetpotato to combat poverty and malnutrition in sub-Saharan Africa through a comprehensive initiative. Acta Horticola. 2011;921:171–9.
24. Global and Regional Advocacy for Small Producers (GRASP). Investing in agriculture: implementing the 2003 Maputo Declaration of the African Union; 2009. Available online at: http://www.search4dev.nl/document/175578; The Hague: 2009.

Index

V.R. Preedy et al. (eds.), *Handbook of Food Fortification and Health: From Concepts to Public Health Applications Volume 1*, Nutrition and Health, DOI 10.1007/978-1-4614-7076-2,

J

K

U

V

MIX
Papier aus verantwortungsvollen Quellen
Paper from responsible sources
FSC® C105338

If you have any concerns about our products,
you can contact us on
ProductSafety@springernature.com

In case Publisher is established outside the EU,
the EU authorized representative is:
Springer Nature Customer Service Center GmbH
Europaplatz 3, 69115 Heidelberg, Germany

Printed by Libri Plureos GmbH
in Hamburg, Germany